OUR GLOBAL ENVIRONMENT

OUR GLOBAL ENVIRONMENT

A HEALTH PERSPECTIVE

FIFTH EDITION

ANNE NADAKAVUKAREN

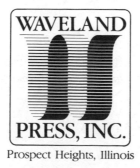

WAVELAND
PRESS, INC.
Prospect Heights, Illinois

For information about this book, write or call:
Waveland Press, Inc.
P.O. Box 400
Prospect Heights, Illinois 60070
(847) 634-0081
www.waveland.com

Contents

Preface

Our Global Environment: A Health Perspective is intended as a text for introductory level courses in environmental health or human ecology, presenting a broad survey of the major environmental issues facing society at the dawn of the 21st century. The book combines an overall ecological concern with specific elements related to personal and community health, emphasizing the interrelatedness of the two and conveying to students an awareness of how current environmental issues directly affect their own lives.

Commencing with a rudimentary discussion of general ecological principles, the text focuses primarily on our present population-resources-pollution crisis and explains why human health and welfare depend on successful resolution of these challenges. Intended for a one-semester course, the text consists of 16 chapters and is divided into three main sections, each with its own introduction. Discussion within each chapter covers general aspects of the subject in question, while specific illustrative examples are treated in box inserts. In order to give students a perspective on the kinds of actions being taken to deal with identified problems, a brief description of federal statutes dealing with particular environmental issues is included wherever appropriate. Appendices at the end of the book describe the various federal agencies dealing with environmental and health issues and list names, addresses, and web addresses of major nongovernmental environmental organizations for the benefit of those students who wish to obtain further information or to become actively affiliated with such groups. The ability of citizens to influence public policy is stressed throughout the book, a basic purpose of the text being to provide students with sufficient information and insight into environmental problems to enable them to understand and participate in the public decision-making processes which will profoundly influence health and environmental quality in the decades ahead.

I would like to express my sincere gratitude to those who helped me make this book possible: to Heinz Russelmann, former Director of the Environmental Health Program at Illinois State University, whose encouragement, suggestions, and painstaking review of the manuscript were of invaluable assistance; to my colleagues Dr. Steve Arnold (now Chairman of the Department of Environmental Health at New Mexico State University) and Dr. Thomas Bierma whose critical review of the sections on noise and radon was extremely helpful; to Dr. Sharron LaFollette for her careful review and comments on the chapters dealing with air pollution and toxic substances; to Becky Anderson whose classroom experience using the text enabled her to give valuable suggestions on content and scope of this revision, especially on issues pertaining to ecology and biodiversity; to Dr. Kenneth Jesse, Professor of Physics (retired) at Illinois State University, for his painstaking review and valuable suggestions on matters pertaining to ionizing radiation; to Drs. Anthony Otsuka and Herman Brockman, Professors in the Biological Sciences Department at Illinois State University, for their insightful comments on the sections dealing with mutations and cancer; to former colleague Phil Kneller, now at Western Carolina University, and to Tom Anderson of the McLean County Health Department for their suggestions and review of material on foodborne disease; to Linn Haramis at the Illinois Department of Public Health for his review of the passage on Lyme Disease; to Dr. Gregory Crouch, Associate Director of the Department of Environmental Health and Safety at Indiana University, for his valuable input on risk assessment and related topics; to Dr. Michelle Covi, Director of the Ecology Action Center in Normal-Bloomington for her review of the chapter on ecological principles; to Laurie Prossnitz, Waveland Press, whose friendly cooperation and painstaking editorial efforts have been sincerely appreciated; to Neil Rowe, publisher of Waveland Press, for his cooperation and help; and especially to my husband and daughters for their loving support and understanding during the course of this project.

Anne Nadakavukaren

PART 1

People, Progress, and Nature

Is Conflict Inevitable?

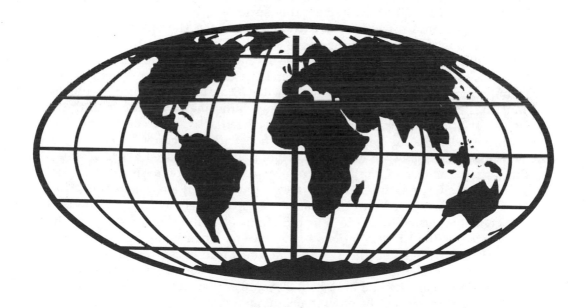

Only within the moment of time represented by the present century has one species—man—acquired significant power to alter the nature of his world.
—Rachel Carson

Human beings, as a species, are unquestionably the dominant form of life on earth today. Inhabiting every continent, roaming the seas, exploring space, creating glittering cities and festering slums, taming rivers, bringing water to the desert, harnessing the atom, tinkering with the gene—people often deceive themselves into believing they are all powerful, creatures apart from the rest of nature. Yet a half-million years of cultural evolution cannot alter the fact that humans, like all other living organisms, are inextricably bound up in the web of interdependency and interrelationships that characterize life on this planet. Human health, well-being, and indeed survival are ultimately dependent on the health and integrity of the whole environment in which we live. Today the natural world that we share with all other forms of life on this planet is under unprecedented attack, not by outside forces of evil, as in a science fiction movie, but rather by a wide range of human activities and the sheer pressure of human numbers. Sometimes unwittingly, sometimes with full awareness of the consequences of our actions, we are rapidly altering the basic foundations of the environment that sustains us.

Will the abuses we are currently heaping upon the environment ultimately lead to the collapse of the entire system? This question has been a hot topic of debate for at least the past three decades as levels of pollution, depletion of resources, destruction of land, and the population spiral continue to mount. On June 3, 1992, representatives of 178 nations converged on Rio de Janeiro, Brazil, for an extraordinary 12-day gathering to wrestle with these issues. Political leaders, journalists, and citizen-activists from around the world joined forces to demonstrate their hopes and concerns for the future health and habitability of our planet. More than one hundred heads of state, the largest number of world leaders ever assembled for a single purpose, attempted to forge an international accord to deal with environmental problems so pervasive that they can no longer be solved solely by national efforts.

Widely referred to as the "Earth Summit," the Rio conference, officially designated as the United Nations Conference on Environment and Development (UNCED), marked the second time the world organization had sponsored a major international gathering to focus on environmental concerns. The first such meeting had been held 20 years earlier in Stockholm, Sweden. Coming at a time when the environmental movement was in its infancy, this event stimulated the formation of thousands of grassroots ecological groups around the world and prompted over one hundred nations to establish official environmental agencies to confront national problems of pollution and resource depletion. During the years following the Stockholm conference, global environmental awareness gradually increased, but Cold War tensions and East-West ideological divisions relegated international cooperation on ecological issues to the sidelines.

With the collapse of the Soviet empire in the late 1980s, it has become increasingly obvious that the major division in the world today is not one separating Communists from capitalists, but is rather a North-South split in which the affluent consumer societies of Europe, North America, and Japan view with apprehension the rapidly growing, resource-hungry populations of the Third World who demand their share of the "good life" enjoyed by their neighbors in the industrialized world. It also has become obvious that if the developing nations of Asia, Africa, and Latin America attempt to copy the model of development followed by Western nations, the resulting pollution and depletion of resources would lead to ecological destruction of enormous proportions, affecting the entire planet. Thus the main goal at the Earth Summit was to try to convince the world's governments to abandon development policies that lead ultimately to ecocatastrophe and to adopt instead programs of "sustainable development"—those which balance valid economic considerations with environmental realities, satisfying reasonable human needs without jeopardizing the well-being of future generations. The urgency of the environmental challenge facing the world's people was aptly described by U.N. Secretary-General Boutros Boutros-Ghali, who opened the Earth Summit with an appeal to delegates to redirect their military spending to programs of environmental protection, suggesting that the Rio conference might well be remembered by future generations as the time when humans recognized that "nature no longer exists in the classic sense of the term" but "lies within the hands of man."

The major issues tackled by Earth Summit delegates were global in scope: loss of biodiversity, tropical deforestation, climate change, eradication of poverty. More local concerns dealing with air and water pollution, the toxic wastes trade, rights of indigenous peoples, and a broad host of other concerns were hotly debated, not only by official dignitaries but also by the thousands of citizens from around the world who flocked to Rio as representatives of nongovernmental organizations. Disappointingly, there were several major policy issues on which participants failed to reach agreement—or refused even to address. Conspicuously absent from the main agenda was serious discussion of how to reverse the population explosion that many observers are convinced is the underlying cause of much, if not most, of the pressure leading to rampant environmental degradation. The combined opposition of the Vatican and the conservative Islamic nations to any meaningful deliberation of family-planning strategies was but one of many examples of politics obstructing effective action. North-South wrangling over who should provide the enormous sums (estimated at $125 billion annually) required to clean up pollution and alleviate poverty in the Third World frequently imparted a rich nations versus poor nations aspect to UNCED sessions. Perhaps most disappointing to those who had envisioned the Rio conference as a major turning point in the "race to save the planet" was the obstructionist position taken by the U.S. delegation which, under orders from President Bush, refused to sign an international convention to protect endangered species and fatally weakened the agreement on global warming by insisting that specific targets and timetables for reducing carbon dioxide emissions be deleted from the final document. Most significantly, American refusal to provide a major increase in funding for Third World development and pollution abatement programs guaranteed that many of the lofty goals adopted at the conference would never be realized. While preaching the virtues of sustainable development to Southern Hemisphere governments, the United States and other nations of the North made it clear that they are unwilling to accept economic limits at home to promote global environmental stability. Reflecting his government's position, an American delegate bluntly pointed out that "the United States standard of living is not up for negotiation."

As the conference ended and the participants headed homeward, some disillusioned observers denounced Rio's results as ineffectual, "business as usual," or "a failure to set a new direction for life on earth." The gathering dramatized a vivid rise in North-South antagonism over money and clarified the difficulties of setting aside national differences even when the stakes involved are as fundamental as planetary survival. Nevertheless, most delegates departed with the conviction that Rio had marked the beginning of something very important—a new era of awareness that human development and well-being is inextricably bound to protection of the earth's environment. As Prime Minister Felipe Gonzales of Spain remarked, "Five hundred years ago men set out to discover the size of the earth. At this meeting we discovered its limits."

In the years since the Earth Summit, numerous crises, both domestic and international, have displaced the concerns raised at Rio from the forefront of world attention. Such issues are not forgotten, however. Beyond the glare of media spotlights, the United Nations Commission on Sustainable Development—a body created at Rio to integrate the environment and development activities of the U.N. with those of other agencies and to monitor follow-up on Earth Summit treaty commitments—meets regularly and prods governments to fulfill pledges made. A more "environmentally friendly" Administration was elected in the United States in 1992, expressing commitment to many of the principles articulated at the Rio conference. Among environmentalists, hope was rekindled that the United States would once again be at the forefront of efforts to protect the global environment.

However, the strongest reason for optimism about humanity's chances of reversing the current downward spiral of environmental degradation is the worldwide proliferation of small grassroots organizations made up of committed citizens, working independently on their own local problems but united in their determination to save our natural heritage for future generations. Inspired and energized by the spectacle at Rio, they have recognized that we don't have to sit back as passive spectators to the despoliation of our environment and the impoverishment of our society. They realize that much can be done to limit the impact of advanced technology on the natural world and to incorporate environmental considerations into national policy-making. These activists, ordinary people from all walks of life, have an important message for the rest of us: to a great extent the technical know-how to prevent further deterioration exists—what is needed most is a societal commitment to get the job done. The most important decisions being made in the environmental health arena today are political decisions, balancing ecological concerns with economic and social considerations. Individuals wishing to become involved in protecting and enhancing environmental quality will find their efforts most effective when directed toward influencing environmental policy-making bodies at every level of government. To be a successful ecoadvocate, however, requires a thorough understanding of the nature of our environmental crisis, how the present situation developed, what the human impact of these threats may be, and what actions have already been taken in an attempt to restore and maintain a quality environment. These are the issues this book will attempt to address in the belief that a well-informed, politically active citizenry is an essential ingredient for attaining the worthy goals so eloquently articulated at the Earth Summit.

CHAPTER 1

Introduction to Ecological Principles

Hurt not the earth, neither the sea, nor the trees.

—Bible, Revelations 7:3

When astronauts Neil Armstrong and "Buzz" Aldrin became the first humans to land on the moon and gazed back at their home planet more than 200,000 miles away, they were filled with a sense of wonder at the beauty and uniqueness of Earth. Of all the heavenly bodies of which we are aware, our planet is neither the largest nor the smallest, the hottest nor the coldest, yet it *is* extraordinary in one vital respect—in all the universe Earth is the only planet known to support life. Within that narrow film of air and water which envelops the surface of the globe, extending vertically from the deepest ocean trenches more than 36,000 feet below sea level to about 30,000 or more feet above sea level, exists what ecologists call the **biosphere**—that portion of Earth where life occurs.

For all practical purposes, the physical extent of the biosphere is even more limited than just described. Even though the deep ocean trenches do possess a number of bizarre aquatic species, and certain fungal spores and pollen grains may be found floating in the upper reaches of the atmosphere, by far the greatest number of living things are found in the region extending from the permanent snow line of tropical and subtropical mountain ranges (about 20,000 feet above sea level) to the limit of light penetration in the clearest oceans (about 600 feet deep). Here a vast assemblage of plant, animal, and microbial life can be found—perhaps as many as 10 million different species living today. These species interact both with each other and with their physical environment; over very long periods of time they become modified in response to environmental pressures and, in turn, they themselves modify their physical surroundings.

The first living organisms on Earth (probably forms similar to bacteria) are now thought to have arisen more than 3.5 billion years ago on a planet whose environment was considerably different from that of the present-day world. The life activities of those early organisms, feeding upon and reacting with the chemical compounds in the waters where they first arose, were responsible for the creation of the modern atmosphere, which made possible the emergence of higher forms of life. The first primitive organisms evolved in a world devoid of atmospheric oxygen but rich in carbon dioxide. This carbon dioxide in turn provided a carbon source for the evolutionarily more advanced photosynthetic organisms which could produce their own food by utilizing the sun's energy to convert carbon dioxide and water into carbohydrates, releasing oxygen as a waste product. It was through the action of such photosynthetic organisms that the earth's atmosphere gradually became an oxygen-rich one, permitting the development of the types of life with which we are familiar today. In this way, the life activities of one group of organisms profoundly altered the environment and created conditions that facilitated the emergence of other forms of life. The ability of living things to modify their surroundings and the tendency of other organisms to respond positively or negatively to such changes has been a constant feature of evolutionary progression throughout the ages and remains so today.

Ecosystems

The concept of nature as divided into basic functional units called **ecosystems** reflects scientists' recognition of the complex manner in which living organisms interact with each other and with the nonliving (or abiotic) components of their environment to process energy and cycle nutrients. The concept is admittedly imprecise, since few ecosystems have definitive spatial boundaries or exist in splendid isolation. Adjacent ecosystems commonly influence each other, as when a pond ecosystem is altered by materials washing into it from surrounding terrestrial ecosystems, and certain components (e.g. water birds, insects) may be moving in and out on a regular basis (Smith, 1986). Similarly, the concept of ecosystems is a broad one, its main usefulness being to emphasize the interdependence of the biotic and abiotic components of an area. An ecosystem has no defining size limitations: an abandoned tire casing containing trapped rainwater, microorganisms, and swarms of mosquito larvae can be regarded as an ecosystem; so can a family-room aquarium, a city park, a cornfield, a tidepool, a cow pasture, or, indeed, the entire planet Earth. Any of these widely diverse situations can be considered an ecosystem so long as living and nonliving elements are present and interacting to process energy and cycle materials (Stiling, 1992).

Biotic Community

The most familiar classification system used for grouping plants and animals is one based upon presumed evolutionary relationships—lions, tigers, and leopards being grouped in the cat family; wheat, corn, and rice in the grass family, and so forth. However, ecologists tend to arrange species on the basis of their functional association with each other. A natural grouping of different kinds of plants and animals within any given habitat is termed by ecologists a **biotic community.**

"Biotic community," like "ecosystem," is a broad term which can be used to describe natural groupings of widely differing sizes, from the various microscopic diatoms and zooplankton swimming in a drop of pond water to the hundreds of species of trees, wild flowers, ferns, insects, birds, mammals, and so forth, found in an Appalachian forest. Biotic communities have characteristic trophic structures and energy flow patterns and also have a certain taxonomic unity, in the sense that certain species tend to exist together.

Individuals of the same species living together within a given area are collectively referred to as a **population.** Such populations constitute groups more or less isolated from other populations of the same species. A population within the biotic community of a region is not a static entity but is continually changing in size and reshuffling its hereditary characteristics in response to environmental changes and to fluctuations in the populations of other members of the community.

The community concept is one of the most important ecological principles because 1) it emphasizes the fact that different organisms are not arbitrarily scattered around the earth with no particular reason as to why they live where they do, but rather that they dwell together in an orderly manner; and 2) by illuminating the importance of the community as a whole to any of its individual parts, the community concept can be used by humans to manage a particular organism, in the sense of increasing or decreasing its numbers. Emphasizing biotic communities as a whole, rather than focusing on their constituent species, is helpful also in demonstrating why removing one species from a community (or, conversely, introducing a nonnative species into a community) can often have unintended—and sometimes disastrous—consequences.

European settlement of the sparsely populated North American continent launched a gigantic experiment in human interference with natural ecosystems. One dramatic example of how a stable biotic community can unravel simply by elimination of one of its members is the sad tale of beaver exploitation. In the late 17th century, French traders began trapping these once-abundant mammals, shipping enormous numbers of valuable pelts back to Europe to accommodate the insatiable demands of the hat-making industry. So extensively and heavily were they hunted that within 150 years beavers faced extinction from the Great Lakes region all the way to Oregon and California. Only as their numbers plummeted did the beavers' role within their biotic community become apparent. With the demise of their architects, beaver dams were no longer maintained and eventually washed away. As a result, rates of stream flow sharply accelerated, destroying the spawning beds of fish species which relied on the quiet waters behind the dams for breeding. Marshy areas created by the dams were either drained or flooded, depending on location, and waterfowl populations declined as nesting sites were lost. Flooding increased in frequency and intensity, streamside erosion worsened, and siltation of river channels accelerated. Disappearance of the beaver, perceived by the trappers as a creature that was "going to waste" in the wilderness, thus led to surprisingly far-reaching effects (Ashworth, 1986).

Introducing a nonnative species (i.e. an exotic) into an established biotic community can be every bit as destabilizing as removing a component species. Time and again, accidentally or deliberately, humans have released plants or animals into a new environment only to see them quickly attain major pest

BOX 1-1

Of Orcas and Otters

Nature is full of surprises, one of the latest being the near-disappearance of sea otters from Alaska's western coastline. Equally surprising is the identity of the agent responsible for the unexpected population crash and the demonstration that only a few members of a transient species can have a profound impact in linking interactions across ecosystems.

Playful marine mammals once hunted almost to extinction by fur traders, sea otters (*Enhydra lutris*) experienced a dramatic comeback following adoption in 1911 of an international treaty which prohibited killing of these animals. By the 1970s sea otter populations had recovered to pre-hunting levels in many parts of their historic range, giving conservationists reason to assume that their long-term survival was assured. Rebounding sea otter populations were regarded as good news for coastal marine ecosystems; as a "keystone species" of its biotic community, the sea otter plays a pivotal role in maintaining the health of the near-shore kelp "forests" on which a diverse assemblage of plant and animal species depend. As voracious predators of kelp-eating sea urchins, the otters prevent overgrazing of the giant algae, thereby contributing to overall ecosystem stability.

Until the late 1980s, sea otter populations along Alaska's Aleutian archipelago appeared healthy and thriving, but by 1990 the picture there suddenly and inexplicably began to change. Along a 500-mile stretch of western Alaska, the number of sea otters, which had been estimated at 53,000 in the 1970s, plummeted to just 6,000 in 1997—a 90% decline in population size. Scientists who had been studying the ecology of the area for several decades were initially at a loss to explain what was happening. They knew the animals weren't experiencing reproductive failure because studies of radio-tagged otters showed that birth and survival rates of otter pups remained at normal levels. Aerial surveys conducted by the U.S. Fish and Wildlife Service in 1965 and again in 1992 confirmed that the recent decline in the otter population was widespread throughout the island chain—the otters weren't simply relocating from one area to another. Consequently, the only explanation for the animals' drastic decline was increased mortality—but why? If otters were falling victim to disease or toxic pollutants, then researchers should have observed carcasses washing up onshore, but not even one had been sighted. Starvation was an unlikely explanation, since sea urchins, the otters' favorite food, were in plentiful supply. That left predation as the only plausible cause for rising otter death rates.

In 1991 when one member of the research team observed an otter being attacked and eaten by an orca, or killer whale (*Orcinus orca*), the sighting was regarded as an anomaly; orcas and sea otters had always shared the same waters and no one had ever seen the whales preying on their small, furry neighbors. However, over the next several years more such attacks were documented and gradually the scientists became convinced that a fundamental change in orca behavior was responsible for the dwindling number of otters. Gradually the case against the whales grew more persuasive; on Adak Island, observations revealed that 65% of the otters in easily accessible Kulak Bay disappeared over the course of one year, while in Clam Lagoon, whose entrance from the sea was too shallow and narrow for the orcas to enter, the otter population decline was only 12%. Finally, statistical analyses of what the rate of observed orca attacks was likely to be if killer whales were responsible for the 90% observed decrease in otter numbers yielded a figure almost identical to the number of attacks actually witnessed. The verdict now was beyond doubt—orca predation was the cause of the otter population crash.

Again, however, the question was why? Why would orcas, whose preferred food had always been the much larger, more nutritious harbor seals and sea lions, suddenly begin eating sea otters? As one ecologist studying the phenomenon remarked, it's like "eating popcorn instead of steaks."

The answer to the riddle demonstrates how truly complex are the workings of nature. Since the late 1970s, populations of sea lions and seals have collapsed across the western North Pacific. While the cause of this event remains controversial, the most likely explanation is overfishing by commercial trawlers in the Bering Sea. The decline in perch and herring led directly to the crash in seal and sea lion populations which, in turn, forced killer whales to resort to a diet of otters. Considering the large energy requirements of orcas and the minimal caloric value of an otter, researchers calculate that a single killer whale may consume 1,825 otters per year, a figure which suggests that as few as four orcas may be responsible for the observed otter depopulation along more than 2,000 miles of shoreline!

Unfortunately, the ecological implications of this sad story don't end with the near-disappearance of Alaskan sea otters. With populations of their main predator so depleted, sea urchins in the affected areas are now experiencing a population explosion; hordes of hungry urchins are gobbling up the kelp beds, reducing the density of these underwater "forests" 12-fold in just ten years. If the kelp forest ecosystem collapses, as it is likely to do now that its keystone species (i.e. the sea otters) has been removed, many other components of this biotic community will be affected. Populations of rockfishes, sculpins, and greenlings fish that live within the kelp beds—are likely to decline as their habitat vanishes; starfish, living in the open ocean beyond the kelp but also preyed upon by otters, will probably increase in numbers; seagull populations may remain stable, since those birds can turn to a diet of invertebrates as their preferred fish species dwindle; but less versatile bald eagles—totally dependent on fish—will either starve or go elsewhere as their food supply disappears.

It requires quite a stretch of the imagination to comprehend how catching too many herring in the North Pacific could result in the destruction of kelp forests and the loss of eagles along the Alaskan coast. Nevertheless, the fact that just such a scenario is now unfolding vividly demonstrates the complexity and interconnectedness of biotic communities and illustrates how human activities can set in motion a series of cascading events, culminating in the demise of species we never intended to harm.

References

Estes, J.A., M.T. Tinker, T.M. Williams, and D.F. Doak. 1998. "Killer Whale Predation on Sea Otters Linking Oceanic and Nearshore Ecosystems"; Kaiser, Jocelyn, "Sea Otter Declines Blamed on Hungry Killers." Science 282, no. 5388 (Oct. 16):390, 473-476.

status, usually due to the absence of natural predators which could keep their numbers under control. In the United States, zebra mussels, Asian long-horned beetles, and Africanized ("killer") bees are but the most recent in a host of unwanted aliens to invade our shores—gypsy moths, European star-lings, carp, kudzu, purple loosestrife, water hyacinths, sea lampreys, Formo-san termites—to mention but a few of the most notorious. Elsewhere in the world, exotic species have been equally disruptive; in the Netherlands, six North American muskrats brought to that country in 1906 have, in the absence of natural enemies, multiplied into the millions. Spreading through-out the country via the hundreds of thousands of miles of canals that charac-terize Holland, the muskrats have become major pests by burrowing into and weakening the vital dikes that protect the low-lying country from devastating floods. Along the Mediterranean coast, a Pacific seaweed, *Caulerpa taxifolia*, accidentally released from aquarium tanks at Monaco's Oceanographic Museum, has proliferated from the French Riviera to the shores of Croatia. Wherever it goes, *Caulerpa* crowds out native plant and animal species, pro-ducing a monoculture that threatens to destroy the entire Mediterranean eco-system. Another uninvited migrant native to the east coast of North America, Leidy's comb jelly, was discharged with ships' ballast water into the Black Sea where it has multiplied so rapidly that a single cubic meter of sea water now contains as many as 500 of the tiny animals. Because the jellyfish out-com-petes native fish for the zooplankton both eat, populations of indigenous anchovies and other commercially important fish species have plummeted and the entire Black Sea ecosystem is now on the verge of collapse (Bright, 1998).

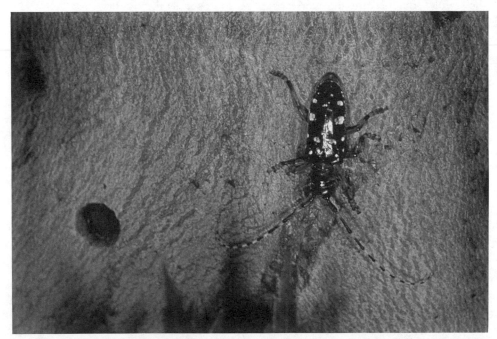

The Asian longhorned beetle threatens many species of hardwood trees, into which they tunnel large holes and then feed. Native to China, Korea, and Japan, the large black-and-white beetle was discovered in Chicago and Long Island in 1998. *[Philip L. Nixon, Illinois Cooperative Extension Service.]*

In our attempts to "control nature" we must never forget that the intricate interdependencies which have evolved over the millennia among the biotic communities of the earth cannot be altered without provoking a corresponding change somewhere else in the ecosystem.

Ecological Dominants

Although all members of a biotic community have a role to play in the life of that community, it is obvious that certain plants or animals exert more of an influence on the ecosystem as a whole than do others. As George Orwell might have put it, "All animals are equal, but some animals are more equal than others." Those organisms which exert a major modifying influence on the community are known as **ecological dominants.** Such dominants generally comprise those species that control the flow of energy through the community; if they were to be removed from the community, much greater changes in the ecosystem would result than if a nondominant species were to be removed. For example, when farmers chop down the dominant hardwood trees in an eastern forest to clear the land for cultivation, the changes produced by this removal (i.e. loss of animal species which depend on the trees for food and shelter, loss of shade-loving plants which proliferate under the canopy, change in soil microbiota, raising of soil temperature, increase in soil erosion, and so forth) are much more pronounced than would be the changes brought about when the farmers' children wander into the forest and pick all of the trilliums and lady slippers they find growing there. In either case, the stability of the ecosystem is upset, but the loss of several species of spring wildflowers, while unfortunate, has much less effect on the forest community as a whole than does the loss of the dominant oaks, maples, and beeches.

In most terrestrial biotic communities certain plants comprise the dominant species because not only do they provide food and shelter for other organisms, they also directly affet and modify their physical environment. That is, they contribute to a build-up of topsoil, moderate fluctuations of temperature, improve moisture retention, affect the pII of the soil, and so on. As a general rule, the number of dominant species within a community becomes progressively fewer as one moves toward the poles and greater the closer the community is to the tropics. While a northern coniferous forest may consist of only spruces or firs, a jungle in Sumatra may have a dozen or more tree species that could be considered dominants. In addition to the effects of latitude on number of dominants in a community, one can also generalize that dominant species are fewer in regions where climatic conditions are extreme, i.e. tundra and deserts (Odum, 1959).

Among animal species in a biotic community, certain **keystone predators** help maintain greater biotic diversity than would exist in their absence. Keystone, or dominant, predators moderate competition among the species upon which they prey, reducing the density of strong competitors and thereby allowing less aggressive competitors to maintain their populations within the community. As described earlier in Box 1-1, stability of the kelp "forest" ecosystem along Alaska's Pacific Coast is maintained by sea otters preying heavily on kelp-eating sea urchins. With urchin population pressures kept at tolerable levels by otter predation, a food supply for other herbivores in that biotic community is maintained and a diverse range of species can flourish. When otter numbers suddenly dropped, the population of sea urchins exploded, overwhelming their competitors and resulting in a sharp decline in the biodiversity of the kelp forest community.

Biomes

The species composition of any particular biotic community is profoundly affected by the physical characteristics of the environment, particularly temperature and rainfall. The kinds of plants and animals one would see while touring Yellowstone National Park would differ significantly from those found on a trek through the Amazon. Ecologists have divided the terrestrial communities of the world into general groupings called **biomes,** areas which can be recognized by the distinctive life forms of their dominant species. In most cases, the key characteristic of a biome is its dominant type of vegetation. We might define a biome as a complex of communities characteristic of a regional climatic zone. Each biome has its own pattern of rainfall, its own seasons, its own maximum and minimum temperatures, and its own changes of day length, all of which combine to support a certain kind of vegetation. Since climatic zones change in a relatively uniform pattern as one moves from the poles toward the equator, the earth's biomes form more or less continuous latitudinal bands around the globe. Starting at the polar regions, let's take a brief look at the major biomes of the earth (note: ecologists list numerous subdivisions of the biomes described here, but for our purposes these general groupings will suffice).

Tundra

The northernmost of the world's land masses, tundra is characterized by permanently frozen subsoil called **permafrost.** In this biome rainfall is quite low, about 8 inches annually, but because the permafrost doesn't allow moisture to penetrate beyond the upper few inches of soil, the tundra in summer is dotted with numerous lakes and bogs—and probably the world's most voracious mosquitoes! The tundra is windy, with only a few stunted trees. The dominant vegetation here consists of moss, lichens, grass, and some small perennials. Animal life is limited in the number of species but very abundant in the number of individuals. These include caribou or reindeer, birds, insects, polar bears, lemmings, foxes, rabbits, and fish. Reptiles and amphibians are absent. The tundra is basically a very fragile environment. Because of the slow rates at which tundra plants grow and decompose (due to the low temperatures and the characteristics of permafrost), the thick, spongy matting of lichens, grasses, and sedges that typify tundra is especially slow to recover from disturbance. Tracks of vehicles or animals can remain visible for decades. Great care must be taken in building on tundra because heat from structures will melt the permafrost and cause uneven settling, which often badly distorts the buildings. Until recently the tundra was relatively unexploited, but with the construction of the Alaska oil pipeline and similar kinds of mineral development in Canada and Siberia, that situation has changed.

Taiga

A Russian word for "swamp forest," the taiga is sometimes called the **northern coniferous forest.** This biome covers much of Canada, Scandinavia, and Russia. As the name implies, the dominant vegetation here consists of conifer trees that have needlelike leaves which stay on the trees for three to five years. These include spruces, firs, hemlocks, and pines. Some deciduous trees such as aspens, alders, and larches are also prominent. In general, the trees are much less diverse in number of species than those in the deciduous forests farther south and the soils have a different kind of humus and are more acid. Precipitation in the taiga is only moderate but, because drainage is poor, lakes, ponds, and bogs are common here. Animals of the taiga include bears, moose, lynxes, weasels, wolverines, and a variety of birds. Because of the huge stands of just one or two species of conifers, the taiga provides an opportunity for periodic outbreaks of pests like the spruce budworm, which can defoliate huge areas of forest. Perhaps because of the lack of diversity of species, taiga populations tend to undergo "boom or bust" cycles fairly regularly.

Temperate Deciduous Forest

This biome occurs in a belt south of the taiga where climate is milder and where rainfall is abundant relative to the amount of evaporation. This is the biome familiar to most of us because it is the one in which Western, as well as Chinese and Japanese, civilization developed. Soil types and elevations vary widely within this biome. Maples, beech, oaks, and hickories are common trees; many species of ferns and flowering herbaceous plants are also found. The deciduous forest has a great variety of mammals, birds, and insects, as well as a modest number of reptiles and amphibians. Because of the annual leaf drop, deciduous forests generate soils rich in nutrients, which in turn support a multitude of soil microbes. When such forests are cleared, the richness of the soils can be maintained if great care is taken to see that their supplies of nutrients and decaying organic matter are preserved (in a sense, raising crops or grazing animals is akin to mining the soil, since the nutrients leave along with the crops, meat, wool, or whatever is removed). All too often, however, short-term careless exploiters have allowed soils to deteriorate or have ignored opportunities to improve them. Unfortunately, economic considerations often lead individuals who are exploiting an ecosystem to use short-term strategies that are disastrous for humanity in the long run.

Grasslands

In regions where annual rainfall is not sufficient to sustain the growth of trees and evaporation rates are high, we find the grasslands of the world. These may be called by different names in various countries: prairie, veldt, savannah, steppe, pampas, llanos. All are characterized by the dominance of grasses and herds of grazing animals. Carnivores also abound, such as coyotes and lions, as do rodents and many species of reptiles. The grassland biome has a higher concentration of organic matter in its soil than does any other biome, the amount of humus in grassland soil being about 12 times greater than that in forest soils. The extraordinary richness of grassland soil has led to the

Figure 1-1 Major Biomes of the World

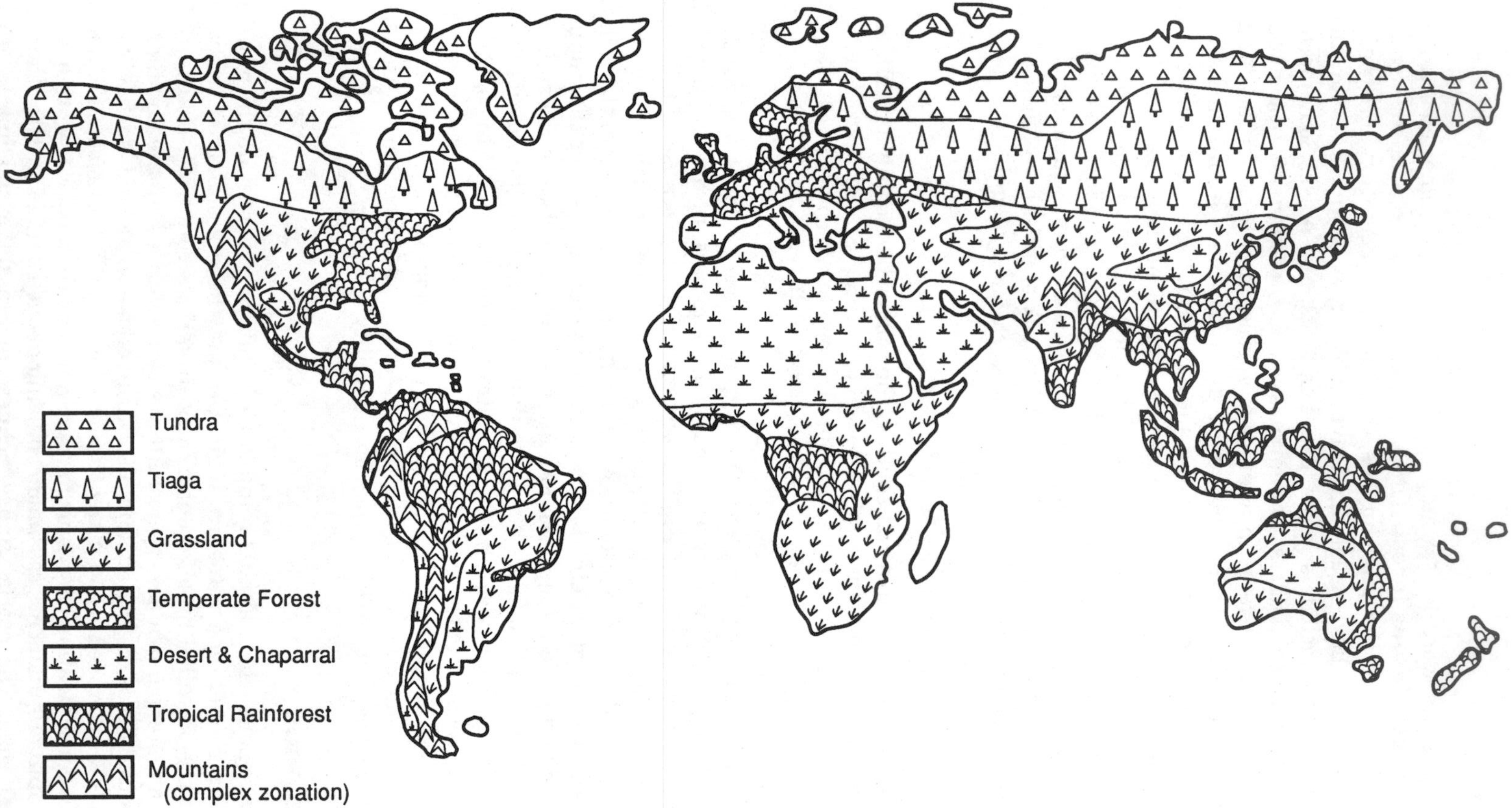

Tundra

Tiaga

Grassland

Temperate Forest

Desert & Chaparral

Tropical Rainforest

Mountains
(complex zonation)

establishment of extremely successful agricultural ecosystems in the grass-land areas. These systems can break down rapidly, however, if careful soil conservation is not practiced. The interlaced roots and creeping underground stems of grasses form a turf that prevents erosion of the soil. When the turf is broken with a plow or overgrazed, the soil is exposed to the erosive influences of wind and water, resulting in such calamities as the "Dust Bowl" of the Great Plains in the 1930s.

Desert

Areas receiving less than 10 inches annual precipitation and featuring high daytime temperatures are classified as deserts. These areas are concentrated in the vicinity of 30° north and 30° south latitude. Lack of moisture is the essential factor shaping the desert biome. Most deserts are quite hot in the daytime and, because of the sparse vegetation and resultant rapid reradiation of heat, quite cold at night. Desert plants and animals are characterized by species that can withstand prolonged drought. Among plants such adaptations include waxy cuticle on stems or leaves, reduction in leaf size, and spiny growths to repel moisture-seeking animals. Plants may appear to be widely spaced, but if their roots were visible, the ground between them would be seen to be laced with a shallow root system to take maximum advantage of any rain that does fall. Proportionately more annual plants are found in the desert biome than in any other; because their seeds often require abrasion or a rain heavy enough to leach out inhibiting chemicals, the desert appears to bloom almost overnight after a heavy rain. For the most part, desert animals are active at night, remaining under cover during the heat of the day. Desert soils contain little organic matter and must ordinarily be supplied with both water and nitrogen fertilizer if they are to be cultivated. Human activities have already produced a great increase in the amount of desert and wasteland, removing many once-productive acres from cultivation. Occasional years of good rainfall cause people to forget that the desert is inherently a very fragile environment.

Tropical Rain Forest

This biome is found in Central and South America, central Africa, and South and Southeast Asia. It is characterized by high temperatures and high annual rainfall; 100 inches or more of annual precipitation is common in this biome. Year-round temperature variation is slight. Tropical rain forests are characterized by a great diversity of plant and animal species and by four distinct layers of plant growth—the top canopy of trees reaching 200 feet or more, a lower canopy of densely intertwined treetops at about 100 feet, a sparse understory, and only a very few plants growing at ground level. A wide variety of epiphytic plants can be found. Both plant and animal species exist in greater diversity in the tropical rain forest than anywhere else in the world, though numbers of individuals of a particular species are usually limited. To most people, the luxuriant growth of a tropical jungle implies a rich soil, and one hears many glowing promises of the agricultural riches to be reaped by turning the Amazon or Congo River basins into farmland. The truth of the situation is far different, however. Tropical forest soils in general are exceedingly thin and nutrient-poor. They cannot maintain large reserves of minerals needed for plant growth, primarily because heavy rainfall and a high rate of water flow through the ground to the water table leach them from the soil. The leaching process leaves large residues of insoluble iron and aluminum oxides in the upper levels of tropical forest soils, a process termed "laterization." With the exception of certain fertile river valleys, primitive slash-and-burn agriculture is the only type suitable to most areas of the tropical rain forest. Unfortunately, this fragile ecosystem is being destroyed more rapidly than any other biome due to human population growth and in some cases, such as in Brazil, as a direct consequence of governmental actions.

It should be noted that in areas where there are substantial variations in altitude, the biomes differ at different elevations. This is primarily because air temperature decreases about 6°C for every 1,000-meter increase in altitude and because, especially in desert areas, rainfall increases with altitude.

This brief survey of biome characteristics should make it obvious that various regions differ in their ability to return to an ecologically stable condition once they have been disrupted by human activities. Thus it should not be surprising that certain practices are far more devastating to the local ecology in some areas than they are in others. For example, strip mining in the flat or gently rolling lands of Illinois, Indiana, and Ohio is certainly disruptive to the environment, yet with proper soil reclamation practices the land can be restored to productive uses once mining has ceased. In the arid regions of the High Plains and Southwest, however, exploitation of fossil fuel reserves by strip mining presents a real threat that the acres thus despoiled could never recover and would remain permanent wastelands.

Ecological Niches

Within any biotic community each species is defined by its own unique position, or **niche,** different from that of any other member of the community and determined largely by its size and food habits. Through the processes of evolution and natural selection, plants and animals have become increasingly better adapted to the specific environments in which they live. In order to reduce competition among species for food and living space, organisms have become more specialized in terms of the foods they utilize, period of the day or night during which they are active, and/or the types of microhabitats they exploit. Thus, in an ecological context, the term niche denotes not simply the physical space that a species occupies but, more importantly, what that species *does* (Pianka, 1988). The **Principle of Competitive Exclusion,** basic to ecological theory, holds that when two species are competing for the same limited resources, only one will survive. Only when the environmental resources in a given community are partitioned among the coinhabiting species by means of niche diversification is direct competition minimized, thus permitting coexistence of species.

The benefits of niche diversification can be well illustrated by several species of lice, which peacefully coexist on a human host by restricting their activities to different anatomical regions. The body louse, notorious in history as the vector of typhus fever, feeds on parts of the body below the neck; the closely related head louse confines its activities to the head and neck. The fact that the two are quite similar in appearance and occasionally interbreed indicates their close relationship, but niche diversification is quite apparent in their different behavioral patterns. Head lice cement their eggs ("nits") to hairs of the scalp, while body lice usually glue theirs to fibers of clothing; in fact, body lice spend most of their time on clothing, coming into contact with the human body only when taking a blood meal. A third type, the crab louse, is morphologically specialized for life among the widely spaced, coarse hairs of the pubic areas. Unlike body and head lice which constantly move about, crab lice tend to settle in one spot and feed off and on for many hours at a time. Through behavioral and territorial specialization, these species avoid competition and thrive in their own unique ecological niche.

In other situations, species may utilize the same physical space but minimize competition by restricting their feeding activities to different times of the day. Within any given area one can find some species which are diurnal (active during the day), such as most birds, grazing animals, primates, and so on; other species which are nocturnal (active at night), including most snakes, many predators such as lions, foxes, owls, and so on; and still others such as deer and rabbits which prefer the in-between hours of dawn and dusk. Structural modifications among species allow animals inhabiting the same general area to utilize different foods. The finches of the Galapagos Islands, immortalized by Charles Darwin, were very similar in appearance and obviously evolved from the same parental stock, but modifications in their beak structure permitted each species to utilize a different type of food—insects, small seeds, medium-sized seeds, or large seeds, depending on the size and shape of beak—and thus to coexist within the same geographic area.

Examples of niche diversification illustrate the fact that throughout evolutionary history ecosystems have become exceedingly complex through increasingly effective adaptation of organisms within any natural community. Such a complex ecosystem is generally quite stable unless something happens to change that environment to which the organisms have become so well adapted. The processes of natural selection and adaptation are too slow to permit the vast majority of organisms to adjust quickly to such radical changes in their surroundings. As a result, the animal and plant populations in such disrupted situations generally die out or move elsewhere and the previously stable ecosystem collapses or, at a minimum, becomes less varied and less stable.

Limiting Factors

Why do corn plants thrive in central Illinois but not in Norway? Why don't ferns grow in the Mohave Desert? Why is the poison produced by the botulism bacterium *(Clostridium botulinum)* sometimes present in canned green beans but never in fresh ones? The reason why living things occur and thrive where they do depends upon a variety of conditions. Sometimes those conditions are quite obvious: summer temperatures in Norway are not hot enough nor is the growing season long enough to produce a bountiful corn harvest; lack of water and shade make survival of ferns impossible in a desert environment. In some cases the factors which control where a plant or animal lives are not quite so apparent: *Clostridium botulinum* can multiply and produce its deadly toxin only in an environment where oxygen is absent; hence it may present a threat in improperly canned foods, but seldom in fresh ones.

Environmental conditions that limit or control where an organism can live are called **limiting factors.** Obviously not every factor in an organism's environment is equally important in determining where that plant or animal can live. Components that are relatively constant in amount and moderately abundant are seldom limiting factors, particularly if the individual in question has a wide limit of tolerance. On the other hand, if an individual has a narrow limit of tolerance for a factor that exists in low or variable amounts, then that factor might indeed be the crucial determinant in where the organism can live. For example, most higher forms of life require a plentiful supply of oxygen to carry out their metabolic activities. Nevertheless, even though oxygen is essential, because it is so abundantly present and readily available to most land plants and animals (with the exception of some parasites and organisms living underground) it is almost never a limiting factor in terrestrial communities. On the other hand, lack of oxygen can definitely be a limiting factor for a number of aquatic organisms. The larvae of certain insects such as mayflies and caddisflies, as well as important game fish such as brook trout, simply die or move elsewhere when levels of dissolved oxygen in a waterway drop below a critical point.

Although the Native Americans who taught the Pilgrims to bury a dead fish in each hill of corn must have intuitively understood the concept, the idea of limiting factors was first formulated in 1840 by the German biochemist Justus Liebig while studying problems of fertility in agricultural soils. Liebig was experimenting with the use of inorganic chemical fertilizers in place of manures then currently in use and found that crop yields were affected not so much by the nutrients needed in large quantities—such as carbon dioxide and water, since these were generally present in plentiful supply—but by some mineral, such as copper, needed in minute amounts but lacking from particular soils. From this observation he proclaimed his famous **Law of the Minimum**, stating that "the growth of a plant is dependent on the amount of foodstuff which is presented to it in a minimum quantity." Succeeding generations of ecologists have expanded Liebig's concept to include not only mineral nutrients but also such things as light, temperature, pH, water, oxygen supply, and soil type as possible limiting factors to the distribution of organisms.

Further investigations revealed a complicating fact: when some factor other than the minimum one is available in very high concentrations, this may moderate the rate at which the critical one is used. For example, plants growing in the shade require less zinc than those growing in the sun. Thus shade-grown plants are less affected by a zinc-deficient soil than are plants of the same species growing in full sunlight. Also, some organisms can substitute a chemically similar nutrient for one that is deficient, as can be seen in certain mollusks that partially substitute strontium for calcium in their shells when amounts of calcium are low.

To make matters more complex, by the early 20th century it became clear that the old adage, "If a little bit is good, then more must be better," was quite untrue so far as the needs of living things were concerned. The concept of the Law of the Minimum was broadened by the American ecologist Victor Shelford, who demonstrated that too much of a limiting factor can be just as harmful as not

BOX 1-2

Frog Watch

The grotesquely deformed frogs discovered in a Minnesota pond by middle school students on a 1995 field trip gave biologists, already dismayed by the crashing populations of once-abundant amphibian species, one more cause for worry. Since 1989, when the alarm was first raised at an international conference about the decline or disappearance of frogs, toads, and salamanders in many far-flung parts of the world, it has become increasingly clear that something more insidious than natural cyclical fluctuations in population size is threatening the existence of these creatures. Until the mid-1990s, concerns among frog-watchers focused solely on the problem of dwindling numbers as scientists scrambled to find a causative agent. However, when the Minnesota observations were followed by a flood of similar reports from across the United States and Canada—tales of legless frogs or frogs with extra legs, frogs with eyes on their backs, frogs with suction-cup fingers growing out of their sides—it became obvious that massive deformities, as well as population decline and disappearance, were wreaking havoc on amphibians over a vast geographic area.

The plight of these animals should be a cause for concern to everyone, not just to naturalists, because amphibians, and especially frogs, are considered "sentinel" species—the first members of a biotic community to show the effects of environmental pollution. Like the caged canaries whose deaths provided an advance warning of the presence of toxic gases to underground miners, vanishing or misshapen frogs may be indicators of impending ecological catastrophe.

It's easy to understand why environmental contaminants would be logical suspects at a time when amphibian populations are under siege. Laying their eggs in water, spending their early months as free-swimming tadpoles, and subsequently moving onto the land as adults, frogs and toads are exposed to a wide range of pollutants. The fact that tadpoles and adults feed at different trophic levels makes the animals uniquely vulnerable to toxins entering the food chain. Their thin, moist skin offers little protection against contaminants such as heavy metals or other pollutants that can easily pass into their bodies from surrounding soil or water. The search for a single, unifying explanation is unlikely to be successful, nor is it known if the twin problems of deformities and population decline are even related. Nevertheless, recent research has yielded clues as to what may be happening and suggests that a variety of forces are to blame.

On the deformity question, researchers have been surprised to discover that the cause appears to be a natural one rather than the originally suspected pesticides or toxic pollutants. In research published in the spring of 1999, a team at Stanford University demonstrated that a type of parasitic flatworm, the trematode *Ribeiroia*, is capable of infecting tadpoles and provoking the types of limb abnormalities found in many California frog populations. While media accounts of this research proclaimed the mystery solved, many scientists caution that trematodes, while an important part of the solution, are probably not the answer to all amphibian deformities and express doubt that any single cause can explain all the problems reported.

Explanations for amphibian disappearances, as opposed to deformities, are more varied and controversial.

Indeed, some scientists continue to argue that reported population crashes are but temporary fluctuations in normal up-and-down cycles. However, the majority viewpoint is that the observed declines are too numerous and widespread to be attributed solely to natural causes. There are, of course, many places where frog populations remain stable and thriving; eastern North America and Europe are little affected by downward trends reported elsewhere. The three major "hotspots" of amphibian decline, where numbers have plummeted since 1980, are western North America (one-third of California's 30 species are in serious trouble); Central America; and northeastern Australia (Queensland). Search for a common environmental "smoking gun" has proven elusive; more than a decade of scientific investigation has shown that there is no single culprit.

In many, perhaps most, areas habitat destruction is the obvious cause for amphibian decline. When marshes are drained to construct shopping centers or when paddy fields are converted to golf courses, frogs disappear. Equally devastating for some native frog populations has been the introduction of exotic (i.e. nonnative) species which out-compete or eat up the original inhabitants. In California, the introduction of nonnative bullfrogs in lowland areas caused a precipitous decline in endemic species as the larger frogs proved more aggressive competitors for the existing food supply; similarly, when previously fish-free streams in the Sierras were stocked with nonnative trout and salmon, the newcomers decimated local frog populations by feasting on frog eggs and tadpoles. Overharvesting of frogs for human consumption also can have a dramatic impact. In southern India, Bangladesh, and Malaysia there is widespread exploitation of these tasty amphibians to meet foreign demand for frogs' legs as a gourmet food. It's estimated that French diners alone consume some 3,000–4,000 metric tons of imported frogs' legs annually—an amount requiring the sacrifice of 60–80 million frogs.

More problematic are the causes of amphibian decline in many seemingly undisturbed regions of the world. In Costa Rica's Monteverde Cloud Forest Reserve, for example, hordes of the brilliantly beautiful golden toad used to emerge from underground burrows during the breeding season, delighting naturalists who traveled from near and far to witness the spectacle. In 1987, thousands of toads participated in the age-old ritual; in 1988 only one was spotted and since then none have been seen. Today it's estimated that fully 50% of the frog species inhabiting the park in the early 1980s have vanished. In 1998 researchers discovered, to their surprise, that a previously innocuous chytrid fungus was attacking frogs in regions as far apart as Costa Rica and Australia, causing massive skin infections that resulted in suffocation of the animals. Why a formerly harmless rain forest fungus should suddenly become a destructive pathogen has yet to be explained. Speculation focuses on impairment of the amphibians' immune system, perhaps induced by reduction in moisture levels caused by global warming.

In the Pacific Northwest where populations of the Cascades frog and western toad had been declining since the 1980s, yet another environmental agent has been identified as the likely villain—ultraviolet light, whose intensity has been increasing as the earth's protective layer of stratospheric ozone thins. Researchers at Oregon State University have demonstrated that amphibian eggs laid in open, shallow water in mountain streams and lakes were failing to hatch because of UV-B damage to the embryos' DNA. Further investigations revealed that while some amphibian species produce sufficient amounts of the protective enzyme photolase to repair DNA damage, those species experiencing the most dramatic declines do not. The Pacific treefrog, whose eggs contain six times as much photolase as western toad eggs, continue to thrive while the latter species is on the verge of disappearing.

The list of environmental threats currently confronting frogs and their kin is thus long and diverse, from habitat loss to parasites, exotic predators, pathogenic fungi, and ultraviolet light. While natural causes now appear to be responsible for many frog deformities and extinctions, human interference with ecosystems further contributes to their plight. Amphibians have been hardy enough to have survived and prospered for the past 350 million years, but whether they can continue to share the planet with *Homo sapiens* remains to be seen. For skeptics who

question all the fuss about small slimy creatures of little economic value and limited emotional appeal, David Wake, a biologist at Berkeley responds, "If frogs and salamanders are dying off in synchrony, there's a message there for us. They survived whatever wiped out the dinosaurs and they have thrived through the age of mammals. If they start to check out now, we'd better take it seriously."

References

Johnson, Pieter T.J., et al. 1999. "The Effect of Trematode Infection on Amphibian Limb Development and Survivorship." *Science* 284 (April 30):802–804.

Blaustein, A.R., et al. 1997. "Ambient UV B Radiation Causes Deformities in Amphibian Embryos." *Proceedings of The National Academy of Sciences* 94, no. 25 (Dec. 9):13735-13737.

Blaustein, Andrew R., and David B Wake. 1995. "The Puzzle of Declining Amphibian Populations." *Scientific American* (April):52-57.

enough. Organisms have both an ecological maximum and minimum, the range in between these two extremes representing that organism's limits of tolerance.

Limits of Tolerance

Subsequent investigations in regard to tolerance ranges have revealed a great deal about why certain species live where they do. Not surprisingly, those plants and animals that have a wide range of tolerance for all factors are the ones that have the widest distribution. However, some organisms can have a wide tolerance range for some factors but a narrow range for others, and thus their distribution will be accordingly more limited. Not all stages of an animal's or plant's life cycle are equally sensitive to the effect of limiting factors. Among many spore-forming bacteria, for example, high temperatures that would be almost instantly fatal for actively growing cells have no effect on the spore stage unless the duration of exposure is fairly long. In general, the most critical period when environmental factors are most likely to be limiting (i.e. when the range of tolerance is narrowest) is during the reproductive period. Susceptibility of the young to conditions that adult organisms could tolerate with little difficulty is well established in regard to one of our major environmental problems at present, that of acid rainfall. The low pH levels that are blamed for the near-total disappearance of many species of fish in lakes throughout eastern Canada, northeastern United States, and parts of Scandinavia have been shown to be lethal to fish eggs and fingerlings, but not to adult fish. Thus the effects of acid rain on aquatic life are much less dramatic than the effects of, for example, a chemical spill into a river. Rather than a massive, immediately visible (and smelly!) fish kill, the fish in an acidifying lake simply fail to reproduce and become less and less abundant, older and older, until they die out completely. Other examples of the vulnerability of the reproductive stage include the observations that while adult cypress trees can grow either on dry ground or with their bases continually submerged in water, cypress seedlings can only develop in moist, unflooded soil. Similarly, some adult marine animals such as blue crabs can tolerate fresh water that is slightly salty and so are frequently found in rivers some distance upstream from the sea. Their young, however, can thrive only in salt water, so reproduction and permanent establishment of these organisms in rivers cannot occur. Just as the very young of lower forms of life display less tolerance to environmental extremes than do adults, the same situation applies with humans. Many widespread environmental toxins have been shown, some in tragic ways, to have a much more devastating effect on developing fetuses and young children than on adults. The drug thalidomide and organic mercury are just two substances that have been ingested by pregnant women with no harmful effects on themselves but with disastrous results on their unborn children. Levels of air pollution that are largely ignored by the adult population can cause severe respiratory distress in infants and children. It's important for us to keep in mind the qualifications to the range of tolerance concept when we hear official assurances that exposure to this or that substance is "safe." What is safe for one segment of the population may be far from safe for others.

Energy Flow Through the Biosphere

Living things are dependent for their existence not only on proper soil and climate conditions but also on some form of energy; a basic understanding of the flow of energy through an ecosystem is fundamental to the study of how that system functions.

The ultimate source of all life activities, from the unfolding of a flower bud to the 100-meter dash of an Olympic athlete is, of course, the sun. Some 93 million miles (150 million km) from the earth, the sun emits vast amounts of electromagnetic radiation which, traveling through space at a rate of 186,000 miles (300,000 km) per second, takes about nine minutes to reach the earth's surface. There is no energy loss as the sun's radiation travels through space, but since its intensity decreases inversely as the square of the distance from the sun, the amount of solar radiation intercepted by the earth is but one two-billionth of the sun's total energy output. On this seemingly tiny portion all life on earth depends. More than half the incoming radiation is unusable by living things, however. Electromagnetic radiation consists of several different wavelengths. Of the total amount of energy received from the sun, 9% is in the form of short-wave, high-energy ultraviolet rays; 50% is in the form of long-wave, infrared waves (heat waves); and 41% is visible light. Only those wavelengths within the visible spectrum, particularly those in the red and blue range, can be absorbed and utilized by green plants. These, through the process of photosynthesis, convert solar energy into the energy of chemical bonds. The complex and still not fully understood mechanism whereby plants harness certain wavelengths of sunlight and use this energy to join molecules of carbon dioxide and water to form the simple sugar glucose, releasing oxygen in the process, makes the existence of all higher forms of life possible. The transfer of this captured energy from organism to organism is basic to the functioning of ecosystems. Before examining the paths of energy flow, however, let us take a brief look at some physical laws that control and limit the amount of energy available to living things.

Laws of Thermodynamics

An understanding of many problems in both environmental science and energy technology depends on a basic conception of the principles that govern how energy is changed from one form into another. Known as the first and second laws of thermodynamics, these principles can be summarized as follows:

The First Law of Thermodynamics. Sometimes called the Law of Conservation of Energy, it states that energy can neither be created nor destroyed, even though it may be changed from one form into another. **Solar energy** that is absorbed by rocks or soil or water on the earth's surface is converted into **heat energy** which, because of temperature differentials and the earth's rotation, gives rise to winds and water currents that are a form of **kinetic energy.** When such kinetic energy accomplishes work such as the raising of water by wind, then it has been changed into **potential energy,** so-called because the latent energy of a water droplet in a cloud or at the top of a dam can be converted into some other kind of energy when it falls. In the same way, light energy absorbed by the chlorophyll molecules in a leaf is converted into the potential energy of chemical bonds within carbohydrates, proteins, and fats. As light energy passes from one form to another, it may appear that most of it is eventually lost or consumed (how often have we heard references to that misnomer, "energy consumption"?). This is a misconception, however, for if one maintained a global balance sheet it would show that all the energy that enters the biosphere as light is reradiated and leaves the earth's surface in the form of invisible heat waves. The form of energy leaving the system is different from the incoming radiation, but no energy has been either created or destroyed during its passage through the biosphere.

The Second Law of Thermodynamics. This law states that with every energy transformation there is a loss of usable energy (that is, energy that can be used to do work). Put another way, all physical processes proceed in such a way that the availability of the energy involved decreases (note that the availability, not the total amount, of energy is what decreases—the latter would be a violation of the First Law). The Second Law introduces the concept of **entropy,** the idea that all energy is moving toward an ever less available and more dispersed state. This process will continue until all energy has been transformed to heat distributed at a uniform temperature throughout the solar system—at which point the stable state will have been achieved.

The Second Law has some interesting implications concerning ecological relationships. Perhaps the most important of these is the fact that no type of energy transformation is ever 100% efficient—there will always be a significant loss of usable energy whenever energy is transferred from one organism to another. This explains why we need a continued input of energy to maintain ourselves and why we must consume substantially more than a pound of food in order to gain a pound of weight. In addition, because a given quantity of energy can be used only once, the ability to convert energy into useful work cannot be "recycled." Thus energy, unlike the essential minerals and gases, moves in a unidirectional way through ecosystems, becoming ever more dispersed and eventually being degraded to heat. Bearing these fundamental physical laws in mind, let's now take a more detailed look at the flow of energy through the biotic community.

Food Chains

Although overly simplistic, the concept of a **food chain** is useful for conveying a general understanding of how energy moves through ecosystems. Basically, a food chain involves the transfer of food energy from a given source through a series of organisms, each of which eats the next lower individual in the chain. In terms of energy flow, the living components of the ecosystem can be subdivided into three broad categories:

1. Producers—the green plants that convert the sun's energy into food energy. On land the major producers are the flowering plants and the conifers; in water they are mainly the diatoms, microflagellates, and green algae.

2. Consumers—animals; primary consumers are the herbivores and secondary consumers are the carnivores.

3. Decomposers—primarily bacteria and fungi, some insects. Decomposers are essential for recycling detritus back into the soil where it is once again available for use by producer organisms. No community could exist very long without decomposers.

There are basically three types of food chains. The most familiar of these, called a **grazing food chain** (or "predator chain"), may be typified by a grass-rabbit-fox association which starts with a plant base and proceeds from smaller to larger animals. Less conspicuous but equally important is the **detritus food chain,** where dead organic matter (detritus) is broken down by microorganisms, primarily bacteria. Small animals eat particles of this detritus, securing energy largely from assimilation of the energy-rich bacteria. The small animals, in turn, become a source of energy for larger consumers. A prime example of a detritus food chain accounting for a substantial portion of an ecosystem's energy flow can be found in the salt marsh habitat of many coastal areas. Here plants such as marsh grass die and are washed into estuaries where they are decomposed by microbes into finely divided particles which are then consumed by such primary consumers as fiddler crabs and mollusks. These, in turn, may be eaten by secondary consumers such as raccoons, water birds, or other crabs.

A variation on grazing food chains can be seen in certain **parasitic chains,** in which energy flows from larger to smaller animals (e.g. dogs which provide an energy source for fleas which in turn are fed upon by parasitic protozoans). In energy terms, however, there is no fundamental difference between a parasitic food chain and a grazing food chain, since a parasite is basically a "consumer."

Ecological Pyramids

Through the interactions of the community, a unidirectional flow of energy occurs from producers to primary consumers to secondary consumers, and so on. Each of these stages in a food chain is called a **trophic level.** It should be noted that placement of an organism into one trophic level or another depends on what that organism *does,* not to which species it belongs, since individuals of the same species may feed at different trophic levels, depending on factors such as age or sex. A male mosquito, for example, is an herbivore (primary consumer), dining on plant juices and nectar, while his mate would be classified as a carnivore (secondary consumer) when she takes the blood meal essential for egg laying. Similarly, while grazing animals such as cattle and horses are strict vegetarians as adults, their young thrive on a diet of mother's milk, making them, in effect, secondary consumers.

To describe the relationships among members of various trophic levels, ecologists frequently use the concept of **ecological pyramids.** If we examine a food chain in terms of its animal and plant constituents, it becomes apparent that these forms can be arranged into what is called a "pyramid of numbers." At the bottom of the pyramid are multitudes of energy-producing plants, then a smaller number of herbivores that feed upon them, then a still smaller number of primary carnivores, followed by an even smaller number of secondary carnivores. The animals at the top of the heap, the final consumers, are usually the largest in the community, while those organisms at the bottom of the pyramid, the producers, are usually the smallest, but much more abundant. In addition, the organisms at the lower trophic levels usually reproduce more rapidly and more prolifically than those higher up, so there is seldom danger of a predator eating itself out of its food supply. It should be noted, however, that in those cases where the size of the producer organisms is very large and the size of the primary consumers is small (e.g. a cherry tree being munched upon by hundreds of caterpillars), the shape of the pyramid of numbers may be inverted.

Just as the number of individual organisms in a community is generally greatest at the lower trophic levels, so the living weight, or **biomass** (measured as dry weight per unit area), is generally greatest at the producer trophic level. In the same way, biomass of the primary consumers will be greater than that of the secondary consumers, so the ecological biomass pyramids used to portray weight relationships among trophic levels will often look identical to numbers pyramids. Biomass, which in effect is an indicator of the amount of energy stored within an ecosystem, varies widely from one type of biotic community to another. For example, the amount of biomass in a tropical rain forest far exceeds that in a comparable area of abandoned field, while open ocean water is relatively poor in terms of biomass.

Although biomass pyramids, like numbers pyramids, usually have a broad base and tapered apex, in those situations where the organisms at the producer level are much smaller than the consumers, the shape of the biomass pyramid may be upside-down. This occurs because the "standing crop biomass" (the total dry weight of organisms present at any one moment in time) that can be maintained by a steady flow of energy in a food chain depends to a large extent on the size of the individual organisms. The smaller the organisms are, the greater is their metabolic rate per gram of biomass. Thus the smaller the organism, the smaller the biomass which can be supported at a given trophic level; in the same way, the larger the organism, the larger the amount of biomass at any one point in time. This is why in, say, an aquatic ecosystem the biomass of the blue whale would be far greater than the biomass of the microscopic diatoms and zooplankton on which it feeds. The biomass pyramid that illustrates the energy relationships in such a situation would be an inverted one. This doesn't mean that the producer organisms are defying the laws of nature; it simply reflects the fact that the tiny phytoplankton have very high metabolic rates and that they reproduce much more rapidly than do whales, having complete turnovers in their populations within very short time periods.

Whereas pyramids of numbers tend to exaggerate the importance of small organisms and pyramids of biomass often understate their role, pyramids of energy give the best picture of energy flow through a food chain, showing what actually is happening within the biotic community. As was mentioned earlier, light energy from the sun is captured by green plants and stored in the form of chemical bonds in the molecules of starch, glucose, fats, and so forth. However, as the Second Law of Thermodynamics states, only a portion of the energy stored by one trophic level is available to the next higher one, since a considerable amount is lost at every stage of transformation. Thus when cows graze in a pasture, some of the chemical bond energy in the grass is converted into the muscle tissue which represents stored food in the cow. The largest portion of energy derived from the grass, however, is lost in the form of waste heat during respiration. A lesser amount is lost as unassimilated food materials in feces or urine and as organic material which is not eaten by the next higher trophic level (i.e. just as people do not eat every part of a cow or pig, so many animals leave certain parts of their prey unconsumed; such "rejects" constitute an energy loss to the food chain).

At each transfer of energy within a food chain, approximately 90% (sometimes a bit more, sometimes less) of the chemical energy stored in organisms of the lower level is lost and therefore unavailable to the higher level. Since the total amount of energy entering the food chain is fixed by the photosynthetic activities of plants (and plants are less than 1% efficient, on the average, in converting solar energy into chemical energy), obviously more usable energy is available to organisms occupying lower positions in the food chain than to those at higher trophic levels. Expressing this concept in simpler terms, one might say, for example:

10,000 lbs. corn → 1,000 lbs. beef → 100 lbs. human

By moving humans one step lower in the food chain, ten times more energy becomes directly available:

$$10,000 \text{ lbs. corn} \rightarrow 1,000 \text{ lbs. human}$$

In very simplified terms, this explains why countries like China and India are largely vegetarian. In order to produce enough food to sustain many millions of people, such nations cannot afford the luxury of wasting the amount of energy involved in raising animals for meat. Some people feel that at a time when massive food shortages are a fact of life in many parts of the world, Americans have a moral responsibility to abstain from our predilection for corn fed beef and use midwestern farmlands to produce crops that humans can eat directly. From another viewpoint, the above equation indicates why

Figure 1-2   Food Pyramid

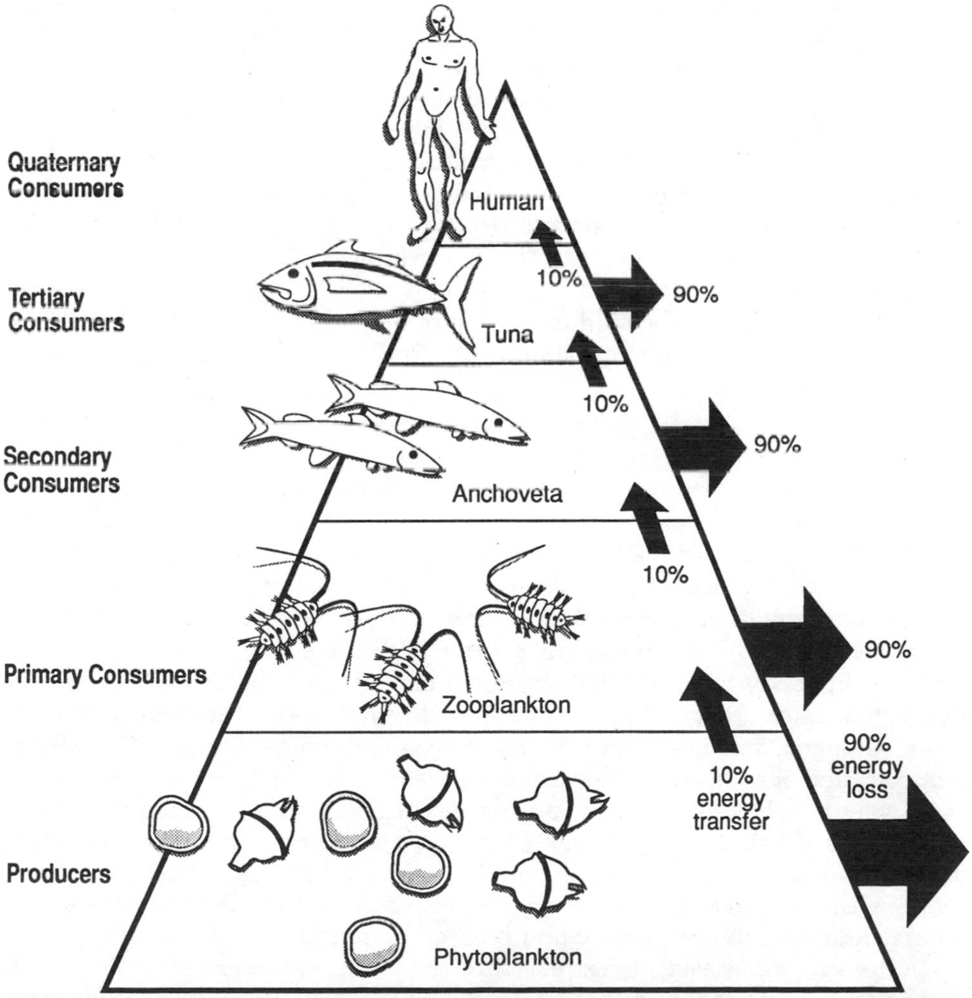

Quaternary Consumers — Human

Tertiary Consumers — Tuna

10%   90%

Secondary Consumers — Anchoveta

10%   90%

Primary Consumers — Zooplankton

10%   90%

10% energy transfer   90% energy loss

Producers — Phytoplankton

populations which, because of their habitat, are almost exclusively dependent on meat as a food source cannot permit their numbers to grow very large. One important factor contributing to the small population size of Eskimo groups is that these people exist as top carnivores of a relatively long food chain:

$$\text{diatoms} \rightarrow \text{zooplankton} \rightarrow \text{fish} \rightarrow \text{seals} \rightarrow \text{Eskimos}$$

Such energy flow patterns indicate that if Americans want to retain meat as a major component of their diet, they cannot permit population levels to increase substantially.

The preceding observations should make it readily apparent that food chains are limited by energy considerations to no more than four or five trophic levels. A food chain of unlimited length is a physical impossibility, because the higher the feeding level, the less energy there is available within a given area. An animal that is a high-level consumer must range over wide areas in order to find enough food to support itself. Eventually the point is reached where the energy required to secure the food is greater than the energy obtained by eating it. At such a point no more organisms can be supported and the upper limits of the food chain have been reached.

Of course in most real communities the actual structure of trophic levels is much more complex than the food chain concept portrays. A "food web" would be a more accurate depiction, since many organisms feed on many different species and in some cases on more than one trophic level. Humans, for example, can be quaternary or tertiary consumers by eating fish, secondary consumers when dining on roast turkey, or primary consumers when munching on peanut-butter sandwiches. The many interlocking food chains tend to promote stability for organisms at the higher levels, providing them with alternative food sources should one or more of the prey species become less abundant. In general, the more complex the food web, the more stable the ecosystem is likely to be.

Biogeochemical Cycling

Every home gardener who maintains a compost pile in the backyard intuitively understands the basic principles of biogeochemical cycling. All living organisms are dependent not only on a source of energy, but also on a number of inorganic materials that are continuously being circulated throughout the ecosystem. These materials provide both the physical framework that supports life activities and the inorganic chemical building blocks from which living molecules are formed. When such molecules are synthesized or broken down, changed from one form into another as they move through the ecosystem, the elements of which they are composed are not lost or degraded in the same way in which energy moving through a food chain becomes unusable. Indeed, the manner in which inorganic materials move through ecosystems differs fundamentally from the movement of energy through those same systems in that matter, unlike energy, is conserved within the ecosystem, its atoms and molecules being used and reused indefinitely.

The cycling of earth materials through living systems and back to the earth is called **biogeochemical cycling.** Of the 92 naturally occurring chemical elements, about 40 are essential to the existence of living organisms and hence are known as **nutrients.** Some of these nutrients are fairly abundant and are needed in relatively large quantities by plants and animals. Such substances are termed **macronutrients** and include carbon, hydrogen, oxygen, nitrogen, phosphorus, potassium, calcium, magnesium, and sulfur. Others that are equally necessary but are required in much smaller amounts are called **trace elements.** These include such substances as iron, copper, manganese, zinc, chlorine, and iodine. The perpetuation of life on this planet is ultimately dependent on the repeated recycling of these inorganic materials in more or less circular paths from the abiotic environment to living things and back to the environment again. Such cycling involves a change in the elements from an inorganic form to an organic molecule and back again. Biogeochemical cycles are important because they help retain vital nutrients in forms usable by plants and animals and help maintain the stability of ecosystems.

Organisms have developed various adaptations to enable them to capture and retain nutrients. As we have seen in our discussion of biomes, plants in both the tropical rain forest and in desert regions have widespread, shallow root systems that permit them quickly to absorb water and the mineral nutrients that it carries in dissolved form before these can be lost through rapid run-off, competition from other organisms, or evaporation. In the tropical rain forest, for example, virtually all the mineral nutrients are retained in plant tissues and the topsoil of this biome is extremely nutrient-poor. If nutrient cycling did not occur, amounts of necessary elements would constantly decrease and would make the development of stable plant and animal populations impossible, since there is no constant addition to the source of nutrients from outside (as there is of energy in the form of sunlight).

There are basically two types of biogeochemical cycles—gaseous and sedimentary—depending on whether the primary source for the nutrient involved happens to be air and water (gaseous cycle) or soil and rocks (sedimentary cycle).

Gaseous Cycles

The elements moved about by gaseous cycles, primarily through the atmosphere but to a lesser degree in water, recycle much more quickly and efficiently than do those in the sedimentary cycle. Gaseous cycles pertain to only four elements: carbon, hydrogen, oxygen, and nitrogen. These four constitute about 97.2% of the bulk of protoplasm and so are of vital importance to life. An examination of two of these, the carbon and nitrogen cycles, gives an idea of the complexity of gaseous cycles.

Carbon Cycle. Carbon atoms are the basic units of all organic compounds and hence, along with water, could be considered the most important component of biological systems. The principal inorganic source of carbon is the carbon dioxide found in the atmosphere and dissolved in bodies of water (the concentration of carbon dioxide dissolved in water is about 100 times greater than the amount present in the atmosphere; for this reason, carbon dioxide is much more accessible to aquatic organisms than to species living on land). Another large source of inorganic carbon lies in storage within deposits of fossil fuels—coal, oil, gas—but the largest amount of all occurs in the form of carbonate sediments such as limestone, formed under the seas and gradually uplifted during slow geologic processes.

Carbon is made available to living organisms through the process of photosynthesis, whereby green plants utilize solar energy to combine carbon dioxide and water, ultimately producing carbon-containing simple sugars. These constitute the basic building blocks for the synthesis of all other organic molecules. Animals obtain the carbon they need by eating plants and resynthesizing these into new carbon-containing compounds. Completion of the cycle, the breakdown of organic molecules to release inorganic carbon dioxide, is accomplished by several different pathways: 1) through the processes of respiration, whereby plants and animals take in oxygen and release carbon dioxide as a waste product; 2) through the decay of dead organisms or of animal wastes, whereby bacteria and fungi decompose the carbon-containing organic molecules, releasing large amounts of carbon dioxide through their respiratory activities; 3) natural weathering of limestone; and 4) by the combustion of organic fuels (coal, oil, gas, wood). The last of these sources of inorganic carbon is causing growing concern among scientists who note that while the amount of atmospheric carbon remained relatively stable for millions of years, it has been increasing steadily since the onset of the Industrial Revolution and particularly accelerated during the 1900s.

Nitrogen Cycle. The major reservoirs of nitrogen in the ecosystem are the 78% of free nitrogen gas that makes up our atmosphere and the nitrogen stored in rock-forming minerals. Atmospheric nitrogen, however, is biologically inert and cannot be utilized as such by most green plants. In nature, gaseous nitrogen is returned to the soil and converted to a form accessible to plants in one of two ways.

1. Lightning passing through the atmosphere can convert nitrogen to nitrogen oxide; when nitrogen oxide is dissolved in water it can be acted upon by certain bacteria in the soil which convert it into nitrate ions that can be absorbed by plant roots.

2. Fixation of atmospheric nitrogen by *Rhizobium sp.* bacteria which live in symbiotic association with leguminous plants inside root nodules, converting nitrogen to nitrates; certain species of free-living soil bacteria and some cyanobacteria also have the ability to fix free nitrogen into nitrates.

Of these two methods, fixation of atmospheric nitrogen by bacteria is by far the most significant way of making nitrogen available to other organisms. To complete the nitrogen cycle, nitrogenous wastes in the form of dead organisms, feces, urine, and so forth, are decomposed to ammonia by other types of soil bacteria; ammonia in turn is acted upon by nitrifying bacteria which form more nitrates. Such nitrates may be taken up again by plants or further broken down by another group of microorganisms called de-nitrifying bacteria, which act upon nitrates to produce free nitrogen that is once again returned to the atmosphere.

Since the early 20th century, natural processes of cycling nitrogen have been supplemented by human activities, which have more than doubled the annual rate at which fixed nitrogen enters the land-based nitrogen cycle (little is known about nitrogen cycling in the oceans). Industrial nitrogen fixation for fertilizer production constitutes the largest human addition of new nitrogen to the global nitrogen cycle; burning of fossil fuels releases gaseous forms of nitrogen into the atmosphere from their long-term storage in geological formations; and still-expanding cultivation of such leguminous crops as soybeans and alfalfa further increases nitrogen releases to the global environment (Vitousek et al., 1997). The adverse ecological consequences of such massive new additions of nitrogen will be discussed in subsequent chapters.

Sedimentary Cycles

Many of the elements that are essential for plant and animal life occur most commonly in the form of sedimentary rocks from which recycling takes place very slowly. Indeed, such sedimentary cycles may extend across long periods of geologic time and for all practical purposes constitute what are essentially one-way flows. In comparison with gaseous cycles, sedimentary cycles seem relatively simple. Iron, calcium, and phosphorus are examples of nutrients whose cycling occurs via the basic sedimentary pattern. A brief look at the phosphorus cycle will give an idea of the transformations involved.

Phosphorus Cycle. Phosphorus, a key element in the nucleic acids DNA and RNA, as well as a component of the organic molecules that govern energy transfer within living organisms, occurs principally in the form of phosphate rock deposits. Smaller, though locally significant, amounts occur where quantities of excrement from fish-eating birds accumulate (e.g. the guano deposits on islands off the coast of Peru) or in deposits of fossil bones. When such phosphate reservoirs are exposed to rainfall, phosphorus ions dissolve and can be absorbed by plant roots and incorporated into vegetative tissue. At the same time, much phosphorus is effectively lost from the ecosystem through run-off to the sea. Animals obtain the phosphorus they need by eating plants. When animals excrete waste products or when they die and decay, phosphates are returned to the soil where they once again become available for uptake by plants or are lost by downhill transport into the sea. Within shallow coastal areas some of this phosphorus is taken up by marine phytoplankton, which constitute the ultimate source of phosphorus for fish and sea birds. However, much of the phosphorus entering the sea is carried by currents to the deeper marine sediments where it is inaccessible to living organisms and may remain locked up for millions of years until future geologic upheavals. The large amounts of phosphate being produced commercially today for use as fertilizers come from the mining of phosphate rock. Unfortunately, much as in the case of oil or coal, such phosphate deposits constitute an essentially nonrenewable resource, since the processes responsible for their creation occurred millions of years in the past.

The fact that the general pattern in sedimentary cycling is a downhill one, where materials tend to move through ecosystems into relatively inaccessible geologic pools, poses some interesting implications for the stability of ecosystems. The loss of soluble mineral nutrients from upland areas to the lowlands and oceans is curbed only by local biological recycling mechanisms which prevent downhill loss from outpacing the release of new materials from underlying rocks. Such local recycling depends upon the return of dead organic material to the soil where breakdown and reuse of materials can occur. Human disruption of this process through widescale removal of potential nutrients (e.g. by logging, which removes trees that would otherwise have died and decayed in place; grazing of livestock which consume local resources but whose flesh, wool, bones, and so on will be disposed of elsewhere) accelerates the impoverishment of certain ecosystems where essential mineral nutrients are already in short supply. In such situations the lowlands are not benefitted either, for the increased flow of materials they receive generally pass into the sea and out of biological circulation before they can be assimilated. Concern about the long-range stability of ecosystems demands that we begin to pay more careful attention to the biological recycling of inorganic materials that move in sedimentary cycles.

Change in Ecosystems

The fact that ecosystems undergo dramatic change over vast periods of time is now well accepted. Geologists have shown us how mountains are worn down and washed to the seas, forming thick layers of underwater sediments that eons later may be uplifted by immense tectonic pressures to form new mountains; deserts expand and retreat as rainfall patterns shift; and periodically great glacial ice sheets move southward, changing the face of the earth. As land forms and climate change, it is not surprising that the biotic communities within the affected ecosystems change also. It is now recognized that the biotic communities in past geologic eras differed greatly from those existing today. What is less well understood is that present ecosystems have a dynamic quality of their own, their component communities changing in an orderly sequence within a given area, a process known as **ecological succession.**

Succession

On May 18, 1980, Mount St. Helens volcano in southwestern Washington State exploded in a blast that obliterated the lush fir and hemlock forests that had blanketed its slopes for centuries. The collapse of the mountain's north face triggered an avalanche of mud and rocks that swept 15 miles down the Toutle River Valley, burying everything in its path under a 140-foot layer of volcanic debris. Observers surveying the scene at the time might understandably have wondered whether life could ever return to a scene of such devastation, yet within a year perennial wildflowers such as fireweed were blooming on the ash-laden mountainside. Year by year, the avalanche-affected area has become progressively greener. By the early 1990s, ecologists studying the area reported that 83 of the 256 plant species known to have been present prior to the eruption were once again thriving. While researchers concede that a return to anything resembling normal conditions will take more than a century (the area in the vicinity of the crater itself still remains virtually barren), the process of regeneration is well underway (Wilford, 1991).

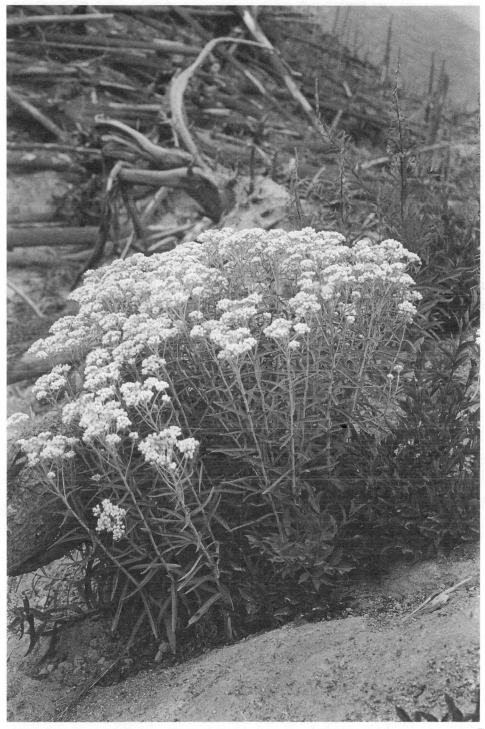

Wildflowers blooming against a backdrop of volcanic debris are indications of the regeneration that has occurred since Mt. St. Helens erupted in 1980. *[Scott Shane]*

BOX 1-3

Golfing Isn't "Green"

Golf is the world's fastest-growing sport, with an estimated 49 million players around the globe, and golf-course construction is the world's fastest-growing type of land development—and that's bad news for the environment.

Modern golf courses bear scant resemblance to the Scottish links introduced by King James, the "father of golf," some 500 years ago. The first courses in Scotland were laid out on pastures, grass-covered marshes, sand dunes, and mudflats, presenting players with the challenge of overcoming natural obstacles. Golf course design changed little over the centuries until the modern era, when the growing addiction to the sport throughout the former British Empire resulted in large tracts of land being reserved expressly for golf course development. With the popularity of golf booming worldwide in recent decades and with golfing facilities increasingly tied to tourism and upscale residential development, modern golf courses have become highly engineered landscapes whose construction requires the use of heavy equipment that completely disrupts and destroys the natural environment. The fact that "golf tourists" demand spectacular views as a scenic backdrop to their game means that courses today are, with increasing frequency, being built in ecologically fragile settings, including acreage in a protected Vietnamese rainforest, Arizona's Sonoran Desert, high in the European Alps, and in the mountain highlands of Malaysia. Construction in such locations not only obliterates many local plant and animal populations but also often results in excessive soil erosion, landslides, and flooding downstream.

When golf courses are not built on mountainsides, in rain forests, or other inherently vulnerable settings, they are often developed on agricultural land where they displace farmers and adversely affect local food production. In Thailand, where golf resorts catering to Japanese tourists have mushroomed over the past decade, two-thirds have been developed on former farmlands; as a result, golf is blamed as the leading cause of rural landlessness in that country. In situations where developers are unable to persuade local agriculturists to sell their land, they may buy up all surrounding parcels and then deny holdout farmers access to their plots. The amount of displacement caused by these developments can be significant, particularly in developing tropical countries where golf courses are generally constructed in tandem with luxury hotels or homes and other recreational facilities.

Unfortunately, golf's adverse environmental impacts don't cease once grass is planted and play begins. Successful cultivation of the varieties of grass preferred by golfers requires prodigious amounts of fertilizers and pesticides—that perfect emerald green doesn't come naturally! Putting greens especially demand chemically intensive care, characterized as they are by shallow-rooted grasses that are particularly susceptible to insect and fungal pests. In spite of their relatively limited area, putting greens account for a disproportionate share of the groundwater contamination associated with golf courses because they are underlain with permeable sand rather than soil, allowing fertilizers and pesticides easy access to aquifers. In comparison with agricultural applications, the amounts of insecticides and herbicides used to keep golf course turf green and healthy are enormous—approximately seven times as much per acre as used by U.S. farmers, eight times more per hectare than farmers apply in Japan. Such heavy chemical use poses serious environmental threats; in addition to polluting groundwater, chemical runoff from golf courses may contaminate nearby lakes and wetlands or poison wildlife. In 1985 an insecticide, diazinon, used for controlling turfgrass pests was blamed for the deaths of 700 Atlantic Brant geese that had walked on a recently treated New York golf course (as a result, the EPA has banned the use of diazinon on American golf courses). Of even greater concern is the impact golf course chemicals may be having on human health. While a direct cause-and-effect relationship has yet to be definitively established, Japanese doctors, surveyed in 1991, concluded that 125 suspected poisonings in that country were associated with golf course chemical exposure. In the United States, the National Association of Golf Superintendents is funding research to explore a possible link between long-term contact with turfgrass pesticides and health problems among greenskeepers, caddies, and players.

Water consumption is another problematic issue associated with golf courses, particularly in arid regions. The proliferation of lush, green golf course oases in the midst of America's desert terrain is a growing cause for concern to water managers and environmentally concerned citizens alike. In some parts of the United States, golf courses are now being irrigated with partially treated human wastewater to reduce demand on public drinking water supplies. While such an approach makes sense from the standpoint of water conservation, it can, depending on the level of wastewater treatment, lead to contamination of nearby surface streams or lakes with fecal coliform bacteria, as well as nitrate and phosphate pollution.

In a few places golf course developers and superintendents have attempted to mitigate some of these problems by adopting techniques of Integrated Pest Management; the European Golf Association has agreed to adopt environmental guidelines, and several years ago the Chinese government ordered a ban on new golf courses. Nevertheless, with 350 new golf courses being built around the world each year, added to the 25,000 (nearly 16,000 in the U.S.) already in existence, golf will continue to exert a negative influence on the global environment.

References
Mitchell, Jennifer. 1998. "The Tigers." World Watch 11, no. 1 (Jan/Feb):2.

Platt, Anne E. 1994. "Toxic Green: The Trouble With Golf." World Watch 7 no. 3 (May/June):27-32.

The gradual replacement of one biotic community by another over time is termed **succession.** While the sequence of events following the Mount St. Helens eruption provides one of the most dramatic recent illustrations of the process, numerous examples of succession in action can be seen all around us. While a casual glance at the plants and animals living together on a vacant city lot or an abandoned pasture may suggest an environmentally stable situation, such an impression is deceptive. If one could observe the same scene over a period of many years, it would be obvious that the composition of the area's biotic community, as well as the physical environment itself, is slowly but surely changing in a directional manner toward a relatively stable, self-perpetuating stage called the **climax community.** Depending on the particular location involved, the changes might take thousands of years or be completed within decades, but in any case the process of change would follow a definite sequence.

The concept can be more easily understood by examining, step by step, the mechanisms of succession in a specific situation. Imagine that a retreating glacier has left behind a barren landscape of scoured bedrock or glacial till. Will the surface of the rock remain lifeless forever? Of course not; over a period of time, perhaps thousands of years if the climate is cold and dry, faster if it is warm and wet, changes in the biotic community occupying the surface of the rock will change it beyond recognition.

At first the only factors that can change the nature of the rock's surface are physical ones. Rain falls, combining with carbon dioxide in the air to form a dilute solution of carbonic acid. Bit by bit, this gradually begins to wear down the rocky surface. If the climate is a northern or temperate one, freezing and thawing may occur, helping to split the rock further. Wind erosion may also play a part. Algal and fungal spores or plant seeds will be carried to the site by air currents or by animals passing through the area, and colonies of lichens or other hardy plants establish themselves on the rock surface. The life processes of these organisms hasten the deterioration of the rock, and when the plants die, their dead organic matter contributes toward building up a thin layer of soil. These **pioneer plants** of the first stage of succession generally are small, low-growing species that can tolerate severe climatic conditions (e.g. intense sunlight, wide fluctuations in daily temperature, periodic wetting and drying), produce large numbers of spores or seeds annually, grow rapidly, and have short life cycles. While pioneer plants are quite tolerant of adverse physical conditions, they are generally intolerant of other organisms. For example, once lichens have helped to corrode rock, create a small amount of soil, and maintain better moisture conditions, mosses take over and crowd out the lichens. These may form a dense cover, attracting insects and other small invertebrates. The mosses continue to build up deposits of organic matter and soil as more rock is broken away and as the old mosses and lichens die. The most significant change these organisms can produce in an environment is that created by their own dead bodies. As decayed organic material accumulates, erosion of the rock slows down, but herbaceous plants move in and assume dominance. Insects and other arthropods will be the main form of animal life at this stage, but some small mammals and reptiles may be present also. Eventually shrubs and tree saplings will establish themselves, and since the taller plants furnish shade and act as a windbreak, the moisture conditions of the soil and near-soil atmosphere improve and temperature fluctuations at soil level become less extreme. Gradually the shrubs become the dominant plants, shading out many of the annual herbaceous species. Correspondingly animal types change also, insects perhaps becoming fewer but bird species increasing in number. As the shrub stage matures, sapling trees begin to predominate. Shade-loving plants proliferate under the canopy. The large trees that characterize the late stages of succession in forest ecosystems are long lived species that grow slowly and tend to persist for an indefinite period of time if environmental conditions of the area remain more or less constant.

This relatively stable, self-perpetuating assemblage of species represents the climax community. Of course in reality a change in environmental conditions, especially climate, is not unusual, and natural events such as fires, high winds, earthquakes, or pest outbreaks (or unnatural events such as lumbering or grazing) can create a mosaic of successional stages within a given region. It is important to note that during the successional process it is not only the composition of the biotic community that is constantly changing through time—the physical environment is being substantially altered as well. Thus succession represents a dynamic process in which abiotic factors influence the plants and animals of the community, and these, in turn, modify the physical habitat.

The preceding examples of succession beginning when pioneer organisms colonize an area formerly devoid of life is referred to as **primary succession.** A less extreme but far more common situation is that of **secondary succession.** In this case, succession proceeds from a state in which other organisms are still present; new life doesn't have to start from scratch, so to speak. Even in cases where the disturbed area may appear quite barren, roots, rhizomes, or dormant seeds lying underneath the soil surface quickly initiate the process of revegetation, joined by migrant species from outside the area taking advantage of the altered conditions. In the case of Mount St. Helens, for example, buried seeds and roots gave rise to new shoots pushing through the volcanic debris as erosion thinned the overlying ash. Examples of secondary succession are legion—abandoned Vermont farmland reverting to forest, revegetation of Yellowstone National Park after the devastating fires of 1988, untended suburban lawns growing up in weeds. In such cases succession begins at a more advanced stage but proceeds, like primary succession, in a directional, more or less predictable manner toward the climax community (Stiling, 1992).

Thus far we have only referred to terrestrial succession, but the same concept applies to most enclosed bodies of water as well. A newly formed lake (e.g. one left behind by a retreating glacier) will generally have clear water with little or no vegetation or debris. Gradually silt and dead materials are deposited on the lake bottom. The sides of the lake may also be eroded by wave action and thus help fill in the deeper parts of the basin. Around the edges of the lake rooted aquatic plants such as water lilies and pickerel weed, rushes, cattails, and so forth, become established. With the accumulation of dead organic material, the supply of nutrients necessary for the growth of algae and microorganisms is increased and they flourish accordingly, providing a food source for fish and other large animals. This process of nutrient enrichment is called **eutrophication.** The speed with which this phenomenon occurs is greatly accelerated when human-produced substances such as phosphate detergents, chemical fertilizers, or sewage is introduced. Eventually, as the lake becomes more completely filled with sediment, the whole area is converted into a marsh. Terrestrial grasses and moisture-tolerant plants subsequently move in, converting the marsh into a meadow, and finally the grasses are displaced by trees, resulting in a climax community. The length of time required for such succession to take place varies widely, depending on such variables as the original depth of the basin, the rate of sedimentation, and other physical conditions which affect the growth of organisms. It should be mentioned in passing, however, that not all aquatic succession results in

Figure 1-3   Primary Succession

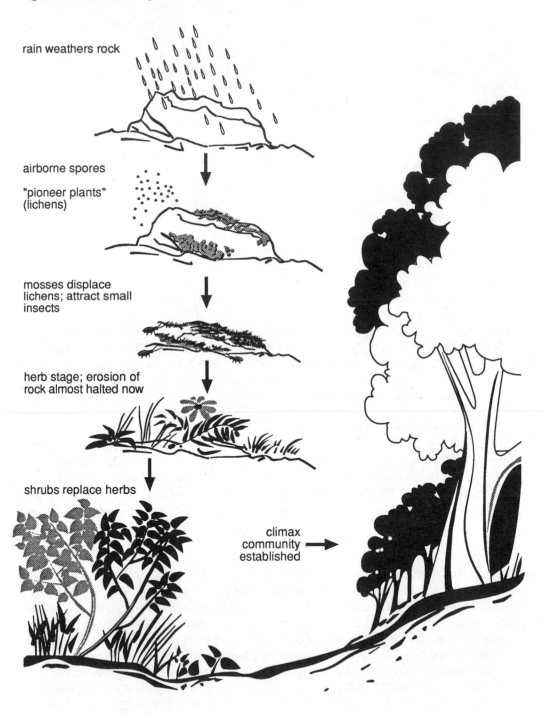

rain weathers rock

airborne spores

"pioneer plants"
(lichens)

mosses displace
lichens; attract small
insects

herb stage; erosion of
rock almost halted now

shrubs replace herbs

climax
community
established

Figure 1-4   Aquatic Succession

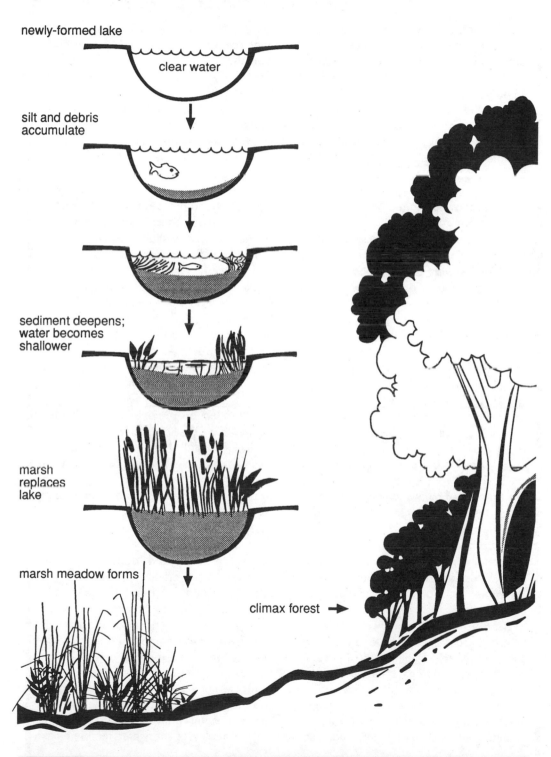

newly-formed lake

clear water

silt and debris
accumulate

sediment deepens;
water becomes
shallower

marsh
replaces
lake

marsh meadow forms

climax forest →

BOX 1-4

Going, Going... Gone?

"Eco-catastrophe" is not an overly dramatic term for the environmental and human tragedy currently being played out in the not-so-long-ago fertile lands of Central Asia. Once a part of the Soviet empire, the now-independent republics of Uzbekistan and Kazakhstan are beset with declining harvests, powerful dust storms, climate change, and diminishing biodiversity—all consequences of misguided agricultural policies that are slowly destroying the region's key natural resource, the Aral Sea.

A vast inland body of fresh water fed by the Syr Darya and Amu Darya rivers, the Aral Sea was once the fourth largest lake in the world. For centuries the influx of river water was just sufficient to offset water losses from the lake due to high evaporation rates, and the size of the Aral remained relatively stable. However, in the early 1960s decisions made in Moscow led to the rapid expansion of irrigated agriculture throughout the Aral basin in an all-out effort to boost production of the region's "white gold"—cotton. As increasing amounts of water from the Syr Darya, Amu Darya, and their tributaries were diverted to thirsty cotton fields, the amount of inflow available to replace water losses in this naturally arid region steadily declined. By 1989 parts of the sea had become so shallow that its basin divided into two separate parts; by the late 1990s the Aral had shrunk by 50% of its former area and had lost 73% of its volume.

The Aral's water quality, as well as its quantity, has steadily deteriorated over the past decades. Salt-laden runoff from improperly irrigated farmlands has increased the salinity of the lake to the point where most of its native fish species have disappeared and a once-thriving commercial fishing industry has collapsed. The lake's environment has now been so adversely altered that experts fear the damage may be irreversible. Even if diversions of water for irrigation were drastically reduced to permit flows into the sea to double, the Aral would continue to shrink to one-sixth of its size in 1960 and its salt content would rise to four times that of ocean waters.

Surrounding land areas have suffered as severely as the Aral itself. As the margins of the sea recede, the salt-encrusted exposed sea bottom has provided a seemingly inexhaustible source of toxic sand that is feeding dust storms so large and powerful that they are regularly tracked by Russian cosmonauts in orbit. Some of these storms may deposit their load as far as 1,200 miles away, but the greatest amount falls on areas within the Aral basin where up to half a ton per acre of salts and sand poison farmlands—and farmers' lungs—each year.

The moderating effect the Aral has long exerted on regional climate is also diminishing as the sea shrinks ever smaller. Rainfall has become less frequent, temperature extremes more pronounced. The frost-free growing season in parts of the basin has now diminished to less than the minimum 200 days essential for cotton cultivation, threatening the region's economic viability. Irrigation diversions and faulty drainage practices have adversely impacted the Aral watershed far from the sea itself. Wetlands adjacent to the rivers, as well as floodplain forests, have dried up and vanished, as have many of the wildlife species which inhabited them. Salinization of soils, caused by excessive application of water without adequate drainage, has brought dissolved salts to the soil surface and significantly reduced crop yields.

The quality of the water remaining in

the rivers has deteriorated to the point that it threatens the well-being of humans as well as wildlife. Run-off of phosphates, nitrates, and ammonia due to heavy fertilizer applications and contamination of drinking water supplies with toxic pesticides, chemical defoliants, and sewage is blamed in part for the scandalously high rates of infant mortality, maternal deaths, psychological disorders, and general poor state of health throughout the region. In one of the poorest areas of Uzbekistan, 97% of the women are now suffering from anemia—the highest rate in the world. Thyroid and kidney problems, as well as liver cancer, have risen sharply since the early 1980s. Some observers warn that unless immediate steps are taken to halt the use of dangerous pesticides, provide safe drinking water, and reverse pollution of the rivers, the region may become uninhabitable. In response, the World Bank in 1997 approved a $75 million loan to Uzbekistan for investments in water and sanitary infrastructure to improve rural water supply and health in the Aral basin.

Can the Aral be saved? In 1988 the USSR's top hydraulic engineer incautiously remarked that "it is time for all the wailing to stop. The case is closed, and the people here will have to learn to live without the sea." Not everyone is willing to surrender without a fight, however. In the late 1980s Uzbek nationalists demanded that certain Siberian rivers flowing into the Arctic Ocean be diverted southward to replenish the dwindling water reserves of the Aral. While such a massive water redistribution scheme was ultimately rejected, there has been growing awareness that a solution to the problems of the Aral basin will require developing new attitudes toward water use and reevaluating economic development policies. The breakup of the former Soviet Union has made implementation

of programs to save the Aral even more problematic. The president of Kazakhstan has been especially bitter that the fledgling nations of the region have been left on their own to deal with the environmental deterioration of the Aral basin, while the cotton whose production is largely responsible for the current situation still is shipped to the European part of the former USSR where 10 million jobs are dependent on its use. Early in 1993, leaders of the newly independent republics of Central Asia met in Tashkent where they adopted a resolution to create an international fund to address the problems of the Aral Sea. Unfortunately, by the end of the decade, in spite of numerous visits by foreign advisory groups, virtually nothing had been accomplished and some authorities were suggesting a mass relocation of people living in the communities that once surrounded the sea. Living conditions have become so bad that the Peace Corps will no longer station representatives in the area and the United Nations also has reduced the number of its personnel. Local people wryly joke that if everyone visiting the region to advise on how to solve its problems brought a bucket of water with them, the Aral Sea would be full again—a sad commentary on the mood of hopelessness and disillusionment prevailing in a human-made disaster area.

References

Becker, P. J. 1999. Peace Corps Volunteer, Kazakhstan, personal communication.

Feshbach, Murray, and Alfred Friendly, Jr. 1992. *Ecocide in the USSR*. Basic Books.

Frederick, Kenneth D. 1991. "The Disappearing Aral Sea." *Resources*, no. 102 (winter).

Kotlyakov, V. M. 1991. "The Aral Sea Basin: A Critical Environmental Zone." *Environment* 33, no. 1 (Jan/Feb).

the establishment of a terrestrial climax community. In cases where the body of water is very large and deep or where there is strong wave action, a stable aquatic community may form and undergo no further change.

Although the later stages of succession are characterized by biotic communities better able to withstand adverse environmental conditions and more stable in terms of species composition and population, humans have generally preferred to utilize the types of communities characterized by the earlier stages of succession. In aquatic ecosystems, for example, the desirable food and game fish such as trout, bass, and perch are all found in the clear, well-oxygenated water of deep, non-eutrophic lakes or in swiftly flowing streams. The carp that thrive in waters at a more advanced successional stage are less highly regarded. In relation to land communities, the development of agriculture and pastoralism have resulted in humans exerting increasingly effective efforts to maintain succession at an early, simplified stage. By replacing natural biotic communities with large expanses of just a few species of crop plants and through the attempt to eliminate such competitors as insects, rodents, and birds, agricultural humans have further simplified biotic communities, often undermining the stability of ecosystems in the process.

The stresses that humans are today imposing upon natural ecosystems extend far beyond the biological simplification of agricultural communities, however. The toxic pollutants being discharged into the air and water in unprecedented amounts are subjecting biotic communities to pressures with which they are evolutionarily unequipped to cope. Perhaps even more serious, the sheer increase in numbers of humans and their domestic animals is creating physical pressures that in many parts of the world are changing ecosystems in ways which are severely detrimental, not only to the biological communities which inhabit them but to human long-term interests as well.

References

Ashworth, William. 1986. *The Late Great Lakes: An Environmental History.* Alfred A. Knopf.

Bright, Chris. 1998. *Life Out of Bounds: Bioinvasion in a Borderless World.* New York and London: W.W. Norton.

Odum, Eugene P. 1959. *Fundamentals of Ecology.* W. B. Saunders.

Pianka, Eric R. 1988. *Evolutionary Ecology.* 4th ed. New York: Harper & Row.

Smith, Robert L. 1986. *Elements of Ecology.* 2d ed. New York: Harper & Row.

Stiling, Peter D. 1992. *Introductory Ecology.* Prentice Hall, Inc.

Vitousek, P.M., J. Aber, R.W. Howarth, G.E. Likens, P.A. Matson, D.W. Schindler, W.H. Schlesinger, and G.D. Tilman. 1997. "Human Alteration of the Global Nitrogen Cycle: Cases and Consequences." *Issues in Ecology,* no. 1 (Spring). Ecological Society of America.

Wilford, John Noble. 1991. "The Gradual Greening of Mt. St. Helens." *New York Times,* Oct. 8, B9.

CHAPTER 2

Population Dynamics

The command "Be fruitful and multiply" was promulgated, according to our authorities, when the population of the world consisted of two people.
                                   —William R. Inge (1931)

"Standing room only" is a phrase used only half in jest to describe the possible human predicament on this finite planet if present growth rates continue unchecked indefinitely into the future. Population projections based on a continuation of current growth rates reveal that within a few centuries, every human on the planet would have just one square meter of land, excluding polar ice caps, on which to live; if the world's present population size were to double twenty times, each individual would have to make do with just 0.7 millionth of an acre of arable land (Rohe, 1998). Obviously such figures represent an exercise in the absurd. Common sense observation of the world around us reveals that when populations of any organism explode, be they swarms of migratory locusts, tent caterpillars, or lemmings marching toward the sea, something, sooner or later, brings that population back into a state of relative equilibrium with its environment. There is no reason to suppose that humans, any more than locusts, caterpillars, or lemmings, can defy the laws of nature by multiplying indefinitely. Certain ecological principles govern the ways in which populations change in size. The study of such changes, or population dynamics, is of great practical importance to those who wish to predict or control the population size of other organisms or, even more important today, to forecast trends in human population growth and, if possible, guide such growth into ecologically sustainable patterns.

Population Attributes

As we saw in chapter 1, a biotic community is made up of populations of a number of different species that are bound together by an intricate web of relationships, interacting with each other and with the physical environment.

Any population, be it leopard frogs in a farm pond, lions on the Serengeti Plain, or humans overcrowding Spaceship Earth, exhibits certain measurable group attributes which are unique to that population. Such group attributes include birth and death rates, age structure, population density, spatial distribution, and so forth. Knowing what these characteristics are for any given population is helpful in predicting how that population will change in response to changes in the environment.

Basically, assessing dynamic changes within a population largely revolves around keeping track of additions to that population from births and immigration and of losses from the same group due to deaths and emigration. Age structure of the population also must be taken into account in those species, such as *Homo sapiens*, where generations tend to overlap.

Limits to Growth

More than one hundred years ago Charles Darwin observed in his *Origin of Species* that all organisms have a tendency to produce many more offspring than will survive to maturity. Indeed, in nature a given population of organisms tends to maintain relatively stable numbers over a long period of time. Although a single oyster may produce up to 100 million eggs at one spawning, an orchid may release a million seeds, or one mushroom may be responsible for hundreds of thousands of fungal spores drifting through the air, nevertheless, the world has not yet been overwhelmed with oysters, orchids, or mushrooms. Even much less prolific species theoretically could give rise to staggering numbers of offspring. Darwin himself cited the example of the slow-breeding elephant (gestation period of 600–630 days), showing that the progeny from a single pair would number 19 million after 750 years, assuming that all survived to reproductive age.

Obviously the increase of populations as described above could only occur in a situation where no forces act to slow the growth rate—a scenario that is virtually nonexistent in the real world, at least for any extended period of time.

The maximum growth rate that a population could achieve in an unlimited environment is referred to as that population's **biotic potential.** In reality, of course, no organism ever reaches its biotic potential because of one or more factors which limit growth. Such limiting factors include food shortages, overcrowding, disease, predation, and accumulation of toxic wastes. Taken together, the environmental pressures that limit a population's inherent capacity for growth are termed **environmental resistance.** Environmental resistance is generally measured as the difference between the biotic potential of a population and the actual rate of increase as observed under laboratory or field conditions (Odum, 1959).

Population Growth Forms

Earlier in this century a number of population biologists were curious to discover what would happen to a population if most of the usual factors of environmental resistance were removed. They devised carefully controlled laboratory experiments to chart growth curves for populations where limitation of resources, predation, parasites, and other factors that normally contribute to high death rates would not come into play. Their findings revealed that populations exhibit characteristic patterns of increase that biologists call **population growth forms.** Experimentation with a wide variety of organisms has revealed two basic patterns, described as the S-curve and the J-curve.

S-Curve

A classic study in population dynamics was carried out by the Russian, G. F. Gause, in 1932 using a population of the protozoan, *Paramecium caudatum*. Gause placed one paramecium into an aquarium with a broth of bacterial cells suspended in water to provide a food supply and then carefully observed the subsequent growth of that population. He found that numbers of paramecia increased rather slowly for the first few days, then increased very rapidly for a period; finally the rate of increase began to slow and gradually leveled off as the upper limits of growth were reached and a steady-state equilibrium was achieved. The growth pattern thus revealed is that of an S-curve (sigmoid curve). The upper limit of such a curve, called the **upper asymptote,** indicates that point at which increased mortality has brought birth and death rates into balance once again (in the case of Gause's paramecia, increased mortality was due to overcrowding in the culture and the inability of the constant food supply to support all the organisms). The population density at the upper asymptote thus represents an equilibrium level between the biotic potential of that population and the environmental resistance. Thus the upper asymptote of the S-curve is often referred to as the **carrying capacity** of that environment—the limit at which that environment can support a population.

J-Curve

The sigmoid growth pattern discussed above, typical of populations as diverse as microorganisms, plants, and many types of birds and mammals as well, results from the gradually increasing pressures of environmental resistance as the density of population increases. Another type of population growth form, more dramatic because it frequently results in the population "crashes" that attract widespread journalistic attention, can be represented by a J-curve. In this type of situation population growth increases at rapid exponential rates up to or even beyond the carrying capacity of the environment. The environmental resistance becomes effective only at the last moment, so to speak, and as a result populations that have overshot the carrying capacity suffer severe die-backs. This pattern is frequently seen in many natural populations such as lemmings, algal blooms, and certain insects. It should be apparent that the early phases of growth represented by S- and J-curves are identical: a preliminary "lag" phase, during which time the rate of increase is relatively slow, followed by a logarithmic, or exponential, growth phase during which not only do the actual numbers grow rapidly, but the rate of increase also increases (in the manner of compound interest). Thus, a J-curve basically can be considered an incomplete S-curve since the sudden imposition of limit-

Figure 2-1

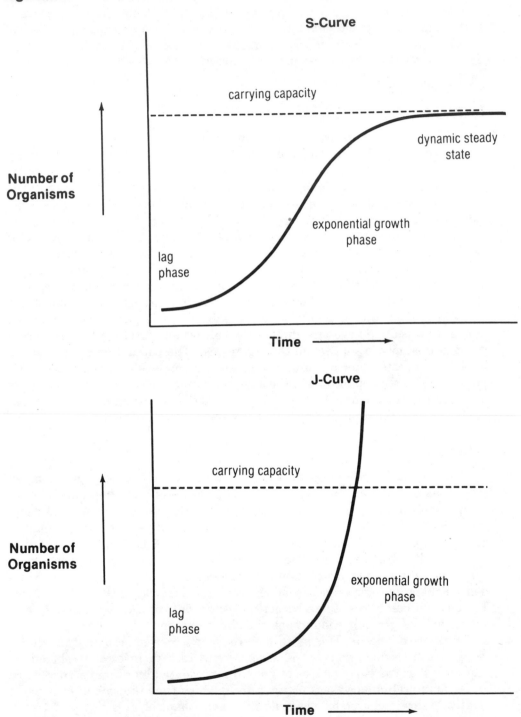

ing effects halts growth before the self-limiting effects within a population become apparent.

Homeostatic Controls

Food shortage, excess predation, and disease are not the only factors which can cause populations to decline. Extensive research has shown that a number of self-regulating factors, or **homeostatic controls,** in the form of behavioral, physiological, and social responses within a population are also very important in controlling its size. Each population appears to have an optimal density, and if this optimum is exceeded a number of stress-related responses become evident. For example, it has been observed that among the snowshoe hares of northern Canada, population crashes occur at regular 9–10 year intervals even in the absence of predators, disease, or human hunting pressures. Researchers have found that during the rapid die-off phase of these oscillations, large numbers of hares suffer a stress-induced degeneration of their livers, resulting in inadequate glycogen reserves. The animals may then exhibit "shock disease," lapsing into convulsions, coma, and ultimately death (Farb, 1963).

Classic studies on the effects of overcrowding in rats have shown that even when abundant food is present, self-regulating mechanisms induce population crashes when rat populations exceed a certain density. When crowded, rats begin to exhibit abnormally hostile behavior; social interactions become pathological and fighting intensifies, often with fatal results to one of the combatants. Some individual males become hyperactive and hypersexual, attempting to mate without the customary courtship rituals and often mounting males, nonreceptive females, and juveniles indiscriminately. Pregnant females under crowded conditions frequently abort; if the young are born alive they are frequently killed by the mother or die as a consequence of neglect. It has been suggested that the cause of such deviant behavior can be traced to the effects of crowding-induced stress on the functioning of the endocrine system, which regulates hormone levels in animals. Whether the rats' response to crowding is indicative of what we can expect among human populations as our species continues to increase is open to question, but there are those who point to rising levels of violence and aggression in many parts of the world as ominous portents.

Human Population Growth

Insights gained from laboratory studies of microbial populations have an importance far transcending mere academic interest. The exponential curves tracking the growth of paramecia in biologists' aquaria or of migratory locusts in the Sahel have a parallel in the growth patterns that typify many human societies today. The fact is that during the 20th century—and particularly during the last 50 years—the human species experienced an unprecedented population explosion, with growth rates resembling those depicted on a J-curve. Although the average *rate* of growth has begun to decrease slightly since peaking in the early 1970s (perhaps indicating that humans are S-curve rather than J-curve organisms?), in terms of absolute numbers the annual increase to the world's total population is now 78 million, considerably more than the 70 million or so added each year when the "population explosion" was headline news (UNFPA, 1999). Many informed observers strongly contend that the most critical environmental issue facing humanity today—and perhaps the most difficult to tackle—is overpopulation. The explosive growth of the human species is arguably the most significant development of the past million years. No other event, geological or biological, has posed a threat to earthly life comparable to that of human overpopulation. We have little hope of significantly reducing other types of environmental degradation if present rates of population increase are not reversed.

Until very recently, people who warned of an impending population-resource crunch or advocated even the mildest measures to restrain birth rates were either ridiculed, castigated, or ignored. One of the earliest to voice alarm was British clergyman-economist Thomas Malthus who, some two hundred years ago, argued that the rapid population growth his country was then experiencing was a prelude to mass misery. Demonstrating that population grows geometrically (2, 4, 8, 16, 32) while agricultural production increases only arithmetically (1, 2, 3, 4, 5), Malthus contended that population would always tend to outpace additions to the food supply, thereby condemning the bulk of humanity to a marginal standard of living and frequent bouts of famine, war, and disease. Although Malthus' "dismal theorem" stimulated a great deal of discussion at the time, his views were soon discounted when improvements in British agricultural technology and the opening of the American prairies to grain production resulted in food supply increases far exceeding the number of new mouths to be fed. As a result, Malthus' warnings were largely dismissed and forgotten. The prevailing attitude throughout the 19th century and well into the 20th viewed population growth as a desirable phenomenon, enhancing a nation's productivity, wealth, and power. Indeed, as late as the 1930s, the main population concern in the United States was that the temporary dip in the American birth rate experienced during the Depression years might indicate a worrisome *shrinking* of U.S. population size!

However, after World War II, and especially since the 1960s, concerns that population growth rates were excessive began to be expressed, first by a handful of far-sighted individuals and private organizations, later by national governments and international agencies. Such concern was precipitated by the awareness that intensive efforts to improve living standards and ensure national stability in the newly independent developing nations were largely being nullified by the rapid population growth they were experiencing. Today the vast majority of Third World governments regard their rate of population increase as too high and have adopted policies aimed at stabilizing numbers as quickly as possible. Unfortunately, such efforts should have been launched decades earlier; the momentum of growth is now so enormous and the existing population base so large, that the ability of some countries to curb growth before national carrying capacity is surpassed is very much in doubt. In order to understand why the seriousness of our current population crisis was recognized so belatedly and why there's such a sense of urgency now, we need to look at some demographic facts.

BOX 2-1

International Migration: Seeking a Better Life

Up-or-down changes in birth or death rates have been the main determinants of fluctuations in population size over time. In recent decades, however, another factor has become a key player—migration across national boundaries. At the dawn of the 21st century, tens of millions of people are traveling hundreds, even thousands, of miles from their homelands in search of a better life for themselves and their children. In so doing, they are having a profound impact on the demographic situation of the receiving country, not only in terms of age structure (most migrants are young adults) and gender balance (primarily male in such receiving areas as the Persian Gulf and southern Africa), but also in terms of sheer population size.

Not counting refugees, the United Nations estimates that by the mid-1990s at least 120 million people were living outside their country of birth, up from 75 million in the mid-1960s. While approximately half of all international migrants are moving from one Third World country to another, in terms of demographic effects the impact of international migration is most keenly felt in the nations of the developed world. On average, for eign-born residents now comprise approximately 5% of the total population in the richer nations—a figure that rises as high as 31% in tiny Luxembourg and over 18% in Switzerland. In the United States, in-migration has totaled over a million newcomers annually throughout the 1990s (offset somewhat by 270,000 leaving the country each year); as a result, 9% of the U.S. population today is foreign-born. Immigration is significantly altering the ethnic composition of Canada as well; for every 1,000 Canadians, five new immigrants enter the country each year, most of them from Asia. Can-ada currently ranks among the 15 countries with the highest net migration rates in the world, even though in terms of sheer numbers, the U.S. receives four times as many immigrants.

Reasons for the vast population shift are numerous, but can be roughly divided between economic and noneconomic considerations, further influenced by the interaction among "push," "pull," and network factors. The millions of Mexicans and Central Americans leaving their native lands for "El Norte" weren't attracted by the better weather but by the prospects of higher wages and a more secure economic future. Similarly, the mass migration of Turks to Germany to take advantage of that nation's guest-worker program or of Indians and Pakistanis to the oil-rich but labor-short emirates of the Persian Gulf were prompted by the "push" generated by poor economic conditions at home and the "pull" of active worker recruitment efforts by receiving country governments. Over time, migrant flows to specific foreign destinations are reinforced by networking, whereby earlier emigrants facilitate the later migration of family members and friends by providing them with information, temporary lodging, even financial assistance. Such networking helps explain the preference of certain immigrant groups for a particular destination; e.g. Moroccans and Algerians to France, Turks and Yugoslavs to Germany, West Indians to the U.K., and Filipinos to the U.S. Noneconomic factors also play an important role in establishing networks; several of the associations cited above were established during the colonial era or developed because certain countries have more generous policies regarding political asylum or social welfare.

Noneconomic forces encouraging international migration include, most notably, war and political or religious persecution. The influx of Vietnamese into the U.S., due to the Communist takeover of South Vietnam in 1975, is a classic example. The Soviet invasion and occupation of Afghanistan led to the flight of millions of refugees into neighboring Pakistan and Iran during the 1980s. A similar scenario unfolded in 1994 when Rwandan Hutus fled en masse across the border into Zaire (now Congo), Tanzania, and Uganda in fear of retaliation from a victorious Tutsi army bent on avenging the genocidal murder of Tutsi civilians. Fear of political repression and persecution has sent Cubans to Miami, Sri Lankan Tamils to Europe, Hong Kong Chinese to Australia and Canada. Its promise as a haven from religious persecution of Jews has resulted in Israel's having one of the world's highest annual net immigration rates, with over 30% of present-day Israelis born somewhere else.

The impact of immigration on receiving countries—and the reception accorded the new arrivals—has varied from country to country. Already the "welcome" mat is being withdrawn in some northern and western European nations where immigration has become a hot domestic policy issue and has given rise to far-right political movements with a distinctly anti-foreign flavor. In the United States, always a nation of immigrants, the present high rate of immigration has generated concern that hardworking new arrivals might drive down wages, take away jobs, or, conversely, go on welfare and become a burden to American taxpayers. The impact of immigration on ethnic mix has been an issue as well; since 42% of legal immigrants in recent years are from Latin America and

another 34% from Asia, immigration will inevitably change the ethnic composition of America—and of Canada, Australia, Germany, and other nations.

Perhaps one of the most profound consequences of high immigration rates is the long-term effect on the ultimate population size of the receiving nations. Already the impacts are becoming apparent in low-birth-rate western European countries where 88% of their growth today is due to immigration. In Germany, characterized by extremely low fertility and a negative growth rate, *all* population growth now is a result of immigration. In the United States, where fertility rates among native-born citizens hover around replacement level, immigration accounts for about one-third of the annual population increase. By 2050, 82 million of the projected 383 million people living in the United States (more than 20% of its population) will be persons who entered the country since 1991 or their children. Past assumptions that U.S. population growth rates would soon mirror those of western Europe and that this country would achieve zero population growth early in the 21st century have now been abandoned, thanks to the impact of immigration.

In many countries around the world, governments now view their immigration levels as too high; nevertheless, given a likely intensification in the years ahead of the push/pull factors, transboundary migration seems certain to continue.

References

Martin, Philip, and J. Widgren. 1996. "International Migration: A Global Challenge." *Population Bulletin* 51, no. 1 (April), Population Reference Bureau.

World Resources Institute. 1998. *World Resources 1998-99: A Guide to the Global Environment*, 147–149.

Historical Trends in Human Population Growth

Assuming that the first humans appeared on earth between 1.5 million and 600,000 years ago, we can estimate that somewhere between 60 and 100 billion people have inhabited the planet at some time. Today the earth supports about 6 billion human inhabitants—close to 6% of all who have ever lived. We don't have enough information to estimate accurately what populations were before A.D. 1650, but we can make some educated guesses based on circumstantial evidence (e.g. number of people who could be supported on X square miles by hunting and gathering, by primitive agriculture, and so on). On this basis, it's been calculated that the total human population in 8000 B.C. was about five million people. By the beginning of the Christian Era, when agricultural settlements had become widespread, world population is estimated to have risen to about 200–300 million, and increased to about 500 million by 1650. It then doubled to one billion by 1850, to two billion by 1930, and to four billion by 1975; by 1987 world population passed the 5 billion mark, hit 6 billion late in 1999, and continues to climb. Thus not only has world population been increasing steadily (with minor irregularities) for the past million years, but the rate of growth has also increased.

Figure 2-2   Trends and Projections in World Population Growth, 1750–2050

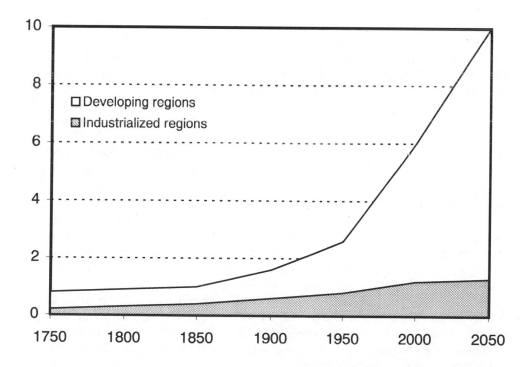

Source: World Resources Institute, based on data from U.N. Population Division, *Long-Range World Population Projections: Two Centuries of World Population Growth, 1950–2150* (1992).

Doubling Time

Perhaps the best way to describe growth rate is in terms of **doubling time**—the time required for a population to double in size. During the period from 8000 B.C. to A.D. 1650, the population doubled about every 1,500 years. The next doubling took 200 years, the next 80 years, and the next, 45 years.

Historical evidence indicates that the increase in human numbers did not occur at a steady, even pace but rather that three main surges occurred. The first took place about 600,000 years ago with the evolution of culture (developing and learning techniques of social organization and group and individual survival); the next occurred about 8000 B.C. with the agricultural revolution; and the most recent began about 200 years ago with the onset of the industrial-medical-scientific revolution (Ehrlich, Ehrlich, and Holdren, 1977). Bearing in mind that changes in the size of populations occur when birth and death rates are out of balance, one can reasonably conclude that each of these spurts indicates that the story of human population growth is not primarily a story of changes in birth rates, but of changes in death rates. Let's now take a closer look at some of the demographic facts that help to explain our current population dilemma.

Birth Rates, Death Rates, and Fertility Rates

Birth rates are generally expressed as the number of babies born per 1,000 people per year. Prior to the Industrial Revolution, birth rates in every society typically were in the 40–50 per thousand range. Today the birth rate gap between nations has widened dramatically, exemplified by Latvia and Bulgaria's 8, the world's lowest, and with a high of 54 in the West African nation of Niger. Indeed, in recent years a nation's birth rate can be looked at as a crude barometer of its level of economic development, since the most prosperous, most technologically advanced countries generally are characterized by low birth rates.

Death rates are calculated in the same way as birth rates, representing the annual number of deaths per 1,000 population. Birth and death rates are frequently referred to as "crude" rates because they don't reflect the wide variations in age distribution within a population—a fact that might result in misleading conclusions when comparing statistics from different countries. For example, the fact that Jordan has a death rate of 5 per thousand population while the death rate in Germany is 10 might lead one to assume that Jordanians enjoy better health care and a higher standard of living than do Germans. Such an assumption would be erroneous, however, since the reason for Jordan's apparent advantage is that nearly half the Jordanian population (41%) is under the age of 15—an age cohort everywhere typified by a low likelihood of death. Germany, on the other hand, is characterized by an aging population; only 16% of Germans are under 15, while 15% are over age 65 (compared to just 2% in Jordan). Even with excellent medical care, death rates are bound to be higher in a predominantly middle-aged to elderly population than in one primarily composed of the very young.

Total fertility rates (TFR), representing the average number of children each woman within a given population is likely to bear during her reproductive lifetime (assuming that current age-specific birth rates remain constant),

Table 2-1   Doubling Time of World Population

Date	Estimated Human Population	Doubling Time (in years)
8000 B.C.	5 million	1500
A.D. 1650	500 million	200
A.D. 1850	1 billion	80
A.D. 1930	2 billion	45
A.D. 1975	4 billion	36

perhaps give a clearer picture of reproductive behavior than do crude birth rates. Although *world* TFR has been gradually falling in recent decades to its present level of 2.9, the wide discrepancies in national fertility rates are illustrated by countries such as Niger, whose total fertility rate of 7.5 is currently the world's highest, and by Hong Kong, whose total fertility rate of 1.1 suggests a preference for one-child families on that crowded island (Population Reference Bureau, 1999).

Growth Rates

Since birth rates represent additions to a population and death rates represent subtractions, a change in population size is represented by the difference between the two, i.e. by the **growth rate** (sometimes called the **rate of natural increase**). Growth rates, which do not take migration into account, can be calculated quite simply by subtracting the death rate from the birth rate. Take the case of Pakistan, for example: with a 1999 birth rate of 39 and a death rate of 11, the growth rate of Pakistan's population will be 39 minus 11, or 28 per 1,000 population. However, because growth rate is expressed as a percentage (i.e. per 100), not per 1,000 as in birth and death rates, Pakistan has an annual growth of 2.8%.

Growth rate is the critical factor to look at to get a quick impression of what is happening to a particular population. It is entirely possible that a country could have a traditionally high birth rate and still have a relatively low growth rate if the death rate is high also. In fact, just such a situation was characteristic of most human societies in the world until only a few hundred years ago.

When the average person hears that Pakistan has a population growth rate of 2.8%, the number in question may fail to make an appropriate impact, since most of us find it difficult to conceptualize what a 2.8% growth rate means in human terms. Besides, 2.8% really doesn't sound like very much! However, when expressed in terms of doubling time, the importance of growth rates takes on a new perspective. By calculating the annual growth rate of a population and then referring to a conversion table, we can learn what the doubling time of that population will be:

BOX 2-2

Will AIDS Defuse the Population Bomb?

Current statistics are horrifying enough: by 1999, there were 33.6 million people worldwide infected with the human immunodeficiency virus (HIV), the virus that causes AIDS; another 16.3 million had already died of the disease. Adding to the human tragedy are the 11.2 million AIDS orphans, children who have lost a mother or both parents to AIDS before they reached the age of 15. Unfortunately, public health officials fear that the grim toll exacted since HIV/AIDS was first described in 1981 represents but the "tip of the iceberg" in terms of future disease and death. In spite of extensive public information efforts and millions of dollars poured into medical research, the epidemic shows no signs of abating. To the contrary, HIV/AIDS has become a **pandemic**—global in scope—affecting virtually every country in the world. In regions such as central Africa, the Caribbean, and North America where the disease has been well-established since the early 1980s, the infection continues to rage; in areas previously spared, HIV/AIDS is now spreading rapidly. In Africa, rural hinterlands where the majority of the population lives are now experiencing rates of HIV infection nearly as high as those characterizing urban centers for more than a decade. HIV/AIDS is proliferating in eastern Europe and has been reported from areas as far-flung as Greenland and tiny island nations in the Pacific. Particularly threatened are the nations of southern and southeast Asia, especially India, Burma, and Thailand, where 6 million people are estimated to have become infected within the last few years. Health officials predict that in the decades ahead there will be more AIDS cases in this region than anywhere else in the world.

Just as the geography of HIV/AIDS is expanding, the sociology of the pandemic is volatile and dynamic as well. Population subgroups formerly thought to be at low risk of infection are now experiencing an alarming increase in disease rates. Once confined primarily to homosexual men and intravenous drug abusers, HIV/AIDS prevalence is rising dramatically among women and infants as heterosexual contact becomes the main route of transmission in many countries; of those persons currently infected, 14.8 million are women and 1.2 million are children under 15.

These realities have health experts forecasting an explosion in HIV infection rates in the years immediately ahead, with young men and women under the age of 25 destined to comprise 60% of new victims. While no country is immune, HIV infection rates and AIDS deaths have stabilized or declined in industrialized nations in recent years, while the epidemic continues to wreak havoc in the poor countries, where victims' inability to pay for expensive drug regimens means a certain death sentence. The disease has been particularly devastating to the nations of sub-Saharan Africa, where 83% of all AIDS deaths have occurred thus far. Infection rates in the region as a whole reached an unprecedented 7.4% in 1998 (compared with 0.6% in the U.S. and Canada and 1.0% worldwide), but are much higher in certain cities or countries. In Nairobi, Kenya, 25% of the adult population is HIV-positive (the Kenyan health minister earlier predicted that by the year 2000 every hospital bed in his country would be needed for AIDS patients), while in Harare, Zimbabwe, the figure tops 30%. In Botswana, where HIV/AIDS appeared later than in many other African countries, a quarter of the population between the ages of 15 and 49 (40% of all pregnant women) is now thought to be infected; infection rates are soaring in South Africa as well.

In the context of such an exponential rate of increase, it seems relevant to question whether AIDS may provide an example of one of those forces of environmental resistance acting to bring a halt to what seems to be a runaway rate of population increase in Africa. Since heterosexual relations constitute the major route of transmission in African countries, AIDS' demographic implications are a subject of considerable speculation. If women of childbearing age sicken and die while still relatively young, total fertility rates obviously will be lower than they would have been in the absence of AIDS. Similarly, if child mortality rises because HIV-positive mothers are transmitting the virus to their babies *in utero* or in breast milk, overall growth rules should be affected.

Whether AIDS-influenced declines in growth rates will be large enough to cause an actual decrease in population size—or even a leveling off—in African countries that are currently growing at rates averaging close to 3% annually is doubtful, however. Data from Uganda, one of the first countries to be hard-hit by the HIV/AIDS epidemic, yield no evidence that the disease is having any noticeable influence yet on fertility rates. Indeed, in 1999 Uganda reported a 2.9% growth rate, a figure which, if maintained, would lead to a doubling of the population in just 24 years. This situation can be explained, at least in part, by the fact that death due to AIDS generally doesn't occur until 8–10 years after infection with the HIV virus. If a woman acquired her infection soon after becoming sexually active in her late teens or early twenties, she could still live long enough to bear a number of children.

Some observers have even suggested that Africa's AIDS epidemic could actually lead to *higher* fertility if it encourages women to marry at an earlier age when the likelihood of HIV infection presumably is less (in general, the younger a woman marries, the more children she is likely to bear during her lifetime). Rising death rates among both children and young adults could prompt women to have more children in compensation. Although AIDS may reduce fertility to some extent (i.e. AIDS may prevent the additional births which would have occurred were the woman to live a normal life span), researchers predict that the impact of such a decline will simply be to lower present growth rules in certain African countries to somewhere between 0.5 to 2% annually early in the next century—rates that still represent relatively rapid growth. Botswana and Zimbabwe, however, may be exceptions to the general rule; the very high infection rates there prompt U.S. Census Bureau demographers to predict that those two countries may indeed experience slightly negative growth by 2010.

While much remains to be learned about the association between HIV/AIDS and fertility, population experts generally agree that in spite of the tragic humanitarian aspects of the disease, African populations will continue to grow for the foreseeable future—not as rapidly as they would in the absence of AIDS, but grow nevertheless.

References

Halweil, Brian. 1998. "HIV/AIDS Pandemic Far From Over." *Vital Signs 1998*, Worldwatch Institute.

"The United Nations on the Impact of HIV/AIDS on Adult Mortality in sub-Saharan Africa." *Population and Development Review* 24, no. 3 (Sept. 1998).

GROWTH RATE	DOUBLING TIME
0.5%	140 years
0.8%	87 years
1.0%	70 years
2.0%	35 years
3.0%	24 years
4.0%	17 years

Thus, with an annual growth rate of 2.8%, the population of Pakistan, already at 147 million, will double in just 25 years. In human terms this means that *just to maintain present standards of living* everything in Pakistan needs to be doubled in 25 years—food production, provision of jobs, educational facilities, medical personnel, public services, and so forth. Whether such a Herculean task can be accomplished remains to be seen; certainly the leaders of Pakistan (and of a great many other nations whose doubling times are similarly brief) face a formidable challenge in the decades ahead, especially at a time when the "revolution of rising expectations" has created a grassroots demand for improved living standards, not just maintenance of the status quo.

Figure 2-3   Population Size and Rate of Growth

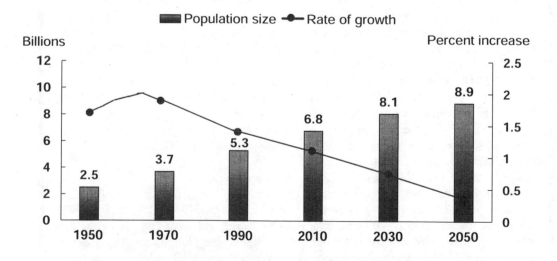

Worldwide, 1950-2050

Source: Used with permission of Population Reference Bureau. Based on data from *U.N. World Population Prospects: The 1998 Revision*, 1998 (medium scenario).

Table 2-2   1999 Population Data for Selected Countries

Region or Country	Population* (millions)	Birth Rate	Death Rate	Growth Rate, %	Doubling Time-yrs.
World	5,982	23	9	1.4	49
AFRICA	771	39	14	2.5	28
Egypt	66.9	26	6	2.0	35
Ethiopia	59.7	46	21	2.5	28
Ghana	19.7	39	10	2.9	24
Nigeria	113.8	43	13	3.0	23
South Africa	42.6	27	11	1.6	43
Kenya	28.8	35	14	2.1	33
Congo, Dem. Rep. of	50.5	48	16	3.2	22
ASIA	3,637	23	8	1.5	46
Bangladesh	125.7	27	8	1.8	38
China	1,254.1	16	7	1.0	73
India	986.6	28	9	1.9	37
Iraq	22.5	38	10	2.8	25
Japan	126.7	10	7	0.2	318
Philippines	74.7	29	7	2.3	31
Thailand	61.8	18	7	1.1	61
Turkey	65.9	22	7	1.5	46
Vietnam	79.5	22	7	1.5	46
LATIN AMERICA	512	24	6	1.8	38
Argentina	36.6	20	8	1.2	58
Brazil	168	21	6	1.5	45
Colombia	38.6	26	6	2.0	34
Cuba	11.2	14	7	0.7	103
Mexico	99.7	27	5	2.2	32
Nicaragua	5.0	38	6	3.2	22
Peru	26.6	28	6	2.2	32
Venezuela	23.7	25	5	2.0	34
NORTH AMERICA	303	14	8	0.6	119
Canada	30.6	11	7	0.4	162
United States	272.5	15	9	0.6	116
EUROPE	728	10	11	-0.1	–
France	59.1	12	9	0.3	210
Germany	82.0	10	10	-0.1	–
Hungary	10.1	10	14	-0.4	–
Italy	57.7	9	10	-0.0	–
Poland	38.7	10	10	0.1	1,155
Russia	146.5	9	14	-0.5	–
Spain	39.4	9	9	0.0	1,980
Sweden	8.9	10	11	-0.1	–
United Kingdom	59.4	12	10	0.2	423

*(mid-1999)

Source: Population Reference Bureau, 1999 World Population Data Sheet.

BOX 2-3

Demographic Disaster in Russia

Increased longevity, low infant mortality, a general across-the-board improvement in health indicators—all these are assumed to be facts of life in a modern industrial nation. Hence the puzzlement and dismay among demographers and public health officials to find that just the reverse is occurring in one of the developed world's largest nations. Russia currently holds the dubious distinction of being the only country in history to have witnessed, year after year since the mid-1960s, a drastic decline in male life expectancy, as well as a marked rise in infant mortality rates.

Throughout the 1990s, the average life span for Russian men fluctuated just above or just below 60 years, dropping to a shocking 57 in 1994—less than the comparable statistic for men in some developing nations (e.g. India, Bolivia, Egypt), and considerably lower than the 72 years life expectancy enjoyed by their American contemporaries (or the 71 years typical for Russian *women*).

During these same years, death rates among infants also were much higher than in other industrialized nations; by the late 1990s, 17 out of every 1,000 Russian babies were dying before their first birthday, compared to 7 in the U.S. and just 4 in Norway and Japan.

Conditions weren't always this bad. Although at the beginning of the 20th century Russian life expectancy was a dismal 32, well below the then-47 year average life span in France and the U.S., improving living conditions gradually raised longevity in Russia to 43 in the years immediately prior to World War II. Following the war, rapid gains in life expectancy were achieved, thanks to Soviet efforts to control infectious disease, investments in social services, and improvements in housing and nutrition. By 1965 Russian life expectancy was almost on a par with that of the Western democracies—64.3 years for men and 73.4 for women. By the late 1960s, however, progress slowed as health gains achieved largely through use of new antibiotics leveled off and as cardiovascular disease and cancer (the so-called "ills of civilization") replaced infectious agents as the leading causes of adult mortality in Russia. By the late sixties, the health gap between Russia and the West inexorably began to widen.

While infant mortality rates and the generally poor state of health among Russian children are cause for serious concern (some medical authorities estimate that only 20% of Russian children can be classified as "healthy"), it is the sharp decline in adult male life expectancy that has attracted the most attention.

Health statistics reveal that heart disease, stroke, and injuries are the leading causes of death among Russian adults, with cancer claiming many lives as well, but such facts by themselves don't explain *why* rates are so high. Alcohol abuse has long received most of the blame, its consequences linked to increased mortality both directly (stroke, cirrhosis of the liver, and alcohol poisoning) and indirectly (automobile and industrial accidents, high blood pressure, some intestinal cancers). Indeed, the alcohol consumption level in Russia is among the highest in the world, at 14 liters/capita of pure alcohol each year. Unlike the situation in France, where annual liquor consumption levels are comparable to those in Russia, Russians don't "wine and dine" but rather indulge in heavy binge drinking of vodka or a potent home-brew called samogon, usually with little or no accompanying food to temper the impact. This practice results in more rapid onset of drunkenness, a greater tendency to violence or serious accidents, more strokes, heart attacks, and fatal alcohol poisonings (caused by drinking a critical amount of vodka or other strong liquor within a relatively short time period). Moreover, the widespread consumption of samogon and other substitutes for state-produced alcoholic beverages further increase a drinker's risk of poisoning. Reports abound of Russians quaffing everything from stolen ethanol to various technical alcohols to cologne and aftershave lotion! Though figures can't be substantiated, Russian authorities estimate that samogon constitutes anywhere from 30–60% of total Russian alcohol consumption, a dismayingly high percentage since home-brew is frequently contaminated with toxic substances. Even liquor in the state stores may be tainted; a Moscow survey found that nearly 40% of the content of alcohol sold there was falsified, perhaps explaining autopsy results showing that a number of alcohol poisoning victims had a high concentration of toxic elements in their blood.

Nevertheless, in spite of the overwhelming evidence pointing to excessive drinking as the leading factor contributing to premature death among Russian men, alcoholism alone can't explain the doubling of male death rates witnessed since the mid-1980s. To some extent the deteriorating health care system—short of medicines, basic supplies, and starved for funds as a result of Russia's on-going financial crisis—bears a portion of the blame. High-fat diets and heavy cigarette smoking also play a role, particularly in terms of escalating cardiovascular problems and cancer rates. High levels of stress caused by the uncertainties of life in post-Soviet Russia are undoubtedly taking a toll. Beyond that, suspicions are now focusing on the decades of environmental abuse heaped on Russia's land, water, and people by a government pursuing production at any cost. A legacy of nuclear bomb-making and careless radioactive waste disposal has left thousands of contaminated sites in the midst of heavily populated areas; discharge of toxic wastes from factories and power plants continues to pollute air and waterways at levels far higher than those permitted in Western countries; exposure of farmers to huge amounts of dangerous pesticides and of industrial workers to toxic chemicals—all may be contributing to the general decline in Russia's state of health, though demonstrating a direct link is problematic.

Whatever the explanation, it's a mystery that needs to be solved as soon as possible, since the challenge of restructuring Russia's society and economy can scarcely be met if such a large proportion of its citizens continue to die at the time of life when they should be most productive.

References

National Research Council. 1997. *Premature Death in the New Independent States*. Washington, DC: National Academy Press.

Feshbach, Murray. 1995. *Ecological Disaster: Cleaning Up the Hidden Legacy of the Soviet Regime*. New York: The Twentieth Century Fund Press.

Population Explosion

With a basic understanding of what birth, death, and growth rates imply, let us now turn our attention to the crucial question of why growth rates have so accelerated during the past several generations. Surveying the history of human population growth (an admittedly risky enterprise, particularly for the prehistoric period), we can say with a fair degree of certainty that birth rates throughout the world were uniformly high until relatively modern times. (Recently some anthropologists doing research among contemporary hunter-gatherer societies have forwarded the idea that, prior to the agricultural revolution, birth rates among primitive peoples were lower than among subsequent agricultural societies. This they attribute to environmental restraints causing such groups to attempt to space the births of their children). That women in many societies continue to bear children at traditionally high levels can be readily perceived by glancing at the current birth rates of most of the nations of Africa and some in Asia and Latin America as well.

With birth rates having apparently held steady during most of human history, we must look then to changes in death rates to explain why growth rates have shot upwards. Each of the three major changes in human lifestyle mentioned earlier effected a decline in the death rate. Cultural advances among prehistoric humans probably reduced the death rate to some slight degree, but the consequences of this cultural evolution were minor compared with the changes wrought by the agricultural revolution. The increase in food supply, the more settled mode of existence, and the general rise in living stan-

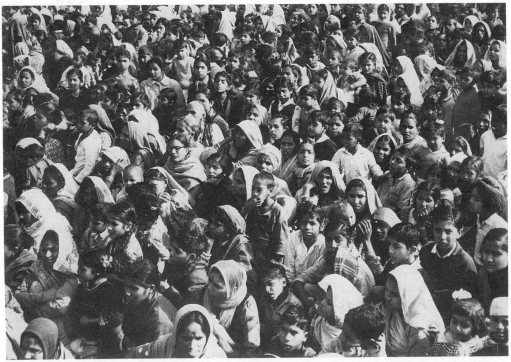

India's population crisis is fueled by a growth rate that could lead to a doubling of its current size in just 37 years. *[Agency for International Development]*.

dards are thought to have reduced mortality rates and increased life expectancy to some degree over that of primitive peoples.

Even so, the gains were gradual until about 200–300 years ago when improvements in public sanitation, advances in agriculture, and the control of infectious disease resulted in a precipitous decline in death rates, particularly in regard to infant and child mortality.

The growth in human numbers that resulted from these improved conditions was not, of course, a steady, uninterrupted rise. Wars, famine, and disease provoked periods of sharp population declines among localized groups. Certainly the most spectacular reversal of the overall growth trend was the impact of bubonic plague (the notorious "Black Death" of the Middle Ages) on the societies of Europe. Plague first reached the Continent in A.D. 1348 and within two years had killed approximately 25% of the total population. Successive outbreaks of the disease continued to sweep across Europe during the next several decades, during which time the population of England dropped by nearly one-half (two-thirds of the student body at Oxford University died during one episode of plague), and many regions in both Europe and Asia were similarly decimated. Nearly constant warfare and the disease and famine that frequently accompanied such conflict also had a negative influence on population growth. Particularly devastating in terms of civilian suffering was the Thirty Years' War (1618-1648), during which time it is estimated that as many as one-third of the inhabitants of Germany and Bohemia died as a direct result of the war. Outside of Europe, warfare, even prior to the World Wars of the 20th century, resulted in enormous loss of life. Conquest and subjugation of Native American civilizations by European colonizers, tribal warfare in Africa, the Moghul invasion of Hindu India, and centuries of internal strife in China resulted in high death rates and sometimes severe depopulation within the affected groups. Perhaps the most extreme example of a population being decimated by warfare involves the most bloody, savage war ever fought in South America. This five-year conflict, which ended in 1870, pitted the combined forces of Brazil, Uruguay, and Argentina against those of Paraguay. The result was virtual extinction for the Paraguayans, whose army was outnumbered 10 to 1 and included 12-year-old boys fighting alongside their grandfathers. Within a five-year period, the population of Paraguay dropped from an estimated 525,000 to 221,000, of whom slightly less than 29,000 were men. A new generation of Paraguayans was sired courtesy of the Brazilian army of occupation (Herring, 1960).

Such examples, while tragic in terms of individual suffering, and occasionally disastrous to certain ethnic groups or nationalities (e.g. the total extermination of native Tasmanians by white settlers), nevertheless represented only minor aberrations from the general upward trend. In general, world population has increased more or less steadily, at first quite slowly but subsequently faster and faster from ancient times right up to the present.

Demographic Transition

By the latter half of the 19th century, western Europe began to witness a demographic phenomenon unlike any that had occurred previously anywhere in the world. Toward the end of the 1700s and early in the 1800s, as the

Industrial Revolution began transforming an entire way of life, death rates started to fall gradually in response to a more adequate food supply, improved medical knowledge, better public sanitation, and so forth. As a result, growth rates predictably accelerated, and during the early years of the 19th century western Europe experienced a population boom. This led, among other things, to massive emigration to the Western Hemisphere. By approximately 1850 another rather surprising trend became apparent—throughout the industrializing nations of that era, birth rates began to fall for the first time since the agricultural revolution. The Scandinavian countries (which were among the first to compile accurate demographic records) provide a good example of the changes that were occurring. In Denmark, Norway, and Sweden the combined birth rate was about 32 in 1850; by 1900 it had dropped to 28 and today stands at 12, among the lowest in the world. Elsewhere in western Europe similar declines were becoming apparent. This phenomenon—the falling of both birth and death rates that has characteristically followed industrialization—marked the onset of the **demographic transition**, a trend that accelerated throughout the 20th century. By the 1930s, decreases in the birth rates in some countries had outpaced decreases in death rates, though actual birth rates remained somewhat higher than death rates. Reasons for the demographic transition are still being debated, but the cause for declining birth rates probably centers on the realization by married couples that in an industrial society children are an economic liability; they are expensive to feed, clothe, and educate; they reduce family mobility and make capital accumulation more difficult. In rural areas of Europe, population pressures on a finite amount of land and the modernization and mechanization of farming tech-

Figure 2-4   The Classic Stages of Demographic Transition

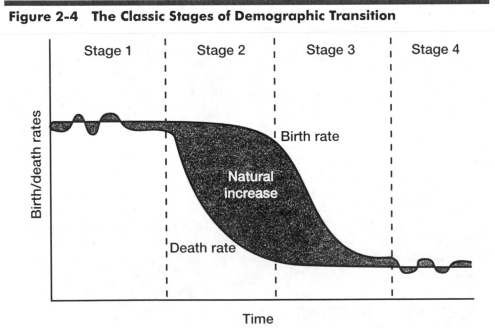

Source: "Population: A Lively Introduction" by Joseph A. McFalls, Jr. *Population Bulletin* 53, no. 3 (Sept. 1988). Used with permission of the Population Reference Bureau.

niques, which reduced the amount of manual labor needed, combined to bring about a reduction in rural birth rates also. In addition, during the late 1800s and into the 20th century, a trend toward marrying at a later age undoubtedly contributed to the decreasing birth rates.

The decline in both birth and death rates that marked the demographic transition in western Europe became noticeable in both eastern Europe and North America several decades later. Although birth rates in the latter have still not fallen as low as those in the nations where the demographic transition began, the trends are quite clearly in the same direction.

Incomplete Demographic Transition

In the nations of Asia, Africa, and Latin America where traditional societies were only marginally influenced by the dynamic economic and social changes occurring in Europe and North America, demographic patterns changed very little until early in the 20th century. In the areas under the control of imperial powers, improvements in public sanitation and an imposed peace between formerly warring factions within the subject nations permitted a gradual increase in population levels. This gradual decline in death rates took a quantum leap in the years immediately following World War II as modern drugs and public health measures were exported from the industrialized nations to the Third World countries. Virtually overnight, the widely applauded introduction of "death control" into traditional cultures produced the most rapid, widespread change known in the history of population dynamics. The situation in Sri Lanka (formerly Ceylon) is a good case in point.

Prior to World War II, a major killer in many tropical countries was the mosquito-borne parasitic disease, malaria. In Sri Lanka a malaria epidemic during 1934–1935 may have been responsible for half the deaths occurring in the country that year (Sri Lanka had a death rate of 34 during that time period). Not only did many victims die outright, but many others were so debilitated by their bouts with the recurring cycles of chills and fever that they became more susceptible to other illnesses. Thus malaria was a contributory cause of death in some cases and a primary cause in others. In 1945, at the end of World War II, the death rate in Sri Lanka stood at 22. One of the great technological innovations to rise out of the war was introduced into Sri Lanka—the synthetic chemical insecticide DDT. Widescale spraying with DDT brought rapid control over the mosquitoes, with a corresponding plunge in the incidence of malaria. As a result, the death rate on the island was cut by more than half within a decade and has continued to drop since then to its present low of 7. Thus, the number of Sri Lankans has soared upwards.

Victory over malaria, yellow fever, smallpox, cholera, and other infectious diseases has been responsible for similar decreases in death rates throughout most of the underdeveloped world. This trend has been most pronounced among children and young adults. Since 1960, according to a World Bank report, the number of children who die before reaching their fifth birthday has declined by two-thirds, thanks to greater public access to standard immunizations and oral rehydration therapy for treating diarrheal diseases (Altman, 1993).

A typical example is Tunisia, where the child mortality rate (deaths of children under age five per thousand live births) plummeted from 210 to 99 in the brief five-year period between 1965–1970. The child mortality rate in Tunisia has continued to drop, albeit not quite so dramatically as during the 1960s, and now stands at 43, one-fifth the level of just a generation ago. Not surprisingly, the population size of Tunisia doubled between 1960 and 1990 (Kennedy, 1993).

This decline in death rates is different in kind from the long-term slow decline that occurred throughout most of the world following the agricultural revolution. It is also different in kind from the comparatively more rapid decline in death rates in the Western world over the past century. The difference is that it is a response to a spectacular environmental change in the underdeveloped countries largely through control of infectious diseases, not a fundamental change in their institutions or general way of life. Furthermore, the change did not originate within these countries, but was brought about from the outside. The factors that led to a demographic transition in the West were not and are not present in the underdeveloped nations. Instead, a large proportion of the world's people have moved rapidly from a situation of high birth and death rates to one of high birth and low death rates, a situation referred to as an **incomplete demographic transition.** This, in essence, is the cause of what biologist Paul Ehrlich refers to as the "population bomb."

Thus have we arrived at the present situation, where approximately 95% of annual world population growth is occurring in developing countries that already are finding it difficult to support current numbers, let alone the additional millions projected for the decades immediately ahead.

Demographers have long assumed that societies now experiencing rapid rates of population increase would, like Europe, North America, and several East Asian nations, witness a significant decline in birth rates as rising incomes and better living conditions resulted in a general desire for smaller families. However, after witnessing more than 50 years of explosive population growth in many developing countries, some observers are beginning to question whether a demographic model based on Western world experience is appropriate to explain what is happening in Africa, Asia, and Latin America. While recent birth rate declines in some of these countries (most notably in China) have been encouraging news to advocates of population stabilization, the fact remains that fertility rates are still well above replacement level throughout the developing world. While population experts agree that growth cannot continue indefinitely, a "just-in-time" completion of the demographic transition is not divinely preordained. Given their already huge population base, developing nations that fail to reduce birth rates sharply in the years immediately ahead are likely to find the sheer pressure of human numbers overwhelming their natural life-support systems long before cultural and economic changes are reflected in a demonstrated preference for two-child families. As demands for food, water, fuel, and living space continue to escalate, the resource base itself will inevitably be degraded and consumed. The decline in incomes and living standards which will occur as a consequence of exceeding the local environment's carrying capacity may well trigger a rise in death rates and thrust affected societies backward into the high birth/high death rate situation characteristic of the pre-demographic transition era.

Age Structure

It's relatively easy to comprehend the significance of birth and death rates so far as population growth is concerned, but there are other characteristics of a population that are important also.

Age structure refers to the number of people in different age categories within a given population. In countries where populations are growing rapidly because of high birth rates and declining death rates, a large percentage of the population is made up of young people; in many Third World countries nearly half the population is under the age of 15. In western Europe, by contrast, there are proportionately many more people in the middle and older age groups. In countries where children comprise a large segment of the population, there hasn't been time yet for individuals born during the period of "death control" to reach the older age groups where death rates are higher than those of the younger age categories. In most of these countries the greatest decreases in death rates among infants and children occurred in the late 1940s and the large numbers of children born in that period reached their peak reproductive years in the 1970s. Their children, in turn, are further inflating the lower tiers of the population structure. Eventually either population control will lower birth rates in these countries, or famine, disease, or other factors will once again increase mortality rates. In the absence of such calamities, death rates in the extraordinarily young populations of the underdeveloped nations may temporarily fall below those of the industrialized countries.

Figure 2-5 Age Distribution in More and Less Developed Countries

Population structures by age and sex, 1995

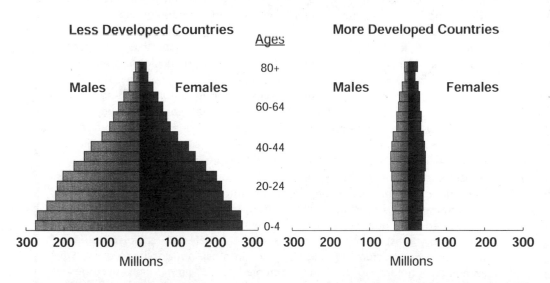

Source: Used with permission of Population Reference Bureau. Based on data from U.N., *The Sex and Age Distribution of World Populations: The 1998 Revision,* 1998 (medium scenario).

BOX 2-4

Global Graying

While leaders of the developing nations struggle to meet the needs of still-growing populations, their counterparts in the industrialized world are facing an entirely different problem: a disproportionate and rapidly increasing percentage of elderly citizens as the "baby bust" generates ever-smaller cohorts of young people. Thanks to improved health care, nutrition, and general standard of living, today's elderly are experiencing a degree of longevity unprecedented in human history. Global life expectancy has lengthened more in the last 50 years than it did throughout the previous 5,000. Until the onset of the industrial era, only 2–3% of people born lived beyond age 65; today that figure is 14% and rising. By 2030, the United Nations estimates that fully one-quarter of the planet's population will be in the "senior" category.

While "global graying" is underway in virtually every country (e.g. China's elderly population is increasing 7 times faster than the population as a whole; between 2000 and 2027, the percentage of Chinese senior citizens will double, from its current 10% to 20%), nowhere are the effects more acutely felt at present than in Japan and Europe. Characterized by plummeting birth rates and excellent health care, those countries have been witnessing a steady decline in the proportion of young people within their populations while increased longevity is simultaneously swelling the ranks of the elderly. The statistics are truly astounding: Italy now has more citizens over 60 years old than it has under the age of 20—the first nation in history to experience such a transformation in age structure. In what one commentator refers to as the "Floridazation" of the developed world,

many countries will soon attain the 19% elderly population that already characterizes the "Sunshine State"; among those soon to reach that benchmark are Italy in 2003; Japan in 2005; Germany in 2006; and both France and the United Kingdom in 2016 (higher fertility rates in the U.S. and Canada will postpone their year of reckoning until 2021 and 2023, respectively). By 2025, half of all Italians will be over 50 years of age and one-third of Japanese will be over 80!

So why should these trends cause any concern? After all, humans have always considered long life among the greatest of blessings and for years environmentalists and population control advocates have preached the virtues of small family size. Now that these goals have been attained, at least in some countries, why isn't there universal rejoicing? Certainly from an ecological standpoint the news *is* good, since all of the countries in question could be considered overpopulated in terms of their environmental impact. Any reduction in population size can only improve congestion, levels of pollution and consumption, and impact on ecosystems. Worries about global aging trends focus primarily on economic and sociopolitical considerations, with some analysts predicting that this unprecedented demographic age shift promises to become the overriding economic and political issue of the 21st century.

Paramount among the issues involved is the impact of burgeoning numbers of elderly pensioners on retirement benefit systems. Like the U.S. Social Security System, the "safety net" social programs in place in most industrialized nations were created at a time when average life expectancy was less than the legal retirement age and when the ratio of young workers to retired persons was heavily weighted toward the former group. Most social security schemes, in essence, borrow from today's workers to support today's retirees. However, as the retired population grows larger and larger and the proportion of young people in the population shrinks, the economic burden on working-age men and women will become increasingly heavy. Today throughout the industrialized world there are three working taxpayers for every retired person. However, unless national retirement systems are radically reformed, by 2030 there will be only 1.5 workers for every pensioner—and in negative-growth countries like Italy and Germany the ratio will be just 1:1. "How to Save Social Security" is already a hot political issue in the United States, but the dilemmas confronting Europe and Japan are even more urgent. With lower birthrates, more rapidly aging populations, larger public pension benefits, and weaker private pension systems than in the U.S., Europeans and Japanese will be hard pressed to preserve social programs and a high standard of living. Experts predict that to meet existing old-age benefit commitments, within the next 30 years developed nations cumulatively will have to spend an extra 9-16% of GDP; if health care obligations are added to this figure, then the financial costs of global aging to developed nations will be in the multi-trillion dollar range. Fears are that this unprecedented burden could destabilize the global economy, threatening financial and political institutions worldwide.

Global graying presents national security concerns as well. Whether developed countries remain able to maintain their military commitments in light of a shrinking pool of potential soldiers and sailors is as yet an unanswered question. Pressure to relax immigration restrictions to ease worker shortages could mount in some countries, in turn creating more strife and political turmoil in areas where an ethnic imbalance is already provoking nationalistic resentment.

In an effort to forestall such problems, several European nations, most notably France and Sweden, have implemented economically costly incentives to encourage childbearing. For the most part, however, such programs have had minimal long-term effects on fertility in societies where young women frequently view children as impediments to a career and an expensive inconvenience.

Whether or not current developed-world attitudes become more pronatalist in the future (and there's no indication they will), global graying is inevitable in the decades ahead because the elderly of 2050 have already been born. The implications of this trend—for society, the economy, and for the environment—will be profound in ways we can now only dimly foresee. As Nicholas Eberstadt, a demographer at the American Enterprise Institute remarked:

"What is happening now has simply never happened before in the history of the world. . . . If these trends continue, in a generation or two there may be countries where most people's only blood relatives will be their parents."

References

Peterson, Peter G. 1999. "Gray Dawn: The Global Aging Crisis." *Foreign Affairs* 78, no. 1 (Jan/Feb): 42–55.

Mitchell, Jennifer D. 1997. "Global Population Growing Older." *Vital Signs 1997.* Worldwatch Institute.

Specter, Michael. 1998. "Population Implosion Worries a Graying Europe." *New York Times* (July 10), p. A1.

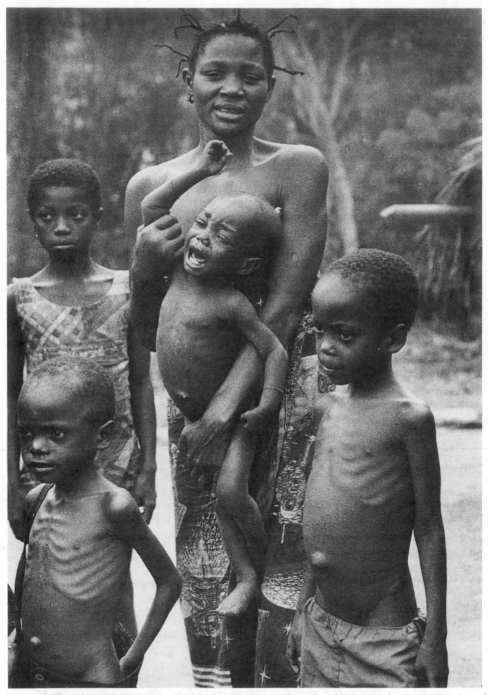

In many Third World countries children make up nearly 50% of the population, indicative of the explosive growth potential in those nations least able to provide for a rapidly growing population. *[Agency for International Development]*

One of the most significant features of age structure in a population is the proportion of people who are economically productive (arbitrarily considered to be those persons between 15 and 59) in relation to those who are dependent on them. The proportion of dependents in the underdeveloped countries is much higher than in the developed nations, presenting an additional heavy burden to those countries as they struggle for economic development. The high percentage of people under 15 is also indicative of the explosive growth potential of their populations. In most developing nations this percentage is 35–40%, while in Gaza children comprise fully 50% of the population! By contrast, the percentage under 15 in most industrialized countries is 20%. In the United States, for example, there are two people of working age for every one who is too young or too old to work; in Mexico and Nigeria there is only one. Thus, underdeveloped countries have a much greater proportion of people in their pre-reproductive years. As they grow up and marry, the size of the childbearing faction of the population will increase tremendously and their children will further inflate the size of the youngest age groups. The existence of such large numbers of young people means that even if great progress were made immediately in reducing the number of births per female in those countries, it would still be some 30 years before such birth control could significantly slow down population growth.

Urbanization

The "urban explosion," referring to the tremendous population increase in metropolitan areas, has been one of the most marked phenomena related to the overall growth of human populations during the past century. Urbanization is, of course, one of the oldest of demographic trends, having its roots in the small settled communities made possible by an agricultural way of life. The first true cities are believed to have arisen in Mesopotamia about five or six thousand years ago, but growth of urban areas proceeded rather slowly during the millennia that followed. Increase in urban populations depended almost entirely on an influx of new residents from the surrounding countryside. Due to extremely poor sanitary conditions and crowded living conditions, mortality rates in these urban centers were higher than birth rates, and not until recent times have urban centers become self-sustaining in terms of population growth.

The advent of the Industrial Revolution gave a tremendous impetus to the growth of cities, and the rate of increase has continued to accelerate ever since. As an example of the great population shift that has occurred, consider the change in rural-urban ratios in the United States: in 1800 a mere 6% of all Americans lived in an urban area: the number of city dwellers increased to 15% by 1850 and to 40% by 1900. In 1999, 75% of the U.S. population lived in cities. [Note: in the United States, "urban" is defined as any community with a population of 2,500 or more. Different countries use different cutoff points to distinguish "urban" from "rural" populations, complicating the comparison of urbanization statistics from various parts of the world. For example, while American demographers utilize the 2,500 figure, their colleagues in Iceland consider a village of 200 as "urban"; in Italy the corresponding number is 10,000, while in densely populated Japan, a community is considered "urban" only when its population surpasses 50,000! (Haub, 1993)].

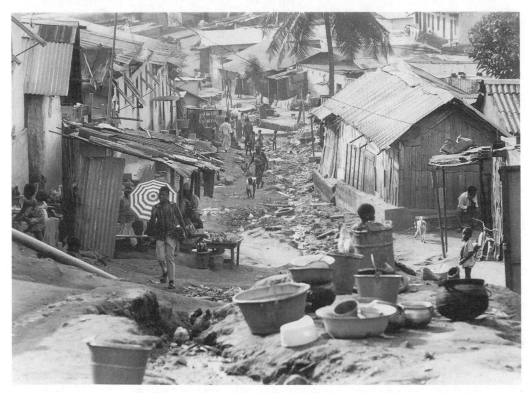

Much of the urban population growth in Third World cities occurs in slum areas like this, where residents lack access to even the basic rudiments of a decent standard of living. *[UN/DPI]*

In the world as a whole, population increased by a factor of 2.6 during the years between 1800 and 1950; during that same time period the number of people living in cities over 20,000 population grew from 22 million to over half a billion—a factor of 23. In the largest cities (100,000 or more) of the industrialized countries, the growth was even more rapid, increasing by a factor of 35. By 1950, 29% of the world's people lived in cities; by 1999 the percentage of urban dwellers in the world had risen to 45 and is expected to surpass 50% by 2005 (Population Reference Bureau, 1999).

In recent years this urban expansion in the developed world has slowed somewhat, but since 1900 has accelerated at a great rate in the nations of Asia, Africa, and Latin America. While the annual urban growth rate was just 0.7% between 1990–1995 in the more developed regions of the world, cities in the developing nations grew by 3.4% each year during the same period. By 2025 the world's urban population is projected to surpass 5 billion—double what it was in the early 1990s. If such forecasts prove accurate, almost two-thirds of humanity will be city dwellers in just 25 years. Of that increase, 90% is taking place in the developing world, particularly in the cities of Asia and Africa (Latin American populations are already 73% urbanized). As of the year 2000, the developing nations boasted 17 of the world's 20 largest cities, each with a population of 10 million or more. Such growth is already having a staggering impact on the ability of those municipalities to provide even the rudiments of a decent standard of living. Much of the population growth in

Table 2-3   World's Largest Cities in A.D. 2015

Rank		Population (in millions)
1.	Tokyo, Japan	28.80
2.	Bombay, India	26.22
3.	Lagos, Nigeria	24.61
4.	Sao Paulo, Brazil	20.32
5.	Dhaka, Bangladesh	19.49
6.	Karachi, Pakistan	19.38
7.	Mexico City, Mexico	19.18
8.	Shanghai, China	17.97
9.	New York, USA	17.60
10.	Calcutta, India	17.31
11.	Delhi, India	16.86
12.	Beijing, China	15.57
13.	Metro Manila, Philippines	14.66
14.	Cairo, Egypt	14.42
15.	Los Angeles, USA	14.22
16.	Jakarta, Indonesia	13.92
17.	Buenos Aires, Argentina	13.86
18.	Tianjin, China	13.53
19.	Seoul, Korea	12.98
20.	Rio de Janeiro, Brazil	11.86

Source: United Nations Population Division, *Urban Agglomerations, 1950–2015 (The 1996 Revision)*, United Nations, New York.

Third World cities occurs in the euphemistically labelled "uncontrolled settlements"—slum areas and shantytowns spreading like ugly cancerous growths around the periphery of almost every large city in the developing world. Estimates indicate that between 30–60% of the people in developing world cities currently live in substandard housing (WRI, 1996). These uncontrolled settlements are growing even faster than the urban areas as a whole, with the consequence that in the years ahead an ever-larger segment of Third World urban populations will be living in the squalor and hopelessness that characterize these shantytowns.

In most cases the trend to the cities seems to be caused by the hope for a better, more comfortable life, and though most migrants continue to live in abject poverty, nearly all seem to prefer to remain there rather than return to the deprivation of their rural home villages. Ironically, recent studies have shown that, contrary to migrant expectations, the quality of life in many Third World cities today is worse than it is in the rural areas they left behind (Brockerhoff and Brennan, 1998). Throughout the developing world, poverty is increasingly becoming an urban phenomenon. At the beginning of the 21st century, approximately half of the world's poorest people—some 420 million—are living in urban settlements. Historically, urbanization seems to have the universal effect of breaking down the traditional cultures of those who migrate to the cities, where anonymity is the main feature. The overwhelming majority of urban dwellers in the Third World are migrants who have brought their peasant culture with them. They generally lack the specialized education and skills required to penetrate the city's complex social web. Migrants inevitably find that their limited skills make them incapable of contributing to the economy and consequently they are scarcely any better off than before. Many migrants form modified village societies within the city and thus tend to transfer aspects of village culture to the city. This may explain why the reproductive rates and attitudes of these city dwellers closely resemble those of their rural relatives.

The rapid increase in the populations of Third World cities presents a number of very serious problems that government officials are going to find extremely difficult to manage. Two of the most pressing needs, if disease outbreaks are to be prevented, will be the provision of safe drinking water and sewage disposal. During the 1980s impressive gains were made in bringing water and sanitation services to urban residents in the developing nations. By 1990, approximately 500 million more city dwellers worldwide had access to adequate drinking water than was the case in 1980; similarly, those served by sewerage projects increased by close to 300 million (Briscoe, 1993). Nevertheless, because of the huge influx of rural migrants into the cities during those years, the number of urban residents *lacking* such services continued to increase. In the mid-1990s, at least 220 million people still had no source of safe drinking water near their homes; many who did have a tap within 100 meters of their house had to share it with as many as 500 other people or had to cope with an intermittent supply, since many communal water taps only function for a few hours daily. In Rajkot, India—a city of 600,000 population— tap water runs for only 20 minutes per day (Bhart, 1994). In general, in the uncontrolled settlements of Third World cities, per capita water availability may be 3–10 times less than in more affluent sections of the same city, a fact which has serious implications for health and sanitation in those areas. Provision of services for disposal of human wastes is lagging even further behind. More than 450 million urban residents of developing countries don't have access even to simple latrines, having to resort to roadside ditches or open spaces. Other families share poorly maintained, often overflowing, privies with 100 or more neighbors. Bombay, the world's third-largest city, needs an estimated half-million public toilets, yet by the mid-1990s had only 200 (Brown et al., 1998). Exposed, untreated human wastes in the midst of densely populated areas pose a direct public health threat, but on-going efforts to meet the sanitary needs of developing world cities are being overwhelmed by the continually growing number of residents to be served. Municipal officials might be forgiven for wondering if they were on a treadmill— having to run faster and faster just to remain in place!

As urban populations continue to expand, provision of such basic services will undoubtedly lag even further behind, increasing the threat of epidemic disease and worsening already serious problems of water pollution. Air quality, already at critical levels in many Third World cities, will continue to deteriorate as the number of old, poorly maintained automobiles and pollutant-emitting motorbikes, scooters, and motorcycles continue to rise. Pressures on municipal authorities to provide jobs, housing, transportation, and social facilities will mount inexorably within the coming years and will present those societies with economic and environmental challenges which may prove impossible to meet.

Population Projections

The obvious question to anyone looking at a graphic representation of human numbers soaring toward infinity on the upswing of a J-curve is, "How long can this continue?" and "Where will population stabilize?" The inherent assumption, and one which is validated by the results of numerous animal experiments in population dynamics, is that such growth rates cannot continue forever. Statistical evidence indicates, in fact, that the world population annual growth rate peaked at about 2% in the early 1970s, declining gradually since then to its present 1.4%. Nevertheless, although a growth rate decrease is good news, in terms of absolute numbers population size will continue to increase significantly for many decades due to the world's enormous population base and the large proportion of young people in developing countries. Talk of a population "explosion," common during the 1970s and 1980s, has been replaced by the metaphor of a giant freight train, slowing a bit, but still traveling dangerously fast with heavy momentum. Describing the current demographic situation, John Bongaarts of the Population Council remarked, "We're climbing uphill, and it's going to take a while to unwind this process. We're not going to stop any time soon" (Borenstein, 1998).

The United Nations, an organization logically quite interested in future world growth patterns, regularly publishes projections of population size for the next several decades. Such projections are not just extrapolations of present trends, but take into consideration trends in fertility, mortality, migration, and so on (they do not consider the possibility of major disasters such as a nuclear war, however). The United Nations presents several sets of projections, all of which assume that there will be some lowering of fertility rates (a substantial drop in fertility is assumed for the low projection, a less significant decline for the high projection) in regions where these are currently quite high. The most widely used medium range projection presupposes a continued steady decline in death rates, with total fertility rates stabilizing at the replacement level (i.e. an average of two children per family) by the year 2055. Given these assumptions, the United Nations' "best guess" for ultimate world population size is just under 11 billion to be reached sometime between 2150–2200. However, if fertility rates deviate even slightly from the replacement level figure presumed for the medium-range estimate, the size of world population at the time of stabilization will be dramatically different from the 11 billion figure cited above. For example, if world fertility drops slightly *below* replacement level (as it has already done in Japan, Hong Kong, and many European countries) to an average of 1.5 children per couple, world population could fall to 3.6 billion by 2150. Conversely, if fertility worldwide remains slightly *above* replacement level at an average 2.5 children per family, world population in 2150 will reach 27 billion and continue climbing. Quite obviously, the childbearing decisions of millions of individual couples will have an enormous impact on total world population size at the time growth eventually levels off. As mentioned before, the U.N. projections displayed in Figure 2-6 all assume some reduction in current fertility rates. Not represented, because U.N. demographers are convinced that human reproductive behavior *will* change, is a "constant fertility" projection that assumes fertility rates will remain constant at approximately 3 children per couple for the next century and a half. Under that scenario, the earth's human population would exceed an incredible 296 billion people by 2150 (UNFPA, 1996).

While both the United Nations and the World Bank are proceeding on the debatable assumption that world population growth will stabilize approximately two centuries from now, widely divergent fertility patterns in different areas of the world guarantee that some regions will achieve population stability long before others do. Italy, Spain, Portugal, Greece, Slovenia, and Sweden have already reached zero population growth (ZPG), while several countries, including Germany, Russia, Ukraine, Hungary, Bulgaria, and Latvia, actually have negative growth rates. Similarly, in Japan, where the average number of children born during a woman's lifetime is now just 1.4, population size will soon peak at a level only slightly higher than present numbers and then begin a slow decline as deaths among the large cohorts of elderly Japanese outnumber births (Yanagashita, 1993).

Looking at population projections on a regional basis, the countries of Asia will experience the largest increase, adding almost 3 billion people to the 3.5 billion already inhabiting that crowded continent. India alone, growing by 18 million annually, is expected to surpass China to become the world's most populous nation by the mid-21st century. Africa, currently boasting the world's highest growth rates, will nearly quadruple its population size by 2150. Together, Africa and Asia will account for fully 80% of the world's total population at the time of stabilization. Latin America is currently growing at

Figure 2-6   World Population Growth, Actual and Projected, 1950–2050

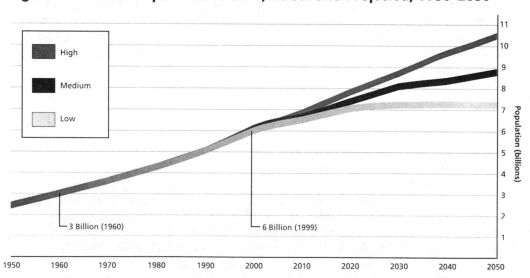

Source: United Nations. 1998. *World Population Prospects* (The 1998 Revision).

BOX 2-5

China: Demographic Billionaire

When the world population growth rate fell from a record-high 2% in the early 1970s to its present 1.4% (although official government figures cite an annual growth rate of 1%, independent experts insist the higher figure is more accurate), some media commentators optimistically hailed the end of the population explosion. If they had examined the statistics more carefully, however, they would have noticed that the downturn was not due to an across-the-board decline in births throughout the world, but rather to some remarkable changes occurring in the planet's demographic giant, the People's Republic of China. Home to one out of every five people on earth, China has always exerted a disproportionate influence among nations on global population trends. To paraphrase an old adage "when China sneezes, the world gets pneumonia"—at least in demographic terms. The fact that world population growth rates have fallen slowly but steadily over the past 30 years is due in large part to the rapid decline in Chinese birth rates; elsewhere in the developing world annual population growth still averages 2%.

Since 1970 China has undergone a demographic transition unprecedented for the speed with which it was carried out. During the years immediately following the 1949 revolution, Chinese mortality rates plummeted as peace was restored and improvements in health and living standards became widespread. As a result, population growth rates rose sharply, averaging more than 2% annually for the next 25 years. Although China's population was already well in excess of 600 million by this time, there was little official concern about overpopulation. Chairman Mao Zedong cheerfully proclaimed that "of all things in the world, people are most precious" and voiced orthodox Communist doctrine by proclaiming that "revolution plus production" would enable China to provide adequately for the needs of a growing population. In response, Chinese parents continued to indulge their preference for large families. By 1970, China's population had passed the 800-million mark, with no signs of a slowdown. By this time, however, the heady optimism expressed by national planners in the 1950s and 1960s had abated. Production figures and living standards were lagging, the economy was stagnant, and the question of how to support a population heading toward 1 billion yielded no easy answers. National leaders, who could no longer pretend to believe that a large, growing population was a blessing, launched a program of "Strategic Demographic Initiatives" (SDI) to curb fertility. By advocating *wan, xi, shao*—later marriage, longer interval between pregnancies, and fewer children per mother Chinese leaders pursued a goal of slowing the growth rate sufficiently to enable the nation to deal with existing population-related problems more effectively. At the time SDI was introduced in the early 1970s, there was no intention of halting growth or reducing population size—the idea was merely to slow the pace of increase. By the late 1970s, however, Communist Party officials had formulated new economic targets that would be unattainable so long as the country's population size continued to grow. Accordingly, the Chinese government developed an official policy position stating that China should not exceed a population maximum of

1.2 billion by the end of the century and should then strive to reduce total numbers to an ultimate population size more appropriate to the nation's carrying capacity—around 700 million. To achieve this goal, Chinese planners in 1979 adopted the now-famous one-child-per-family policy, an idea which, ironically, they seem to have picked up from Zero Population Growth (ZPG) advocates in the United States. Interestingly, by the time the one-child policy was adopted, Chinese birth rates had already fallen to the lowest levels ever recorded in that country; by promoting the concept that "One is not wanting, two are good, and three are excessive," China succeeded in lowering the national fertility rate from six in 1950 to three in 1979. Implementation of the more stringent one-child policy had only a limited additional impact on China's demographic statistics. By the mid-1980s, less than 16% of Chinese couples had signed "Only Child Glory Certificates"—contracts guaranteeing preferences in housing, education, and employment so long as the couple had only one child.

In spite of the new policy, by the early 1980s the phenomenally rapid decline in birth rates that China had witnessed during the previous decade had leveled off and by 1982 began inching upward again, thanks largely to passage of legislation lowering the legal age for marriage and to the breakup of agricultural communes, which motivated farmers to produce more home-grown labor. The fact that by the 1980s women born during the "baby boom" of the 1960s were entering their prime reproductive years further stimulated a modest upswing in birth rates at that time. By 1982, China's population passed the 1 billion mark and hopes for stabilizing growth at 1.2 billion quickly faded.

Although recent official figures cite a current average nationwide fertility rate just under 2.0, with government leaders pronouncing themselves "satisfied" with the country's demographic situation, independent researchers are not so sanguine. Those observers conclude that the actual total fertility rate (TFR) has remained fairly steady around 2.5 since the mid-1980s and, at the close of the century, is again beginning to rise. Ironically, the latest upswing has been prompted in part by a newly prosperous Chinese economy that has persuaded millions of Chinese couples that they can now afford to have that second or third child. Equally significant in undermining China's one-child policy have been the numerous exceptions granted in its implementation. Members of officially designated minority groups, as well as couples living in rural areas (representing approximately 80% of China's land area and 87% of all births) are exempt from compliance. While one-child families have become increasingly common in Chinese cities, resistance to the idea of stopping after one—particularly if that one was a girl—has been especially strong in agricultural areas where manual labor is required. In rural villages characterized by age-old social attitudes and where a male heir is still viewed as essential to ensure his parents' immortality, abstaining from childbearing after producing just one daughter is virtually unthinkable; as one village mother declared to an interviewer, "Having sons is what women come into the world for."

Nevertheless, significantly fewer Chinese sons and daughters are coming into the world than in generations past, thanks to the Herculean efforts of family planning providers and the wholehearted support of China's government. Throughout that vast nation, family planning workers go door-to-door, disseminating birth control information while stressing the benefits of small families.

Contraceptives have been distributed free to married couples since 1974 and the percentage of users is among the highest in the world—by 1999, 83% of married couples in China were practicing contraception, compared with just 76% in the U.S. and 44% in other developing nations. China today has more than 40 contraceptive factories, producing condoms, contraceptive pills, IUDs, and vaginal foam suppositories. In upgrading its contraceptive technology, China has received significant financial assistance from the United Nations, much to the chagrin of some American legislators who have blocked U.S. funding for the international agency to protest anecdotal reports of coercive abortion policies or forced sterilizations targeted against women who had already borne their quota of babies.

Those who resist supporting China's on-going efforts to improve and modernize its population control program should consider the implications of that program's failure. If China's estimated TFR of 2.5 remains unchanged, population in the People's Republic could soar to 2.5 billion in less than a hundred years. Even accepting the official TFR of 2.0, without further reduction in birth rates, China's population will reach 1.5 billion by late in the 21st century—double the number Chinese authorities believe is a sustainable population size, given the country's resource base. The historic demographic experiment being conducted in China today will be followed with extreme interest by all who realize that the ultimate size of world population will be determined to a considerable extent by the success or failure of China's attempt to tame the population monster.

References

Tobias, Michael. 1998. *A Paradox Of Souls: China; World War III. Population And The Biosphere At The End Of The Millennium.* New York: Continuum Publishing.

Tien, H. Yuan, et al. 1992. "China's Demographic Dilemmas." *Population Bulletin* 47, no. 1 (June).

a rate second only to Africa. In 1960 there were approximately equal numbers of Latin Americans and North Americans. At the end of the 20th century there were 500 million people living south of the Rio Grande, 300 million to the north. Population size in Latin America is expected to reach nearly one billion by 2150 while numbers in North America, by contrast, are expected to total approximately 414 million at that time, less than half the size of our southern neighbors. Only Europe, among major geographical regions, is projected to experience population decline in the years ahead. European populations, which now total slightly over 700 million, are projected to fall gradually to just under 600 million by the time world population growth stabilizes (U.N. Population Division, 1998).

Obviously, making global population projections is a risky business, with accuracy of forecasts depending not only on the childbearing decisions of millions of individual couples but also on trends in mortality rates. A number of demographers fear that an increase in death rates may be as influential in curbing growth as a decrease in birth rates. Already there is evidence that in widely scattered areas of the developing world child mortality rates are rising due to increasing levels of malnutrition. There is a real danger that mounting human pressures on already overtaxed ecosystems may cause a collapse in the food-producing capabilities of many regions. While most long-range projec-

Figure 2-7   Population of the Major Regions of the World, 1998 and 2050

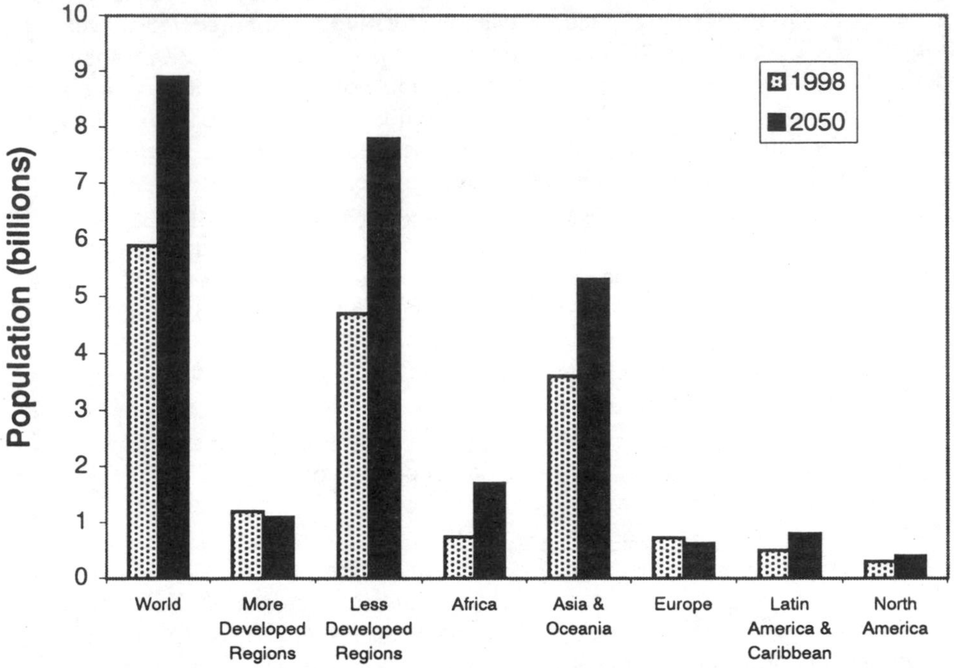

Source: United Nations. 1998. *World Population Prospects* (The 1998 Revision).

tions show global population growth halting between 2150–2200, the ability of natural ecosystems to support another doubling of world population has been questioned. Since 95% of the expected increase will occur in the poorest countries, many observers insist that population growth needs to be stabilized long before it reaches the theoretical levels projected by the United Nations. Recognizing the enormous cooperative effort needed to resolve humanity's demographic dilemma, 1,670 scientists from 70 countries have signed a population stabilization statement drafted by the Union of Concerned Scientists, declaring that:

> Fundamental changes are urgent if we are to avoid the collision our present course will bring about. . . if vast human misery is to be avoided and our global home on this planet is not to be irretrievably mutilated (Tobias, 1998).

References

Altman, Lawrence K. 1993. "Big Health Gains Found in Developing Countries." *New York Times*, July 7.

Bhart, Arunkumar. 1994. "Rajkot Chronic Scarcity." *The Hindu Survey of the Environment 1994* (May 31):113–117.

Borenstein, Seth. 1998. "State of World Population: Fate Rests with Record-Size Generation." *Population Press* 5, no. 1 (Nov/Dec):5.

Briscoe, John. 1993. "When the Cup is Half Full: Improving Water and Sanitation Services in the Developing World." *Environment* 35, no. 4 (May).

Brockerhoff, Martin, and Ellen Brennan. 1998. "The Poverty of Cities in Developing Regions." *Population and Development Review* 24, no. 1 (March): 75–114.

Brown, Lester, Michael Renner, and Christopher Flavin. 1998. *Vital Signs 1998: The Environmental Trends that Are Shaping Our Future.* Worldwatch Institute. New York: W.W. Norton.

Ehrlich, Paul R., Anne H. Ehrlich, and John P. Holdren. 1977. *Ecoscience: Population, Resources, Environment.* W. H. Freeman and Co.

Farb, Peter. 1963. *Ecology, Life Nature Library.* Time Inc.

Haub, Carl. 1993. "Tokyo Now Recognized as World's Largest City." *Population Today* 21, no. 3 (March).

Herring, Herbert. 1960. *A History of Latin America* Alfred A. Knopf.

Kennedy, Paul. 1993. *Preparing for the Twenty-First Century.* Random House.

Kraft, Michael E. 1998. "World Population Trends." *Population Press* 5, no. 1 (Nov/Dec):6–7.

Odum, Eugene P. 1959. *Fundamentals of Ecology.* W. B. Saunders Company.

Population Reference Bureau. 1999. *World Population Data Sheet.*

Rohe, John F. 1998. *A Bicentennial Malthusian Essay: Conservation, Population and the Indifference to Limits.* Traverse City, MI: Rhodes & Easton.

Tobias, Michael. 1998. *World War III: Population and the Biosphere at the End of the Millennium.* New York: Continuum.

U.N. Population Division. 1992. *World Urbanization Prospects.*

———. 1998. "World Population Projections to 2150." *Population Newsletter,* no. 65 (June).

United Nations Population Fund (UNFPA). 1996. "The State of World Population 1996."

———. 1999. "The State of World Population 1999."

World Resources Institute (WRI). 1996. *World Resources 1996–97.* New York: Oxford University Press.

———. 1998. *World Resources 1998–99.* New York: Oxford University Press.

Yanagashita, Machiko. 1993. "Slow Growth Will Turn to Decline of the Japanese Population." *Population Today* 21, no. 5 (May).

CHAPTER 3

Population Control

We want better reasons for having children than not knowing how to prevent them.

—Dora Russell
English feminist (1925)

Studies of population dynamics clearly indicate that no population can sustain limitless growth, raising the as-yet unanswered question: what will eventually bring a halt to still-climbing human numbers? Basically, one of two factors could effect a drop in growth rates: a decrease in birth rates or an increase in death rates. Either change would result in a narrowing of the gap between births and deaths that has been responsible for the unprecedented growth in human population during the past century. A decrease in the death rate caused the population explosion, and a number of demographic experts gloomily predict that a reversal of this trend in the future will bring a halt to further growth. They point to an observable rise in infant mortality rates due to the increasing frequency of malnutrition; to the possibility of global pandemics as population densities increase; and to the growing likelihood of military confrontations as nations compete for dwindling resources.

However, no rational individual would advocate starvation, epidemics, or war as a means of ending the population explosion. The humane approach to a very real problem lies instead in attempts to reduce growth by lowering birth rates to the point at which they will be in approximate equilibrium with death rates, thereby achieving a stabilization of population size, popularly referred to as ZPG (zero population growth).

Early Attempts at Family Limitation

Although most traditional cultures have consistently encouraged prolific childbearing, records indicate that during stressful periods of famine, war, or civil upheaval many couples throughout history have attempted in various

83

ways to prevent unwanted births. While some of the methods employed were based on nothing more than superstition, others were moderately effective and continue to be used today.

One of the oldest documented means of contraception, referred to in the Old Testament story of Onan (Genesis 38:9), is that of withdrawal (*coitus interruptus*), whereby the man withdraws his penis from the vagina prior to ejaculation. Since a keen sense of timing is essential to the success of this method, withdrawal has the highest failure rate of any major method of birth control, but it does have the advantage of requiring no drugs or devices nor access to medical personnel for its use—and it costs nothing. Where couples are highly motivated not to have children, it can be fairly successful and, in fact, is believed to be the method by which European couples substantially reduced birth rates in that part of the world during the early years of the demographic transition. Even today, an estimated 38 million couples world-wide continue to rely on withdrawal as a means of preventing unwanted births. In developing countries it may account for as much as 9% of contraceptive practice; in modern Turkey it remains the most common method of birth control (Rogow and Horowitz, 1995). In the past, the popularity of withdrawal prompted numerous attacks on the method by certain disapproving segments of society. Some doctors declared that the practice would lead to both physical and mental illness, but such admonitions fell largely on deaf ears. One 40-year-old German farmer, warned of the dire consequences of indulging in *coitus interruptus,* calmly retorted, "I don't believe that. Otherwise everybody would be sick."

Crude barriers to the cervix, similar in concept to the modern diaphragm or cervical cap, were used by women in ancient Egypt who fashioned such devices out of leaves, cloth, wads of cotton fibers, or even crocodile dung!

Herbal concoctions have been used for both contraceptive and abortive purposes for thousands of years. The modern era's contraceptive pill, along with hormonal implants and injectables, are but the most recent in a venerable line of antifertility drugs widely employed in ancient and medieval societies as well as in folk cultures right up to the present time. Although it long was fashionable to dismiss such brews as totally useless, recent research has found that some of the plants used are, in fact, remarkably effective in preventing pregnancy, while others are powerful abortifacients. The contraceptive properties of drugs extracted from such plant materials as pomegranate rind, black pepper, ivy, cabbage flowers, and willow bark were described in Greek and Roman medical literature almost two thousand years ago. Pennyroyal *(Mentha pulegium)*, a member of the mint family, was widely used for centuries to induce abortions, as was rue *(Ruta graveolans)*, which has both abortifacient and contraceptive properties. In recent decades the results of a number of studies and field observations confirm that certain plant substances do indeed exert an antifertility effect (a phenomenon first noticed in relation to spontaneous abortions or a failure of ovulation among grazing animals when feeding on certain plants). Preliminary research has confirmed many of the claims made by ancient medical authorities and efforts are now on-going in a number of countries, especially India and China, to conduct clinical and laboratory tests of traditional drugs believed to possess contraceptive properties (McLaren, 1990; Riddle, 1992).

The use of condoms dates back at least to the 16th century when a fine linen sheath worn on the penis during intercourse was recommended as a means of preventing the spread of venereal disease. By the 17th century condoms made of lamb intestines, tied shut at the end with a ribbon, were introduced for the express purpose of preventing conception and by the 18th century were reportedly available for use by patrons at all the finer houses of prostitution in Europe (some versions were also made of silk!). With the advent of vulcanized rubber in 1844, a truly effective and relatively cheap (advertised at $5 per dozen in 1850) male contraceptive became available for the masses. Nevertheless, rubber condoms were not widely used until World War I when they were distributed among the troops as protection against venereal disease (Stokes, 1980; McLaren, 1990).

Other birth-control practices with a similarly long history include douching (flushing out the vagina with a water solution immediately after intercourse), almost totally ineffective in spite of its popularity; and breast-feeding of infants, quite an effective means of suppressing the onset of ovulation following childbirth and thereby helpful in spacing pregnancies. In fact, prior to the advent of modern contraceptives, breast-feeding was the chief tactic employed by women to prevent an unwanted second pregnancy soon after childbirth. A survey conducted in Bangladesh revealed that, on average, each month of breast-feeding increases the birth interval between babies by about 0.4 months (Weiss, 1993; Kleinman and Senanayake, 1984).

When such birth-control methods failed, as they frequently did, women commonly resorted to abortion, a very ancient practice believed to have been the most prevalent method of family limitation throughout history.

As a last resort, unwanted children in past centuries frequently fell victim to infanticide—the deliberate killing of babies, particularly girl babies, immediately after birth. This practice was quite common in ancient Greece and in several Asian countries up until fairly recent times, especially during periods of famine or civil upheaval.

Modern Family Planning Movement

The origins of the modern family planning movement in the United States can be traced to the publication in 1832 of a contraceptive textbook, *Fruits of Philosophy,* written by Dr. Charles Knowlton. Dr. Knowlton won renown as the first person in this country to be jailed for advocating birth control. The development of the diaphragm in the 1840s further stimulated public interest in contraceptive techniques and although proponents of birth control were viciously persecuted by so-called "societies for the suppression of vice," the resultant notoriety only enhanced sales of birth-control literature. Open discussion of sex or reproductive matters was still taboo during those years of Victorian morality, however, and an "establishment" backlash against the growing birth-control movement was reflected in the passage in 1873 of the Comstock Law, a federal mandate that prohibited sending birth-control information or devices through the mail, such items being defined as "obscene."

Toward the end of the 19th century, the burgeoning feminist movement lent support to the concept of family planning, stressing the health burdens imposed on women by too many children born too close together. An outstand-

BOX 3-1

The "Morning-After Pill" Comes of Age:
Emergency Contraception

In September 1998, the U.S. Food and Drug Administration put its seal of approval on the Preven Emergency Contraception Kit, thereby legitimizing use of a birth-control method that had been acknowledged by medical practitioners with "a wink and a nod" for years. The need for a so-called "morning-after pill" (more accurately termed a **postcoital contraceptive**, since it can be used effectively any time up to 72 hours after unprotected intercourse) is apparent from a glance at U.S. statistics for unwanted pregnancy. In spite of near-universal access to a wide range of highly effective methods of birth control, each year approximately 3.5 million American women experience unplanned pregnancies; of these, an estimated 1.7 million are blamed on contraceptive failure (e.g. condoms that break, pills that were forgotten, an IUD accidentally expelled). In situations like these, as well as in cases of rape, drunkenness, or careless neglect, an emergency after-the-fact contraceptive has enormous potential to prevent unwanted pregnancies and drastically reduce the incidence of abortion.

Though their existence has been a well-kept secret, there's nothing really new about postcoital contraceptive drugs. As early as the 1920s, researchers had discovered that natural estrogenic hormones extracted from ovarian tissue could interfere with mammalian pregnancies—a finding quickly put to practical use by veterinarians who administered estrogens to pedigreed dogs and horses that had mated with unpedigreed partners. In the 1960s physicians in the Netherlands copied the veterinarians' approach and administered estrogens to a young rape victim—the first case of deliberate emergency contraceptive use documented in the medical literature. During the next several decades a number of different hormonal formulations for oral postcoital contraception were investigated in laboratories around the world, most of them focusing on high-dose estrogens or, as in the case of Preven, a combined estrogen-progestin regimen. Several of these products have been on the market in Europe and Asia for a number of years, long before most American women had even heard of their existence.

By the late 1970s, a nonhormonal emergency contraceptive, a copper-releasing IUD, was developed (currently being marketed as Paraguard T380 A). Acting to produce changes in the uterine lining that prevent implantation of a fertilized egg, the copper IUD can be inserted up to 7 days following unprotected intercourse and is 99.9% effective in preventing pregnancy. This device has the added benefit of providing worry-free contraceptive protection up to 10 years following insertion.

The emergency contraception kit that ultimately received FDA's blessing is available only by prescription and is relatively inexpensive (costing about $20 at the time it was introduced). The kit consists of four emergency contraceptive pills (ECPs), each containing 0.25 mg of levonorgestrel and 0.05 mg of ethinyl estradiol—the same chemicals found at lower concentrations in ordinary birth control pills. Accompanying the pills are a patient information booklet and a urine pregnancy test. The patient is instructed to take the pregnancy test and, if results are negative, to take two of the pills immediately, following with the remaining two pills 12 hours later. When used as directed within 72 hours after intercourse, the pills' effectiveness in preventing pregnancy is estimated at about 75%—not as good as conventional contraceptives used before or during intercourse, but certainly better than nothing. The most common side effects associated with use of Preven are nausea and vomiting. Such problems are largely absent in a progestin-only ECP called "Plan B" that received FDA approval in July 1999. Unlike RU 486, marketed as an abortifacient, ECPs will not cause abortions or birth defects if the woman using them is already pregnant. Depending on timing of administration, the pills work by preventing or delaying ovulation, or by inhibiting the implantation of a fertilized egg.

Unfortunately, despite the obvious need, women still encounter many obstacles in obtaining accurate information and in accessing the pills within the 72 hour window of effectiveness. Pharmaceutical companies have shied away from ECPs for fear of being targeted by anti-abortion groups who erroneously equate emergency contraception with abortion. Even FDA approval has not resulted in vigorous advertising efforts to increase public awareness of ECPs. On college campuses—source of much of the demand for emergency contraception—student health centers vary widely in the extent to which they inform prospective clients of ECP availability. Some advertise aggressively through student newspapers, fliers, and on the Internet while others, particularly at church-affiliated institutions, provide ECPs only when specifically requested by students. The fact that most student health centers offer emergency contraception only on weekdays from 9 a.m. to 5 p.m. greatly restricts access when quick action is most urgently needed. For this reason, some proponents advocate making ECPs available through vending machines; others advocate giving pharmacists the authority to dispense them, an action already taken by the State of Washington.

Anecdotal evidence suggests that emergency contraception is still underused both by women who need it and by health care providers. Some observers estimate that 5 million women would use ECPs each year if they knew the pills were available and where to obtain them. Similarly, they estimate that if ECPs were sold over the counter, rather than by prescription only, the demand could be in excess of 13 million courses annually. In light of the 3.5 million unwanted pregnancies in the United States each year, as well as the nearly 1.4 million abortions—most of which never would have occurred if emergency contraceptive services were more widely utilized, the need to raise awareness and dispel the misinformation surrounding this issue is all too apparent.

References

American Medical Association. 1998. "Emergency Contraception Kit Approved." *Journal of the American Medical Association* 280, no. 17 (Nov. 4):1472.

Ellertson, Charlotte. 1996. "History and Efficacy of Emergency Contraception: Beyond Coca-Cola." *Family Planning Perspectives* 28, no. 2 (March/April):44-48.

Ellertson, Charlotte., et al. 1997. "How Many U.S. Women Need Emergency Contraception?" *Contemporary OB/GYN* 42, no. 10:102-104, 108.

ing pioneer of family planning in America was Margaret Sanger, a nurse in New York City who was appalled by the extent of poverty due to over-large families and the rate of maternal death due to abortion among the people with whom she worked. Recognizing that the Comstock Law prevented such people from obtaining the contraceptive information they so badly needed, she launched a personal crusade to overturn that legislation. In 1914 Sanger founded the National Birth Control League and began publishing a monthly magazine, *The Woman Rebel,* containing birth-control information—which the Post Office therefore refused to distribute. The following year she circulated a more comprehensive birth-control pamphlet, *Family Limitation,* which also violated the Comstock Law. Sanger was indicted for this action, but the indictment was subsequently dropped. In 1916 Mrs. Sanger opened the first birth-control clinic in America, in a section of Brooklyn, New York. For this offense she was arrested and served 30 days in prison, but the resulting public outcry led to a gradual easing of legal restrictions against the family planning movement.

Mrs. Sanger traveled extensively throughout the country, seeking to persuade both the medical profession and the public at large of the importance of facilitating access to birth control. By 1932 the Birth Control League had established 80 clinics throughout the United States; in 1937 the American Medical Association officially endorsed birth control; finally, by 1938, two major court cases resulted in the overthrow of the Comstock Law and, in effect, made it possible for doctors to prescribe contraceptives to patients (except in Connecticut and Massachusetts where contraceptives remained illegal under state law until the 1960s). In 1942 the National Birth Control League and its affiliated clinics became Planned Parenthood Federation, with Margaret Sanger as honorary chairperson (League of Women Voters Education Fund, 1982).

Birth Control—Its Health Impact

Over the years the services offered by Planned Parenthood have expanded to include premarital counseling and fertility assistance in addition to the original intent of providing birth-control information to married women. However, the basic rationale of all family planning work in America— today as in 1916 when the first clinic opened its doors—is to promote the health and well-being of mothers and children by preventing unwanted births. Because of the threat which uncontrolled fertility poses, both to maternal health and to that of infants, it is generally accepted today that no community health program can be considered complete if it fails to provide ready access to birth-control devices and information.

Enhancement of maternal and child health through family planning is largely related to one of three basic parameters: 1) age of the mother, 2) interval between births, and 3) total number of births during a woman's reproductive lifetime. A brief examination of each of these factors reveals how uncontrolled fertility has a major impact on mortality and morbidity rates among both women and infants.

Age of Mother

Although the average woman is fertile from her early teens until her late 40s, the biologically optimum period for childbearing is much shorter, extending from approximately 20 to 30 years of age. In fact, research suggests that becoming pregnant is increasingly difficult as women approach middle age. The ability to conceive appears to peak at age 31 and declines steadily every year thereafter. From a safety standpoint, mothers either younger or older than this optimum age span run an increased risk of difficulties or death during pregnancy and childbirth, and their infants are statistically more likely to die than are babies of mothers in their 20s.

Teenage mothers, whose reproductive organs are not yet fully developed, are more likely to die during childbirth than are women in their prime reproductive years. In addition, babies of young mothers have a tendency to be born premature or underweight, factors which greatly increase their susceptibility to infectious diseases and malnutrition. Studies have revealed consistently higher infant mortality rates among babies born to mothers under age 20 as compared to those born to mothers in their late 20s.

Among women over 35, pregnancy poses an increased risk of complications during childbirth. Studies of pregnant women aged 44 and older reveal considerably higher rates of medical complications such as high blood pressure and diabetes compared to women in their 20s and 30s; women in the over-44 cohort also are much more likely than younger mothers to have a Caesarean delivery (Dulitzki et al., 1998). Mothers over 35 are more likely than younger women to bear a child with congenital disorders such as Down's Syndrome (however, a recent Canadian study of more than half a million births revealed no greater risk of nonchromosomal birth defects among babies born to older mothers than among infants whose mothers were younger). In addition to concerns regarding birth abnormalities, mothers in their 30s and 40s have reason to worry about the general health of their babies. Up to age 30, a pregnant woman has an 89% likelihood of delivering a healthy baby; this level of assurance diminishes by 3.5% for each additional year of maternal age (Baird, Sadnovnick, and Yee, 1991; van Noord-Zaadstra, 1991).

Interval Between Births

Short birth intervals have long been recognized as an important factor contributing to infant mortality. Studies conducted in rural India demonstrated that babies born less than two years after a previous birth were 50% more likely to die before their first birthday than were babies born after a birth interval of more than two years. Researchers working with the U.S. Agency for International Development in Bangladesh report that efforts to encourage women to space their pregnancies had a greater impact on reducing infant mortality than did childhood immunization campaigns or oral rehydration therapy.

For years public health workers assumed that short birth intervals were equally harmful to the health of the mother. A condition called "maternal depletion syndrome," characterized by premature aging, weakness, and anemia is frequently observed among undernourished women in poor societies, where teenage marriage is often followed by about 20 years of uninterrupted pregnancy. Anemic women may indeed be at heightened risk of dying during or soon after childbirth due to their lower tolerance for blood loss. If one pregnancy quickly follows another, the intervening period may be too short for an anemic woman to make up the blood loss experienced during the earlier birth, thus increasing her risk of death due to hemorrhage or childbed fever during the next delivery. However, a study conducted in Bangladesh could find no evidence to support general claims of a direct link between birth intervals of less than two years and enhanced risk of maternal mortality. Short birth intervals, without question, pose real concerns regarding survival prospects of the baby; however, contrary to popular belief, it cannot be demonstrated that having several babies close together increases a woman's own likelihood of dying during pregnancy or childbirth (Ronsmans and Campbell, 1998).

Total Number of Births

Contrary to the popular notion that mothers with large numbers of children give birth "as easy as rolling off a log," statistics reveal that such women are especially prone to problem pregnancies and death during childbirth. Indeed, the total number of babies born to a woman during her lifetime can have a significant impact on her general state of health.

Generally speaking, a woman's second and third births are the safest; the first birth carries slightly greater risk statistically because it will reveal any physical or genetic abnormalities in the parents that could cause problems. With the fourth pregnancy, risk of maternal death, stillbirth, and infant death begins to rise, increasing sharply with the birth of the fifth and every succeeding child. Health workers in Bangladesh report triple the number of deaths among women giving birth to their eighth child as among those bearing their third. Degree of risk depends to a considerable extent on the socioeconomic status of the mother, the greatest hazards being faced by women from the lowest income groups. However, even among well-fed, affluent women, every birth after the fourth involves an increased degree of danger for both mother and child.

Significantly higher rates of infant and child mortality among higher-order births in poor families seem to be due primarily to poor nutrition, as the limited amount of food available must be divided among many mouths. Unlike their older siblings, the latest born children must survive on reduced average portions during those early years when they are most susceptible to the effects of nutritional deficiency (Eckholm and Newland, 1977).

Thus a family-planning program that provides contraceptive protection for teenage women, women over 35, mothers who have already borne three or more children, and women who have recently given birth can make a very positive contribution to improving public health.

Contraceptive Safety

In assessing the health impact of family planning, one must of course take into account possible risks posed by contraceptive use. There has been considerable controversy in recent years regarding the safety of the birth-control pill and the intrauterine device (IUD), raising public concerns and causing potential contraceptors to turn to less reliable methods or to abandon attempts at birth control altogether. What indeed are the risks and benefits of the most commonly used contraceptives? A brief summary of the most popular methods used in the United States indicates that although various adverse side effects may accompany the use of contraceptives for some women, all common means of contraception entail fewer risks than do pregnancy and childbirth.

Hormonal Contraceptives

Such contraceptives are made of synthetic substances similar to the hormones that occur naturally in women's bodies. They prevent pregnancy by inhibiting ovulation.

Birth-Control Pill.   Among American women aged 15–44 currently practicing contraception, approximately 27% use "the Pill," making this the second-most popular method of birth control in the U.S., ranking just slightly below female sterilization. Available either as a combination pill (containing both estrogen and a progestin) or as a "mini-pill" containing progestin only, oral contraceptives, when used correctly, are 97–99% effective in preventing pregnancy. Since the early 1960s when the birth-control pill first became available, safety concerns centered around a possible increased risk of cardiovascular disorders such as blood clots, which could lead to a stroke or heart attack. For this reason medical authorities feel that a decision to use oral contraceptives should be made only after consultation with a health professional, and currently in all Western nations a doctor's prescription is required for the purchase of birth-control pills. Nevertheless, the results of extensive epidemiological research on oral contraceptive safety over nearly four decades of pill use indicate that women over 40 are the only group for whom pill use poses a greater health threat than does childbearing; among this group an increase in cardiovascular problems suggests the advisability of discontinuing pill use in favor of other contraceptive methods. However, for younger women, with the exception of those who smoke or have certain medical conditions (e.g. a history of blood clots, heart problems, cancer of the breast or female organs), medical evidence supports the view that the Pill is quite safe. Moreover, during the period they are taking contraceptive pills, users experience certain health benefits, including significant protection against ovarian and endometrial cancer, pelvic inflammatory disease, iron-deficiency anemia, and fibrocystic breast disease. In addition, women who use oral contraceptives have a lower risk of developing ovarian cysts. Persistent fears that women who use contraceptive pills might be at greater risk of developing cancer later in life were laid to rest in 1999 with the publication of results from a 25-year investigation of British women who had used oral contraceptives. The study convincingly demonstrated that ten years after they stopped taking contraceptive pills, the women experienced no higher risk of dying of cancer or stroke than did women who had never used oral contraceptives—good news for the 300 million women worldwide who have used the Pill at one time or another (Beral et al., 1999).

BOX 3-2

"Your Turn, Jack!"

For the past 40 years, contraceptive research has focused almost exclusively on female methods of birth control. In part this is due to the persistent assumption that men are reluctant to use a systemic method of contraception—and that women are reluctant to trust them to do so in a consistent, reliable manner! Pharmaceutical companies historically have shied away from developing contraceptive drugs that might diminish male libido and have preferred to concentrate on the female reproductive system, free from such worries. To some extent, limited research efforts into new approaches to male contraception reflect the reality that sperm production, continuing without interruption from puberty until death, is much more difficult to interrupt physiologically than is ovulation. Nevertheless, with approximately a third of all contracepting couples worldwide already utilizing male methods of birth control (vasectomy, condoms, and withdrawal), there is ample evidence that many men are willing to share the responsibility for avoiding unwanted births.

For the past several years, a top priority of the World Health Organization (WHO) has been to find an effective, acceptable, reversible, and preferably long-acting hormonal contraceptive for men. At long last, it appears that researchers may be on the brink of success. A spokesman for WHO's Human Reproductive Programme announced early in 1999 that, if all goes well, at least one hormonal male contraceptive could be available within 5–7 years.

Various forms of the male hormone testosterone comprise the experimental drugs receiving the most serious scrutiny. Several different testosterone compounds are now being tested (e.g. testosterone enanthate, testosterone undecanoate, testosterone buciclate), both with and without accompanying synthetic progestogens. These compounds appear able to block sperm production by disrupting normal hormonal stimulation of the testicles without reducing sex drive or adversely interfering with sexual performance. Various formulations of these drugs are also being investigated, including a daily pill, a once-every-three-months injection, and a subdermal implant that remains effective for one year. While it is assumed that most men would prefer long-lasting preparations, having an assortment of options available to suit individual needs and preferences is regarded as most desirable.

In terms of effectiveness, tests with testosterone enanthate in the early 1990s indicated that the hormone was at least as effective as the female contraceptive pill. Unfortunately, the fact that it had to be administered as a once-per-week injection diminished its user acceptability. Clinical trials on testosterone undecanoate, in the form of a two-month injection, are now underway in China and Indonesia; early results indicate no adverse side-effects in terms of sexual function. WHO is most optimistic, however, about the prospects for a testosterone buciclate-progestogen combination that will be administered as an every-three-months injection. Human testing is now underway for this product as well.

While most male contraceptive research currently focuses on hormonal methods, investigations also are proceeding on a natural chemical, triptolide, extracted from a Chinese medicinal herb. Recognition of the possible contraceptive value of the plant, *Tripterygium wilfordii*, came from chance observations that Chinese men who had been using the herb for two months or more to treat rheumatoid arthritis or psoriasis had become infertile. Investigations are now ongoing to determine the drug's mode of action.

Since many women, for one reason or another, experience problems with currently available methods of female birth control, there is an obvious need for long-lasting, effective male contraception as one more option in the "cafeteria approach" to the provision of family planning services. Experience in many countries has shown, time and again, that the greater the number of birth-control choices offered, the more couples are likely to become contraceptive acceptors. It appears that male hormonal contraception is an idea whose time has come.

Reference
Bonn, Dorothy. 1999. "Male Contraceptive Research Steps Back into Spotlight." *The Lancet 353*, no. 9149 (Jan. 23) :302.

Norplant. First approved for use in the United States in December, 1990, Norplant has been hailed as the most radical new form of birth control since the Pill—an extremely safe, nearly 100% effective contraceptive for women weighing less than 150 pounds. Consisting of six small progestin-containing capsules inserted by a health care professional just below the skin of the upper arm, Norplant continuously releases a small amount of contraceptive hormone into a woman's body over a five-year period, providing a consistently high level of protection without any further action on the part of the woman or her partner. A completely reversible method, Norplant begins providing protection within 24 hours after insertion; if at any time during the five-year period of use a woman decides she would like to have a baby, the capsules can be removed in a minor surgical procedure and fertility is immediately restored. Norplant has an excellent safety record, although during the first year after implantation some users experience minor side effects such as irregular menstrual bleeding, weight gain, acne, or rashes. In general, women whose medical condition precludes pill use should avoid Norplant also.

One problem that has emerged regarding Norplant is the difficulty some users encounter in having the implants removed, a process that requires a trained physician. In some cases, medical personnel lack the skill to perform the removal efficiently and painlessly. In other situations, care providers have refused to remove the implant when requested because of the cost or because the provider felt the woman involved should not be exposed to a possible pregnancy. Of the 56 countries where Norplant has now been approved for use, only in Indonesia are large numbers of women currently opting for this method, possibly because among traditional cultures in Bali and western Java it was considered beautiful for women to insert gold or silver needles under their skin. Although the percentage of American contraceptive users choosing Norplant remains quite low at just 1.3%, among those who choose the implant the vast majority report a high degree of satisfaction.

Depo-Provera. A relatively new birth-control option for American women, this injectable contraceptive was approved by the FDA in 1992 after more than 20 years of use in over 90 countries worldwide. Administered as an injection in the arm or buttocks every three months, Depo-Provera fills a need for women who want the reliability of hormonal contraceptives without having to worry about forgetting to take a daily pill. Depo-Provera is a synthetic form of progesterone that works by inhibiting ovulation, and it is 99% effective in preventing pregnancy. Worldwide, more than 30 million women have taken the drug since it was first introduced in 1969 and its overall safety record is good. Side effects among women receiving a Depo-Provera injection are similar to those experienced by Norplant recipients or users of the progestin-only "mini-pill"; in addition, about half the women who use Depo-Provera for a year or more experience amenorrhea (no menstrual period).

Surgical Sterilization

The most widely adopted method of family limitation in the United States, sterilization is a logical alternative for those who have already attained their desired family size. Currently, sterilization is the contraceptive method of choice for almost 39% of contracepting couples, with nearly 11% opting for sterilization of the male partner, 28% for the female procedure. Vasectomy, or male sterilization, is a simple operation involving an incision in the scrotum to cut or block the vas deferens (tubes which carry semen from the testes to the penis) and accounts for slightly more than a third of the sterilizations performed in the United States each year. Vasectomy most often is performed under local anesthesia in a doctor's office, the entire procedure generally taking less than 30 minutes. In rare cases minor postoperative infections may develop, but in general male sterilization is among the safest of all birth-control methods. Female sterilization, or tubal ligation, entails a slightly higher degree of risk since it involves sealing off the fallopian tubes—an operating room procedure done under general anesthesia. Although major complications are rare, they occur in an estimated 1.7% of cases. Sterilization, both male and female, is more than 99% effective in preventing pregnancy and ends any further expense, fuss, or bother related to contraceptive use. However, sterilization is a permanent method of birth control and such a decision should not be made lightly. Efforts to date at reopening the vas deferens or fallopian tubes have met with minimal success, so sterilization should be regarded as irreversible.

Intra-uterine Device (IUD)

Once among the most popular forms of contraception in the United States and still widely relied upon by women in other countries (particularly in China and Russia where it is the most common method of birth control), the IUD today is the method of choice for less than 1% of contracepting American women. Indeed, by the mid-1980s IUDs had nearly disappeared from the marketplace, withdrawn by manufacturers fearing legal liability for alleged harmful side effects of the device (a situation brought about by thousands of lawsuits against the A. H. Robins pharmaceutical firm, charging that the company's Dalkon Shield had caused numerous cases of bleeding, pelvic infections, and resultant infertility among users). Nevertheless, physicians and manufacturers consider most IUDs both safe and reliable. Currently two types of IUD are being marketed in the U.S.—the Paragard T 380 A, effective for 8–10 years, and Progestasert, a hormone-releasing IUD that must be replaced yearly. Among malnourished, anemic women IUD use has sometimes been correlated with increased blood loss during menstruation. For healthy, well-fed women, however, IUDs are as safe as the Pill and nearly as dependable. The major problem associated with IUD use is an increased risk of pelvic inflammatory disease (PID) which, if severe, can result in permanent infertility. IUDs are not recommended for women who have never been pregnant and in general are considered most suitable for young women in mutually monogamous relationships (PID incidence is highest among women with several sex partners) who want no more children but are not yet ready for an irreversible surgical sterilization.

Spermicides

Spermicidal foams, creams, suppositories, or gels must be inserted into the vagina within an hour before intercourse and must be replenished if intercourse is repeated. They act to form both a physical and chemical barrier to sperm and are available without a prescription. While few problems are associated with spermicides (those who experience a burning sensation or irritation should avoid them), their effectiveness when used alone is only 70–80%.

Barrier Methods

Barrier methods employ some device that prevents the egg and sperm from uniting, thus preventing fertilization.

Vaginal Contraceptives. Diaphragms, cervical caps, sponges, and the recently introduced female condom all work by keeping egg and sperm apart. (The polyurethane female condom is also intended to provide some protection against sexually transmitted disease, but medical authorities caution that for best protection, male latex condoms are preferable.) When used with spermicides, vaginal contraceptives have few, if any, adverse effects and are moderately effective at preventing pregnancy. Both the sponge and the female condom have an estimated failure rate of about 1 in 4; the cervical cap and diaphragm are somewhat more trustworthy, with failure rates ranging from 6% for a diaphragm used with spermicide to 18% for the cervical cap.

Condoms. Like the vaginal contraceptives, condoms cause no adverse health effects other than an occasional allergic reaction to rubber among some individuals. Used alone, their reliability is significantly less than pills or IUDs, but in combination with vaginal contraceptives and in situations where legal, early abortion is available, they offer the safest means, other than sterilization, of totally effective fertility control. The third most commonly used contraceptive method in the United States today, the condom is being actively promoted by health agencies not only for birth-control reasons but also as an

Table 3-1   Birth Control Guide

Efficacy rates given in this chart are estimates based on a number of different studies. They should be understood as yearly estimates, with those dependent on conscientious use subject to a greater chance of human error and reduced effectiveness. For comparison, 60 to 85 percent of sexually active women using no contraception would be expected to become pregnant in a year.

Type	Estimated Effectivenes	Risks	STD Protection	Convenience	Availability
Male Condom	About 85%	Rarely, irritation and allergic reactions	Latex condoms help protect against sexually transmitted diseases, including herpes and AIDS	Applied immediately before intercourse	Nonprescription
Female Condom	An estimated 74–79%	Rarely, irritation and allergic reactions	May give some protection against sexually transmitted diseases, including herpes and AIDS; not as effective as male latex condom	Applied immediately before intercourse; used only once and discarded	Nonprescription
Spermicides Used Alone	70–80%	Rarely, irritation and allergic reactions	Unknown	Applied no more than one hour before intercourse	Nonprescription
Sponge	72–82%	Rarely, irritation and allergic reactions; difficulty in removal; very rarely, toxic shock syndrome	None	Can be inserted hours before intercourse and left in place up to 24 hours; used only once and discarded	Nonprescription
Diaphragm with Spermicide	82–94%	Rarely, irritation and allergic reactions; bladder infection; very rarely, toxic shock syndrome	None	Inserted before intercourse; can be left in place 24 hours, but additional spermicide must be inserted if intercourse is repeated	Rx
Cervical Cap with Spermicide	At least 82%	Abnormal Pap test; vaginal or cervical infections; very rarely, toxic shock syndrome	None	Can remain in place for 48 hours, not necessary to re-apply spermicide upon repeated intercourse; may be difficult to insert	Rx

Source: *FDA Consumer,* September 1993.

Type	Estimated Effectivenes	Risks	STD Protection	Convenience	Availability
Pills	97%–99%	Blood clots, heart attacks and strokes, gall-bladder disease, liver tumors, water retention, hypertension, mood changes, dizziness and nausea; not for smokers	None	Pill must be taken on daily schedule, regardless of the frequency of intercourse	Rx
Implant (Norplant)	99%	Menstrual cycle irregularity; headaches, nervousness, depression, nausea, dizziness, change of appetite, breast tenderness, weight gain, enlargement of ovaries and/or fallopian tubes, excessive growth of body and facial hair; may subside after first year	None	Effective 24 hours after implantation for approximately 5 years; can be removed by physician at any time	Rx; minor outpatient surgical procedure
Injection (Depo-Provera)	99%	Amenorrhea, weight gain, and other side effects similar to those with Norplant	None	One injection every three months	Rx
IUD	95–96%	Cramps, bleeding, pelvic inflammatory disease, infertility; rarely, perforation of the uterus	None	After insertion, stays in place until physician removes it	Rx
Periodic Abstinence (NFP)	Very variable, perhaps 53–86%	None	None	Requires frequent monitoring of body functions and periods of abstinence	Instructions from physician or clinic
Surgical Sterilization	Over 99%	Pain, infection, and, for female tubal ligation, possible surgical complications	None	Vasectomy is a one-time procedure usually performed in a doctor's office; tubal ligation is a one-time procedure performed in an operating room	Surgery

effective prophylactic against the spread of AIDS and other sexually transmitted diseases.

Natural Family Planning

Frequently referred to as the "rhythm method" or "periodic abstinence," this approach to birth control carries no health risk but has a consistently high failure rate. To utilize this method, a woman attempts to determine when she is ovulating by charting daily bodily functions such as basal temperature (i.e. temperature when the body is at its lowest level of metabolic activity, usually measured before getting out of bed in the morning) and by examining her cervical mucus. The problem is that many women experience monthly variations in their menstrual cycle, making accurate calculation of the fertile period problematic. In addition, the abstinence from sexual activity during fertile periods which must be rigorously observed by couples using natural family planning requires a high degree of motivation and cooperation between partners and can significantly limit the number of days each month when couples can have intercourse free from fear of unwanted pregnancy.

The success of the family planning movement in the United States is evident from surveys which reveal that among sexually active women at risk of an unwanted pregnancy, fully 95% are using some method of birth control. In an age when sexual activity seems to be as popular a pastime as it ever was, an even more convincing indicator of contraceptive usage is the fact that the average number of children per U.S. couple is now just two, one of the lowest figures in our history. Apparently most Americans now agree with the family planning sloganeers who affirm that "A small family is a happy family" (Piccinino and Mosher, 1998).

Family Planning in the Third World

Whereas the birth-control movement in the United States and Europe grew out of the conviction that health and social considerations demanded that women receive help in regulating their fertility, the impetus for family planning in most Third World countries grew directly out of concerns over the high rates of post-World War II population growth and the awareness that this "population explosion" would impede their rate of economic development. Only after family-planning programs had been launched did Third World governments attempt to justify their support for such efforts on the basis of protecting maternal and child health and of guaranteeing couples the means for regulating the spacing and number of their children. This superficial shift in emphasis constituted a publicly acceptable rationale for reconciling the interests of the nation with those of individuals.

In most cases, the initial promoters of family planning in the Third World were private organizations such as International Planned Parenthood Federation, the Ford and Rockefeller Foundations, and the Population Council. By the 1960s, however, even earlier in some countries, national governments were becoming increasingly active in establishing their own family-planning programs, usually in conjunction with their ministries of health.

Generally they were assisted by the private organizations mentioned and, in later years, by the U.S. Agency for International Development and such United Nations agencies as the World Bank and the U.N. Fund for Population Activities (UNFPA). Funds, both governmental and private, allocated for family-planning work increased sharply after the mid-1960s, but even today constitute a very small percentage of most national budgets. Today the vast majority of developing countries have some sort of family-planning program in operation. How effective those programs are in reducing national birth rates will in large part determine the success of such countries in raising living standards and ensuring a bright future for their people.

Spreading the Word

Since the main impetus for implementing family planning came from central governments or outside agencies rather than reflecting grassroots interest, as was the case in North America and Europe, success required intensive efforts to reach all elements of society, the majority of whom lived at subsistence level in rural areas, often isolated from adequate medical care and frequently illiterate. Such people had to be made aware of the existence of fertility-regulating methods, provided with regular access to the same, and convinced that it was in their own best interest to use them.

In pursuing this goal, family-planning workers in Third World countries adopted methods radically different from those used in Western nations. Mobile units in the form of specially equipped vans or buses have been essential in carrying health workers and equipment into villages far from any hospital. Trained field workers actively attempt to recruit contraceptive acceptors, meeting with women's groups, farmers, and so on, to persuade them of the advantages inherent in limiting family size. Considerable reliance has been placed on mass media communications. Advertisements in newspapers, on radio, and in cinemas regularly stress the benefits of small families while roadside billboards or posters on buses, in train stations—even painted on the hides of farm animals—proclaim such messages as "Two or Three—Enough!" Some governments have attracted participation by offering gifts to contraceptive acceptors. In India thousands of men agreed to vasectomies in order to receive a free transistor radio; in Thailand the government has sponsored free distribution of condoms at sporting events or all-expense paid tours of Bangkok's temples for rural men agreeing to sterilization!

Most Third World programs, like those in the West, offer a choice of birth-control methods and generally include information on child-spacing, nutrition, and child-care along with contraceptive services. Some also enlist the services of midwives, teachers, or other respected community leaders to act as distributors of contraceptives, particularly pills and condoms, thereby giving these influential individuals a vested interest in the success of such programs.

Motivation—The Key to Success

Efforts to reduce birth rates in developing nations have met with mixed results, though general trends have been encouraging. With the exception of

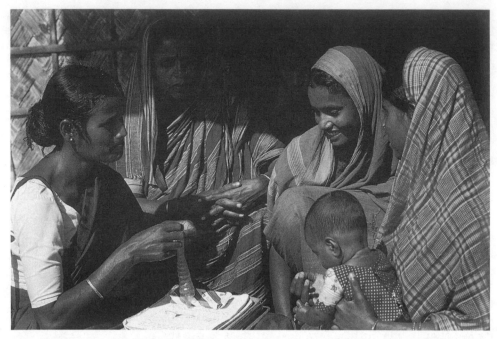

A community health worker in Bangladesh demonstrates condom use to local women. Such workers also provide child nutrition and family planning advice. *[Mark Edwards/Still Pictures]*

the countries of sub-Saharan Africa, where fertility remains at traditionally high levels (a current average of 6 children per mother), birth rates have declined significantly in recent decades. Today in the developing nations as a whole, average family size is 3–4 children and more than 50% of all married couples employ some form of contraception. A number of surveys conducted over the past 25 years have shown that the vast majority of women in the developing world are aware of the existence of at least one modern method of contraception. Nevertheless, a sizable proportion of these women—including many who told interviewers they wanted no more children—were, for one reason or another, not practicing contraception. To some extent, failure to use contraceptives is related to easy access; not surprisingly, contraceptive use was higher in communities where a family-planning clinic or other source of contraceptive supplies was close by—a particularly important factor among people using either pills or condoms. A far more important determinant in contraceptive practice, however, is motivation—the desire of couples to limit family size. In many parts of the developing world economic and social factors interact to perpetuate the traditional attitudes toward childbearing. For very practical reasons, many Third World couples have concluded that although two or three children per family might be in the best interest of society, they want and feel they need a significantly larger number themselves. In the absence of coercion, when individual and societal needs conflict, personal desires generally prevail.

Factors contributing to this continued preference for large families among many Third World couples include high infant mortality rates, the

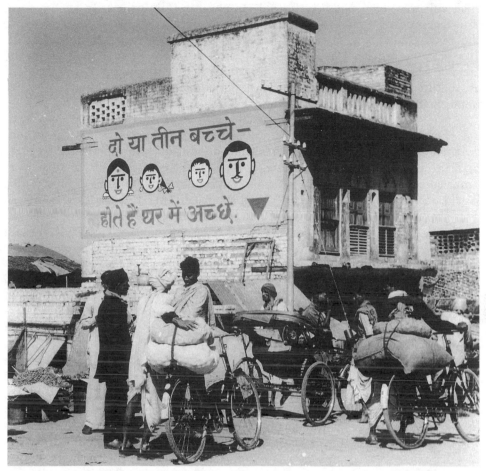

Wall paintings and billboards throughout India carry the family-planning message. This sign with the symbolic family of four bears the slogan, "Two are enough!" *[Agency for International Development]*

view of children as "social security," the desire for sons, and the low educational and economic status of women.

High Infant Mortality Rates. Although the drop in infant and child death rates was a major factor in fueling the explosive growth of Third World populations, such rates are still substantially above the levels prevailing in developed countries. In many parts of Africa, for example, infant death rates are over 100, compared to 7 in the United States and 3.8 in Japan. At the personal level, surveys have found that wherever childhood deaths are common, it is extremely difficult to convince parents to limit themselves to two births. For this reason, sharply lowering infant and child mortality rates is regarded as one of the key components in any population control program.

Children as "Social Security." In most Third World countries, lack of extensive social welfare programs means that most parents are dependent on their grown children for financial support in their post-retirement years. In such cultures, responsibility for elderly parents falls primarily on the sons; thus a couple may feel the need to produce at least two or three boys to ensure their being adequately provided for in old age. In addition, even young children may be regarded as financial assets, since their labor is needed on the farm or around the home. In such situations an additional baby is not viewed as another mouth to feed but rather as an additional pair of hands to gather wood, tend livestock, haul water, and so forth. (Dasgupta, 1995).

Desire for Sons. Many family-planning program administrators fear that the preference for sons rather than daughters will keep fertility rates high in many developing countries. Son preference is apparent in surveys of American couples but is even more pronounced among parents in most Third World nations. In such cultures, doubt about whether they will have enough boys concerns parents who are asked to produce no more than two or three offspring. A woman's status, even the stability of her marriage, is dependent on her having sons. To some extent, such preferences are based on economic concerns: sons can support parents in old age while daughters are a financial liability, often requiring an expensive dowry at time of marriage. A fertility preference study conducted in Nepal found that although more than 80% of the couples surveyed named two to three children as the ideal family size, a substantial majority of both husbands and wives would opt for one extra child in order to achieve their preferred number of sons; almost half of the husbands and a third of the wives indicated their willingness to have more than twice the number of children they really wanted in order to attain the desired number of sons (two was the most commonly designated number of boys wanted). While over two-thirds of the couples questioned said they'd like to have one daughter, none had any desire to go beyond their stated ideal family size if the first two children were boys (Mahler, 1997).

The bias in favor of sons has taken a tragic twist in recent years, with a noticeable rise in female infanticide in several countries. After promulgation of the one-child policy in China—where the age-old view that "more sons mean more happiness" still prevails—numerous cases were reported of newborn girls being murdered by parents who hoped that a second try would produce a boy. More recently, parents' efforts to ensure the birth of male offspring have been given a major boost by the advent of a modern device whose impact is revolutionizing Asian societies—the ultrasound scanner. In Korea, China, India—indeed throughout Asia—ultrasound and other medical technologies like amniocentesis are being used not to detect developmental abnormalities but to learn the sex of the fetus. And if it's a girl, women often opt for abortion. By the early 1990s, more than 100,000 ultrasound scanners were in use in China; even illiterate peasants in remote villages are now aware of the existence of machines that can tell the sex of an unborn child. In India, the widespread practice of aborting female fetuses led authorities in Bombay to prohibit prenatal tests for women under age 35 unless they had a family history of birth defects (an earlier survey conducted in that city's hospitals revealed that of 8,000 abortions performed, all but one were of female fetuses). While the use of medical procedures for sex selection has generated sharp criticism among some commentators in India, others defend the practice on the grounds that it is preferable for a woman to have abortions rather than produce six or seven children in hopes of having one or two boys. Citing the abuse often directed at Indian wives who bear too many daughters, one physician defended the practice of sex selection as a "lesser evil," declaring that "it is better to have feticide than matricide." Ironically, with the exception of a few vague warnings in the official press about future "bachelor villages" where wives will be a scarce commodity, few Asian parents today seem concerned about the social consequences of a population where young women are vastly outnumbered by young men. While some government officials recognize the problem and are trying to curtail use of ultrasound scanners, the devices are now so widespread, corruption so rampant, and the desire for sons so strong that curbing the abuse of medical technology is likely to prove impossible (Riley, 1997; Kristof, 1993).

Low Educational and Economic Status of Women Birth rates today are highest in those parts of the world where women have little schooling and where opportunities for paid employment outside the home are few. In such societies, a woman's worth is measured in terms of her childbearing abilities. Such women, striving to maintain favor with their husbands and in-laws, are unlikely to respond favorably to the idea of family limitation. In addition, illiterate women or women with only an elementary education are less likely than their better educated sisters to have heard about modern contraceptive techniques or to know how to use them. Surveys indicate that providing women with at least a secondary school education is one of the most effective ways of reducing the birth rate in developing countries. In general, fertility drops noticeably as the level of female education increases, primarily because educated women tend to marry later, have greater opportunity for

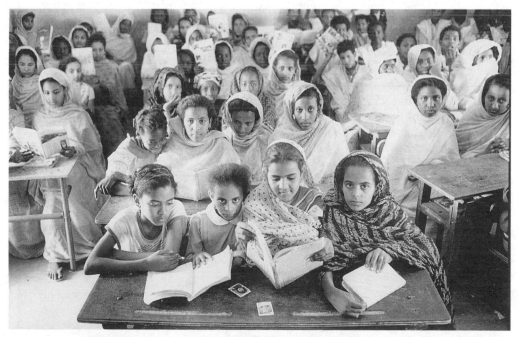

Providing young women with at least a secondary school education is one of the most effective ways of reducing birth rates in developing countries. *[Jorgen Schytte/Still Pictures]*

BOX 3-3

The Elusive Quest for ZPG:
India's Family-Planning Program

According to the *Guiness Book of World Records*, the most common family name on the face of the planet is Chang—not particularly surprising since every fifth person in the world today is Chinese. However, a generation or so hence the Changs may cede their preeminence to the **Patels** or **Singhs** or **Mehtas** as India overtakes China as the world's most populous nation. Indeed, with an annual growth rate hovering around 2% and with 36% of its people still in their pre-reproductive years, India could well surpass the two billion mark before population growth halts.

India's continued rapid pace of growth is ironic since it was one of the first countries in the world to concede that high rates of population increase were hindering national development. Soon after independence from colonial rule in 1947, the Indian government adopted an official policy goal of lowering fertility rates to replacement level in order to achieve a stable population size. At that time India's population was under 400 million, increasing by about 7 million a year. By the late 1990s, the annual increment of growth approximated 18 million, with total population size reaching one billion by the year 2000. How is it that after more than 50 years of trying to stabilize growth, Indian leaders see their country poised to become the world's demographic superpower? A look at the strengths and weaknesses of the Indian family-planning program illustrates the challenges inherent in an effort to bring about behavioral change in a traditional Third World society.

Although officially launched in 1951, India's family-planning program got off to a slow and unimpressive start. Vastly underfunded during its early years, the new program was confined to providing services at urban clinics and relied exclusively on the promotion of periodic abstinence (rhythm method)—an unreliable form of birth control and particularly inappropriate in a culture where high levels of illiteracy rendered the concept of "safe" and "unsafe" periods mysterious indeed. The government's efforts floundered along, making little headway and receiving only perfunctory attention from national leaders until the results of the 1961 census revealed an unexpected surge in the population growth rate from a relatively moderate 1.5% during the 1940s to almost 2% during the 1950s. Alarmed, national leaders expanded program activities into the previously unserved rural areas where three-fourths of India's people live. They also initiated a mass media effort, employing catchy slogans and billboard advertising to promote the small family ideal. Throughout the 1960s, IUD insertions were the focus of government family-planning efforts. Unfortunately, widespread reports of complications (not uncommon among anemic or malnourished women) and lack of adequate follow-up care led to a sharp decline in IUD acceptance by the end of the decade.

When the 1971 census results revealed still-rising rates of population growth, the government responded with additional measures, prohibiting the marriage of girls under 18 (a law that has been nearly impossible to enforce) and enacting one of the Third World's most liberal abortion laws (interestingly, there has been virtually no public controversy in India over the issue of legalized abortion; however, the practice is not very common).

With the failure of the IUD effort, family-planning strategies shifted to an emphasis on male sterilization. Prizes or cash awards were offered to men who agreed to undergo vasectomy, and early statistics appeared impressive. However, a closer look at sterilization figures revealed that a significant percentage of vasectomy clients were men whose wives were in their forties or older—well beyond their prime reproductive years. In 1975 the vasectomy campaign took a fateful (and fatal) turn when the powerful and politically ambitious son of then-Prime Minister Indira Gandhi decided to espouse population control as a high-priority personal commitment. During a two-year period of emergency rule, when usual democratic procedures were suspended, lower-level officials attempted to curry favor with Gandhi by harassing and sometimes coercing thousands of men to submit to vasectomy in an effort to achieve regional sterilization quotas. During these months male government employees frequently were denied promotions, desired transfers, food ration cards, and various other benefits unless they could produce a vasectomy certificate. Rumors spread of men being rounded up in railway stations and forcibly sterilized. In some rural areas, wary villagers slept in their fields at night, fearing police raids during which all men captured would be vasectomized. Some Indian states at this time seriously debated legislation that would have made sterilization mandatory for any couple with three or more children. From 1976-1977 the number of men with vasectomies jumped from 2.7 million to 8.3 million, but at the grassroots level opposition to the campaign of forced sterilization was mounting, occasionally erupting into riots and demonstrations. When general elections were held in 1977, the Gandhi government was decisively defeated, largely as a result of public anger at the excesses committed in the name of family planning.

The debacle of the coerced sterilization effort represented a devastating setback to India's family-planning program; contraceptive usage plunged to less than 6% of Indian couples following the demise of the Gandhi administration. For years afterwards, government officials for the most part distanced themselves from any active association with birth-control efforts, seldom going further than to support maternal and child health services. In a semantic break with the past, the name of the program was changed in the 1980s to "family welfare program," and in yet another about-face, the contraceptive emphasis shifted from male to *female* sterilization. In fact, currently 9 out of every 10 sterilizations performed in India is a tubectomy.

From the early 1980s to the present, government support and funding for population control programs has waxed and waned, depending on the administration in power. Although some progress has been made in raising the percentage of married women using contraception to approximately 41% in the late 1990s (but only to 16% among the highest fertility age cohort, women between 15-29), the program nevertheless is characterized by several glaring weaknesses that must be resolved if national goals are ever to be attained.

Overreliance on sterilization as the chief means of limiting fertility is the main reason for the program's negative public image; fully 75% of all contracepting couples rely on sterilization. Family-planning workers spend an inordinate amount of time recruiting clients in order to meet sterilization targets set by the central bureaucracy, and the fact that they receive a cash bonus for each client recruited provides temptation for abuse.

The near-absence of alternative reversible contraceptive options essentially means that the needs of young couples who would like to postpone childbearing or to space intended births are largely neglected. While in theory the government program provides four contraceptive choices—sterilization, IUDs, condoms, and pills—in fact only sterilization and IUDs have been routinely available throughout the country. Birth-control pills and condoms can be readily obtained in urban areas but are difficult to find in many rural regions.

Another serious deterrent to public acceptance of family-planning services is the widespread perception that clinic staff are discourteous to clients and unwilling to provide follow-up care to the patients they so eagerly recruit for sterilization. At some clinics, women giving birth to a second or subsequent child report considerable pressure to agree to sterilization before returning home; in a few cases, new mothers have had IUDs inserted without their knowledge or consent. While the quality of health care providers in India is generally quite high, many rural clinics are staffed by inexperienced doctors fresh out of medical school, most of whom received minimal training in family planning or public health. Physicians' lack of knowledge regarding correct use and possible side effects of reversible birth-control methods, particularly the contraceptive pill and new hormonal implants and injectables, is a major deterrent to increasing contraceptive use.

The virtual absence of an effective public education effort geared to the special informational needs of a semiliterate or illiterate audience is another weakness of the program. Although mass media advertising has created nationwide awareness of the concept of family limitation, there is an enormous unmet need for educational materials on specific contraceptive methods and for trained workers who can convey such information in language clients can understand.

Finally, perhaps the most essential element in achieving India's population goals is improving the status of Indian women. By expanding girls' access to education (only 39% of females in India are literate, compared to 64% of males), supporting programs to encourage later marriage, and increasing opportunities for female employment, the government could help to create a cultural climate conducive to fertility reduction. Evidence that such a transition is possible even in the absence of marked economic development can be seen in the case of Kerala, a state at the southwestern tip of India where 93% of women are literate, contraception is practiced by 80% of couples, and the two-child family is the norm. It will require a major restructuring of India's family-planning program and a major commitment of additional funding to extend the fertility reduction achievements of Kerala to the rest of the country. However, given the mounting social and environmental pressures posed by the demographic nightmare, India's leaders have no choice but to redouble their efforts to reach the stabilization goal proclaimed a half century ago.

References

Conly, Shanti R., and Sharon L. Camp. 1992. *India's Family-Planning Challenge: From Rhetoric to Action*. Country Study Series #2, The Population Crisis Committee.

Tobias, Michael. 1998. *World War III: Population and the Biosphere at the End of the Millennium*. Continuum Press.

employment outside the home, are more aware of the advantages of smaller family size, and understand how to practice contraception more effectively. The mother's education level is even more strongly correlated with improved childhood health and nutritional status. Women who have primary schooling or higher are much less likely to see their children die than are women who never attended school; children whose mothers completed high school or college are much less likely to be underweight or short for their age in comparison with children whose mothers are less educated (Riley, 1997).

Such factors support the contention of many demographers that broad-based social and economic changes must precede or accompany population programs in developing nations if population growth is ever to be stabilized; simply making contraceptives more widely available will not be enough to overcome traditional biases that favor large families.

Population Policy: Moving Beyond Birth Control

Since the inception of both private and government-sponsored family planning programs in the 1950s and 1960s, efforts have focused on increasing the availability of contraceptives while simultaneously trying to encourage their use. Numerous surveys conducted in many countries during these years demonstrated that many women were continuing to have more children than they desired, often because of misperceptions about the health effects of certain contraceptives, excessive cost of obtaining supplies, insufficient choice of contraceptive methods, or other problems related to access. Building new clinics and expanding social outreach programs seemed like the most straightforward approach to dealing with a problem that government leaders were beginning to view as increasingly urgent. By the 1980s, public opinion in many developing countries was supportive toward stabilizing growth rates and many Third World governments had begun implementing vigorous efforts to increase the percentage of couples practicing contraception. A declaration by delegates to the United Nations-sponsored International Conference on Population, held in Mexico City in 1984, for governments to make family planning services "universally available" was hailed as a significant achievement by population control advocates.

During those same years, however, feminists and others concerned about women's health issues and civil rights were growing increasingly critical of national programs' single-minded focus on distributing contraceptives, often with no follow-up and apparently with little concern for the welfare of the women they were recruiting as contraceptive acceptors. Particularly in Asian countries (India and China being notable examples), family planning programs were target-driven, with administrators' job security based on how many IUDs their staffs inserted within a month or how many sterilizations they performed. Such quota systems inevitably lead to violations of patients' rights—sometimes to outright coercion—and critics charged that the emphasis on numerical goals diminished the quality of services provided.

In 1994 when the United Nations convened its third decennial international population conference in Cairo, Egypt, a grassroots insistence that contraceptives alone are not the answer to the world's population dilemma persuaded planners of the need for a radical change in focus. Reflecting the new emphasis, the name of the event itself was changed to the International Conference on Population and Development (ICPD), highlighting the conviction of those attending that only in conjunction with broad-based development initiatives to improve health, reduce poverty, and improve the status of women could fertility rates be reduced further. Attracting delegates from 180 different countries, as well as representatives of 1,200 nongovernmental organizations, many of them women's advocacy groups, the Cairo conference was the most comprehensive international meeting ever held on the population issue. While agreeing that both family planning *and* economic development are essential for reducing population growth rates, delegates for the first time acknowledged that empowerment of women will be a crucial factor in stabilizing world population size. Moving away from the past emphasis on people-counting and birth control, the Programme of Action coming out of Cairo was based on the premise that population programs should focus on individual needs, not on numerical targets. Endorsed by all but a few of the 180 national delegations participating, the Programme of Action lists fully 243 goals to be achieved by 2015. Among the most important are the following:

1. To provide universal access to a full range of safe and reliable family-planning methods and related reproductive health services.

2. To reduce infant mortality rates to below 35 per 1,000 live births and child mortality rates (i.e. deaths of children under age 5) below 45.

3. To achieve a maternal mortality rate below 60 deaths per 100,000 live births.

4. To increase life expectancy at birth to more than 75 years (or to more than 70 in the countries currently experiencing high mortality rates).

5. To achieve universal access to and completion of primary education; ensure the widest and earliest possible access by girls and women to secondary and higher levels of education.

To carry out this ambitious program will require a sustained commitment by national governments, as well as many billions of dollars to implement the called-for reproductive health programs. Achievement of the designated goals is also incumbent on wrenching changes in lifestyle and cultural norms in societies reluctant to alter age-old traditions regarding gender roles (Ashford, 1995). Whether the promise of Cairo will be realized in an era of dwindling development dollars, when women's opportunities remain severely constrained in many countries, and at a time when the developing world is beset by pressing economic problems remains to be seen.

References

Ashford, Lori S. 1995. "New Perspectives on Population: Lessons from Cairo." *Population Bulletin* 50, no. 1 (March).

Baird, P. A., A. D. Sadovnick, and I. M. L. Yee. 1991. "Maternal Age and Birth Defects: A Population Study." *Lancet* 337:527.

Beral, Valerie, Carol Hermon, Clifford Kay, Philip Hannaford, Sarah Darby, and Gillian Reeves. 1999. "Mortality Associated With Oral Contraceptive Use: 25-Year Follow up of Cohort of 46,000 Women From Royal College Of General Practitioners' Oral Contraceptive Study." *British Medical Journal* 318, no. 7176 (Jan. 9): 96–100.

Dasgupta, Partha S. 1995. "Population, Poverty, and the Local Environment." *Scientific American* 272, no. 2 (Feb) 40–45.

Dulitzki, M., D. Soriano, E. Schiff, A. Chetrit, S. Mashiach, and D. S. Seidman. 1998. "Effect of Very Advanced Maternal Age on Pregnancy Outcome and Rate of Cesarean Delivery." *Obstetrics and Gynecology* 92, no. 6 (Dec): 935–939.

Eckholm, Erik, and Kathleen Newland. 1977. "Health: The Family Planning Factor." *Worldwatch Paper* 10, Worldwatch Institute.

Kleinman, R. L., and P. Senanayake. 1984. *Breastfeeding, Fertility, and Contraception.* IPPF Medical Publications.

Kristof, Nicholas D. 1993. "Peasants in China Discover New Way to Weed Out Girls." *New York Times,* July 21.

League of Women Voters Education Fund. 1982. *Public Policy on Reproductive Choice.* No. 286 (July).

Mahler, K. 1997. "Strong Son Preference Among Nepalese Couples May Outweigh Their Desire For Smaller Families." *International Family Planning Perspectives* 23, no. 1 (March).

McLaren, Angus A. 1990. *A History of Contraception.* Basil Blackwell, Ltd.

Piccinino, Linda J., and William D. Mosher. 1998. "Trends in Contraceptive Use in the United States: 1982-1995." *Family Planning Perspectives* 30, no. 1 (Jan/Feb): 4–10.

Riddle, John M. 1992. *Contraception and Abortion from the Ancient World to the Renaissance.* Harvard University Press.

Riley, Nancy E. 1997. "Gender, Power, and Population Change." *Population Bulletin* 52, no. 1 (May).

Rogow, Deborah, and Sonya Horowitz. 1995. "Withdrawal: A Review of the Literature and an Agenda for Research." *Studies in Family Planning* 26, no. 3 (May/June): 140–150.

Ronsmans, Carine, and Oona Campbell. 1998. "Short Birth Intervals Don't Kill Women: Evidence from Matlab, Bangladesh." *Studies in Family Planning* 29, no. 3 (Sept):282–290.

Stokes, Bruce. 1980. "Men and Family Planning." *Worldwatch Paper* 41. Worldwatch Institute.

Van Noord-Zaadstra, B. M. et al. 1991. "Delaying Childbearing: Effect of Age on Fecundity and Outcome of Pregnancy." *British Medical Journal* 302:1361.

Weiss, Peter. 1993. "The Contraceptive Potential of Breastfeeding in Bangladesh." *Studies in Family Planning* 24, no. 2 (March/April).

CHAPTER 4

The People-Food Predicament

Famine seems to be the last, the most dreadful resource of nature. The power of population is so superior to the power in the earth to produce subsistence for man, that premature death must in some shape or other visit the human race.

—Thomas Malthus
"An Essay on the Principal of Population" (1798)

The fierce debate sparked by Malthus' gloomy pronouncements over two centuries ago continues to reverberate today as policymakers and scientists argue about the planet's ability to meet the nutritional needs of additional billions of people in the decades ahead. Viewpoints vary widely, with many experts expressing cautious optimism that improvements in agricultural technology, coupled with declining birth rates, guarantee that future generations will be adequately fed. Other less sanguine observers insist that current trends are already seriously undermining the long-term sustainability of world agriculture and fisheries while simultaneously increasing the number of mouths to be fed.

The wide divergence in outlook stems from personal assumptions regarding future trends in human fertility, world economic growth, environmental degradation, and agricultural productivity—assumptions that may ultimately prove correct or radically off-base. Until relatively recently, remarkable gains in agricultural productivity worldwide provided ample grounds for optimism that one day in the not-too-distant future, no child would go to bed hungry nor any family worry about the next day's meal. From 1950 until 1984 the world's farmers were successful in producing increased quantities of food more rapidly than the world's parents were producing babies. During this period world grain consumption per person increased by 38% in spite of spiraling population figures, resulting in impressive nutritional gains in many formerly food-short regions of the world. Global trends were somewhat misleading, however, since the world food production averages to a large extent reflected an enormous and disproportionate increase in North American crop yields during those years. These figures masked grimmer statistics showing that in many of the rapidly growing developing nations, per capita increase in food production had halted by the late 1950s due to high rates of population increase. Until the mid-1980s, global averages continued to convey the impression that all was rosy on the food front. Throughout this period, world grain harvests increased by almost 3% annually (compared with a world population growth rate at this time of about 2%). During the 1970s the resource-intensive technologies of the Green Revolution resulted in a major boost in Third World agricultural production; by the early 1980s news of huge crop surpluses dominated the farm pages of newspapers and laments of a worldwide "grain glut" were heard from Chicago to Melbourne. Even Western Europe, reliant on food imports for the past 200 years, became a grain exporter during those golden years.

By the mid-1980s, however, some worrisome trends were becoming evident. After nearly 40 years of steady growth in world food output, a significant slowdown became apparent in many of the world's most populous countries. In India, grain production has been stagnant since 1983—at a time when India's population continues to increase by 18 million yearly; in China, agricultural output has dropped since 1984's peak harvest; Indonesia and Mexico have witnessed a leveling off of their production, while in Japan, Taiwan, and South Korea grain output has been declining for years. In contrast to the 3% annual increases in grain harvests that characterized the period between 1950 and 1984, during the 1990s world grain output grew by just 1% a year—while world population figures continued to climb at a 1.4% annual rate. This gap between grain production and people production means that food availability *per capita* has actually declined in recent years. In 1997, for example, world grain harvests hit a record high of 1,881 million tons. However, if this amount were evenly distributed among all the world's people, it would amount to 322 kilograms per person—fully 6% less than the all-time high of 342 kilograms represented by the 1984 harvest when global population had not yet reached 5 billion.

Of course, livestock production and fisheries also contribute significantly to human diets. Mirroring the per capita increase in grain harvests, production of beef and mutton tripled between 1950 and 1990; since then, a lowering of rangeland productivity due to overgrazing has resulted in a leveling off in production, with future increases unlikely unless more feed grains are diverted to livestock. Meat production overall continued to grow by more than 2% annually in the late 1990s, thanks largely to big increases in poultry production, as well as to a continued expansion in the market for pork, the world's most popular red meat. Growth in world fisheries, which witnessed a near-quintupling of the annual catch between the early 1950s and the early 1990s, now appears to be at or near its maximum sustainable yield; many stocks of preferred table fish species have already been fished to commercial extinction and marine biologists fear we may have already exceeded the carrying capacity of the world's oceans (Brown et al., 1999, 1998).

While many national leaders tend to blame adverse weather conditions for food shortfalls, the true causes are more complex: loss of good cropland to erosion and nonfarm uses, inefficient agrarian structures, lack of investment in agriculture by city-oriented government officials, cutbacks in agricultural research, and *too many people*.

Factors Influencing Food Demand

While it is obvious that the total yield of the world's croplands, pasture-lands, and fisheries constitutes the world's food *supply*, assessing food *demand* is slightly more complicated. **Population growth,** not surprisingly, is the single largest factor in determining food demand. Since 95% of the world's population increase is occurring in the countries of Asia, Africa, and Latin America, food supply problems currently are most acute in these regions. An additional factor must be considered in assessing food demand, however. **Rising personal incomes** that have characterized the economic development of most industrialized countries since the Second World War have greatly added to world food demand. This is not because the typical American, Swede, or Japanese eats tremendously greater quantities than the average Peruvian, Pakistani, or Sudanese, but because higher incomes gener-ally translate into an increased demand for high-quality foods, particularly meat and dairy products. As you will recall from our discussion of trophic lev-els and energy transfer (chapter 1), it requires from two to ten times as much grain to produce a pound of human flesh from meat as it would if that same grain were eaten directly, due to inescapable inefficiencies of energy conver-sion. (Some animals are more efficient converters than others, however. The grain demand imposed by eating poultry is far less than that of eating beef, for example, since producing a pound of chicken requires just three pounds of feed grain, while it takes seven to ten pounds of grain to produce a pound of beef.) Currently nearly 40% of world grain production is utilized for livestock feed; with analysts predicting that world meat consumption is likely to increase at a 1.8% annual rate for the next twenty years, pressure on grain supplies will correspondingly increase (Pinstrup-Andersen, 1997).

Perhaps nowhere does the pent-up consumer craving for animal protein have more explosive potential than in the People's Republic of China, where rapid economic growth is bringing hitherto undreamed-of prosperity to the world's most populous nation. Visiting China in the late summer of 1993, a *New York Times* reporter questioned a villager on how changing conditions were affecting him personally. Offering a revealing insight on how newfound wealth can boost food demand, the farmer replied, "Overall life has gotten much better. My family eats meat maybe four or five times a week now. Ten years ago we never had meat" (Kristof, 1993). The rapid rise in personal incomes in East Asia and in many developing nations during the past decade is having a profound impact on both the type and amount of food people in those countries eat. As the people of China—and elsewhere—shift from prima-rily vegetarian to more heavily meat-based diets, world grain demand will grow even faster than mere population figures would suggest.

Extent of Hunger

Determining the number of hungry people in the world today is a rather tricky business. Certainly there is a quantum difference between the teenager coming home from school complaining, "When's dinner, Mom? I'm starving!" and a Somali child with stick-like limbs and protruding abdomen, dying of acute malnutrition. In an attempt to establish some basis for comparison, the Food and Agriculture Organization (FAO) of the United Nations has devised a concept called the **basal metabolic rate** (BMR). The BMR is defined as the minimum amount of energy required to power human body maintenance, not including energy required for activity. On this basis, the FAO considers anyone receiving less than 1.2 BMR food intake daily to be undernourished. Using this rather conservative figure (some authorities feel the cut-off point should be raised to 1.5 BMR), the FAO estimates that 841 million people in the developing nations currently suffer from protein-calorie malnutrition, receiving insufficient food to develop their full physical and mental potential. Hunger, of course, is not equally shared among nations or even within nations. The vast majority of the world's hungry people inhabit the South Asian countries of India, Pakistan, and Bangladesh, parts of Southeast Asia, Africa south of the Sahara, and the Andean region of South America—all regions where rates of population growth continue to be high. Nevertheless, pockets of hunger can be found even within many affluent societies. In the United States malnutrition is distressingly common among the poor, the elderly, migrant farm workers, and Native Americans.

In developing nations as a group, as many as one-third of all children under 5 years old are malnourished, a figure that rises as high as two-thirds in India and Bangladesh. The World Health Organization estimates that every day 19,000 children die as a result of malnutrition and related ailments; malnutrition is the direct or indirect cause of more than half the deaths of children under age 5 in Third World countries (WHO, 1997). Women, too, are at disproportionate risk of malnutrition. This situation exists because within households in many cultures men, being the primary workers and providers, are served the best food before the rest of the family eats. Children and women, including both pregnant and nursing mothers, whose nutritional needs in proportion to their size exceed those of men, subsist on whatever remains. In such situations, girl children frequently receive less than boys, since males are more highly regarded (Riley, 1997).

The hunger issue most frequently impinges on the public consciousness during periods of severe famine, generally caused by prolonged droughts, floods, or wartime upheavals. During recent years, media coverage of starving children and anguished parents in Somalia, Angola, Sudan, and Ethiopia have kept us grimly aware of human suffering during times of calamity elsewhere in the world. Such periodic episodes of famine, tragic though they are, do not represent the world's major hunger problem at present, however. Rather, the chronic, undramatic, day-after-day undernutrition of those who know that, good harvest or poor, their bellies will never be full constitutes today's most serious food supply dilemma.

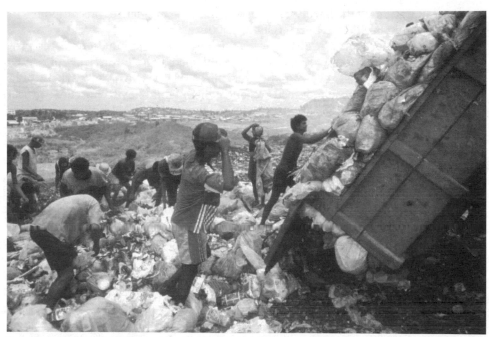

Scenes from a city garbage dump in Recife, Brazil, where men, women, and children search daily for items that can be eaten or sold. *[G. Bizzarri/FAO photo]*

Causes of Hunger

The existence of more than 800 million severely malnourished people seems paradoxical when one considers that during the 1990s the world's farmers, ranchers, and fishers produced enough food to supply every human on the planet with 3,800 calories per day—more than enough for good health (Bender and Smith, 1997). Most commentators similarly conclude that resources exist to meet the food demands of the projected world population well into the 21st century and even to reduce existing levels of malnutrition. If this is so, why are so many people today suffering from inadequate diets? The current situation is caused largely by two factors: **uneven distribution** of food and **poverty**.

Although global averages suggest that there should be enough food for everyone, as was stated earlier many of the areas where hunger is endemic are regions where there is a widening gap between food production and population growth; only imports from food-surplus areas prevent the problem from worsening further. However, as human numbers continue to climb, more equitable distribution of existing resources may not suffice—particularly if a high-quality diet rather than caloric content alone is the goal. Researchers at Brown University calculate that an even apportioning of the current world harvest, without any diversion of grain for livestock fodder, would provide an adequate vegetarian diet to a world population of six billion people—a milestone passed in 1999. A diet comparable to that currently consumed by South Americans, consisting of about 15% animal products, could be evenly distributed to four billion. To provide everyone with a typical North American or European-style diet (about 30% of calories derived from animal products), world population could barely exceed two billion—one-third the number currently dwelling on Planet Earth (Chen, 1990).

On a more practical level, however, the most basic explanation for the prevalence of hunger is poverty. Even in chronically food-short countries, the rich eat quite well. By contrast, even in the wealthiest nations, where markets bulge with a veritable cornucopia of foods, people who lack money to purchase groceries go hungry. Today, according to World Bank estimates, 1.3 billion people live in absolute poverty, earning less than the equivalent of $1 per day. These "poorest of the poor" include farmers whose land holdings are too small to be economically viable, rural landless laborers, and urban residents of the rapidly growing squatter settlements ringing many Third World cities. For these hungry people, and for two billion more who are only marginally better-off, an increase in world food production will mean little unless corresponding social and economic improvements increase their ability to purchase food for their families.

Poverty's role as a determinant of hunger was clearly evident during the 1967 drought in Bihar, a state in eastern India threatened with severe famine due to near-total crop failure. Food aid rushed into the area by the United States and other donors was credited with averting large-scale loss of life, and interviews with villagers after the crisis was over revealed that many of them ate better during this period of natural disaster than at any other time in their lives. Why? Because the donated wheat was distributed to the needy free of charge and all received a share. During normal times the poorer segments of society lacked money to buy sufficient food in the marketplace and so went hungry. As George Verghese, editor of the *Hindustan Times* and information advisor to Prime Minister Gandhi during the famine eloquently described:

> For the poorest sections of the society, 1967, the Year of the Famine, will
> long be remembered as a bonus year when millions of people, especially the
> children, probably for the first time were assured of a decent meal a day . . .
> in a "normal year," these people hover on the bread line. They are beyond
> the pale, nobody's concern, they starve. In a famine year, they eat. Their
> health is better and the children are gaining weight. For them this is a year
> of great blessing. This is the deep irony, the grim tragedy of the situation.

Most observers are confident that until 2025 at least there will be adequate food to meet the demand of those who can afford to pay for it. For those who cannot, the outlook is less promising. In a number of the poorest countries, food production is falling farther and farther behind increasing food demand as their populations continue to grow. If their economies are unable to generate the foreign exchange necessary to purchase food from abroad, nutritional levels are likely to suffer. Free food aid and other forms of development assistance from the wealthy industrialized countries have declined substantially in recent years, further increasing the vulnerability of the world's poorest people. Food insecurity is expected to increase significantly in sub-Saharan Africa and South Asia during the first decade of the 21st century, with large proportions of the population in those regions too poor to purchase food at prevailing prices. Political instability, regional conflicts, greater variability in agricultural production due to climate change—all could have an impact on food price fluctuations that will determine who eats and who goes hungry (Pinstrup-Andersen, 1997).

Health Impact of Hunger

Stressing the national security aspect of world hunger, the Presidential Commission on World Hunger issued a report some years ago stating that:

Hunger has been internationalized and turned into a continuing global issue, transformed from a low-profile moral imperative to a divisive and disruptive factor in international relations. The most potentially explosive force in the world today is the frustrated desire of poor people to attain a decent standard of living. The anger, despair, and often hatred that result represent a real and persistent threat to international order.

Malnutrition

Political instability may be a worrisome consequence of hunger, true enough, but an even more fundamental reason for trying to eliminate hunger is its adverse impact on public health and well-being. Even during years when acute famine is absent, inadequate caloric intake has a significant impact on death rates. Among the poor in Third World countries, malnutrition is the number one health problem and is the major factor responsible for the wide gap in infant mortality rates between developed and less-developed societies. Chronic undernourishment, harmful at any age, is particularly devastating to young children. If children receive less than 70% of the daily standard food requirement, their growth and activity fall below normal levels; if food deprivation is prolonged, stunted physical development becomes irreversible and adult size is correspondingly reduced. As a result, their work performance is affected, particularly if they are employed in manual labor (work performance in both agriculture and industry has shown a positive correlation with increased body size and height). Even more ominous than the link between malnutrition and decreased physical development, however, is the finding that severe malnutrition in children, especially very young infants, results in a permanent stunting of brain development, characterized by a decrease in the number of brain cells and an alteration of brain chemistry. Studies have shown that if a nutritional deficiency occurs just before or immediately after birth, the baby will suffer a 15–25% reduction in number of brain cells. If malnutrition afflicts the developing fetus and continues to persist in the post-natal period, the child's complement of brain cells will be lowered by 50–60%.

Even milder cases of malnutrition can result in lowered performance on tests designed to measure learning and sensory abilities. Extensive research has been conducted in India, Indonesia, Latin America and elsewhere, comparing intelligence levels of school-age children who had been malnourished during their first years of life but subsequently recovered with other children from similar socioeconomic backgrounds who had not experienced similar nutritional deprivation. The former group, though to all appearances in perfectly good health, exhibited, on average, significantly lower I.Q.s and had much greater difficulty learning to read and write than did the children who had been adequately fed. Malnutrition, by reducing bodily defenses, also greatly increases a child's susceptibility to infectious diseases. Common childhood ailments such as diarrhea and measles are much more likely to prove fatal to an undernourished child than to a well-fed one. The fact that young-

BOX 4-1

Feeding China

Just as population control programs in China have a disproportionate demographic impact on ultimate world population size, so the success of China's farmers and agricultural scientists in further boosting Chinese crop yields will determine the ultimate stability—or turmoil—of global grain markets. Since the mid-1990s, a major concern has been growing among policymakers and agricultural economists over China's continued ability to feed its still-growing population. Implications of that question are profound, since if the answer is "no," the inevitable follow-up query is "then who will?"

Until quite recently, the general assumption has been that China has always been largely self-sufficient in food and will continue to be so. Historically, food imports have represented a miniscule proportion of total consumption; in 1990 China imported just 6 million tons of grain while producing 340 million. The technologies of the Green Revolution were eagerly adopted in China, and Chinese agriculture today is highly productive. So why are some analysts pessimistic? A number of converging trends suggest possible trouble in the years ahead.

On the demand side of the equation, **continued population growth** is a factor. Although China has achieved a remarkable lowering of fertility rates within the past several decades, its current population of 1.3 billion is expected to reach 1.5 billion by 2020. More people equals greater food demand. Further adding to the pressure is the **growing affluence** of Chinese consumers. China's booming economy and rapid pace of industrial development have dramatically raised living standards for millions of Chinese citizens. With money in their pockets, these consumers are opting for higher-quality diets, including meat, fish, eggs, and dairy products (especially ice cream!) that formerly were too expensive to eat on a regular basis. Between 1978–1994 meat consumption increased 5-fold and continues to rise. Even if population growth were to halt completely, the escalating demand for animal protein would significantly increase grain demand to support livestock production (meats favored by Chinese consumers—primarily pork—are not raised on rangelands as in the case of U.S. beef cattle but are almost exclusively grain-fed). Grain also is being diverted to the brewing of beer, for which newly affluent Chinese have acquired a taste. China has now surpassed Germany to become the world's second largest beer-drinking nation, after the U.S.

While food demand is thus inexorably increasing, the ability of Chinese agriculture to produce an adequate supply is looking more and more problematic. Some of the factors pointing to a downturn in total grain harvests include:

1. **Farmland conversion.** The rampant industrialization that has brought a new measure of prosperity to many parts of China has also inevitably resulted in the loss of good farmland. Unfortunately, only one-tenth of China's total land area is cultivable, and most of this good land lies along the country's eastern and southern coasts—exactly where most of China's new factories, roads, and housing are being constructed. In addition, a growing population and rising personal incomes are further increasing pressure on scarce land resources as villagers build new or bigger homes and city dwellers acquire automobiles. More cars require more land for roads, parking lots,

and service stations; massive highway construction projects are underway, consuming broad stretches of productive cropland. In some of the most prosperous sections of the country, golf courses, private villas, shopping centers, and tennis courts are sprouting up in fields where rice once grew. Chinese planners might well heed the lament of U.S. land preservationists that "asphalt is the land's last crop."

2.   **Stagnating grain yields.** Like most major agricultural nations, China is approaching the upper limits of the potential inherent in hybrid seeds and nitrogen fertilizer inputs. As the world leader in fertilizer use, China, like the U.S., has appeared to have reached the point of diminishing returns. Topsoil loss due to wind and water erosion also is adversely affecting efforts to increase per hectare yields. As a result, after enjoying a phenomenal 7% annual increase in production during the early 1980s, gains during the 1990s dropped to just 0.7% annually, below the rate of population growth.

3.   **Dwindling water supplies.** Extensive use of irrigation is credited for much of the yield increase achieved by Chinese farmers in recent decades. Currently 70% of the grain produced in China is grown on irrigated land. However, soaring water demand by Chinese industry and populous urban areas is creating competitive pressure for the country's limited supply, and Chinese agriculture appears to be the loser. Northern China, with two-thirds of the nation's farmland, has but one-fifth of its water resources. Diversion of irrigation water to urban and industrial consumers, along with over-pumping of groundwater that has caused some wells to go dry, is forcing many farmers either to revert to less-productive dry land farming or to abandon their fields altogether. In some regions where adequate water is still available to farmers, industrial wastewater discharges have polluted the water so badly that it can't be used for irrigation. Some experts now regard water scarcity as the most urgent threat to China's food security.

If future food demand in China exceeds the domestic supply, Chinese leaders will undoubtedly fill the gap by purchasing food from abroad. Indeed, China seems to be following the same course traced by Japan, Taiwan, and South Korea several decades earlier as those nations industrialized and became major food importers. The difference, of course, lies in the sheer size of potential Chinese demand. Although there is considerable controversy among economists regarding the likely magnitude of China's need for food imports 30 years hence, some analysts argue that the amounts could be staggering. Prompted by a report issued by the Worldwatch Institute, which first raised the alarm, the National Intelligence Council (NIC)—an umbrella group representing all U.S. intelligence agencies—commissioned a group of scientists to conduct an interdisciplinary assessment of China's food prospects. The initial conclusions of that study, issued jointly by the NIC and CIA in January 1998, stated that by 2025 China would, in all likelihood, need to import 175 million tons of grain. Such a projection is sobering indeed, since the entire amount of grain available for export on a worldwide basis has remained relatively stable at about 200 million tons annually for the past 20 years. A great many countries, most of them poor developing nations, rely on large grain imports to feed their growing populations. The fear among NIC members and many other informed observers is that if China becomes the dominant grain importer, demand pressures will drive up prices to the point that poor countries could no longer afford to buy. The resulting social unrest and political upheaval provoked by food shortages in Third World cities could pose serious threats to the national security of many countries.

Confronted by this scenario, many people assume that the leading grain exporters will happily respond to this situation by boosting production to meet marketplace demand while increasing their own earnings. Unfortunately, prospects for doing so are dim. Currently, the world grain trade is dominated by just five major producers: the United States, Canada, Australia, the European Union, and Argentina. The U.S., which supplies about half of all grain traded internationally, has seen little, if any, increase in per capita grain production since the early 1980s. With projections indicating there will be an additional 60–65 million Americans to feed in 2025 than there were in 2000, any increased production by U.S. farmers is likely to be eaten up at home. Limited water resources make it unlikely that Canada or Australia will be able to increase crop yields and the outlook for future growth in European harvests—already at record levels—is similarly bleak. Only Argentina appears capable of doubling its exportable surplus, but since current Argentine exports now average only 20 million tons annually, this increment is but a tiny fraction of what will be needed if NIC projections prove accurate.

Chinese leaders angrily dispute the alarming scenario described here, insisting their grain imports will remain quite modest. One high-ranking agricultural official even insists that China will have large grain *surpluses* by 2025. Analysts at the International Food Policy Research Institute similarly dismiss concerns about feeding China. Only time will tell who's right, but the debate provides one more reminder that we are truly living in a global economy where seemingly unrelated happenings in one country can have a dramatic impact on the daily lives of ordinary citizens half a world away.

References

Brown, Lester R. 1995. "Who Will Feed China?" *Worldwatch Environmental Alert Series*, W.W. Norton.

Brown, Lester R., and Brian Halweil, 1998. "China's Water Shortage Could Shake World Food Security." *World-Watch* 11, no. 4 (July/Aug):10-21.

sters in poor countries are several hundred times more likely to die of measles than are children in more affluent societies is indicative of malnutrition's impact on infection rates.

Malnutrition takes its toll among older children and adults as well. Undernourished people lose weight and become less able to combat infections or environmental stress. They thereby become less economically productive and less able to care for their families (however, while adults suffering temporarily from severe food deprivation may become listless and apathetic, unable to engage in strenuous physical labor, they seldom experience the permanent damage characteristic of childhood malnutrition). At greatest risk, of course, are pregnant and lactating women. Such women, if malnourished, run a significantly higher risk of miscarriage or premature delivery than do adequately fed mothers. If they manage to carry their babies full-term, the child is likely to suffer from low birth weight (one of the most frequent causes of infant mortality) or to be stillborn (Sasson, 1990). The old myth that nursing mothers draw on their own nutritional reserves to provide top-quality food for their infants is untrue—the milk of undernourished mothers is lower than normal in vitamins, fat, and protein content.

Nutritional Deficiency Diseases

To be well-nourished implies not only an adequate caloric intake, but also a proper balance of carbohydrates, fats, proteins, vitamins and minerals. If amounts of any of these are insufficient, certain deficiency symptoms may become apparent even when all other vital nutrients are in adequate supply. Some of the more common deficiency diseases include the following.

Kwashiorkor. The single largest contributor to high child mortality rates in Third World countries, kwashiorkor is a protein deficiency disease that affects millions of children in tropical areas, particularly in Africa. Kwashiorkor most frequently develops in babies who are weaned early and given only starchy, low-protein foods such as rice, cassava, or bananas to eat—common baby foods in many tropical regions. Symptoms of mild kwashiorkor include discoloration of the hair and skin (in dark-haired children, hair may assume a reddish cast), retardation of physical growth, development of a protruding abdomen due to accumulation of fluids, and a loss of appetite. In more severe cases the hair may fall out painlessly in tufts, digestive problems arise, fluid collects in the legs and foot, muscle wastage and enlargement of the liver may occur, and the child becomes listless and apathetic. Once this stage of the disease is reached, death is likely unless the child receives medical attention. In its milder forms, however, the effects of kwashiorkor are reversible and generally disappear as the child becomes older and is given a more varied diet.

Marasmus. The second of the two most commonly observed deficiency diseases among children, marasmus is an indication of overall protein-calorie deprivation. Most frequently striking babies under one year of age, especially those no longer being breast-fed, marasmus often occurs after the child has been suffering from diarrhea or some other disease. Victims of marasmus can be distinguished by their thin, wasted appearance, with skin hanging in loose wrinkles around wrists and legs and eyes appearing unusually large and bright because of the shrunken aspect of the rest of the body.

Xerophthalmia (Blindness). Vitamin A deficiency, a public health problem among the poor in more than 60 countries, is the single most important cause of childhood blindness in developing nations. Lack of vitamin A, seldom a concern among those whose diet includes eggs, dairy products, and green leafy vegetables, can result in a drying of the eye membranes or a softening of the cornea. Such conditions lead first to night-blindness and, if not treated, to total blindness of its victims. In areas such as South and Southeast Asia, Africa, Central America, Haiti, and northeastern Brazil an estimated 250 million preschool children suffer from vitamin A deficiency; at least 5 million develop xerophthalmia each year and, of these, approximately half a million go blind. Scientists have confirmed that not only can vitamin A deficiency lead to blindness, but it also is an important determinant of child mortality due to its deleterious effect on the immune system. The micronutrient stimu-

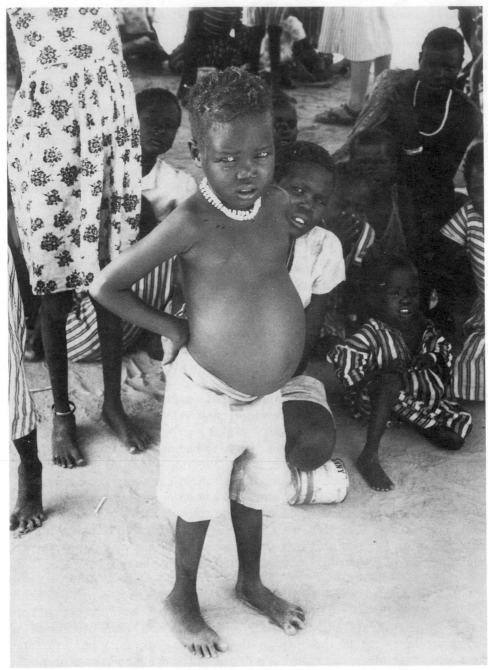

This child exhibits the protruding abdomen characteristic of kwashiorkor sufferers. [R. Bafa-lis/U.S. Agency for International Development]

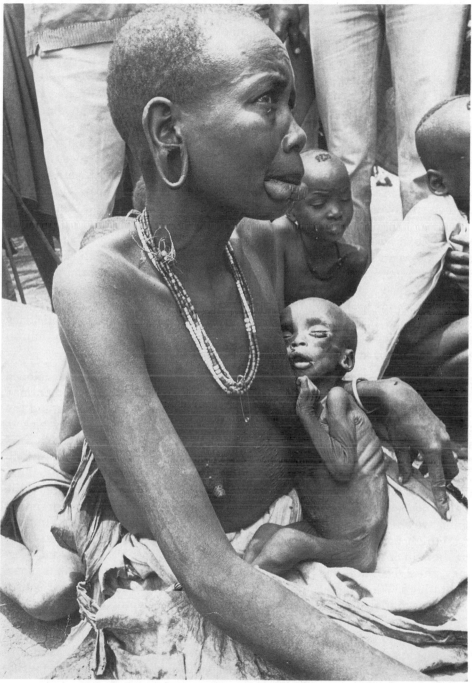

Victims of marasmus, an overall protein-calorie deprivation, can be identified by their thin, wasted appearance. *[World Vision]*

lates maturation of white blood cells, which aid the body in fighting disease; its deficiency provokes changes in the mucous membranes lining the respiratory, gastrointestinal, and urinary tracts, rendering them less effective in protecting the body against invading pathogens. Studies conducted among Indonesian preschoolers suffering from night blindness have shown that these children were 4 to 12 times more likely to die than their nonaffected peers, apparently due to their greater susceptibility to respiratory and diarrheal infections.

Efforts to combat vitamin A deficiency have focused on three alternative approaches. Educating parents to provide their children with foods rich in vitamin A seems to offer the best long-term solution to the problem; such an approach can also include promotion of home gardening to grow vitamin A-rich foods in regions where they aren't locally available in the marketplace or are too expensive. Supplying children with mega-doses of vitamin A in capsule form twice a year has proven to be an easy-to-implement, cost-effective approach to reducing child mortality rates among children at high risk of vitamin A deficiency. A third approach involves fortifying some common dietary constituent such as sugar or monosodium glutamate (MSG) with vitamin A, a strategy that has been moderately successful in Latin America and parts of Southeast Asia. In the long run, however, eliminating vitamin A deficiency depends on reducing levels of poverty and raising living standards so that all families can enjoy an adequate and nutritious diet (Potter, 1997).

Anemia. Iron deficiency anemia is very common in the less-developed countries where 20–25% of children, 20–40% of women, and 10% of men may suffer from this disorder, caused primarily by strict vegetarian diets and the prevalence of parasitic worm infections. Anemia is characterized by lack of energy and low levels of productive activity. It is especially dangerous—and especially common—in pregnant women, where anemia increases the likelihood of maternal death, premature delivery, or stillbirth. Repeated pregnancies rapidly drain a woman's reserve supplies of iron; in India, where the problem is more severe than anywhere else in the world, 88% of pregnant women are anemic. Iron deficiency anemia is held responsible, at least in part, for the high female mortality rate in that country. While women need three times as much iron as men to replace losses during menstruation and pregnancy, their food intake is generally lower than that of their husbands, sons, and brothers. While increasing the consumption of red meat (the best source of easily assimilated iron) among poor women in developing nations may not be a practical option due to religious prohibitions or lack of purchasing power, the frequency of iron deficiency anemia could be significantly reduced by supplying ferrous salt tablets to pregnant and lactating women, as well as to children, living in areas with a high prevalence of this deficiency disease (WHO, 1997; Sasson, 1990).

Goiter. An indicator of iodine deficiency, goiter affects approximately 655 million people worldwide, resulting in a disfiguring enlargement of the thyroid gland on the front or side of the neck. Lack of iodine can have more serious implications than goiter alone, however. Iodine deficiency is the world's single most important cause of preventable brain damage and mental retardation, affecting approximately 26 million people. Iodine deficiency in pregnant women can result in irreversible brain damage to the fetus, resulting in babies being born dwarfed and mentally retarded. Iodine deficiencies are most common in the Himalayan foothills, the Andean Mountain area of South America, and parts of central Africa. Goiter has largely been eliminated in the United States by the simple expedient of adding iodine to table salt (Levin, 1993).

Other deficiency diseases that are much less common today than they were in the past due to fortification of dietary staples with the missing vitamin or mineral include: scurvy (vitamin C), beri-beri (thiamine-vitamin B1), pellagra (niacin), and rickets (vitamin D).

Prospects for Reducing World Hunger

When confronted with stark pictures of starving babies or cold statistics on the growing prevalence of malnutrition, the typical reaction among most Americans is to say, "let's do something about it!"—send a donation to CARE or OXFAM, eat a vegetarian meal once a week, write a letter to a congressional representative urging a "yes" vote on the next food aid bill. Certainly there has been no shortage of suggestions as to what might be done to ease the population-food crunch. Some of the approaches being tried have real merit, as well as limitations, while others are merely wishful thinking. It's important that the public have some understanding of the key elements in the ongoing debate as to how best to eradicate hunger, since this issue is certain to assume even greater urgency in the years ahead. Some of the most frequently mentioned ways of increasing the world food supply are discussed in the following sections.

Expanding the Amount of Land Under Cultivation

From the beginning of the Agricultural Revolution right up to the early 1950s, increasing acreage put to the plow was the major, often the only, way of increasing food supply. Expanding the amount of cultivated land was accomplished by clearing forests, terracing mountainsides, or building irrigation systems—all of which permitted hitherto unproductive lands to be farmed. During the 1950s the Soviet Union vastly increased its agricultural acreage by opening up the "virgin lands" of Kazakhstan; at the same time the Chinese completed some major irrigation networks, substantially expanding their cultivated acreage and making it possible to raise two to three crops per year on the same land. Since that time, significant increases in highly productive farmland have been quite limited. The hard truth is that the world's prime farmland is in finite supply, and after approximately 10,000 years of agricultural expansion most good land is already being cultivated. Since the 1950s most of the additional land cleared for farming has been so-called "marginal land"—land which, because of its poor soil, erodability, or steep slope is incapable of sustaining moderately good yields over any extended period of time. Farmers who today are moving onto marginal lands, desperately trying to eke out a living for their families, do so only because the better lands are already overcrowded. The additional food that such lands will contribute to world harvests is negligible and the long-term ecological damage caused by removing the natural vegetative cover from such lands may eventually have an adverse impact on better lands elsewhere.

Some optimists look hopefully to regions of South America and Africa where nearly half of the yet-undeveloped land suitable for agriculture is located. However, such lands are far from current markets and lack the transportation infrastructure necessary for viable agricultural development. The huge amount of capital investment that would be required appears at present to be far beyond the financial capabilities of the nations involved. Moreover, increasing cultivated acreage in a few land-abundant regions is unlikely to provide additional food or benefits for land-scarce countries. In the world's two most populous nations, China and India, opportunities to expand farmland acreage are virtually nonexistent (Bender and Smith, 1997).

When assessing the contribution that additional farm acres could make to the total world harvest, commentators frequently overlook the other side of the coin, i.e. the substantial amounts of good cropland that are currently being lost every year to erosion, desertification, salinization and water-logging of irrigated fields, and urban development. It is now recognized that the increase in world food production witnessed during the 1970s and early 1980s was achieved in part by plowing marginal lands unsuitable for sustained cultivation and by over-irrigating, which has resulted in drastic drawing-down of groundwater reserves in many areas. Today in many of the major grain-producing areas of the world, the cropland base is beginning to shrink as highly erodible lands are abandoned. According to a survey conducted by the International Soil Reference and Information Center, 10% of the earth's vegetative surface is at least moderately degraded and more than 22 million acres have been converted to virtual wastelands. Global averages understate the problem in regions such as Central America and Mexico, where the percentage of seriously degraded land is as high as 24%, compared to 5% in North America. On moderately degraded lands reforestation is theoretically possible, though the cost of such an undertaking might be prohibitive. Extremely degraded soils—those on which the soil's biotic functions have been destroyed—cannot be reclaimed. The following chapter will examine these trends in more detail, but it is important to bear in mind that while most of the lands currently being added to our agricultural base are marginal acres, those being lost are, for the most part, prime croplands that will never be returned to production.

Increasing World Fish Catch

When one considers that 71% of the earth's surface is water, it's understandable that many people, confronted with the prospect of impending food shortages, look to the oceans as the source of apparently limitless high-quality animal protein. Such optimism seemed justified during the years between 1950-1989, when total world fish catch soared from about 22 million tons annually to 89 million tons—a four-fold increase that, even at a time of unprecedented population growth, resulted in a doubling in the per capita availability of seafood. Since fish provide approximately 20% of all the animal protein consumed by humans on a worldwide basis, this bounty from the sea raised hopes for substantial progress in combating malnutrition if the 2 million ton/year increase in global fish catch could be sustained. During the

1990s, annual world fish catch fluctuated slightly up and down, reaching a new high of 93 million tons in 1996 (figures do not include harvests from fish-farming). This apparent continued rise in ocean fish catch, however, obscures the fact that the increase in tonnage is a result of fishers hauling in many species formerly regarded as "trash fish." Stocks of species traditionally regarded as desirable table-grade fish—Atlantic cod, swordfish, haddock, orange roughy, bluefin tuna—are in sharp decline, with some nearing commercial extinction. The Food and Agriculture Organization (FAO) of the United Nations has designated 11 of the world's 15 major fishing grounds as seriously depleted and reports that 70% of the major fish species are either fully exploited or overexploited. For the one billion people worldwide who rely on fish as their main source of protein—and for the 200 million fishers whose livelihood depends on the commercial viability of ocean fisheries—current trends are ominous. At present about 80 million metric tons of fish are available for direct human consumption annually; FAO predicts that population growth will increase the demand to 110–120 million tons by 2010. Unfortunately, FAO expects world fish catch to plateau at current levels or to decline, resulting in a growing gap between supply and demand. Such a gap will inevitably lead to higher prices. Already 83% by value of the world's fish harvest is exported to affluent consumers in Japan, the U.S., and other industrialized nations. In the decade ahead, rising prices sparked by rising demand will further boost fish exports from developing nations, leaving fewer fish for local consumers and making fish protein less and less affordable for low-income families (WRI, 1998; Brown et al., 1999).

While the main factor affecting sustainability of ocean fisheries is over-exploitation (see Box 4-2), marine pollution is having an impact as well. It has not yet been possible to demonstrate a decline in the abundance of entire species in the open sea due solely to pollution, but experiments have shown that toxic contaminants such as hydrocarbons, heavy metals, and synthetic organic compounds—all common water pollutants—can kill or injure aquatic organisms. In the coastal waters that constitute some of the world's most productive fishing grounds, nutrients, primarily nitrates and phosphates from sewage discharges or farmland runoff, constitute the most extensive and serious pollution problem. A large area of sea bottom in the Gulf of Mexico offshore from New Orleans is now a virtual "dead zone," thanks largely to agricultural runoff from Midwestern farmlands. The decline of Chesapeake Bay's crab and oyster harvest, once among the world's richest, can be traced to contamination from runoff as well. Shellfish are particularly susceptible to pollution of near-shore areas; if not directly killed by toxic contaminants, they are often declared unmarketable because of the health threat they pose to human consumers.

Development activities that destroy coastal habitats, particularly coastal marshes, mangroves, and sea grasses, also play a role in reducing populations of ocean fish because many commercially important species depend on coastal or estuarine waters for survival during some phase of their life cycle. Burgeoning urban populations along most of the world's coastlines are rapidly increasing development pressures in these areas, yet few countries are managing such growth in a manner that will protect the ocean's biotic resources.

Figure 4-1

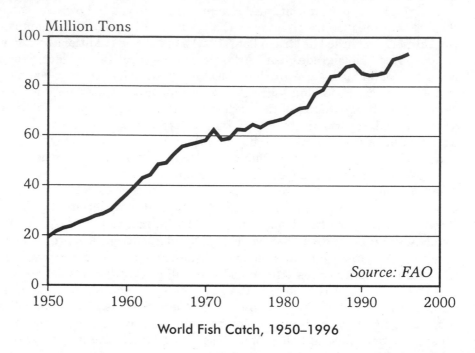

World Fish Catch, 1950–1996

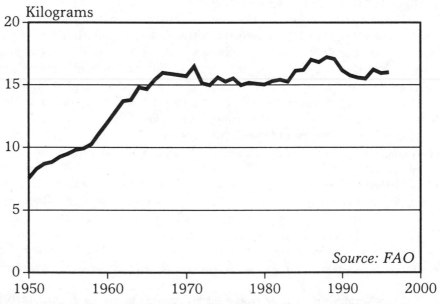

World Fish Catch Per Person, 1950–1996

Source: Brown, Lester R., Michael Renner, and Christopher Flavin. 1998. *Vital Signs 1998*. Worldwatch Institute. Used with permission.

Table 4-1 Peak Harvest Year of High-Value Fish

Fishing Area	Year of Maximum Harvest	Recent Harvest (000 metric tons)	Maximum Harvest (000 metric tons)
Atlantic, Northwest	1967	1,007	2,588
Antarctic	1971	28	189
Atlantic, Southeast	1972	312	962
Atlantic, Western Central	1974	162	181
Atlantic, Eastern Central	1974	320	481
Pacific, Eastern Central	1975	76	93
Atlantic, Northeast	1976	4,575	5,745
Pacific, Northwest	1987	5,661	6,940
Pacific, Northeast	1988	2,337	2,556
Atlantic, Southwest	1989	967	1,000
Pacific, Southwest	1990	498	498
Pacific, Southeast	1990	459	508
Mediterranean	1991	284	284
Indian Ocean, Western	1991	822	822
Indian Ocean, Eastern	1991	379	379
Pacific, Western Central	1991	833	833

Source: Food and Agriculture Organization of the United Nations. 1997. *The State of World Fisheries and Aquaculture—1996.*

Aquaculture

In contrast to the rather gloomy outlook for the capture fisheries, fish harvests from **aquaculture** (fish-farming) have been growing rapidly. Production from fish farms exceeded 23 million tons in 1996—triple the amount harvested in the mid-1980s. At present, one out of every four fish eaten worldwide is farm-raised. For some species, the numbers are even more impressive: 30% of shrimp; 40% of salmon, oysters, and clams; and 65% of freshwater fish consumed today are products of aquaculture. In China, the world leader in aquaculture, output more than doubled (to 12.8 million tons) between 1990–1995. Today China, Japan, India, Thailand, Korea, Indonesia, and the Philippines all obtain a substantial portion of their seafood products from aquaculture. In the United States, aquaculture now accounts for just 2% of total world production but is expanding rapidly. Already aquaculture accounts for most of U.S. catfish and crayfish production and is the main source of the salmon supplied by American supermarkets.

While as much as a third of the wild fish catch is used to make fish meal and fish oil, farmed fish go directly to human consumers. It is anticipated that any future increases in fish consumption will have to come from aquaculture, since there is little hope of further increasing ocean fish catch. Unlike capture fisheries, however, aquaculture demands significant resource inputs. Fish farms require considerable amounts of land and water, both of which must be diverted from other types of agricultural production. Concerns over cropland loss to fish production has already prompted Chinese authorities to restrict

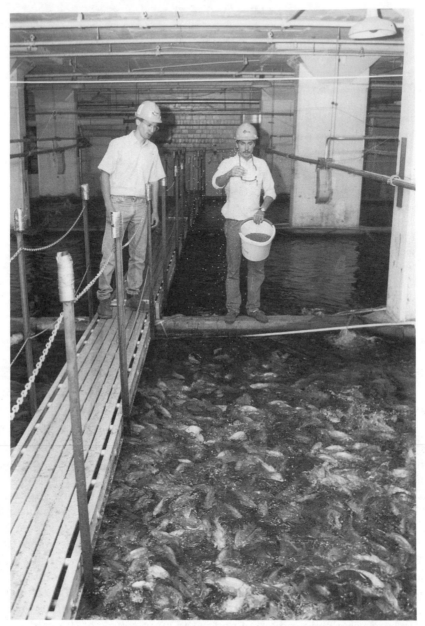

Aquaculture (fish farming) provides 23% of the total world fish harvest. Species that can be successfully raised include catfish, crayfish, salmon, trout, and tilapia (shown above). *[Archer Daniels Midland]*

future farmland conversion to aquaculture. Additionally, farmed fish, unlike those caught on the open seas, must be fed by those who raise them. Fortunately, fish are among the most efficient energy converters, requiring about two pounds of feed to gain one pound of flesh. Ironically, the growth of fish farming has intensified pressures on ocean fish stocks because 10–15% of all

BOX 4-2

Fishing Down the Food Chain

They that go down to the sea in ships
that do business in great waters.
—Psalms 107:23

Thus sang the ancient psalmist, but if present trends in the capture fisheries persist, those who go down to the sea a generation or two hence may do little business indeed. From the legendary cod fisheries of Georges Bank to the salmon runs of the Pacific Northwest, catastrophic declines in marine fish stocks threaten thousands of commercial fishers with economic ruin. In recognition of the dire state of affairs, delegates from virtually every fishing nation met in Rome in February 1999, at the urging of the United Nations' Food and Agriculture Organization (FAO), and promised to make substantial reductions in their fishing fleets in order to control overfishing.

Although in terms of tonnage the world fish catch has remained relatively stable at record-high levels for the past decade, the *kinds* of fish being caught by today's highly modernized fleets are no longer the top predators of the ocean food chain, but are instead lower trophic level species that are being exploited simply because the larger, more valuable fish have disappeared. Since the 1980s, low-value fish species have accounted for almost three-quarters of the overall increase in world fish catch. This rampant, worldwide "fishing down the food chain" is impoverishing marine ecosystems and, if the experts are correct, will inevitably lead to the widespread collapse of ocean fisheries.

So what is to blame for this sad state of affairs? Although a number of factors are imposing stress on marine ecosystems, the most obvious explanation is overfishing. Since the 1950s, new fishing methods have revolutionized one of the world's oldest commercial enterprises. Fishers are employing such military technologies as radar, allowing them to navigate in dense fog, and sonar, which makes it possible to "see" schools of fish deep under the water. Satellite positioning systems enable ships on the open sea to sail within 50 feet of a desired location (e.g. fish breeding grounds) and satellite weather maps indicating water temperature give clues as to where fish will be traveling. Aircraft spotters work in conjunction with some fleets to locate concentrations of fish. Increasingly efficient "floating factories"—huge ships that both harvest and process fish at sea—have greatly increased the catch of nations like Russia, Poland, and Japan. In doing so, however, they threaten the long term viability of the industry by harvesting young and mature fish indiscriminately.

In the 1980s and early 1990s such widescale capture was facilitated by the use of enormous driftnets that stretched 5–50 kilometers through the water, suspended at or near the surface by floats. Hanging vertically like giant curtains, driftnets were ruthlessly efficient in snaring any hapless fish that attempted to swim through the mesh. Utilized primarily by Japanese, Korean, and Taiwanese fishers, driftnets were roundly condemned by the United Nations' General Assembly because of their propensity to capture nontarget fish, birds, turtles, and marine mammals, primarily dolphins. For this reason, driftnets were ultimately banned by the world community (though some continue to be used), but were promptly replaced by another destructive fishing technique. Thousands of ships from many nations, the U.S. included, now employ long lines, machine-baited and bearing thousands of hooks each, to catch wide-ranging ocean fish species such as swordfish, sharks, and tuna. Typically stretching 20–40 miles (sometimes as much as 80 miles), the lightweight monofilament lines from just one large vessel may bear tens of thousands of hooks. Their efficiency has taken a heavy toll on the species being fished. Scientists contend that numbers of Atlantic swordfish are now but 58% of those necessary to maintain a viable population over the long term and the decline continues. Current stocks have but 2–3% of the number of reproducing adults found in unexploited swordfish populations. Fishing pressures are now so intense that 80–90% of the individuals within some fish populations are removed each year. As a result, according to the FAO, 60% of the world's 200 most important commercial fish stocks are in serious danger.

As the large predator fish become commercially extinct, fishers have little choice but to shift to less valuable species lower on the food chain. Since these species are smaller but more numerous, this transition at first yields large catches such as those witnessed during the 1990s. However, if fishing persists, the cycle of overfishing will again lead to depletion, forcing fishers to move still further down the food chain until there's nothing left to harvest but plankton.

Although the problems inherent in overfishing are well understood and widely publicized, few effective actions have been taken to reverse the situation. Fisheries management traditionally has focused on maximizing the catch of economically important species by every means possible, even when the ultimate result of such efforts is the collapse of the fishery. Governments have exacerbated the problem by subsidizing the purchase of new or upgraded fishing vessels. These subsidization programs complicate the newly declared intention of the global fishing community to reduce fleet size; political barriers to doing so are formidable, especially in Europe where subsidies have been extremely generous. International policies of open access to marine resources have further encouraged a global free-for-all in the race to harvest the remaining riches of the sea. Regulations, even when agreed upon in international treaties, are frequently disregarded by fishers, who view their activities as a right, not a privilege. Where restrictions have been imposed, poaching is common and penalties are minimal.

Nevertheless, desperate times give rise to desperate actions and in recent years governments have begun to impose bans on fishing in some areas to forestall total collapse of endangered stocks. The complete ban on fishing the Grand Banks off Newfoundland and the quotas limiting catches in European Union waters are cases in point. However, bans currently are in effect for less than 1% of all the world's fishing grounds and researchers are convinced that many more protected areas must be created if catastrophe is to be averted. By setting aside large "no-take" areas where fish populations can rebuild within functioning marine ecosystems, governments may yet provide hopes for recovery. Failure to take such action could well mean that future generations of those who go down to the sea in ships will return with empty nets.

References

Pauly, Daniel, Villy Christensen, et al. 1998. "Fishing Down Marine Food Webs." *Science* 299, no. 5352 (Feb. 6):860–863.

Safina, Carl. 1995. "The World's Imperiled Fish." *Scientific American*, (Nov):46–53.

fishmeal obtained from capture fisheries is fed to farmed fish. Currently, Chinese scientists are hard at work developing a yeast-based protein supplement that can replace more than half the fishmeal component of aquaculture feeds. Nevertheless, like every other enterprise, aquaculture has its economic and environmental costs (WRI, 1998; Brown et al., 1998).

Reducing Post-Harvest Food Losses

Implementation of better methods of handling and protecting food between the time it is harvested and the time it appears on the consumer's plate may not sound particularly exciting—rat-proof grain bins are not the stuff of which poetry is made—but, in the short-run at least, such simple, well-understood measures could help to increase the availability of food in the marketplace. Each year enormous amounts of harvested foods are lost to pests and spoilage, particularly in tropical countries. Rats, birds, insects, and molds all consume or render unfit for human use large amounts of stored foods which would otherwise have been available for people. Cultural practices are partially responsible for such losses. In many countries grains are stored in the open or in easily penetrated sacks or bins. Lack of adequate refrigeration promotes spoilage, while poor transport facilities delay rapid movement of food from fields to consumers, thereby increasing chances of loss or spoilage.

In wealthier countries, consumers' insistence that food be cosmetically perfect results in substantial wastage of harvested crops, particularly fruits and vegetables. Tiny blemishes that in no way affect a food's taste or nutritional value frequently result in its being discarded because it doesn't meet market standards of aesthetic acceptability. Retailing, food service, and personal consumption habits also result in considerable wastage of food. Just these three stages of the marketing process account for the loss of almost 95 billion pounds of food annually in the United States—27% of all food available for consumption (Kantor, 1997). Of course there is no guarantee that less food wastage in rich countries would result in greater food availability for the poor, but some analysts suggest that if food losses could be reduced to 23% worldwide, an amount equivalent to 13% of global consumption would be saved, thereby reducing per capita food demand (Bender and Smith, 1997).

Eating Lower on the Food Chain

Humanitarians are frequently troubled by the apparent inefficiency of converting a substantial portion of the world grain harvest into meat or poultry to satisfy consumers' carnivorous cravings. The same amount of corn, wheat, or oats, they argue, could satisfy the caloric needs of millions of additional people dining on vegetarian fare (to be consistent, they might also target the 10% of the U.S. corn crop diverted to the manufacture of corn syrup, much of which is used for sweetening soft drinks; that same amount of corn could make a lot of tortillas!)

The impact of diverting feed to food, even if fully implemented, might not be as great as proponents suggest, however. It has been estimated that abandoning the use of grain for feed entirely would increase market supplies of food by 20–30% at most (Ehrlich, Ehrlich, and Daily, 1993). If world population continues to grow as projections indicate, the one-time gains achieved by going vegetarian would soon be erased by the continuously mounting food demands generated by more and more people.

Regardless of whether promoting meatless diets would be an advisable or effective approach to increasing food availability, it is not a realistic option. While health concerns are prompting some individuals to reduce their consumption of high-fat animal products, no society in modern times has voluntarily reduced meat-eating by any significant amount. Indeed, as we have seen, the trends in newly affluent areas of the world are in exactly the opposite direction. Contrary to common perceptions, a large portion of feed grain use occurs in the Third World; next to the United States, China is the second-leading nation in terms of amounts of grain fed to livestock, poultry, and fish (USDA, 1992). While consumers might simplify their diets in response to scarcity-induced higher prices, an appeal to altruism—asking diners to forego their steaks and sauerbraten so that strangers far away could enjoy a temporary increase in food supplies—is unlikely to meet with a positive response.

Improving Yields per Acre

Since mid-century the largest gains in world food supply have been obtained not by expanding our cropland base but by dramatically increasing per acre or per hectare (metric unit for land measurement, equivalent to 2.47 acres) yields on existing farmlands. In the United States, corn yields, which had remained stable for almost 70 years, more than quadrupled from 1940 to 1985. Impressive increases in yields were also achieved for wheat, rice, barley, rye, peanuts, and sorghum. In Great Britain, where wheat yields are the world's highest, per hectare wheat production tripled from 1940 to 1984. These enormous gains were accomplished through the application of research and technological improvements gradually developed and perfected since the late 1800s, the major elements of which included new hybrid crop varieties, better farm machinery, tremendous expansion in the use of chemical fertilizers and pesticides, and increased use of irrigation.

The developed nations were not alone in realizing major gains in agricultural productivity during the past several decades. In the late 1960s, twenty years of plant breeding experiments to improve grain yields in tropical and semi-tropical regions resulted in the development of several strains of so-called "miracle wheat" and "miracle rice" which heralded the advent of what commentators have dubbed "The Green Revolution." Within a few years of its introduction, the new hybrid wheat was giving farmers from Mexico to India yields two to three times greater than the best formerly obtained from traditional strains. Since the introduction of the first miracle wheat in India in 1966, that country has more than doubled its wheat production. Pakistan, Turkey, and Mexico were among more than 30 other countries whose farmers eagerly adopted the new technology and witnessed a corresponding surge in their wheat production statistics. Similarly, the miracle rice varieties developed at the International Rice Research Institute in the Philippines have approximately doubled the yields of this grain in situations where the hybrid seeds, along with proper fertilization and adequate irrigation, were employed.

The spectacular gains of the Green Revolution led many political leaders during the early 1970s to relax on the population issue, assuming that continued dramatic increases in food production had erased the Malthusian image of starving millions. Agricultural experts, however, were less sanguine regarding the food-population crunch and warned that it would be a fatal mistake to assume that plant scientists would be able to achieve another quantum leap in crop yields in the foreseeable future. Agronomist Norman Borlaug, "Father of the Green Revolution" and recipient of the 1970 Nobel Peace Prize for his key role in developing miracle wheat, cautioned dignitaries assembled for the awards ceremony in Oslo that his contribution would, at best, buy humankind about 30 years of food security—years which he warned they must use to tame the population monster. Unfortunately, Borlaug's gift of time has largely been squandered; in developed and developing nations alike the gains of the Green Revolution are losing momentum even as population figures continue to climb. The fact that many of the world's farmers are already fully exploiting the technologies which enabled them to double, triple, or even quadruple yields in the years prior to 1984 means that future gains will come in ever-smaller increments and will be increasingly difficult to achieve. Throughout the 1990s, increases in per acre grain yields averaged barely 1% annually, with analysts lamenting the "yield plateau" that now seems to characterize cereal production in most of the world's major grain-growing areas.

Some observers predict that in the not-too-distant future we are likely to encounter an absolute yield ceiling imposed by plants' photosynthetic efficiency. The plant breeders who developed "miracle wheat" and "miracle rice" created these high-yielding genetic cultivars by boosting the proportion of sugars produced by photosynthesis that are diverted to seed production. While traditional varieties converted roughly 20% of these sugars into seeds, Green Revolution cultivars are able to convert over 50%. Scientists estimate that the absolute upper limit of sugar production that could go into seed formation without depriving the plant of energy needed for other vital functions is about 60%. Therefore, the opportunity for further yield gains through conventional breeding programs is extremely limited (Brown et al., 1999).

Similar limits are becoming apparent regarding fertilizer applications. Use of nitrogen fertilizers grew more than nine-fold between 1950–1998 and, along with hybrid seeds, receives much of the credit for the crop yield increases of the past 50 years. However, there are now signs that the Law of Diminishing Returns has set in and crops that have been receiving higher and higher levels of fertilizer applications for many years are approaching the limits of their physiological capacity to utilize nutrients. As an example of this, take the case of fertilizer use in America's "Corn Belt." During the 1950s and 1960s, for every extra pound of nitrogen applied a farmer could expect a yield increase of 15–20 extra bushels of corn. By the late 1970s, that increment was 5–7 bushels and falling. By the 1990s, growth in fertilizer use, both in the U.S. and Europe, had virtually halted, partly due to more efficient application methods but also in response to farmers' recognition that additional fertilizer inputs were not economically justified by the minimal boosts in yields per acre. In developing regions such as the Indian subcontinent where reliance on nitrogen fertilizer is more recent and less intensive, potential for increasing yields through additional fertilizer application still exists. In the longer term, however, the same laws of nature will impose an upper ceiling on production there as well. Unless plant scientists can develop new cultivars of wheat, rice, and corn that are even more responsive to heavy fertilization than those currently being grown, it is unlikely that the slowdown in annual growth of world harvests witnessed during the past decade will be reversed.

Other components critical to the success of Green Revolution technologies—irrigation and chemical pesticides—also may be approaching practical limits. High-yielding varieties can only achieve their maximum potential when supplied with abundant water. Today approximately one-third of all crops harvested come from the 17% of world cropland under irrigation (Ehrlich, Ehrlich, and Daily, 1993). For a number of reasons, the rapid expansion in irrigated acreage which occurred annually from 1950 to 1978 has tapered off since that time to less than 1% a year (Brown et al., 1998). In the absence of irrigation, "miracle grains" perform less well than lower-yielding traditional varieties—another reason why the recent slowdown in grain production is likely to continue. Chemical pesticide use, another factor critical in optimizing yields from new crop strains highly susceptible to insects and fungal pathogens, is also less effective than it was several decades ago. Overuse of these products has promoted development of resistant pest populations that are once again having an adverse impact on agricultural production.

Many people optimistically assume that biotechnology will soon present us with a new generation of super-high-yielding crop plants. Indeed, genetic engineers in both the United States and Japan are now hard at work to develop transgenic plants that have a more efficient photosynthetic apparatus. If successful, such plants could significantly boost crop yields. Scientists caution, however, that their work is progressing very slowly and any practical applications for such research lie years in the future (Mann, 1999). In the short term, biotechnology's main contribution to world agriculture is likely to be the introduction of disease- and insect-resistant crop varieties, as well as crops more tolerant of drought or salt. Such cultivars may boost current yields somewhat, but do not represent the quantum leap in production represented by the Green Revolution's "miracle grains."

For all these reasons, experts seriously doubt that a doubling or tripling of world harvests can be repeated. In most of the world's major agricultural areas farmers have already reaped the full potential offered by "miracle crops"; in regions not yet touched by the Green Revolution, natural conditions such as lack of water resources or inadequate technology transfer may preclude them from ever enjoying its fruits. Even within countries where the new technologies have boosted food self-sufficiency, large areas remain mired in poverty and backwardness—northwest China, the Andean Mountain area, the highlands of Mexico, and large areas of central India are all notable examples. The outlook for improvement is perhaps most clouded in the semiarid regions of sub-Saharan Africa where yields of maize, the most important cereal crop, have remained stagnant at about one ton per hectare since 1961. A few countries in west and central Africa, however, have recently experienced some productivity increases, thanks to the introduction of new maize varieties (Pinstrup-Andersen et al., 1997). Food production in these chronically food-deficit areas could improve, despite maximum *genetic* yield barriers, if the use of existing production technology is further expanded. More on-site research to develop improved seed varieties adapted to local growing conditions, more

Figure 4-2

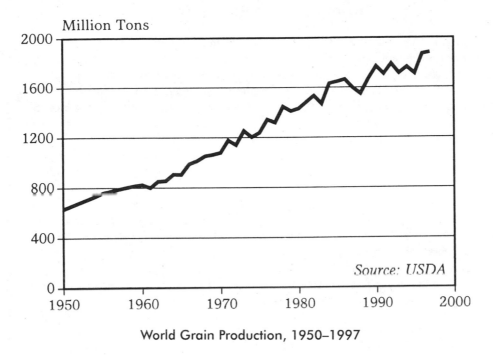

World Grain Production, 1950–1997

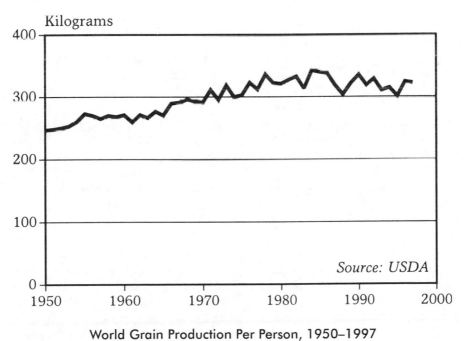

World Grain Production Per Person, 1950–1997

Source: Brown, Lester R., Michael Renner, and Christopher Flavin. 1998. *Vital Signs 1998.* Worldwatch Institute. Used with permission.

BOX 4-3

Shrimp's "Blue Revolution"

In tempura or paella, broiled with garlic butter or boiled in Cajun spices, Japanese and Western diners love shrimp—lots of shrimp! A decade or two ago, netting sufficient quantities of the tasty crustacean to meet market demand was raising serious concerns of overfishing among marine biologists. Not only did they fear for the long-term viability of wild shrimp populations, but they also deplored the environmental damage caused by the methods employed by shrimp fishers. Utilizing trawlers—ships with weighted nets dragged along the sea bottom—shrimpers created ecological havoc on the ocean floor and caused extensive collateral damage to other marine species inadvertently caught along with the target shrimp.

Thus the advent of shrimp aquaculture, shrimp's "Blue Revolution," was initially welcomed as an enterprise that could both ease the environmental stresses posed by ocean shrimp fishing while boosting overall supplies. Begun on a small scale in the 1970s, shrimp farming grew explosively during the two decades that followed. By the mid-1990s shrimp farming had grown into a $6.8 billion industry, raising almost one-third of all shrimp eaten worldwide. Most of this production is based in Asia—in Thailand, India, China, and Indonesia; in the Western Hemisphere, Ecuador is a major producer as well. Unfortunately for consumers in those nations, however, the high price shrimp garners in the international marketplace has made the product too expensive to sell locally. Virtually all the shrimp harvested in developing countries is now exported to more affluent consumers in the U.S. (the world's largest shrimp importer), Japan, and Europe.

From an ecological perspective, shrimp aquaculture has proven to be more detrimental to local environments than early enthusiasts would have predicted. Part of the problem is the location of shrimp ponds, which in most areas are constructed near the seashore to take advantage of a convenient water supply. When built on salt flats or other ecologically-poor areas, the impact was minimal, but in many situations the locations chosen were biologically diverse mangrove thickets or coastal wetlands. Small-scale producers with little capital or expertise were especially likely to set up their facilities in these environmentally sensitive areas, with disastrous consequences. Productive cropland has often been sacrificed to shrimp aquaculture as well; in Thailand almost half the land now used for growing shrimp formerly was used for rice cultivation. When shrimp ponds are no longer productive and are abandoned, the land they occupied is frequently so contaminated with salt and other pollutants it's no longer fit for agriculture.

Farming shrimp, like cultivating any other crop, involves certain inputs that exert an environmental impact. In any given situation, the nature of that impact depends on the method of shrimp aquaculture being employed. Least detrimental are so-called extensive systems that involve low densities of shrimp per unit of water and rely on naturally occurring algae to feed the shrimp larvae. Aquaculturists relying on this method add manure or chemical fertilizer to their ponds to promote algal growth, but provide no additional feed. Intensive systems, by contrast, feature much denser shrimp populations that can only be maintained by regular feeding with fishmeal pellets. Intensive shrimp production thus continues to rely on ocean fisheries.

Intensive shrimp farming also produces a considerable amount of waste in the form of feces, uneaten food, ammonia, phosphorus, and carbon dioxide. Shrimp ponds may gradually become depleted of oxygen as organic wastes decompose on the bottom. When waste materials are periodically flushed out to the sea, serious water pollution can result; in many cases, eutrophication (over-fertilization) of coastal waterways has resulted in troublesome algal blooms and other water quality problems. Contamination of groundwater resources has occurred in areas where shrimp ponds were constructed in sandy soil without proper liners underneath; as salt water seeps downward out of the ponds, underlying aquifers become more saline and unfit as drinking water sources.

Intensive methods of shrimp production also have fostered the spread of viral diseases, creating serious problems for shrimp farmers in a number of countries. In Taiwan, one of the first countries to establish shrimp farms, viral infections among farmed shrimp populations were so devastating that the shrimp aquaculture industry there completely collapsed in the late 1980s. To combat this problem, some aquaculturists have turned to medicated feeds, raising fears among critics that this tactic may lead to the development of a new generation of antibiotic-resistant microbes, with unpredictable effects on the local ecology.

Widespread reports of the environmental damage caused by shrimp farming have led to numerous protests against the industry. In 1997 global activists formed the Industrial Shrimp Action Network, calling for a halt to unsustainable shrimp farming.

Advocates, however, believe that improved shrimp farming practices are already underway and will, once widely adopted, result in shrimp aquaculture being more "green" than ocean shrimp harvesting. Reforms include the prohibition of pond construction in mangrove forests, wetlands, or sandy soil (unless impermeable clay or plastic liners are installed underneath); adopting improved feeding techniques that result in less waste; developing improved feeds that incorporate less fishmeal and more vegetable protein; reducing the use of potentially harmful chemical additives; and establishing better breeding programs to develop more disease-resistant varieties of shrimp. Within the industry, increasing attention is being focused on interrelationships between shrimp farming and the environment and a number of host country governments now require environmental impact statements before new shrimp farms can be developed. Shrimp producers recently formed the Global Aquaculture Alliance, aimed at promoting "best management practices" within the industry. Members of the alliance hope to reward responsible producers and raise consumer awareness through "eco-labeling." Like the "dolphin-safe" labels on tuna cans, labels to distinguish shrimp raised by environmentally friendly methods will, it is hoped, enjoy a marketplace advantage. Since the investments required to alleviate current problems will not always result in increased efficiency, the costs incurred will inevitably be passed on to shrimp consumers. Whether diners will be environmentally conscious enough to pay the premium price "green shrimp" will command remains to be seen. Nevertheless, adoption of sustainable production systems is essential if shrimp farming is to prosper in the decades ahead.

Reference

Boyd, Claude E., and Jason W. Clay. 1998. "Shrimp Aquaculture and the Environment." *Scientific American* (June):58-65.

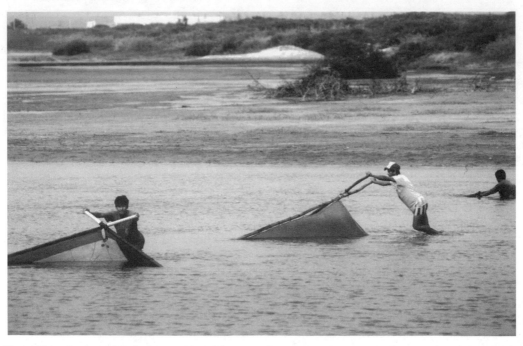

These Ecuadorean shrimp farmers employ special nets to collect shrimp larvae. *[G. Bizzarri/FAO photo]*

attention to efficient water use and proper planting dates, greater emphasis on educational outreach programs to transfer the latest agricultural developments to cultivators in the field, adoption of government financial and economic policies which make it profitable for farmers to adopt new technologies—all offer potential for boosting currently modest yields in some Third World areas. However, continued rapid rates of population growth in those same areas demand that the governments of those nations give priority to modernizing their agricultural sectors in order to realize this potential. In addition, bountiful harvests alone will not eradicate hunger. By the late 1970s the Green Revolution had increased production to such an extent in countries such as India and Pakistan that those nations were declared self-sufficient in food grains; yet millions of their people still suffer the ravages of malnutrition because they are too poor to purchase the food they need.

As we enter the 21st century, humanity is confronted by demographic projections indicating that global population will continue to climb by more than 80 million each year—at a time when growth in per capita food supply has leveled off or even declined in some key areas of the world. While optimists continue to insist that human inventiveness will somehow find the means for feeding future billions of hungry mouths, there are no new technologies on the horizon offering the quantum leaps in food production witnessed during the recent past. With a shrinking cropland base, falling water tables, diminishing impact of chemical fertilizers, and the long-term specter of adverse climatic change in some of the world's most productive agricultural regions (see chapter 11), farmers will be hard-pressed to meet future food demands at prices hungry people can afford. More vigorous efforts at stabilizing population size and reversing land degradation are urgently needed if we are to prove Malthus wrong.

References

Bender, William, and Margaret Smith. 1997. "Population, Food, and Nutrition." *Population Bulletin* 51, no. 4 (February).

Brown, Lester R., Michael Renner, and Christopher Flavin. 1998. *Vital Signs 1998*. Worldwatch Institute, W.W. Norton.

Brown, Lester R., Christopher Flavin, and Hilary F. French. 1999. *State of the World 1999*. Worldwatch Institute, W.W. Norton.

Brown, Lester R., Hal Kane, and Ed Ayres. 1993. *Vital Signs 1993*. Worldwatch Institute, W. W. Norton.

Chon, R., od. 1990. *Tho Hungor Roport: 1990*. The Alan Shawn Feinstein World Hunger Program, Brown University.

Ehrlich, Paul R., Anne H. Ehrlich, and Gretchen C. Daily. 1993. "Food Security, Population, and Environment." *Population and Development Review* 19, no. 1 (March).

Food and Agriculture Organization (FAO). 1974. "State of Food and Agriculture."

Jensen, Neal F. 1978. "Limits to Growth in World Food Production." *Science* 201 (July 28).

Kantor, Linda S., et al. 1997. "Estimating and Addressing America's Food Losses." *Food Review* 20, no. 1.

Kristof, Nicholas D. 1993. "Riddle of China: Repression as Standard of Living Soars." *New York Times*, September 7.

Levin, Henry M., et al. 1993. "Micronutrient Deficiency Disorders." In *Disease Control Priorities in Developing Countries*, edited by Dean T. Jamison et al. Oxford University Press.

Mann, Charles C. 1999. "Genetic Engineers Aim to Soup Up Crop Photosynthesis." *Science* 283, no. 5400 (Jan. 15):314-316.

Pitt, David E. 1993. "Despite Gaps, Data Leave Little Doubt that Fish Are in Peril." *New York Times*, August 3.

Pino, John A., and Andres Martinez. 1981. "The Contribution of Livestock to the World Protein Supply." In *Future Dimensions of World Food and Population*, edited by Richard Woods. Westview Press.

Pinstrup-Andersen, Per, Rajul Pandya-Lorch, and Mark W. Rosegrant. 1997. *The World Food Situation: Recent Developments, Emerging Issues, and Long-Term Prospects*. International Food Policy Research Institute, Washington, DC (December).

Potter, Andrew R. 1997. "Reducing Vitamin A Deficiency Could Save the Eyesight and Lives of Countless Children." *British Medical Journal* 314, no. 7077 (Feb. 1):317–318.

Riley, Nancy E. 1997. "Gender, Power, and Population Change." *Population Bulletin* 52, no. 1 (May).

Sasson, Albert. 1990. *Feeding Tomorrow's World*. UNESCO/CTA.

U.S. Department of Agriculture. 1992. *World Grain Database*.

World Health Organization (WHO). 1997. *The World Health Report—1997*.

World Resources Institute (WRI). 1998. *World Resources 1998–99*.

CHAPTER 5

Impacts of Growth on Ecosystems

> To sustain an environment suitable for man, we must fight on a thousand
> battlegrounds. Despite all of our wealth and knowledge, we cannot
> create a redwood forest, a wild river, or a gleaming seashore.
> —**President Lyndon B. Johnson (1966)**

Certainly the issue of how to feed additional multitudes in the years ahead, when close to a billion of the earth's current inhabitants are malnourished, looms as a monumental task for future world leaders. However, population growth exerts many other socioeconomic and environmental impacts that may be less publicized than famine, yet have a profound influence on human well-being and on the sustainability of planetary life-support systems. In many parts of the world today evidence is mounting that large and still-growing human and livestock populations have already exceeded the carrying capacity of the land itself. In effect, at a time when we are trying to produce more and more from a given land area to sustain increasing numbers of people, the activities of those people are damaging natural ecosystems to the extent that they are becoming incapable of supporting their present population, much less future billions.

Giving evidence of the fact that population growth and ecological degradation are inextricably interrelated are the swelling numbers of **"environmental refugees"**—people seeking refuge abroad due to environmental problems at home. Oxford University ecologist Norman Myers estimates that 25 million people have been forced to leave their place of birth due to water scarcity, depleted soils, deforestation, desertification, or other environmental calamities. Regions most affected by this phenomenon include Central America, India, China, the Horn of Africa, and the Sahel. More ominously, Myers predicts that this number could double by 2010 as population growth in many of the world's poorest countries puts even more pressure on already-stressed local environments. Such vast movements of environmentally displaced persons could become one of the major political and national security issues in the years immediately ahead.

Degradation of Land Resources

*We abuse land because we regard it as a commodity belonging
to us. When we see land as a community to which we belong, we
may begin to use it with love and respect.*
                    —Aldo Leopold, *A Sand County Almanac*

The disruption of natural cycles resulting from human pressures on land
resources is undermining the sustainability of ecosystems in many parts of
the world today. A survey of soil degradation conducted by the International
Soil Reference and Information Center estimates that 10% of the earth's vege-
tated surface is at least moderately degraded, while 9 million hectares (about
22 million acres) are so severely degraded that their original biotic functions
have been completely destroyed (WRI, 1996). Although much of this land is
still being cultivated, some of its natural productivity has been lost and could
be restored only through implementation of expensive national programs to
provide farmers with technical assistance and financial incentives. In the
absence of such efforts, the condition of these lands will only deteriorate further. On those lands classified as "severely degraded," restoration, for all practical purposes, is impossible. The factors responsible for land degradation
include overgrazing of livestock herds, faulty agricultural practices, and deforestation. While the environmental damage provoked by such activities theoretically could occur anywhere, certain natural areas are more vulnerable to
long-lasting destruction than others. Tundra, desert, tropical rain forest, and
arid grasslands are more easily impaired and take much longer to recover
from disruption than does, for example, temperate deciduous forest. Because
several of these areas today encompass the homelands of many millions of
people whose well-being, and indeed survival, depends on the continued productivity of their land, it is important for us to take a closer look at some specific ways in which humans, consciously or not, are radically undermining the
stability of natural ecosystems.

Overgrazing

Of the various activities contributing to soil degradation, none is more
significant than overgrazing. Conditions on 35% of all lands classified as
degraded can be attributed to excessive pressure generated by too many cattle, goats, or sheep (World Resources Institute, 1992). In India, more than half
the land now regarded as "wasteland" was reduced to that status by goats,
allowed by their owners to forage freely prior to slaughter. Municipal authorities in India's capital, New Delhi, have spent millions of rupees to replant
shrubs and grass on hillsides near the city, but in the absence of efforts to control goat populations, such expenditures have been largely wasted (Tobias,
1998). Under natural conditions, grassland communities are well-adapted to a
moderate level of grazing; herds of bison, antelope, wild horses, and so forth,
have for millennia been the dominant animals in the grassland biome, evolving and adapting in conjunction with the native plants on which they are
dependent. However, when livestock managers increase the number of livestock beyond a certain size or when they introduce types of grazing animals

foreign to a particular plant community, the resulting pressure on that community often leads to an unraveling of the ecosystem. The effects of overgrazing are first seen in the declining populations of those plant species least able to tolerate the increased cropping. As these plants disappear, species more tolerant of heavy grazing are then relieved of competition and expand to fill the niche vacated by the more vulnerable types. The loss of the latter, however, results in an overall reduction in the height, biomass, and total coverage of the grassland. If overgrazing persists, even the more resistant native plants will be unable to withstand the pressure and give way to invader weed species that were not members of the original community. Such plants are generally much inferior to the native plants in nutritive qualities and, as a result, the vitality of the herd is adversely affected. Eventually the weeds themselves may be trampled to such an extent that they, too, are reduced in coverage. The soil, thus exposed to the forces of wind and water, may be worn away, leaving a barren mud flat or rocky hillside, devoid of any community (Whittaker, 1975).

While land degradation due to overgrazing is most pronounced in Australia (80%) and in Africa (49%), extensive areas of rangeland in the American West are severely affected as well. Of the approximately 270 million acres of publicly owned rangeland in 16 western states, over 60% are considered to be in unsatisfactory condition, degraded by years of overgrazing and mismanagement. The many native species of fish and wildlife inhabiting these rangelands have been severely affected by the deteriorating ecological conditions; close to 90 animal species on federal lands are now listed as endangered or threatened because of environmental damage provoked by overgrazing. Rangeland riparian habitats—the narrow bands of lush vegetation bordering streams and lakes—have been particularly hard-hit. When oversized herds of cattle or sheep congregate in or along the edge of waterways, they trample and eat vegetation, pollute the water, and damage streambank stability. The resulting soil erosion and sedimentation may result in stream beds becoming shallower, warmer, and more turbid, negatively affecting aquatic life. Overgrazing is now regarded as the leading culprit blamed for the decline of native trout populations in western states.

Soil Erosion

Throughout much of the world, including the rich farmlands of the American Midwest, the fertile topsoil that is the basis of agricultural productivity is thinning at an alarming rate. Around the globe, over 25 billion tons of soil is lost to erosion annually, destroying over a billion acres (430 million hectares) of farmland—about 30% of the land currently under cultivation (Lal and Pierce, 1993; Stutz, 1993). Given the fact that under normal agricultural conditions it takes from 200 to 1,000 years to form an inch of topsoil, such losses could well undermine the productive capacity of farmlands if effective conservation strategies are not implemented. The Food and Agriculture Organization of the United Nations has warned that unless Third World countries give much higher priority to soil erosion control efforts, they could witness a 30% reduction in harvests by the end of the 21st century—at which time their populations will have increased by as much as sixfold over current levels.

Some degree of soil loss is, of course, a natural process and occurs even in

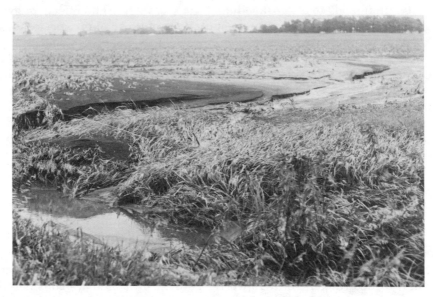

Sheet erosion after heavy rain robs farmland of valuable topsoil and causes water pollution and sedimentation problems in nearby streams and ditches. *[Gary Fak, Soil Conservation Service]*

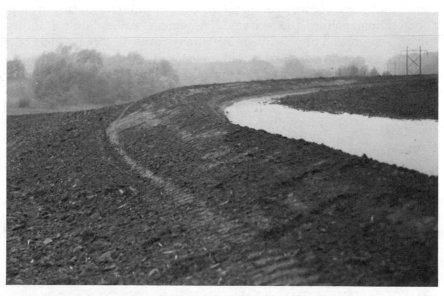

An effective erosion-control method is the construction of grass ridge terraces such as the one pictured here. A terrace reduces soil runoff by shortening the length of the slope and diverting water in a horizontal direction. When planted in perennial grasses, the approximately 10-foot-wide area has the additional benefit of providing valuable wildlife habitat. *[Gary Fak, Soil Conservation Service]*

the absence of human intervention. Poor agricultural practices, however, greatly increase the rate of erosion, and when the amount of topsoil lost exceeds that of new soil formed through the gradual decomposition of organic matter (an amount referred to in agricultural circles as **T-value** or, more simply, **"T"**), then the layer of topsoil becomes thinner and thinner until it disappears completely, leaving only the unproductive subsoil or, in extreme cases, bare rock. Topsoil loss has a direct negative impact on cropland productivity, though in recent decades the relationship between soil erosion and diminishing yields has been largely masked by the greatly expanded use of chemical fertilizers. We have, in a sense, been substituting chemical nitrogen and potash for topsoil in order to maintain good harvests. However, while chemicals can replace nutrients lost through erosion, they can't substitute for the lost organic material necessary for maintaining a porous, healthy soil structure. Some studies suggest that heavy fertilizer use can actually damage the soil by disrupting natural nutrient cycles and predict that in the future per acre yields, even on lands receiving chemical inputs, will begin to drop if erosion trends aren't reversed (Smil, 1991; *Yearbook of Agriculture,* 1981).

Serious erosion control efforts in the United States grew out of the disastrous Dust Bowl years of the mid-1930s when millions of tons of rich Great Plains topsoil were literally "gone with the wind" as a result of drought and unwise cultivation practices. In 1935 the Soil Conservation Service (SCS) was created and Congress funded a major research effort to learn more about the

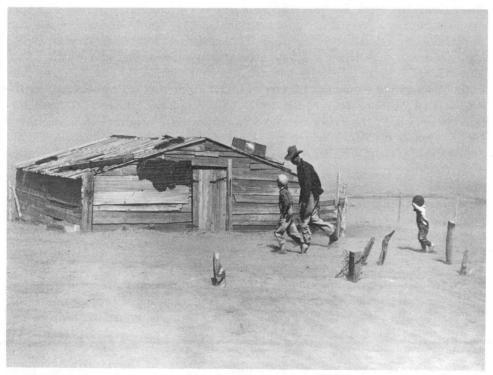

"Dust Bowl" years: an Oklahoma family runs for shelter during one of the numerous sky-blackening storms which afflicted the Great Plains states during the 1930s. *[U.S. Department of Agriculture]*

processes of erosion and effective methods of control. By the 1940s and 1950s soil loss on U.S. farmlands was declining noticeably as American farmers followed the advice of Cooperative Extension advisors ("county agents") or SCS personnel to install terraces, plant windbreaks, contour strip-crop, build grass waterways—whatever method or combination of methods was most suitable to reduce erosion rates on the lands they were cultivating.

By the 1970s, however, soil loss due to farmland erosion once again began to accelerate, reversing the gains of the previous two decades. High commodity prices and the demand for agricultural exports to feed growing populations overseas combined to boost farm production—and promoted record levels of erosion. Citing the link between farm exports and land degradation, an official at the Illinois Department of Agriculture remarked at the time that ". . . for every bushel of corn we ship overseas, we send 1½ bushels of topsoil down the Mississippi River." In the push for expanded production, the traditional practice of crop rotation was abandoned in favor of continuous cropping of corn or soybeans, a practice that greatly increases erosion rates since this leaves the soil surface without any plant cover during a considerable portion of the year. Strong export demand prompted farmers to plow "from fencepost-to-fencepost" to reap the maximum possible profit. By doing so, however, they brought into production much highly erodible land which would have been better left in pasture—and it promptly began to wash away. In the Midwest, fall plowing came into vogue and contributed to substantial amounts of erosion by both wind and water during winter and early spring when fields are bare. By the late 1970s it was evident that soil loss was once again becoming a serious national problem. In 1981 the USDA estimated that the inherent productivity of fully one-third of American farmlands was declining because of high rates of erosion. Efforts were launched at both the state and federal level to reduce soil loss to tolerable levels (i.e. to T-value). The main strategy for achieving this goal was the promotion of **conservation tillage,** a cultivation practice which involves leaving 30% or more of the soil surface covered with the previous year's crop residue. Variants on conservation tillage include **no-till,** in which crops are planted in the undisturbed residue of an old crop; **ridge-till,** where seeds are planted in ridges developed by cultivation of the field during the previous growing season and left undisturbed after the harvest; and **mulch-till,** a situation where crops are planted in a field where the entire surface has been disturbed, but at least the minimum amount of residue remains after planting. These crop residues perform a number of protective functions: cushioning the impact of falling raindrops, decreasing wind access to bare soil, serving as mini-dams to restrict overland runoff from fields, and improving soil characteristics which resist erosive forces. Alone or in combination with such soil conservation measures as terracing or construction of grass waterways, conservation tillage can substantially reduce erosion rates while maintaining or even increasing crop yields. While conservation tillage is not appropriate for all crops, the practice has expanded rapidly during the past two decades, particularly in corn- and soybean-producing areas of the Midwest. According to the USDA's Natural Resources Conservation Service (NRCS), by 1998 37% of cropped land in the U.S. was under some form of conservation tillage—still short of the NRSC national goal of 50% by 2002.

Erosion control efforts in the United States were given a major boost when Congress passed the **Food Security Act of 1985,** creating the **Conservation Reserve Program (CRP).** Under this landmark program, excessive production and soil loss are both being curbed by offering farmers financial incentives to take highly erodible or environmentally sensitive land out of production for 10 to 15 years, converting them to pastures or woodlands. By 1996, over 36 million acres, about 11% of all U.S. cropland, had been enrolled in Conservation Reserve Program contracts. Surveys by the NRCS indicate a 19-ton per acre reduction in soil loss from lands under CRP contract. Modifications to the CRP since its inception in 1985 have broadened the focus of conservation activities. Though CRP's original goal of controlling soil erosion remains a top priority, improving wildlife habitat and water quality are now important components of the program as well. Landowners are encouraged to sign up for high-priority conservation projects such as developing filter strips (areas of grass or other vegetation at the low end of fields that can filter out soil particles or other pollutants suspended in farmland runoff) or windbreaks. The magnitude and far-reaching scope of the Conservation Reserve Program makes it the federal government's single largest environmental improvement program and represents a major success story in reversing soil loss on U.S. agricultural lands (USDA, 1997).

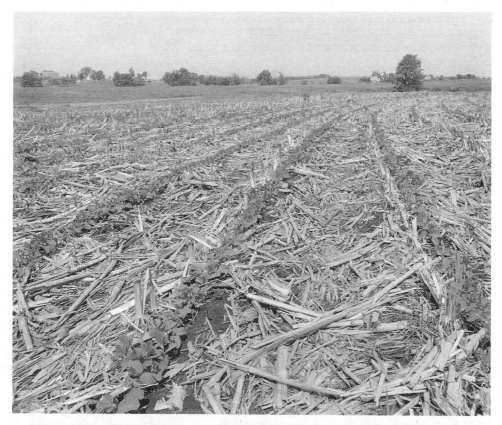

No-till farming: young soybean plants emerge from a field whose surface is protected from erosion by a cushioning layer of corn stubble. *[U.S. Department of Agriculture]*

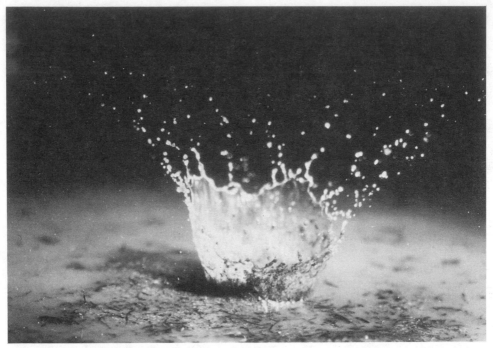

Each drop of rain strikes bare soil like a tiny bomb, propelling soil particles into the air; subsequent overland flow of rainwater across a field carries these loosened particles into waterways, resulting in the annual loss of enormous quantities of topsoil. *[U.S. Department of Agriculture]*

Currently the United States is the only major agricultural nation pursuing systematic efforts to reduce excessive soil erosion, yet outside this country the situation is even more serious. Indian agronomists estimate their country is losing 5 billion tons of topsoil annually, almost double the soil loss in the United States where the cropland area is about the same (Brown, 1988). In Ethiopia erosion is depriving that nation's hard-pressed farmers of 1.5 to 2 billion cubic meters of topsoil every year; as a result, 4 million hectares (about 10 million acres) of Ethiopian highlands are now termed "irreversibly degraded." At the foothills of the Himalayas, in eastern Nepal, 38% of the land area consists of barren fields, abandoned because their topsoil has been lost to erosion (Stutz, 1993). In the lush farmlands of central Chile, the current prosperity may be short-lived because excessive rates of soil loss are undermining agricultural productivity even on the best lands; on the marginal lands where over half the country's peasant farmers live, erosion is seriously depressing crop yields and threatening farmers with large financial losses if current trends are not reversed (Faeth, 1994). In China, soil erosion is endangering increases in crop production desperately needed to feed a still-growing population. In China's northwestern Gansu Province, half or more of all arable land has already been lost to erosion and encroaching deserts. Alarmed by the shrinking resource base, a Canadian scientist who studied environmental problems in China commented, "You can clean up air pollution, but once you ruin your soil it is very difficult to go back. Land is the irreplaceable foundation of China's food production" (Tyler, 1994).

Although soil erosion is the most obvious form of land degradation, other processes may play a role as well. Compaction or crusting of soils may occur as a result of improper methods of mechanical tillage; depletion of soil nutrients results when crops are repeatedly grown on the same land without sufficient fallow periods or, alternatively, the replacement of nutrients through the use of manure, cover crops, or appropriate amounts of chemical fertilizers. Extensive land degradation in arid regions of the world has been caused by poor water management on irrigated fields. Failure to drain such areas adequately can result in the salinization or water-logging of soils. The former process occurs when salts naturally present in certain soils are dissolved by rising water tables under poorly drained irrigated fields and eventually accumulate at the soil surface, poisoning crop roots. Currently between 10–15% of all irrigated lands are plagued by water-logging or salinization. In the case of salt-affected lands, restoration efforts may take generations, with some lands never recovering. In Australia, 10% of the land area is now suffering from salinization and experts there worry that the percentage could grow to 40% within the next 50 years. Other regions threatened by salinization include irrigated areas of Iraq, Turkey, Pakistan, northern India, China, and the American Southwest.

Deforestation

For the last ten thousand years humans have been cutting and burning woodlands at an ever-increasing pace in their quest for additional farmland, fuel, and building material. Forests still cover slightly over one-fourth of the world's land area (excluding Greenland and Antarctica), but recent decades have witnessed a significant decline in both the area covered by forests and in the quality of remaining woodlands. In spite of increased forest protection efforts in many parts of the world, in 1999 the FAO announced that global forest cover is still shrinking by 28 million acres per year. At the end of the 20th century only 40% of lands categorized as "forested" are high-quality **frontier forests**—relatively undisturbed, extensive areas that remain ecologically intact. The remaining 60% consist of secondary forests, tree plantations, open woodlands, and brushlands. Frontier forests today are largely limited to the northern boreal forests of Russia, Canada, and Alaska and to the tropical forests of the northwestern Amazon basin and the Guyana Shield along South America's northern coast. These remaining frontier forests cover scarcely one-third the areas they occupied before human activities set in motion the processes of deforestation that have markedly accelerated within recent decades. As the rate of forest loss accelerates, so do pressures on ecosystems as species loss, soil erosion—even climate change—become increasingly apparent.

Deforestation, defined as the permanent decline in crown cover of trees to less than 10% of its original extent, is regarded as particularly worrisome in regard to tropical forests, where most of the deforestation of the past 30–40 years has occurred. Unfortunately, rates of loss continue to accelerate. Between 1960–1990, one-fifth of tropical forests were destroyed, including over 30% of those in Asia and approximately 18% in Latin America and Africa. Tropical deforestation continued apace during the 1990s. Regional averages for tree loss understate the severity of the problem in certain countries. Just

Figure 5-1   Estimated Tropical Deforestation Rates, 1960-90

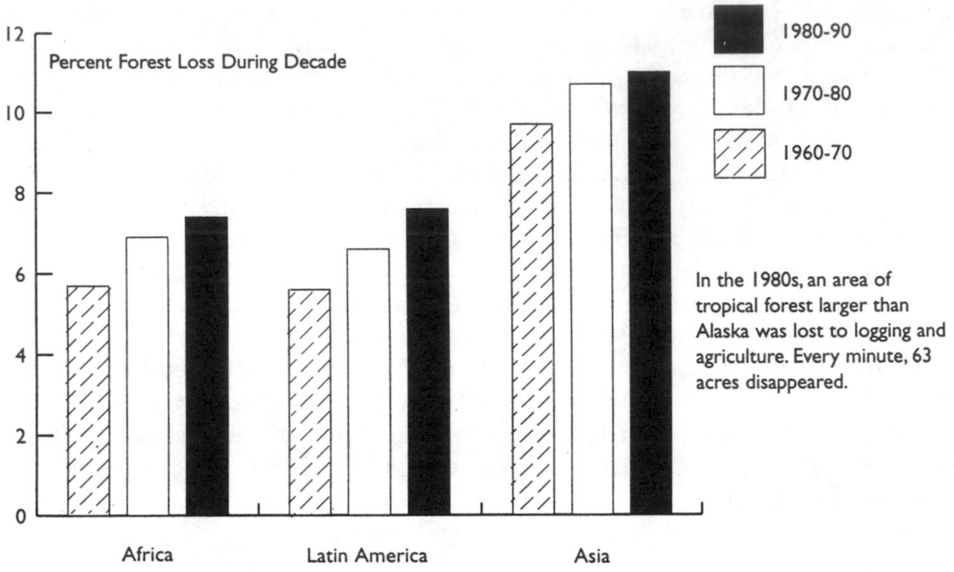

Percent Forest Loss During Decade

■ 1980-90

□ 1970-80

▨ 1960-70

In the 1980s, an area of tropical forest larger than Alaska was lost to logging and agriculture. Every minute, 63 acres disappeared.

Africa   Latin America   Asia

Source: Why Population Matters. Population Action International, 1996.

seven nations experienced over half of all forest lost between 1980–1995: Brazil, Malaysia, Indonesia, Congo, Bolivia, Venezuela, and Mexico (Abramovitz, 1998).

Elsewhere, in the semiarid regions of Asia, Africa, and Latin America where forests have always been scanty, existing forests have almost entirely vanished. Only in Europe and, quite recently, in North America are forests being managed on a sustained-yield basis. In the United States, wooded areas have expanded significantly over the past 50 years, as once-cleared marginal farmlands revert to forest. As a result, the nation's total timber volume has increased by 30%. In Europe as well, the growing stock of wood increased by 25% between 1971–1990 (Moffat, 1998). However, this overall increase in forest biomass obscures the fact that large areas of temperate old-growth forest have been replaced by tree plantations, often comprising but a single species that is grown and harvested within a relatively short time period. Such plantations can be ecologically beneficial for reducing erosion, regenerating degraded soils (e.g. pulpwood plantations in the U.S. Southeast now thriving on abandoned cotton acreage), or providing fuelwood for local consumption. Nevertheless, they are much less biologically diverse than the primary forest ecosystems which once flourished in those regions.

The largest single cause of deforestation today, as in the past, is the **clearing of land for agriculture.** The population pressures behind this trend and the ecological damage caused by exploitation of marginal lands not suited for sustained cultivation have already been described. The Cote d'Ivoire

(Ivory Coast) provides a classic example of such pressures. With an annual population growth rate averaging between 3–4% until quite recently, slash-and-burn farmers have destroyed fully 95% of the forest cover in that West African nation (Tobias, 1998). A second major contributor to deforestation, also a direct result of human population growth, is the **gathering of wood for fuel.** The FAO estimates that approximately half of all wood cut in the world today is used for firewood or for making charcoal. For approximately 90% of the people in the world's less-developed nations, today's true energy crisis is the scarcity of firewood. In most tropical countries wood is used largely for cooking, but in colder climates and mountainous regions it's used for heating as well. Spiralling population growth rates in such nations have boosted demand for firewood to such an extent that trees are being cut at a pace which far outraces nature's ability to grow new ones. As a result, treeless areas around towns and villages throughout Africa, Asia, and Latin America are expanding rapidly as desperate people gather every twig and sometimes even leaves and bark in their never-ending search for fuel.

The problem is particularly acute in semiarid regions where removal of vegetation leaves land at the mercy of wind and water, subject to rapid rates of soil loss. In once heavily forested lands such as Nepal, whole mountainsides are being stripped by villagers who now spend most of the day searching for a supply of firewood which a few decades ago could have been gathered in an hour. The investment in time and physical energy required just to obtain enough fuel to cook the family meal has thus increased tremendously in just one generation. Of greater concern to Nepali officials, however, and to their counterparts in the vast Indian subcontinent to the south is the fact that the progressive denudation of the Himalayan slopes is resulting in a massive increase in soil erosion in this ecologically fragile mountain region. As a result, not only is the productive capacity of the land rapidly decreasing, but also much more frequent and severe flooding is occurring downstream in the river valleys of northern India, Pakistan, and Bangladesh due to greatly increased amounts of runoff in the headwaters area of the Ganges, Indus, and Brahmaputra rivers. The devastating floods that regularly leave millions homeless and kill thousands during the subcontinent's monsoon season represent an "unnatural disaster" caused by increased runoff from the denuded Himalayan watershed upstream and increased rates of siltation in lowland deltas that diminish their water-holding capacity. While severe flooding used to occur perhaps twice in a century, "50-year floods" have become regular events, thanks to progressive deforestation in the Himalayas.

As the supply of fuelwood continues to diminish, prices rise accordingly, imposing additional burdens on already impoverished populations. In the West African nation of Niger, for example, an average laborer's family must spend close to 25% of its income for firewood; in neighboring Burkina Faso the figure may approach 30% (exploitation of forest resources for fuel is more acute in African nations than anywhere else in the world; fully 90% of all the wood harvested in Africa is burned directly or used for making charcoal). Where people can't afford the high cost of wood, women and children spend much of their time scrounging the countryside for anything burnable—dry grass, fallen leaves, animal dung, garbage—a practice that in the long run further degrades the soil which is being robbed of these natural fertilizers. In the

Figure 5-2   Loss of Original Forest Cover by Region

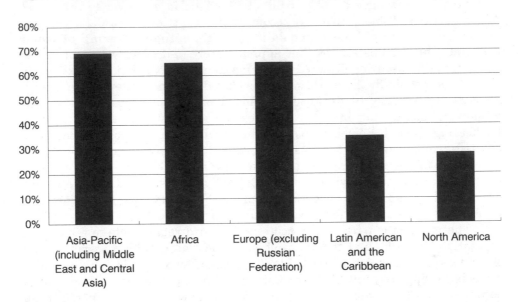

Source: Loh et al., *The Living Planet*, World Wide Fund for Nature, 1998; Population Action International.

industrialized nations, which until about 100 years ago had been just as dependent on wood for fuel as the developing countries are today, the substitution of coal, petroleum products, and natural gas for wood forestalled a growing pressure on their forests for fuel. In the developing world, increasing use of kerosene or bottled gas stoves has slightly eased the burdens on those nations' timber resources among those who can afford them. Unfortunately, for millions of the world's poorest people such wood substitutes remain priced out of reach.

While the clearing of land for subsistence farming and the increasing demand for fuelwood are two of the most prominent factors resulting in destruction of forests on a worldwide basis, in some areas, most notably in Southeast Asia but recently in South America as well, **commercial lumbering** is decimating valuable tropical hardwood reserves in order to supply the increased demands of industrial nations for furniture, plywood, and paper pulp. Until relatively recently, tropical forests largely escaped the logging pressures which earlier had decimated the virgin forests of Europe and North America, primarily because they were sparsely populated and not easily accessible. In addition, in tropical forests commercially valuable tree species are widely dispersed over a broad geographic area, interspersed with many less-desired species, a fact which made their large-scale exploitation economically unfeasible. This situation changed dramatically in the 1960s when mechanization of the timber industry and the arrival of giant multinational lumber companies made possible the ever-more-rapid felling of tropical forests. The methods employed by these companies have been particularly destructive and wasteful; in a typical operation only 10–20% of the trees are cut and removed (i.e. those species with commercial value), but 30–50% of nontarget trees are destroyed in the process. On many tracts, trees are felled by utilizing giant tractors, working in tandem, to drag huge link chains across the forest floor, pulling down everything in their path. This process causes such extensive soil damage that the land may never fully recover. During the 1990s, the use of fire to clear vast tracts of land became the principle means of deforestation in the Amazon and was widely employed in Indonesia as well. In late 1997, fires set to clear new land for rice cultivation and tree plantations burned out of control, spreading through at least 2 million hectares of forest and igniting underground deposits of peat. The fires cast a pall of smoke across much of Southeast Asia for several months, creating serious air quality problems as far away as Malaysia, Singapore, the Philippines, and Thailand (Abramovitz, 1998).

While commercial lumbering in the tropics has taken its greatest toll thus far in Southeast Asia, the near-exhaustion of primary forests in that region has prompted timber barons to shift their attention to South America, particularly to Bolivia, where logging concessions have been granted for more than half that nation's forest lands; to Guyana, where more than 80% of government-owned forests have been leased to wealthy Korean and Malayasian timber companies on terms extremely generous to the Asian firms; and to Chile, where the world's largest remaining expanse of still-pristine temperate rain forest is being felled at an alarming rate to meet the insatiable demands

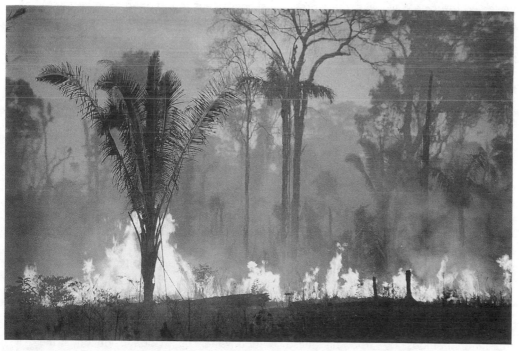

Vast areas of the Amazon rain forest have been destroyed in recent years by fires set to clear new land. *[John Maier Jr./NYT Pictures]*

BOX 5-1
Certification and Eco-Labels: Promoting Healthy Forests

In many parts of the world today commercial lumbering operations are not only ecologically devastating—over the long term they also are unsustainable. Seeking to extract maximum profits as quickly as possible, industrial timber interests from Indonesia to Canada are treating forests like mines, extracting wealth without replenishing it. In tropical regions, less than 0.1% of forests are managed on a sustained yield basis; even Canada, the world's second-largest timber producer and supposed role model for world-class forestry practices, is harvesting its Pacific Coast forests at a rate 20% above sustainable levels.

For many years the response from environmentalists was to urge that tracts of yet-intact woodlands be set aside as protected reserves. While wilderness preservation remains a desirable objective, marketplace demand for forest products continues to grow; in the U.S. alone, wood consumption has doubled since the 1950s. Setting aside all forest lands in the name of conservation simply isn't an option. Consequently, a movement aimed at combining economically viable forest management practices with sound conservation principles has recently been gaining adherents. Based on an approach known as **sustainable forest management (SFM)**, forests are to be managed as intact ecosystems, capable of supplying a wide variety of goods and services for generations to come.

Doing so successfully requires an understanding of how complex forest ecosystems function, using such knowledge to define SFM practices, and formulating methods for applying these principles to the wide variety of forest types and economic systems around the world. Forestry experts, biologists, economists, and several international bodies have been wrestling with these issues for a number of years and have reached a general consensus that sustainable forests should preserve biodiversity, protect water quality, and respect the rights of indigenous peoples to participate meaningfully in forest management programs.

Proponents of SFM realized this new approach would have little appeal to the industrial timber interests who would have to implement it unless a demand could be created for sustainably managed forest products, which usually cost more. Although the differential diminishes over time, it's estimated that initial costs of doing business following SFM principles may be 10–15% higher than using the conventional approach. Many skeptics thus questioned whether SFM-produced lumber would find buyers. By the early 1990s it was evident that a growing number of consumers were indeed willing to pay a premium for "green" wood products, provided they could be assured the timber was grown and harvested in an environmentally responsible manner. They were confused, however, by the plethora of unverifiable and often misleading claims (e.g. "environmentally friendly," "sustainable") employed by marketers. What obviously was needed was an independent third party to evaluate forest management practices and to certify compliance with performance standards. As prestigious an institution as the World Bank endorsed the concept of forest certification, stating that "experience with other products suggests that consumers will modify their behavior substantially if they are given information on the ecological sustainability of the production process."

Responding to the situation, a consortium of foresters, timber producers and traders, environmental groups, organizations representing indigenous forest peoples, and certification institutions joined forces in 1993 to form the nonprofit **Forest Stewardship Council (FSC)**. Established to coordinate the diverse certification programs which were proliferating in a number of countries, as well as to accredit certifiers, FSC is the first international program to be accepted by major retailers and to win public confidence for marketing claims.

Within a year of its inception, FSC adopted a set of principles and criteria describing sustainable forestry management practices and published guidelines for the conduct of field inspections. By 1995 the group had developed a stringent framework for evaluating, accrediting, and subsequently monitoring the certifiers who validate producers' claims of sustainable forest management practices. Certifiers accredited by FSC are authorized to audit operations of timber companies wishing to use the FSC logo (an eco-label for wood products equivalent to the "Good Housekeeping Seal of Approval"). If the petitioning company's entire chain of custody, from forest to processing, meets FSC's high standards, certification will be awarded, along with environmental labeling rights.

For consumers, the FSC logo provides assurance that the wood they are purchasing comes from a sustainably managed forest; retailers carrying FSC-certified timber products are motivated by good business sense and a desire to reap customer good-will; and suppliers trust that FSC certification will provide them with a marketplace advantage and help to distinguish their company from its competitors.

The most favorable response to lumber certification thus far has been in Europe, particularly in Germany, the Netherlands, Belgium, and the United Kingdom. In the latter country, a buyers group that has pledged to phase out marketing of noncertified wood products represents about one-quarter of the British market. FSC-certified timber is making gradual headway in the U.S. as well, though the concept has not yet sparked the general enthusiasm currently enjoyed by recycling programs. In Japan, which purchases more than a third of all raw lumber traded internationally, certified wood products were virtually unknown until quite recently, a situation reflected in many other Asian countries where the lumber business is booming.

While the overall impact of FSC's initiatives remains limited, by 1999 more than 37 million acres of commercial forest lands (4.8 million in the U.S.) had been awarded FSC certification. Perhaps just as important, FSC activities have prompted the establishment of rival industry-based programs that co-opt FSC's goal of improving forest management. Several years ago the American Forest & Paper Association, a major trade group for the pulp and paper industry, launched its Sustainable Forestry Initiative (SFI), which establishes management guidelines timber companies must follow as a condition of membership in the professional organization. Although SFI has no enforcement powers or any specific standards, it does push member companies in the direction of more environmentally responsible practices.

In the long run, success of certification programs in maintaining healthy forests hinges on whether consumers will use their purchasing power to safeguard forest ecosystems. If purchasers refuse to buy wood products not displaying the FSC logo, market demand would give timber producers a strong pocketbook incentive to manage forests sustainably. Despite the minuscule market share captured by FSC-certified companies to date, timber certification is sending a strong signal to the wood products industry. According to the author of a 1995 World Bank report on the subject, while not all companies will upgrade their practices enough to meet FSC's strict requirements, the very existence of such standards has the potential to improve forestry practices around the world.

References
Abramovitz, Janet N. 1998. "Taking a Stand: Cultivating a New Relationship with the World's Forests." *Worldwatch Paper 140* (April).
Wagner, Michael. 1997. "Building Forests, Growing Homes." *Amicus Journal* 19, no. 1 (Spring):17-22.

of Japanese paper producers for wood chips. Environmentalists fully expect to see the same well-documented pattern of land degradation and abuse which have accompanied logging operations in Africa, Malayasia, Indonesia, and Papua New Guinea repeated in South America. In political systems where politicians control the distribution of timber concessions, bribery and corruption ensure the overexploitation of forest resources with minimal regulation of environmental damage. Careless logging practices frequently result in permanent ecological degradation and those charged with enforcing sound forest management practices are either bought off or become totally frustrated by their inability to prosecute loggers whose political connections insulate them from any enforcement actions. Land rights of indigenous forest peoples, 50 million of whom still make their home within the tropical rain forest, are another casualty of commercial logging operations in the tropics. Preexisting tribal claims are seldom considered when timber concessions are granted and native peoples frequently suffer total impoverishment after logging destroys the forest resources which sustained these groups for millennia (Colchester, 1994; Nash, 1993, 1994).

International efforts to promote sustainable timber harvesting in the tropics have been hampered by a North-South divergence of economic interests. At the 1992 Earth Summit in Brazil, attempts to produce a world forestry agreement calling on developing nations to adopt tougher conservation policies to protect tropical forests were stymied by Third World insistence that the industrialized North similarly pledge its members to observe environmentally friendly logging practices in temperate forests. Charges of hypocrisy by developing countries are understandable in light of the unsustainable logging practices of timber companies in the Pacific Northwest. In the Canadian province of British Columbia, where two-thirds of the coastal rain forest has been degraded by logging and development, official government policy since 1945 has been the elimination of all old-growth forest. Logging in the region has more than doubled since the late 1960s and the annual allowable cut is 20% higher than long-term harvest levels. The destructive clear-cutting of the region's rich temperate rain forests has earned British Columbia the pejorative nickname, "Brazil of the North" (Abramovitz, 1998).

The years following the 1992 Earth Summit have seen little meaningful progress in international efforts to combat tropical deforestation, though numerous forums and commissions have been convened to discuss the issue and to urge nations to take action. Environmental groups are skeptical that governments influenced by powerful vested interests are yet prepared to deal seriously with the problems of tropical forest loss.

In Latin America, **cattle-ranching** has imposed additional pressures on threatened forests. In such Central American nations as Costa Rica and Panama, cattle ranching has destroyed more hectares of tropical forest than any other activity—70% of the land formerly covered by trees in both countries is now utilized as pastureland (Coffin, 1993). During the 1980s much of this destruction was driven by the demand for cheap beef to supply fast-food chains in the United States—the infamous "hamburger connection," now largely curtailed. In Brazil, cattle ranching is a major cause of deforestation in the Amazon basin, the largest continuous tract of tropical forest in the world. Since the 1970s, ranchers have cleared more than 10 million hectares of rain forest for pastureland, a practice originally encouraged by generous tax breaks and subsidies from a Brazilian government eager to develop the vast interior of that nation while providing an abundant supply of inexpensive meat for working-class consumers in the country's large coastal cities. In recent years subsidy programs have been terminated, but ranchers continue to clear new pasture as a form of land speculation—a means of obtaining legal title to such lands at a time of rapidly rising property values. Unfortunately, as in the case of agricultural exploitation in Amazonia, grazing pressures on these deforested tracts can be sustained profitably for only a few years. When the fragile tropical soils wear out, their content of phosphorus and other nutrients depleted, ranchers simply move on, burn or cut down more trees, and thus perpetuate the destructive cycle. Although the abandoned pasturelands are subsequently revegetated by invader plant species, the new biotic community bears little resemblance to the original forest either in biomass or in biodiversity. Observations of ecological succession in areas of rain forest denuded by ranching operations suggest that regeneration of such areas to mature forest conditions may require several centuries (World Resources Institute, 1990).

That destruction of the earth's forest cover will have a serious and adverse impact on terrestrial ecosystems—and on their human inhabitants as well—is undisputed. Past history should have taught us that heedless deforestation can lead to excessive erosion rates, decrease the soil's water-absorbing capacity, increase the amount of runoff and flooding, and lead to the transformation of once-productive environments into desert-like conditions. Today we have growing evidence to indicate that loss of forest cover can also lead to local climatic changes, with an increase in temperature and drop in annual rainfall when large expanses of woodland are cleared. More ominous is the possibility that heedless deforestation will hasten the onset of global warming, due to the pivotal role forests play as a "carbon sink," absorbing CO_2, and thereby counteracting the so-called "Greenhouse Effect."

One might suppose that since the consequences of deforestation are well understood, a serious attempt to reverse current trends would be well underway. Unfortunately, in many of the countries most seriously affected reforestation efforts are negligible. Even where the political will exists and funds are available, large-scale tree-planting programs encounter serious difficulties which are inextricably related to the cultural, political, and economic facts of life in rural societies. In many areas saplings planted with high hopes are promptly devoured by overabundant and freely-roaming goats, sheep, and cattle. In some places nomads passing through an area may decimate a village's efforts at reforestation, while in still other areas villagers themselves may uproot young trees because they simply have no other source of fuel. Successful reforestation efforts require extensive administrative efforts to protect the plants for years—efforts which may be politically unrewarding to officials trying to win voters' approval for next year's election rather than a "job well done" 20 years in the future. There have been some reforestation success stories, most notably in India where approximately four hectares of trees are being planted for every one that is deforested. Although these tree plantations, which consist primarily of fast-growing eucalyptus or pine, lack the diversity of species which characterized the native forest cover, they nevertheless provide soil and watershed protection while serving as windbreaks and a renewable source of fuel for local residents.

Ultimately the most serious obstacle to curbing forest loss is the continued rapid growth of human populations in the countries most affected. As a Costa Rican squatter on a partially forested ranch poignantly stated, "By subsisting today I know I can destroy the future of the forest and the people. But I have to eat today" (Hamilton, 1989).

Desertification

That humans can create desert-like conditions on once-productive land has been known, though largely ignored, since the time 2300 years ago when Plato bewailed the ecological fate of his native Attica, writing that "our land, compared with what it was, is like the skeleton of a body wasted by disease. The soft, plump parts have vanished and all that remains is the bare carcass." This sorry situation was brought about by the cutting of forests and overgrazing of livestock, which in that semiarid climate inevitably resulted in erosion of topsoil and the drying up of springs that were no longer being recharged, since rainwater quickly ran off the bare ground rather than percolating through the soil. The formation of cultural wastelands which occurred over two millennia ago in Greece and the lands around the eastern Mediterranean is a process that has so increased in extent during the 20th century that it has been graced with the somewhat unwieldy, though descriptive, term **desertification.** Defined by delegates at the 1992 United Nations Conference on Environment and Development (UNCED) as "land degradation in arid, semiarid, and dry sub-humid areas resulting from various factors including climatic variations and human activities," desertification today is adversely affecting the lives and economic well-being of an estimated 900 million people in over 100 countries. According to a report presented by World Bank officials at the UN-sponsored Convention on Desertification held in Dakar, Senegal, in 1998, economic losses worldwide caused by desertification total more than $42 billion each year.

Contrary to the prevailing image of sand dunes relentlessly sweeping down over green fields and pastures, desertification seldom involves the steady influx of sands along a uniform front. Most often the process is set in motion when climatic fluctuations and abusive land-use practices interact to extend desert-like conditions irregularly over susceptible land. Spots of extreme degradation are especially likely to form around water holes when nearby pastures are heavily grazed and trampled and around towns when people denude adjacent lands in their search for fuelwood. Since desertification first captured world attention in the 1960s and 1970s, it has generally been assumed that population pressures have been the primary cause. Recently, however, data obtained from a decade's worth of satellite photos indicate that climatic variations exert a much more pronounced influence on the expansion of desert-like conditions than do human pressures. In the world's arid grasslands and semi-desert regions, year-to-year fluctuations of rainfall can be moderately destructive to biotic communities even under natural conditions, but in the long run natural processes can correct the imbalance and quickly reestablish pre-drought vegetational patterns. However, when environmental stresses due to normal climatic variation are coupled with pressures created by human activities (e.g. overgrazing, fuelwood gathering, poor cultivation practices), problems of land degradation are seriously aggravated. If such human pressures persist and intensify, they can sharply limit the regenerative capabilities of the land, hindering its recovery even after climatic conditions improve (Hulme and Kelly, 1993; Stevens, 1994).

Whatever its cause, desertification is a process occurring today on an unprecedented scale. The human tragedy embodied in the great dust storms that blackened the skies in the American prairie states during the 1930s is being repeated today in sub-Saharan Africa, where the nomadic herdsmen and their oversized flocks seem to have pushed the carrying capacity of the land beyond the point of no return; in northwest India, the world's most densely populated arid zone and, thanks to the large herds of cattle, camels, goats, etc., also perhaps the world's dustiest area; in North Africa, where excessive rates of soil erosion are accelerating the pace of desertification on lands that were once the granary of the Roman Empire; in China, where sand-break forests are being planted in a desperate effort to combat sandstorms that threaten almost 9 million hectares of agricultural lands and cause direct economic losses valued at approximately $800 million annually; and in the American Southwest, where overgrazing during the past several hundred years may be largely responsible for the formation of Arizona's Sonoran Desert. Many of these areas still have the potential to reestablish their former grassland ecosystems if the constant pressure of overgrazing and overplowing could be lifted, but some have been irreversibly degraded by complete loss of topsoil. If human pressures continue to mount, degradation of arid lands will result in the permanent destabilization of existing ecosystems and a continuing impoverishment of both ecological and cultural conditions. Ecosystems, like civilizations, can decline and fall if pushed too far.

Wetlands Loss

Swamps, bogs, fens, tidal marshlands, pocosins, estuaries, ponds, river bottoms, flood plains, and prairie potholes all fall under the designation of **wetlands,** ecosystems characterized by soils which are inundated or water-saturated for at least a portion of the year and by the presence of certain water-loving plants ("hydrophytes"). In the not-too-distant past, most people viewed wetlands as a nuisance, useful only to frogs and mosquitoes, and thus prime candidates for draining or filling to convert them into more "profitable" areas for farming, mining, or urban development. As a result, over half the wetlands which existed in the contiguous 48 states at the time European settlers first arrived (estimated at more than 200 million acres in A.D. 1600) have now disappeared. Fortunately, the rate of loss has declined in recent years, thanks to federal legislation protecting wetlands. In 1997 the U.S. Fish and Wildlife Service released its decennial estimate on wetlands status and trends, reporting that the average annual net loss of wetlands has dropped by about 60% since 1985, from 290,000 acres per year to a mid-1990s level of 117,000 acres annually. Today, wetlands cover just 5% (104 million acres) of the land surface in the lower 48 states. Alaska has another 200 million acres, with wetlands extending across half the North Star State. Outside Alaska, Florida and Louisiana have the largest remaining expanses of wetlands, though they are also among the states with the highest rates of wetlands loss in recent years. California has lost a greater percentage of its original wetlands than any other state (91%), but Florida has lost the largest number of acres (*America's Wetlands,* 1988; World Resources Institute, 1992). In recent years the significance of this loss has finally begun to be realized, and belated efforts to control wetlands conversion are now underway at both the federal and state level.

Today the importance of wetlands in both ecological and economic terms is unquestioned. Their ability to retain large amounts of water makes them extremely valuable as nature's own method of preventing devastating floods. Not surprisingly, as wetlands along the Mississippi River Valley have been destroyed, the severity and frequency of floods in that region has escalated—a fact made tragically clear during the disastrous flooding along the upper Mississippi River Valley in the summer of 1993. Wetlands provide the major recharge areas for groundwater reserves and also serve as "living filters" for purifying contaminated surface waters as these percolate into the ground. Indeed, taking advantage of wetlands' capacity to act as "nature's kidneys," some communities are now utilizing constructed marshes to treat stormwater or secondary wastewater effluent by directing the flow through **engineered wetlands** where living organisms remove pollutants efficiently and inexpensively. The sustained productivity of commercial fisheries is also heavily dependent on the existence of wetlands. Between 60–90% of fish caught along the Atlantic and Gulf coasts spend at least some portion of their life cycle, usually the vulnerable early stages, in coastal marshes or estuaries. Further inland in the Midwest, the system of lakes, marshes, and prairie potholes extending from the Gulf of Mexico north into Canada provides the major life-support system for millions of migratory waterfowl (half of all ducklings in North America are hatched in the prairie potholes of the Dakotas and Canada). A $1 billion recreational hunting industry, attracting 2.5 million duck hunters each year, is thus totally dependent on preservation of these vital wetlands breeding areas. Wetlands also provide a habitat not only for ducks and geese but for many other bird and mammal species—whooping cranes, river otters, black bears, and so on.

Although some wetlands are lost due to natural causes such as erosion, land subsidence, storms, or saltwater intrusion, human activities account for

Figure 5-3   Percentage of Wetlands Acreage Lost, 1780s–1980s

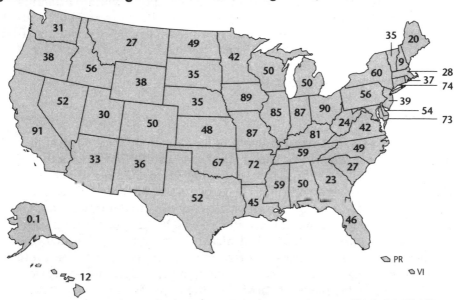

Source: USEPA. 1998. *National Water Quality Inventory: 1996 Report to Congress.* EPA-841-R-97-008.

by far the greatest amount of loss. Draining swamps or bottomlands for agricultural purposes is the leading cause of wetlands destruction. The Fish and Wildlife Service estimates that in spite of federal incentive programs for farmers to preserve wetlands, fully 79% of current wetlands loss can be traced to drainage for agricultural use. Coastal development has also taken a heavy toll of wetlands, particularly along estuaries that provide vital habitat and breeding grounds for many commercially valuable fish and shellfish species. Dredging for canals and port construction, flood control projects, and road building have all had a negative impact on wetlands, as has urban sprawl. In the southeastern states, the clearing and draining of deep-soil swamps for conversion to pine plantations resulted in extensive wetlands loss until 1994, when the EPA banned such activities. While there are no federal laws expressly prohibiting the draining, filling or converting of most wetlands, Congress took a small step toward protecting our remaining wetlands when it included a section in the 1985 farm bill referred to as the "Swampbuster Provision," aimed at discouraging draining of wetlands for agriculture by stating that farmers who do so will lose their farm program benefits. The Conservation Reserve Program, enacted under that same legislation, provided farmers with financial incentives to protect lands taken out of cultivation and thereby fostered the restoration of critical wetlands habitat. Government agencies and private organizations such as the Nature Conservancy and Ducks Unlimited also have worked cooperatively to reestablish habitat for dwindling wetlands species. The success of these efforts, resulting in the restoration of hundreds of thousands of acres of prairie potholes, was dramatically evident by the mid-1990s when breeding populations of waterfowl rebounded to their highest levels since the 1970s (Stevens, 1994).

Since almost three-fourths of all wetlands acreage in the United States is privately owned, the ultimate success of wetlands preservation attempts hinge on efforts by both government and environmental organizations to educate landowners on the intrinsic value of wetlands, to encourage wetlands conservation and restoration, and to provide the technical assistance and financial incentives which will persuade property owners to protect our nation's precious wetland resources.

Loss of Biodiversity

Extinction of a species, like the death of an individual, is a natural process. As fossil evidence clearly indicates, many groups of plants and animals which dominated life on earth in past millennia have died out, only to be replaced by newly evolving organisms. The rise and fall of species throughout the course of earth's history was determined largely by a population's ability to adapt to changing environmental conditions or to become increasingly specialized for life in a particular ecological niche. As evolution proceeded, the number of plant and animal species proliferated as populations dispersed into far-flung geographic regions and adapted to life in a seemingly endless variety of ecological niches. Today biologists have classified approximately 1.8 million species of living things, but estimate that the actual number currently in existence, many yet undiscovered, ranges from 3 to 30 million, the largest number being small creatures living in tropical forests and in the deep oceans. Unfortunately, it is widely feared that many of these species will vanish before their existence is ever noted or recorded.

The sad truth of the present situation is that human actions have greatly accelerated the rate at which species are becoming extinct; indeed, for the first time since the last great die-off at the end of the Cretaceous Period 65 million years ago, species are vanishing more rapidly than new ones are evolving, resulting in a diminishing diversity of life forms. The first recorded animal extinction—that of the European lion—was documented in A.D. 80; more than half of the animal species which have disappeared since that time have become extinct since 1900. Just as human populations have been increasing at an ever-faster pace in recent centuries, so has the rate of species loss. While estimates indicate that over the vast span of geologic time one mammalian species suffers extinction every 400 years and one bird species every 200, the record for the past 400 years shows a dramatic acceleration in the rate of extinction: 58 mammalian species and 115 bird species (World Conservation Monitoring Centre, 1992). Even these numbers don't accurately represent the true toll, especially for recent decades, since, by international agreement, a species isn't classified as extinct until 50 years after its last sighting. In addition, with millions of species still undiscovered and unnamed, it is quite likely that large numbers are quietly disappearing, unnoticed and unmourned (Wilcove, McMillan, and Winston, 1993). By 1996 approximately 25% of mammalian species and 11% of bird species worldwide were threatened with extinction (Tuxill, 1998). When *all* types of organisms are considered—not just the feathered or furry creatures which appeal to human emotions, but the myriads of insects, mollusks, fish, fungi, plants, and other organisms which greatly enrich the diversity of life—then current rates of extinction are even

BOX 5-2

New Hope for the Everglades

The Everglades, Florida's legendary "River of Grass" and the world's largest freshwater marsh, is today one of the most threatened ecosystems in the United States. Under incremental attack for more than a century by humans who have dredged, drained, and diked this once-vast swampland, the Everglades has shrunk to little more than half of its original 4 million acres, stretching from Lake Okeechobee in central Florida more than 100 miles south to Florida Bay. In 1948 Congress authorized the U.S. Army Corps of Engineers to launch the **Central and South Florida (C&SF) Project,** a mammoth multi-purpose water management effort intended to provide flood control, ensure a dependable water supply for urban and agricultural consumers, prevent saltwater intrusion into aquifers, and to preserve conditions beneficial to wildlife, navigation, and outdoor recreation. While the Corps continues to insist that the C&SF Project performed its functions well, making it possible for over 5 million people to live and work in the 18,000 square mile area, many view the Project's ultimate consequences as an ecological disaster.

The insatiable water demands of irrigated agriculture and of cities lining the Sunshine State's "Gold Coast," along with flood control projects and natural droughts, have disrupted the natural sheet flow of water which for millennia sustained the natural rhythms of life throughout the Everglades. The ecological damage caused by this disruption has been further compounded by serious degradation of water quality due to fertilizer-laden drainage from adjacent sugarcane fields. Phosphate pollution in particular has precipitated massive fish kills and algal blooms, as well as the explosive growth of cattails.

Another major threat to ecosystem stability in the Everglades has been the melaleuca tree, an exotic Australian species introduced in 1906 to help drain the swamp; it did its job only too well and, in the absence of natural enemies, is now displacing many of South Florida's native plant and animal species. As a result of this triple onslaught (i.e. drainage projects, pollution, and melaleuca), wildlife populations in the Everglades have plummeted in recent decades—breeding pairs of waterbirds are down 90% from former levels and 33 species of indigenous animals are listed as either threatened or endangered. In the long run, degradation of the Everglades threatens not only flamingoes and alligators but Floridians as well, since the groundwater supplies on which the southern part of the state depends, naturally replenished through hydrologic contact with the Everglades, are not being recharged as rapidly as in the past. Soil resources also are threatened, thanks to drainage projects and intensive agricultural production that have exposed the rich topsoil to oxidation and erosion. Soil loss in these areas has averaged an inch per year since the late 1970s and in some places topsoil now is completely gone.

The slow ecological decline of this invaluable wetland resource has not gone unnoticed; since the early 1900s, activists have loudly protested the activities which, they warned, would destroy the very features that attracted people to South Florida in the first place. By 1947 proponents of preservation were successful in persuading Congress to set aside the southern portion of the giant marshland as Everglades National Park. More recently, the Everglades Coalition, an assemblage of 28 national and local environmental groups, began pressing toward a far more ambitious goal—reengineering, and in some places undoing, the elaborate plumbing system that makes the Everglades the most intensively managed region on earth. The ultimate objective of this effort, as proclaimed in 1983 by then-Governor Bob Graham, was nothing less than to make ". . . the Everglades look and function by the year 2000 more as it did at the turn of the century."

Restoration of the Everglades moved a giant step closer to reality in the fall of 1992 when Congress authorized a Comprehensive Review Study (referred to simply as the **"Restudy"**) of the C & SF Project. Under the joint direction of the Corps of Engineers and the South Florida Water Management District, the Restudy's purpose is to restore the Everglades and Florida Bay ecosystems while providing for other water-related needs of southern Florida. Plans include an $8 billion network of channels and reservoirs that would capture up to 85% of the fresh water currently being discharged to the ocean during the rainy season, storing it in large surface impoundments and in underground aquifers. A portion of this water would then be released during the dry season to flow in a sheet-like fashion through the Everglades to Florida Bay. The remainder of the stored water would be used for irrigation and to meet urban water demands. Once underway, the project is expected to take 15-20 years to complete, with half the funding contributed by the federal government, the remaining half from the State of Florida. This restoration effort represents an historic turning point—the first time ever that a major U.S. public works project (i.e. the Central and Southern Florida Project) has been "undone" for ecological reasons.

Engineering projects alone, however, won't be enough to restore the Everglades to good health. The water quality problems caused by nutrient runoff from 440,000 acres of cane fields and 60,000 acres of vegetable farms present a politically charged dilemma. "Big Sugar" is a powerful force in South Florida, and growers don't take kindly to demands that they control polluted runoff from fields. Court battles pitting agricultural interests against state officials and environmentalists raged through much of the 1990s. In 1994, the Florida legislature passed The Everglades Forever Act, mandating the construction of 40,000 acres of filtration marshes around Lake Okeechobee to reduce phosphate concentrations in farmland runoff. Subsequent disputes over who should pay for this project culminated in a 1997 decision by the Florida Supreme Court that costs of pollution cleanup be shared between sugar growers and state taxpayers, since development and population growth in South Florida have compounded the environmental insults heaped upon the Everglades.

While progress toward the goal of a restored and revitalized Everglades ecosystem will be slow, arduous, and expensive, the task is now underway, offering Floridians and all who love wetlands a realistic hope of one day experiencing "Paradise Regained."

References
Cushman, John H. 1998. "U.S. Unveils Plan to Revamp South Florida Water Supply and Save Everglades." *New York Times*, Oct. 14, p.A12.

Derr, Mark. 1993. "Redeeming the Everglades." *Audubon* (Sept/Oct).

U.S. Army Corps of Engineers, Jacksonville District. 1998. "What Is the Restudy?" *Case Restudy Update*. no. 1 (June).

Figure 5-4 Predicted Percent Decline in Tropical Forest Plant and Animal Species, 1999–2040

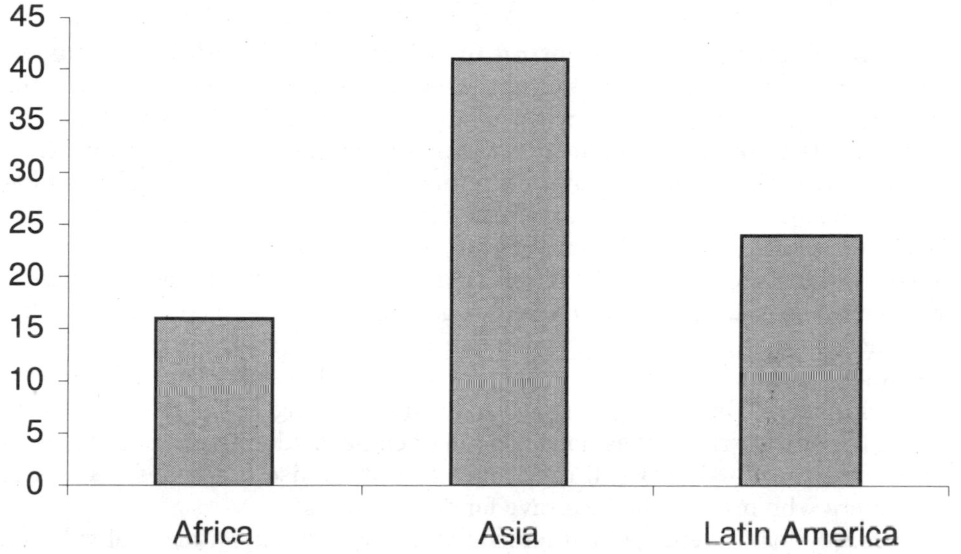

Source: Based on data from Andrew P. Dobson, *Conservation and Biodiversity,* 1996.

more alarming. Harvard biologist E. O. Wilson estimates that in tropical forest areas alone, home to a conservatively estimated 10 million species, the world is currently losing 3 species every hour, 74 per day, 27,000 each year— and the rate of loss continues to accelerate. If present trends of rain forest destruction are not reversed, 10–20% of all rain forest species will be extinct within 30 years—a number equivalent to at least 5–10% of all species on earth (Wilson, 1992).

The magnitude of such a loss is staggering. Species diversity is generally considered a prime determinant of ecological stability; extinction of key species, particularly plant species, may lead to the collapse of whole ecosystems. Less spectacular but equally distressing from a human viewpoint is the prospect of many potentially useful plant species being lost before their food or medicinal value is discovered. Even today, one-fourth of all pharmaceutical products bought by Americans contain active ingredients derived from plant products. The discovery of taxol, a potent anticancer drug derived from the bark of the Pacific yew (formerly regarded as a weed tree in old-growth forests of the Pacific Northwest) is but one of the more recent additions to a long list of valuable medicinal products extracted from forest plants. From a philosophical viewpoint also, the implications of the wholesale destruction of nonhuman life is profoundly disturbing. Over a century ago Thoreau proclaimed that "In wildness is the preservation of the world." Much ethical discussion in recent years has centered around the question of whether humans have the moral right to exterminate another form of life, to abruptly terminate the product of millions of years of evolution. Undeniably, "extinction is forever."

Although the causes of accelerating species loss are by now fairly well understood, reversing the trends which have brought about the current situation will be extremely difficult, particularly in regions where rapidly growing human populations are in direct competition with wildlife. Human pressures on other species can assume a variety of forms:

Direct Killing or Collecting of Wildlife for Food, Pleasure, or Profit. From the Paleolithic hunters who decimated the wooly mammoths and mastodons with primitive weapons to the modern Russian and Japanese fishing fleets that have brought several species of whale to the brink of extinction, predatory humans have totally eliminated a number of bird and mammalian species. Of all the animal extinctions known to have occurred within the past 400 years, the World Conservation Union estimates that nearly one-fourth (23%) were caused by overhunting. Collectors who dynamite reefs to obtain chunks of coral or capture rare tropical fish for sale to aquarium hobbyists; cactus "rustlers" who steal plants from nature preserves to satisfy the growing demand for rare houseplants; African poachers who shoot the endangered rhinoceros for the high profits its horn will bring in the markets of the Orient (powdered rhinoceros horn has long been considered an aphrodisiac in China and the Far East)—all contribute to the demise of species, as do the consumers who provide the incentive for such actions.

In an effort to remove the financial incentives for exploitation of wildlife, conservation groups mustered enough support to secure passage of the 1973 **Convention on International Trade in Endangered Species of Flora and Fauna (CITES).** Meeting twice a year, CITES' governing body regulates international trade in and shipments of specified animal and plant products and flatly prohibits trade in products from endangered species. CITES has received much credit for stemming the slaughter of African elephants after issuing a ban in 1989 on ivory trading (a partial lifting of this ban, effective in 1999, will allow Namibia, Botswana, and Zimbabwe to begin selling limited amounts of ivory to Japan; funds generated by this trade are supposed to be reinvested into wildlife conservation programs and may thus benefit elephant populations in those countries, so long as monitoring of the trade is rigorous enough to exclude illegally harvested tusks). CITES has been less effective in curbing the illicit trade in tiger parts which just in the last few years has resulted in such a precipitous decline in populations of the big cats that many wildlife biologists hold out little hope for the survival of tigers outside of zoos. In countries such as China and Taiwan, virtually every part of the animal's body brings premium prices due to their supposed medicinal benefits: tiger bones for potions to cure rheumatism, tiger whiskers to provide strength, tiger eyes to calm convulsions, and tiger penis, simmered in a soup, to rekindle male sexual prowess among senior citizens (only *wealthy* senior citizens need apply, however—a bowl of tiger penis soup may cost over $300!). The apparent lack of effort on the part of government officials to stem illegal commerce in tiger and rhino products brought strong CITES criticism of both Taiwan and China. Since CITES has no enforcement powers of its own against treaty violators, the U.S., citing authority under the Pelly Amendment, in 1994 imposed trade sanctions on Taiwan. This action marked the first time any government had ever employed trade restrictions against another country specifically to protect endangered wildlife. Stung by the ban on export of their fish and wildlife products to the U.S., Taiwanese officials improved enforcement of their country's wildlife conservation laws and launched a public education effort to inform Taiwanese citizens about the endangered status of animals whose products were being used for medicinal purposes. As a result, Taiwanese trade in illegal wildlife parts fell sharply and in 1996 the situation had improved enough for U.S. sanctions to be lifted.

Unfortunately, trade sanctions imposed by individual countries to protect wildlife may conflict with international agreements to promote free trade, since the World Trade Organization (WTO) regards such unilateral actions as illegal. In 1998 the WTO ruled against a controversial U.S. ban on shrimp imports from certain Asian nations whose fishers refused to install turtle excluder devices on their nets to reduce the accidental by-catch of several species of endangered sea turtles (Tuxill, 1998).

Introduction of Exotic Species. Until relatively recently, the single most important factor accounting for the demise of many plant and animal species has been the accidental or deliberate introduction by humans of nonnative species into environments where such organisms had no natural enemies to curb explosive rates of growth. These alien invaders frequently decimated indigenous species by preying upon them or by outcompeting them for food or living space. The examples are legion: the melaleuca, an Australian tree that is taking over the Everglades; European starlings, which have driven many less-aggressive songbirds from their original range; zebra mussels, which are outproducing and overwhelming native mussel species throughout inland waterways in much of the United States and have caused an estimated $5 billion in damage to water intake pipes (by 1999, just 11 years after a few individuals were accidentally released into Lake St. Clair near Detroit, zebra mussels have spread throughout much of the eastern U.S., south to New Orleans, and as far west as Oklahoma). The fish-stocking programs that have introduced exotic species such as carp, brown and rainbow trout, Atlantic salmon, or Nile tilapia into waterways where they previously didn't exist have put native species under extreme pressure and have driven some to extinction (Bright, 1998). Experts estimate that over two-thirds of the fish extinctions which already have occurred in the United States were caused, at least in part, by the introduction of alien species, while half the fish now on the "endangered" list are thus imperilled because of introduced exotics (Luoma, 1992).

The impact of nonnative species can be seen most dramatically in island ecosystems such as Hawaii, site of fully three-fourths of all known bird and plant extinctions in the United States. The goats, pigs, sheep, rats, and mongooses that came ashore with European settlers in the years after Captain Cook's voyage to the islands in 1778 are the most notorious of approximately 3,900 plant and animal species arriving in Hawaii over the past two centuries. Today, of the remaining native Hawaiian plants, one-fifth are endangered; for native bird species, the proportion at risk rises to nearly half, primarily due to the impact of exotic newcomers. On the Pacific island of Guam, the brown tree snake, a recent arrival from New Guinea, has virtually wiped out native bird populations since it was first introduced some 35 years ago. Nowhere, however, has the impact of alien species been more devastating than in Africa's Lake Victoria, a waterway once renowned for its amazing diversity of cichlid fishes—more than 300 species found nowhere else in the world. In 1959 Nile perch, a type of carnivorous fish growing up to six feet in length, were introduced into the lake by British settlers who thought they would enhance sports fishing opportunities. Within 25 years the invaders had gobbled up so many of the native cichlids that several species disappeared completely; it is expected that eventually over half the native species will become extinct. The demise of the plant-eating cichlids has had far-reaching effects on the Lake Victoria ecosystem, leading to algal blooms, oxygen depletion, and the decline of many other lake species. While the decision to introduce the perch had no malicious intent, the catastrophic results of this act led a team of biologists to observe: "Never before has man in a single ill-advised step placed so many vertebrate species simultaneously at risk of extinction and also, in doing so, threatened a food resource and traditional way of life of riparian dwellers" (Wilson, 1992).

Recognition of the heavy toll exacted by exotic species in the United States is reflected in the 1999 establishment through executive order of an interagency Invasive Species Council. Chaired by the Secretaries of Agriculture, Interior, and Commerce, the group has been charged with developing a broad management plan to minimize the impact of bioinvasions and to prevent their spread. Citing the widespread environmental and economic damage caused by exotic pests, government officials warn that the problem is growing, thanks to rapidly expanding world trade. While some of the species introductions in recent years have been a deliberate result of commercial transactions, most are accidental consequences of the global distribution networks that facilitate international commerce. Exotic species frequently invade new territory attached to the hulls of ships; as stowaways in wooden crates or packing materials; hidden inside unprocessed logs, fruits, or seeds; as unticketed passengers on aircraft; or, most common of all, swimming in the ballast water discharged by ships entering ports. The impact of exotics has been particularly severe on coastal ecosystems. In San Francisco Bay alone, according to a spokeswoman at the Center of Marine Conservation, a new species is discovered entering the bay, on average, every 14 days.

Biologists estimate that in excess of 6,000 exotic plant and animal species have now become permanent residents of the United States; while not all of these bioinvaders cause problems, many are now numbered among our most troublesome pests. A notorious recent newcomer is the Asian longhorned beetle, native to China, Korea, and Japan. Discovered in 1998 in both Chicago and on Long Island, the large, shiny black-and-white beetle poses a serious threat to many species of hardwood trees, especially maples, into which it tunnels and feeds. An aggressive eradication effort is now underway in the localized areas where infestations have been identified and regulations have been imposed requiring that wooden shipping crates from China be heated and chemically treated to kill any beetles they might be harboring.

At the level of international policymaking, stemming bioinvasions is more difficult and complex than curbing trade in endangered species. With the exception of various protocols that categorically exclude exotic organisms from Antarctica, there are no treaties specifically enacted to prevent bioinvasions. The 1992 Convention of Biological Diversity, which emerged from the UN-sponsored Earth Summit that year, requires signatory nations to prevent the introduction of alien species that pose a threat to ecosystem stability but to do so "as far as possible and appropriate"—a qualifying phrase that makes the treaty little more than a weak statement of noble intentions. For the foreseeable future, efforts at mitigating the impact of exotic species will likely remain a combination of port-of-entry inspections, prohibitions or controls of listed problematic species or items (e.g. potentially insect-infested logs from Siberia, non-treated wooden crates from China), and eradication or control programs targeting already established exotic pests. The task is daunting, but biologists are convinced that over the long term controlling exotic species will be just as important for protecting biodiversity as are efforts to save those that are threatened and endangered; indeed, the two activities may be but opposite sides of the same coin (Bright, 1998).

Pollution of Air and Water with Toxic Chemicals. The death of entire aquatic ecosystems due to acid rainfall is but one of the more recent examples of the effect toxic pollutants are having on other forms of life. Particularly since the introduction of the synthetic organic pesticides after World War II, numerous wildlife species, especially carnivorous birds, have suffered sharp population declines, and contamination of rivers, lakes, and estuaries with industrial effluents threaten the sustained productivity of those ecosystems. The problem is even more acute in the developing nations, where environmental laws regulating toxic discharges are either weak or nonexistent and where many of the hazardous pesticides now banned in most industrialized countries are still widely and indiscriminately used (Tuxill, 1998).

The impact of pollution on wildlife was a major topic of international discussion in the summer of 1988 when beaches along Europe's North Sea and the U.S. East Coast were littered with the bodies of dead and dying seals and porpoises. Though the cause of the marine mammals' demise was ultimately determined to be a type of pneumonia, it was theorized that swimming in highly polluted coastal waters weakened the animals' resistance to disease and thereby contributed to their death. More recent casualties have been the beluga whales inhabiting the St. Lawrence River. Once numbering in the thousands, the belugas have dwindled to an estimated population of 500 animals, large numbers of which are afflicted with various types of tumors, ulcers, lesions, cysts, pneumonia, and reproductive problems. Scientists attribute the whales' plight to chemical contamination of the river with mercury, lead, PCBs, and various organochlorine pesticides. Analyses of tissue samples from dead belugas show concentrations of all these chemicals at levels far above those in whales from Arctic waters. One researcher commented that beluga carcasses contain such high concentrations of PCBs that they ought to be regulated as hazardous wastes! (Dold, 1992). While marine mammals and fish are particularly hard hit because of the toxic soup that constantly surrounds them in many waterways, polluted air also is taking its toll on sensitive species. In western Europe fungi appear to be dying off *en masse,* with a 40–50% loss of species in certain areas of Germany, Austria, and the Netherlands. Among those adversely affected are the mycorrhizal fungi which live in symbiotic association with plant roots, promoting the uptake of dissolved nutrients. The fact that these inconspicuous organisms play an important role in the normal functioning of many plant species gives their demise far-reaching significance (Wilson, 1992). Efforts to safeguard human health by curbing pollutant emissions will have a beneficial impact on the health of eco-systems as well.

Habitat Destruction. By far the greatest threat to biodiversity today—and the most difficult to control—is the destruction of those natural areas that wildlife require for breeding, feeding, or migrating. As the pres-sures of expanding populations and economies increase, forests are chopped down, swamps are drained, prairies are put to the plow, rivers are dammed. Some wildlife species can thrive in close proximity to humans; most cannot and perish when their natural habitat is destroyed or reduced in size below a critical minimum.

While there is little disagreement that preservation of biodiversity is a lost cause without a significantly greater commitment to conserving natural habitats, the question of how to maintain the integrity of dwindling expanses of forest, savannah, and grasslands at a time of exponentially increasing human needs is a vexing one for policymakers everywhere. Since 1872 when Yellowstone was established as the world's first national park, the conven-tional approach to preserving wild areas of great beauty or biological richness has been to set aside **protected areas** as wildlife refuges, national parks, or wilderness areas. Today 4% of the earth's total land surface has been thus pre-served in approximately 8,000 protected areas worldwide, their natural wealth safeguarded by limiting human access to such areas. Although in the past this approach has been somewhat successful, particularly in regions such as North America where population pressures are modest, trends suggest that in the years ahead preservation of critical habitat through reliance on govern-ment-established exclusion zones cannot adequately protect biodiversity and is ultimately doomed to failure. This is true for a number of reasons: 1) in most cases, the protected areas are too scattered, small, and fragmented to sustain the long-term stability of their biotic communities; ecologists have amply documented the adverse impact of crowding species into isolated "islands" of woodland or tropical forest, surrounded by a "sea" of farmlands or urban development. The "edge effect" experienced around the periphery of these fragmented habitats (i.e. increased exposure to wind, sunlight, decreased humidity, vulnerability to new predators) may result in the loss of many species highly adapted to life within a narrow range of environmental conditions; 2) many so-called protected areas, particularly those in developing countries, are protected in name only, since governments frequently lack the financial resources, the technical expertise, or the will to enforce their bor-ders. The widescale poaching of endangered rhinos in East Africa or of tigers in India—both legally protected animals—is indicative of the difficulty many poor countries face in trying to safeguard their natural heritage; 3) finally, and perhaps most importantly, the protected area strategy doesn't take into account the fact that humans are an integral part of ecosystems also. Most of the areas set aside for wildlife once sustained the needs of local people who are now forbidden to hunt, fish, or grow crops on lands they once considered theirs to use. As growing human populations press against park boundaries, it will be impossible and, indeed, unjust, to forbid them the use of their own sur-roundings without providing viable alternatives for survival.

Accordingly, within the past two decades a radically different approach to conservation of habitat has slowly gained adherents, an approach which attempts to make local communities both the *beneficiaries* and the *custodians* of efforts to safeguard biodiversity. Referred to as **community-based conservation,** this new concept recognizes that the exclusionary policies of the past, as embodied in the wildlife reserves, cannot be sustained in the face of mounting human poverty and hostility to programs which seem to place greater value on elephants or pandas than on people. Community-based conservation relies on positive grassroots participation, relinquishing the traditional top-down planning by central government officials in favor of involving local people in the planning, design, and implementation of conservation efforts which will benefit them directly and give them a personal stake in the successful outcome of such ventures. Community-based conservation efforts are quietly underway in a number of areas around the world and involve situations as diverse as the "extractive reserves" in Brazilian Amazonia, subsistence farming combined with ecotourism in Papua New Guinea, forest management by community councils in India, or incentive payments to private landowners for fostering biodiversity in England (Wright, 1993).

Another interesting approach to involve local people in wildlife conservation efforts is that of **biodiversity prospecting**—enlisting residents of species-rich tropical countries to assist in the search for plants or animals of potential medicinal, pesticidal, or agricultural value. Several bioprospecting agreements have been signed since the early 1990s between drug companies and national governments or institutes in the developing world (the U.S. National Parks Service has also indicated an interest in similar arrangements involving bioprospecting in such unique ecosystems as the hot springs at Yellowstone National Park). Merck & Co., Inc., the world's largest pharmaceutical corporation, now pays a private non-profit organization in Costa Rica to send the company a steady supply of plant, animal, and microbial specimens to be analyzed for possible medicinal properties. Merck has agreed to pay royalties to its Costa Rican partner, the Instituto Nacional de Biodiversidad (INBIO), for any commercial products developed from Costa Rican specimens. It is assumed that once the biochemically active ingredient of a newly discovered species is identified, it will be possible to mass-produce an identical synthetic compound, thereby avoiding further exploitation of the species in its native habitat. By intimately involving local people in cataloging their country's biodiversity, INBIO gives Costa Ricans an in-depth understanding of their natural heritage and a personal stake in protecting it. Similar arrangements involving other pharmaceutical firms are now in effect in Ghana, Nigeria, and Surinam (Tuxill, 1998).

The shift in focus from preserving wildlife to acknowledging the need to factor human needs into the equation may be the only practical approach to saving as much biodiversity as possible, particularly at a time when human-modified landscapes are relentlessly expanding. Convincing local people that their own well-being can best be ensured by conserving and sustainably using the biological wealth of their surroundings may ultimately be the key to species preservation. Whether motivated by poverty or greed, those who today are engaged in mindless destruction of natural habitat, thereby driving untold numbers of species to extinction, might well consider the words spoken more than 35 years ago by Julius Nyerere, a leader in the African independence movement and the first President of Tanzania:

> The survival of our wildlife is a matter of grave concern to all of us in
> Africa. These wild creatures amid the wild places they inhabit are not only
> important as a source of wonder and inspiration but are an integral part of
> our natural resources and of our future livelihood and well-being.

Protecting Biodiversity: The Endangered Species Act

Since its enactment in 1973, the **Endangered Species Act (ESA)** has
constituted the nation's most effective weapon for ensuring the survival of
native plants and animals. Probably the toughest wildlife protection law anywhere in the world, the ESA prohibits the killing, collecting, harassment, or
capture of any species listed by the U.S. Fish and Wildlife Service (FWS) as
"endangered" or "threatened." It also provides strict protection for the critical
habitat of endangered species and requires FWS to develop recovery programs
for each species listed. In the United States, 1,180 species had been officially
designated as endangered or threatened (478 animals and 702 plants) by
1999, up from just 78 in 1967 when the original endangered species list was
compiled.

While environmentalists hail the ESA for noticeably slowing the pace of
wildlife extinction in the United States, citing as evidence the fact that 60
endangered species have increased their numbers or expanded their range
over the past quarter-century, opponents are working hard to weaken the law
when it comes up for reauthorization. Charging that the Act has excessive
power to supersede individual property rights, hinder economic progress, and
threaten jobs, such disparate constituencies as land developers, Gulf Coast
shrimpers, and loggers in the Pacific Northwest would like to see the Act significantly weakened. These groups raise the question of how much biological
diversity can or should be preserved, especially when the species in question
isn't particularly cute or fuzzy. Some people find it hard to get emotional
about the Colorado squawfish or the scrub plum!

ESA defenders counter-charge the assertion that the Act is blocking the
inexorable march of progress (and profits) by pointing out that, for the vast
majority of protected species, recovery plans seldom provoke conflict. Perhaps
one explanation for increasing antagonism toward ESA is the fact that in
recent years the Act has begun to affect entire regions rather than just isolated projects, as was generally the case in the past. The acrimony in Northwest logging regions in the early 1990s over attempts to save the northern
spotted owl by declaring large areas of old-growth forest off-limits for timber
harvesting prompted vociferous complaints that the ESA favors wildlife over
people.

In fact, contrary to detractors' claims, the Act *does* make an effort to
accommodate societal concerns. Economic considerations are taken into
account to some degree when designations of critical habitat are made; in situations where proposed projects threaten endangered species, the Act requires
that an effort be made to find alternative means of carrying out the activity
without endangering survival of the species in question. In those rare cases
where the conflict is irreconcilable, an official panel (the "God Squad") can
give the green light to projects deemed of sufficient importance, even if this

action constitutes a death sentence for an endangered species.

Even supporters admit, however, that implementation of ESA is in need of improvement. To some extent, problems center around insufficient money and personnel to carry out the intent of the Act. Even more problematic is the cumbersome process of officially listing rare species as threatened or endangered. Frequently the official designation comes so late that populations of the species in question may already be too low to halt the slide into oblivion. In other cases, only costly rescue missions such as captive breeding programs can guarantee long-term survival, when earlier action could have achieved success through less extreme measures. Although studies suggest that a minimum population in the low thousands is a prerequisite for viable vertebrate populations, the average number of individuals remaining in vertebrate groups listed as endangered was just 1,075; for invertebrates it was even lower—999. For plants, the average number of remaining specimens in at-risk populations at the time of official listing is a mere 120, making recovery of such species extremely difficult. Biologists suggest that the minuscule number of species which have rebounded and been removed from the endangered list can be explained by the fact that official designation often comes too late to implement effective recovery plans.

A major test of the ESA's ability to save species while accommodating human needs will unfold in the years immediately ahead. In March 1999, the federal government announced its intent to place seven species of salmon and two species of trout on the endangered list, an act with profound consequences for the Pacific Northwest and particularly for the rapidly growing Seattle metropolitan area. Saving the salmon will be neither easy nor cheap. To reduce the coastal pollution that has severely impacted fish populations, Seattle residents may be forced to curtail use of fertilizers and pesticides and to pay more taxes to upgrade sewage treatment and to acquire land bordering waterways. Developers may face unwelcome restrictions on construction, especially near streams. Residents' utility bills could rise sharply if recovery plans necessitate modifying or removing the hydroelectric dams that have given northwesterners the cheapest electrical rates in the country—but have also closed off salmon access to ancient spawning grounds. Interestingly, initial citizen reaction to the federal announcement has been positive. Unlike the spotted owl whose listing provoked such bitter controversy, salmon are venerated in the Northwest, regarded as an integral part of the regional identity which no one wants to lose. Though some observers are skeptical that salmon recovery efforts can be successfully implemented in an urban area that already is home to 3 million people, others are convinced that a serious salmon restoration program will not only rescue the fish but bring enormous quality of life gains, as well as economic benefits, to people as well. As Seattle Mayor Paul Schell put the case, "In working together to save salmon, it may turn out the salmon saves us" (Verhovek, 1999).

In spite of its limitations, the Endangered Species Act can claim its share of notable success stories. Although over the past 25 years only 11 species have been reclassified as "recovered," a number of others have made a remarkable comeback from near-extinction. These include the bald eagle, which is scheduled for removal from the Endangered Species List in 2000 since its population in the lower 48 states has climbed from just 791 nesting

BOX 5-3

Endangered Reefs

In terms of biodiversity, coral reefs are the rain forests of the sea, home to one-fourth of all ocean species. Unfortunately, these rich marine ecosystems, like their terrestrial counterpart, are now under siege around the globe.

Coral reefs are formed by tiny cnidarian animals, related to sea anemones, that secrete a stony external covering of calcium carbonate around their soft body parts. Over vast periods of time, coral communities slowly grow to cover enormous expanses of shallow ocean bottoms; today living reefs cover about 360,000 square miles throughout the world's tropical seas.

Where they occur, coral reefs provide invaluable ecological services to the millions of people living along adjacent coastlines. Since reefs frequently extend nearly to the water's surface, they help shield shore areas from storm surges and beach erosion. Reef-dwelling fish provide an important food source for local people, comprising 20–25% of the total fish catch in developing countries. In many areas, reefs are a significant source of tourist dollars; some Caribbean island nations derive half their annual revenue from foreign visitors attracted by the recreational attractions of reefs. Degradation of this resource is therefore bound to impose heavy costs, both economic and environmental.

Sadly, such losses now appear inevitable. In at least 93 of the 110 tropical countries possessing coral reefs, reef degradation or destruction has assumed major proportions. A 1998 assessment report by the World Resources Institute estimates that 58% of reefs worldwide are now endangered by human activities, with 27% experiencing high or very high

risk. In Southeast Asia, along the coasts of Indonesia, the Philippines, Vietnam, and Malaysia, fully 80% of coral reefs are threatened, with 55% in the high or very high risk category. Marine biologists regard the situation as an ecological tragedy, since Indo-Pacific reefs are the most species-diverse in the world.

The problem confronting reef ecosystems, from the Indonesian archipelago to the Middle East to the Caribbean are remarkably similar and can be summarized as "too much pressure from too many people." Most significant are pressures related to **overexploitation** and **coastal development**. Overexploitation of reef resources is a direct result of the soaring demand in Asia for live food fish and in North America and Europe for live aquarium specimens. In Southeast Asia approximately $1 billion worth of live reef fish are shipped each year to markets in Hong Kong and elsewhere to satisfy the appetites of wealthy diners willing to pay as much as $225 per *plate* for the lips of freshly killed napoleon wrasse, a highly prized and increasingly rare reef fish. The fact that the fish is now considered endangered only seems to boost its demand among Hong Kong gourmets and the astronomical prices it commands reinforces overfishing pressures on tropical reefs. What makes overexploitation of reef resources particularly damaging are the methods commonly used to capture live fish. Traditional nets or hook-and-line techniques have given way to blast fishing with homemade explosives and to cyanide poisoning. Both methods are illegal and both are devastating to coral. Use of cyanide has been increasing especially rapidly because of the booming live fish export industry. After crushing sodium cyanide pellets into squirt bottles filled with seawater, divers swim among coral formations and squirt the cyanide solution into cavities where fish hide. In most cases, the poison doesn't kill the fish but merely stuns them, making it easier for divers to hand-catch their prey (many fish are weakened by cyanide exposure, however, and die in transit). Although fish are the targets of cyanide-wielding divers, corals and other reef invertebrates frequently fall victim to the poison as well. Numerous fishers and divers attest to the deadly impact of cyanide fishing, reporting that extensive reef areas off the Philippines and Indonesia are now virtually devoid of life.

The impact of overfishing includes both direct physical damage to reefs, especially in areas of blast fishing, and a change in the species composition within reef communities. When certain keystone fish species are removed, major disruptions in the functioning of marine ecosystems may follow. The present sorry condition of reefs off the island of Jamaica provide a case in point. When decades of overfishing drastically reduced populations of herbivorous reef fish, the task of controlling algal overgrowth of the reefs reverted to a species of sea urchin. However, when the beneficial urchins were decimated by an epidemic in the early 1980s, algae populations exploded and killed the coral. Several years later, hurricanes pulverized the dead reefs and today living coral can be found covering but one-tenth the area it formerly occupied off the Jamaican coast.

Coastal development is the second-leading cause of stress on coral communities. Use of dynamite to "mine" coral for construction material, the dredging of harbors, and filling along shorelines for land reclamation all directly destroy or damage reefs. Equally harmful and more widespread are the indirect impacts of sewage pollution and the deposition of silt and sediments onto reefs when runoff from farmlands, construction sites, and recently deforested areas enters shallow coastal waters. Other human activities degrading reef ecosystems include near-shore oil spills and unregulated tourist activities, such as the dropping of boat anchors onto fragile reef formations.

While the factors discussed above constitute the primary forces currently endangering reefs, an even more ominous threat looms on the horizon—global climate change. Coral is exquisitely sensitive to changes in water temperature and most coral communities now live at the upper edge of their temperature tolerance. Since the early 1980s a phenomenon know as **coral bleaching** has become increasingly common throughout the tropics, spurring anxious questions and a great deal of scientific investigation among researchers watchful for early signs of global warming. Coral bleaching, a process in which coral reefs lose their characteristic color and become white in appearance, occurs when the microscopic dinoflagellate algae that live in symbiotic association inside the coral, giving the animals their distinctive color, are expelled due to some sort of environmental stress. While chemical pollution, fluctuations in salinity, and silt accumulation have, on occasions, been shown to induce coral bleaching, only elevated seawater temperature can account for the massive bleaching episodes observed in recent years. The problem was particularly acute and widespread in 1998 when sea-surface temperatures were the highest ever recorded. Damage was especially severe in the Indian Ocean near the Maldive Islands, where up to 90% of the reefs were killed. If scientists who predict that average world temperature will increase by about 2°C within the next 50 years are correct, the future of coral reefs is grim—a 1°C increase is sufficient to cause coral bleaching.

The worsening plight of the world's coral reefs has finally captured the attention of policymakers in many countries and belated actions are finally being taken to limit the damage. More than 80 nations have joined the International Coral Reef Initiative, organized in 1995 to monitor global reef conditions. A number of national governments and local communities are acting to protect and restore coral reefs through such measures as better law enforcement, legal reef protection, environmental education, and improved planning and management. The Philippines, for example, has adopted a program to eradicate cyanide fishing—the only nation to do so thus far. Australia has combined strict enforcement of reef zoning regulations (20% protected, 80% multiple-use) with environmental education to maintain its Great Barrier Reef in good condition. In the United States, a Coral Reef Task Force was created by presidential order in June 1998, and is initiating a number of activities to improve protection of coral reefs around the world. With global surveys documenting a significant deterioration of reef conditions in just the last few years, groups working to save these priceless ecosystems confront a challenging task.

References
Barber, C.V., and V.R. Pratt. 1998. "Poison and Profits: Cyanide Fishing in the Indo-Pacific." *Environment* 40, no. 8 (October):4–9, 28–34.

World Resources Institute. 1998. *World Resources, 1998–99.* Oxford University Press.

pairs in 1974 to 6,000 by 1999; the American alligator, which remains on the "threatened" list despite full recovery only because it is easily mistaken for the American crocodile which *is* still endangered; whooping cranes, peregrine falcons, California sea otters, grizzly bears, black-footed ferrets, the red wolf—all now have a new lease on life, thanks to the Endangered Species Act (World Resources Institute, 1994).

While ESA historically has focused on protecting individual species on a case-by-case basis, a 1982 amendment to the Act established an alternative approach to preserving biodiversity in the form of **habitat conservation planning (HCP).** Devised as a way of striking a balance between pressures for economic growth and habitat preservation, HCP allows landowners to develop property occupied by endangered species if they agree to minimize the loss of critical habitat or offset that loss by providing additional land nearby. While this approach implicitly permits the loss of some members of the endangered species in question, it guarantees that enough critical habitat will be preserved to sustain the remainder of that population indefinitely. Drawing up an acceptable plan may involve years of negotiations among developers, environmentalists, local governments, and Fish and Wildlife Service personnel who supervise the process and must ultimately approve the plan. Nevertheless, both environmentalists and property rights advocates are supportive of the HCP concept, the former seeing it as a way of winning concessions from landowners who might otherwise ignore the law, the latter preferring negotiated plans rather than blanket restrictions on land use.

By early 1999, approximately 240 habitat conservation plans had been approved and an additional 200 were being negotiated. The HCP process has been particularly important in southern California, where intense development pressures on biologically rich natural areas have pitted preservationists against developers for years. In 1993 Interior Secretary Bruce Babbitt worked out an agreement between environmentalists and developers who had been at loggerheads for years over the fate of a diminutive songbird, the California gnatcatcher. Since fewer than 3,000 nesting pairs remained in the 250,000 acres of sage scrub stretching along the Pacific Coast from Los Angeles to San Diego, environmentalists had been demanding the Fish and Wildlife Service list the gnatcatcher as endangered; developers were adamant that such action, automatically triggering prohibitions on the use of valuable real estate, would impose serious economic hardships. Under the HCP brokered by Babbitt, the gnatcatcher was listed as merely "threatened" rather than "endangered," thus permitting a more flexible recovery plan; in return, development interests agreed to protect critical habitat by setting aside up to 12 reserves, an act which benefitted not only the gnatcatcher, but as many as 40 other species as well. Habitat conservation planning has continued to win proponents throughout southern California, particularly in the San Diego area where what has been billed as a model HCP was approved by the city council in 1997. Under the agreed-upon arrangement, specified natural areas adjacent to the city will be acquired and permanently set aside for habitat preservation while other still-open lands will be available for unrestricted development.

While experience with habitat conservation planning is not yet extensive enough to render a verdict on its ability to save species, hopes are high that it provides a means for avoiding bitter confrontations and halting the decline of species long before their situation deteriorates beyond redemption.

References

Abramovitz, Janet N. 1998. "Taking a Stand: Cultivating a New Relationship with the World's Forests." *Worldwatch Paper 140* (April).

Bright, Chris. 1998. *Life Out of Bounds: Bioinvasion in a Borderless World.* W.W. Norton.

Brown, Lester. 1988. "The Changing World Food Prospect: The Nineties and Beyond." *Worldwatch Paper 85* (Oct.).

Coffin, Tristam, ed. 1993. "The Damage Done by Cattle-Raising." *The Washington Spectator* 19, no. 2 (Jan. 15).

Colchester, Marcus. 1994. "The New Sultans." *The Ecologist* 24, no. 2 (March/April).

Dold, Catherine. 1992. "Toxic Agents Found to Be Killing Off Whales." *New York Times,* June 16.

Environmental Protection Agency. 1988. *America's Wetlands: Our Vital Link Between Land and Water.* OPA-87-016 (Feb.).

Faeth, Paul. 1994. "Building the Case for Sustainable Agriculture: Policy Lessons from India, Chile, and the Philippines." *Environment* 36, no. 1 (Jan/Feb).

Hamilton, John Maxwell. 1989. "Rescuing the Bounty of Rain Forests." *The Christian Science Monitor,* Jan. 26.

Hulme, Mike, and Mick Kelly. 1993. "Exploring the Links Between Desertification and Climate Change." *Environment* 35, no. 6 (July/Aug).

Lal, R., and F. J. Pierce. 1991. "The Vanishing Resource." In *Soil Management for Sustainability,* edited by R. Lal and F. J. Pierce. Soil and Water Conservation Society.

Linden, Eugene. 1994. "Tigers on the Brink." *Time,* March 28.

Luoma, Jon R. 1992. "Boon to Anglers Turns into a Disaster for Lakes and Streams." *New York Times,* Nov. 17.

Moffat, Anne Simon. 1998. "Temperate Forests Gain Ground." *Science* 282 (Nov. 13):1253.

Nash, Nathaniel C. 1994. "Vast Areas of Rain Forest Are Being Destroyed in Chile." *New York Times,* May 31.

_____. 1993. "Bolivia's Rain Forest Falls to Relentless Exploiters." *New York Times,* June 21.

Smil, V. 1991. "Population Growth and Nitrogen: An Exploration of a Critical Existential Link." *Population and Development Review* 17, no. 4.

Stevens, William K. 1994a. "Threat of Encroaching Deserts May Be More Myth Than Fact." *New York Times,* Jan. 18.

_____. 1994b. "Prairie Ducks Return in Record Numbers." *New York Times,* Oct. 11.

Stutz, Bruce. 1993. "The Landscape of Hunger." *Audubon* 95, no. 2 (March/April).

Tobias, Michael. 1998. *World War III: Population and the Biosphere at the End of the Millennium.* Continuum Press.

Tuxill, John. 1998. "Losing Strands in the Web of Life: Vertebrate Declines and the Conservation of Biological Diversity." *Worldwatch Paper 141* (May).

Tyler, Patrick E. 1994. "Nature and Economic Boom Devouring China's Farmland." *New York Times,* March 27.

U.S. Department of Agriculture (USDA). 1997. *The Conservation Reserve Program.* Farm Services Agency, PA-1603 (May).

Verhovek, Sam Howe. 1999. "Northwest Confronts Its Growth: Wild Salmon Called Endangered." *New York Times* (March 16), p. A1.

Whittaker, Robert H. 1975. *Communities and Ecosystems.* Macmillan.

Wilcove, David S., Margaret McMillan, and Keith C. Winston. 1993. "What Exactly Is an Endangered Species? An Analysis of the U. S. Endangered Species List, 1985-91." *Conservation Biology* 7, no. 1.

Wilson, Edward O. 1992. *The Diversity of Life.* Harvard University Press.

World Conservation Monitoring Centre. 1992. *Global Biodiversity: Status of the Earth's Living Resources.* Chapman and Hall.

World Resources Institute (WRI). 1990. *World Resources 1990-1991.* Oxford University Press.

_____. 1992. *World Resources 1992-1993.* Oxford University Press.

_____. 1992. *The 1993 Information Please Environmental Almanac.* Houghton Mifflin Co.

_____. 1994. *The 1994 Information Please Environmental Almanac.* Houghton Mifflin Co.

_____. 1994. *World Resources 1994-1995: People and the Environment.* Oxford University Press.

_____. 1996. *World Resources 1996–97: The Urban Environment.* Oxford University Press.

_____. 1998. *World Resources 1998–99: Environmental Change and Human Health.* Oxford University Press.

Wright, Michal, ed. 1993. *The View from Airlie: Community-Based Conservation in Perspective.* Liz Claiborne and Art Ortenberg Foundation, narrative sampling of discussions during workshop held at Airlie, Virginia, week of Oct. 17.

PART 2

Our Toxic Environment

Does Everything Cause Cancer?

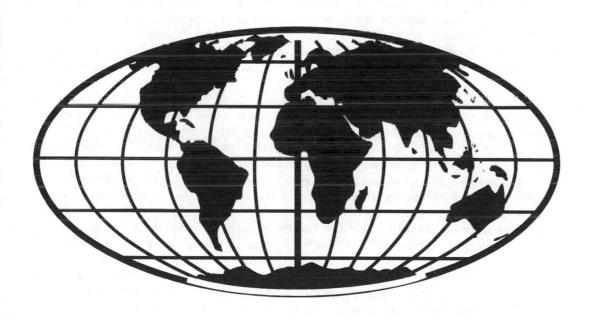

We have met the enemy, and it is us.

—Walt Kelly, POGO (1972)

Newspaper headlines screaming "Ozone Alert!"; a $1 million damage settlement to an asbestos worker's widow; public protests over a leaking hazardous waste dump; migrant workers hospitalized for pesticide poisoning; accidental sewage discharge forcing closure of public beaches—such situations represent but a handful of the issues daily facing modern society in which some aspect of environmental quality has a direct impact on human health.

From primitive times up until the mid-19th century the idea that health and disease were determined, at least in part, by environmental factors was widely accepted (witness the belief that night air precipitated fever and chills). The middle 1800s, however, marked a period of rapid progress in research relating to disease causation. The discovery of the anthrax bacterium by the German microbiologist Robert Koch and his demonstration in 1877 that this organism was responsible for an important human disease revolutionized society's view of health. For the next 70 years virtually all human ailments were blamed on pathogenic organisms such as bacteria, viruses, and protozoans. It was widely assumed that the development of preventative vaccines or curative antibiotics should be our main focus in protecting public health.

More recently, however, recognition of the role that deprivation or stress can play in initiating serious health problems and the sharp increase, particularly in more affluent societies, of the so-called "degenerative diseases" (cardiovascular disease, cancer, hypertension) have led to the realization that good health depends on more than just the absence of disease-causing microorganisms. Some of today's most prevalent ills are increasingly blamed on toxic environmental contaminants—synthetic chemical wastes carelessly dumped in waterways or landfills, products of combustion spewed into the air, pesticide residues and chemical additives in the food we eat. Other illnesses are associated with personal habits that in the broad sense can be considered aspects of environmental quality—smoking, drinking, high-fat diets, lack of regular exercise. Perception of the threat that such factors pose to human well-being provided the main thrust behind the environmental movement of the last 30 years. Preservation—or restoration—of environmental quality means far more than protecting bald eagles or ensuring that the last coastal redwood isn't converted into a picnic table; the prime emphasis among environmental advocates has always been the protection of human health, with the implicit recognition that human well-being is inextricably intertwined with the health and stability of the natural ecosystems of which we form an integral part.

While not a perfect standard, the health status of societies is often measured in terms of life expectancy—the number of years an average individual in that society can expect to live. In terms of longevity, health conditions in the Western world have improved markedly in recent centuries. Whereas in the days of Roman emperors the average lifespan was about 30 years, today in most industrialized countries it has reached 75 years, up from 50 years at the turn of the century (Japanese are currently the world's longest-lived people, with an average life expectancy of 80, compared to 76 in the United States). Among the developing nations average longevity is more variable, ranging from the lower to mid-40s in Afghanistan and some African countries to the mid-70s in parts of Latin America and the Caribbean. Many people, looking at such statistics, assume that the major factor accounting for increased longevity worldwide was the introduction of modern medicines and pesticides that provided the first really effective weapons against many of the infectious epidemic diseases. While medical science undoubtedly played a part in reducing mortality rates, many observers feel that a more fundamental factor was a general improvement in living conditions: better nutritional levels made possible by increased agricultural productivity; improved sanitary conditions as a result of sewer system construction; the provision of safe drinking water supplies; refuse collection; sewage treatment; the enforcement of housing codes, and so forth. Rising incomes, increasing levels of education, mass communications, and improved standards of personal hygiene have also been extremely important determinants in furthering the health advances observed in most parts of the world.

However, we seem to have now reached a longevity plateau and are no longer observing a continued rapid drop in death rates such as characterized the years between 1950–1960. Indeed, longevity is actually declining in Russia, where high levels of pollution, added to the ravages of alcoholism and substandard health care, have caused male life expectancy to fall to 61 years, the lowest for any industrialized country (female life expectancy has remained stable at 72 years). There appears to be general agreement that future gains will come, not so much through new medical discoveries, but when—and only when—essential preconditions of better health are everywhere available. These essential preconditions relate largely to environmental considerations: sufficient quantities of uncontaminated water, elimination of malnutrition, proper handling and disposal of human wastes, control of toxic pollutants, adoption of healthier personal lifestyles. The environmentally induced diseases currently plaguing much of humanity can best be controlled through a strategy of prevention, rather than cure, requiring not only application of technology but also social, political, and behavioral changes. Adopting such a strategy and enlisting the public support necessary to attain the goal of a healthful society require a thorough understanding of the issues and dilemmas involved. The following chapters will delineate the major concerns regarding our increasingly toxic environment and the health implications inherent in our present lifestyle; they also attempt to show that improving human health and enhancing environmental quality are but two sides of the same coin.

CHAPTER 6

Environmental Disease

Environmental illness is simply an incurable disease. There is no cure. It can only be prevented.

—Barry Commoner, 1990

Polluted air and water, excessive levels of noise, sunshine, nuclear weapons fall-out, overcrowded slums, toxic waste dumps, inadequate or overly adequate diet, stress, food contaminants, medical X-rays, drugs, cigarettes, unsafe working conditions—these comprise but a partial listing of the many environmental factors which, through their adverse impact on human health, can be regarded as causative agents of environmental disease. In recent years public concern about rising levels of pollution and environmental degradation has increasingly focused on the question of whether such trends may be influencing disease rates, particularly ailments such as heart disease, cancer, and stroke. If such a connection exists, as virtually all authorities agree it does, then society's response should be clear: most environmentally induced diseases, unlike those caused by bacteria or other pathogens, are difficult to cure but theoretically simple to prevent—remove the adverse environmental influence and the ailment will disappear. In other words, by preventing the discharge of poisons into our air, water, and food, by avoiding exposure to radiation, by refusing to fill our lungs with cigarette smoke or our stomachs with synthetic food colorings, we can protect our health far more effectively and cheaply than we can by desperately searching for an often nonexistent cure after our bodies succumb to a malignancy or degeneration of vital organs or when our children are born deformed. The old adage, "Prevention is the best cure," has never been more true than when applied to environmentally induced disease.

In spite of the fact that environmental factors can affect human health in many ways, the focus of most environmental health concern today in this age of toxic pollutants is on those substances that, in ways not yet completely understood, act at the cellular level to initiate often irreversible changes that

187

BOX 6-1

General Disease Classification

Human disease conditions can be categorized in various ways: infectious or noninfectious; endemic or epidemic; acute or chronic. It is important to have an understanding of the basic nature of any particular disease state in order to know how to respond to the problem in an appropriate manner.

Infectious vs. Noninfectious

Infectious diseases are those caused by pathogenic organisms such as bacteria, viruses, protozoans, parasitic worms, and so on. Infectious diseases can be spread from one person to another by inhalation of airborne pathogens released when an infected person coughs, sneezes or talks; by direct contact with food, water, soil or clothing that has been contaminated with fecal matter or saliva from an infected person; through sexual intercourse or other close physical contact with a diseased individual; or as a result of activities of a nonpathogenic disease-carrier, or vector, such as mosquitoes or body lice which transfer the disease agent from an infected person to a healthy one. Many of the leading killers of the past included such infectious diseases as malaria, smallpox, cholera, typhoid, measles, and tuberculosis.

Noninfectious diseases, currently the major cause of mortality in industrialized societies, are those that are not caused by pathogenic organisms and are not transmitted from one person to another (except in the case of hereditary conditions.) Noninfectious diseases frequently have multiple causes, often related to adverse environmental conditions, and may develop slowly over a number of years. Unlike many infectious diseases which, if survived, are of short duration, most noninfectious diseases are irreversible. Although many can be kept under control with proper medical treatment, few such conditions can be permanently cured. Examples of some of the leading noninfectious diseases include cardiovascular disease, cancer, diabetes, emphysema, sickle-cell anemia, asthma, and cerebral palsy.

Endemic vs. Epidemic

When the causative agent of an infectious disease such as typhoid is carried by many individuals within a population without leading to a rapid and widespread outbreak of illness and a high death rate, the disease is said to be endemic within that population. An epidemic disease, by contrast, involves a sudden severe outbreak of an infectious disease affecting a large number of people. The term "pandemic" refers to an epidemic that is worldwide in extent.

Acute vs. Chronic

Generally used in reference to certain infectious diseases such as smallpox, plague, or cholera which can be quite severe but are of short duration, an acute illness can also be caused by a short-term, high-dose exposure to a toxic substance. In most cases, if the victim survives the initial attack, the effects of the illness are reversible. With chronic conditions (e.g. malaria, tuberculosis, heart disease, cancer, emphysema) the illness is of long duration, often lasting a lifetime, occasionally flaring up, sometimes going into remission, or in some cases, growing progressively worse as the years pass.

can kill or damage the cell in question. Although health damage due to environmental pollutants may be manifested by outward symptoms, research has shown that the action of such contaminants in fact occurs at the level of an individual cell or cells. In spite of its small size, the cell is an exceptionally complex structure—the end product of billions of years of evolution and natural selection in response to existing environmental conditions. Thus it should not be surprising to find that a sudden change in the environment (e.g. exposure to X-rays, synthetic organic chemicals, heavy metals, etc.) to which a cell has become so finely adapted can kill or injure the cell. Cell death, in many respects, is a lesser concern than cell injury because it has no further implications—the cell is dead. Cell damage, on the other hand, has more ominous implications. The subject of extensive scientific and medical research for the past half century, cell damage can be manifested as mutations, birth defects, or cancer.

Mutation

Mutation, defined as any change in the genetic material, is perhaps the most worrisome type of cell damage because of its potential for harming not only the person or organism harboring the mutant cell but, if the mutation occurs in an egg or sperm, unborn generations as well. To understand the significance of mutation, it is necessary to examine the nature of the hereditary material itself.

The most conspicuous organelle in most cells is the nucleus, readily visible under an ordinary light microscope. The nucleus contains threadlike structures called **chromosomes;** each species of plant or animal has its own characteristic number of chromosomes per cell—in humans the normal chromosome number is 46. When cells undergo **mitosis** (cell division), each chromosome splits longitudinally into two daughter **chromatids,** one of which goes into each of the two newly forming cells. Thus the number of chromosomes per nucleus remains constant and the hereditary material contained within the chromosomes is equally shared.

Chemically, each chromosome consists of a single giant molecule of DNA (deoxyribonucleic acid) and associated histone and nonhistone proteins. The DNA molecule itself is composed of two antiparallel strands of alternating units of a five-carbon sugar and phosphate molecules, cross-linked by one of four different nitrogenous bases (adenine, guanine, thymine, and cytosine), and twisted into a helical configuration (see Figure 6-1). The pairing of the nitrogenous bases is quite specific: adenine can pair only with thymine and guanine with cytosine. Along any one strand bases can occur in any sequence, but once the order on one strand is given, the sequence on the antiparallel strand is automatically determined. The adenine-thymine (A-T) or guanine-cytosine (G-C) combination making up each cross-connection is referred to as a **base pair.**

DNA is vitally important to cellular function and is often referred to as the "Master Molecule" because 1) it passes genetic information from one generation to the next and 2) it controls cellular metabolism by giving the instructions for protein synthesis.

The hereditary characteristics are controlled by **genes** along the length

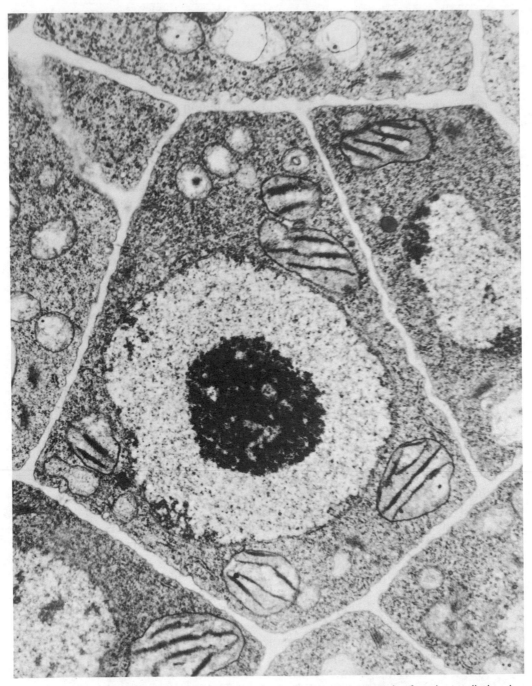

The complexity of cell structure can be seen in this electron micrograph of a plant cell showing such organelles as nucleus, chloroplasts, ribosomes, endoplasmic reticulum, mitochondria, and vacuoles. Environmental toxins act here at the cellular level within organisms. *[Mathew Nadaka-vukaren]*

of the chromosome. In essence, a gene is a section of chromosome consisting of thousands of base pairs (ranging from 1,500 in bacterial DNA to approximately 40,000 in higher organisms). Genes are responsible for the production of proteins necessary for proper cell function. It is absolutely essential that the integrity of the DNA molecule be maintained if the correct information for protein synthesis is to be passed from one generation to the next. Any change within the gene constitutes a mutation.

Types of Mutations

There are three basic types of mutations recognized.

"Point" Mutation (gene mutation). By far the most common type of mutation, point mutations involve a change at the molecular level within a gene. Such a change could consist of the deletion, addition, or substitution of a single base pair or could involve a small portion of a single gene (e.g., a so-called "jumping gene," more properly referred to as a "transposable element"). Any of these changes would result in the "misreading" of the genetic code (the sequence of bases along a DNA strand is all-important; any change can result in the wrong protein being formed). The severity of a point mutation depends on precisely where within a gene the change occurs; it can range from being lethal to causing an almost imperceptible loss of vigor. Point mutations are now known to be responsible for several serious human ailments, including sickle-cell anemia, hemophilia, diabetes, and achondroplastic dwarfism. Though such ailments are tragic for the victim (prior to modern forms of treatment, which are only partially effective, these diseases invariably resulted in death at a fairly early age), many geneticists are more concerned about the accumulation of sub-lethal mutations in populations. Such sub-lethal mutations don't kill their victims outright, but render them less fit than they would otherwise be. Examples of the types of impairment that could result from a sub-lethal mutation include reduced physical or mental vigor, shortened life span, increased susceptibility to disease, or varying degrees of malformation of some organ. Such changes, though possibly debilitating, nevertheless permit afflicted individuals to survive, reproduce, and pass altered genes on to succeeding generations.

Chromosomal Aberrations. These represent gross structural changes in the chromosome, usually caused by the loss or addition of sizeable pieces of a chromosome or the reversing of chromosome parts which frequently occurs during a stage of meiosis (reduction division) when the homologous chromosomes are in synapsis and crossing-over occurs. Although some types of chromosomal aberration seem to have little outward effect, others can have serious consequences. In humans, the translocation of sections of chromosomes 9 and 22 results in a specific chromosomal abnormality (the "Philadelphia chromosome") that results in the development of chronic myelogenous leukemia, a form of cancer. In the majority of cases, loss of a part of a chromosome is fatal to the cell—that is, it represents a lethal mutation.

Figure 6-1   DNA Double Helix

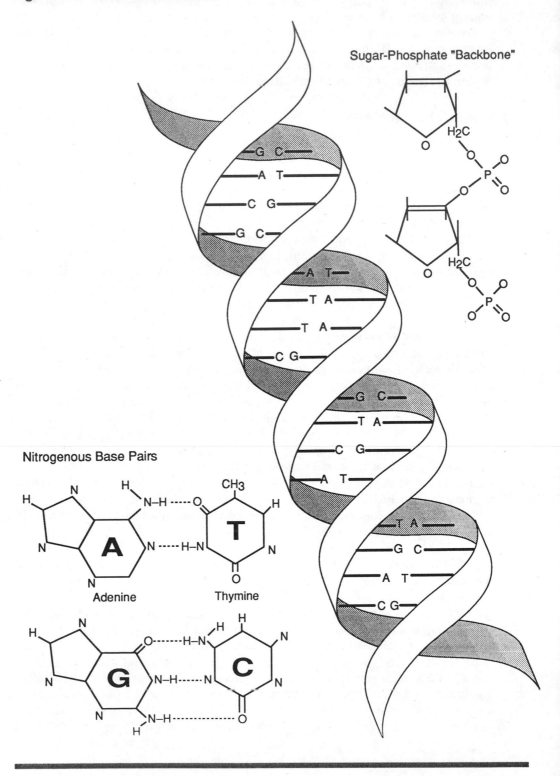

Sugar-Phosphate "Backbone"

Nitrogenous Base Pairs

Adenine   Thymine

Change in Chromosome Number. Caused by the nondisjunction (failure to separate) of paired homologous chromosomes during meiosis, this type of mutation features some cells with more than the normal chromosome number, others with less. In some cases, a change in chromosome number can be lethal. Having three copies (**trisomy**) of chromosome 16 is relatively common in the very early stages of human development; however, none of the fetuses characterized by this condition ever survives to birth. Trisomy of chromosomes 13 and 18 also is seen relatively often in fetuses miscarried during the first few months of pregnancy, but the condition is extremely rare among liveborn infants and almost all of them die soon after birth (Sack, 1999). The best known human ailment resulting from a change in chromosome number is Down's Syndrome. Afflicting about 3 babies out of every 2,000 live births, Down's Syndrome inevitably results in mental retardation (IQ seldom exceeds 70) as well as below-average physical and psychomotor skills. Victims often exhibit heart malformations and respiratory problems, few live beyond the age of 50. Down's Syndrome occurs due to the presence in the victim's cells of 47 chromosomes instead of the normal 46 (to be more precise, three copies of chromosome 21 rather than two). Interestingly, the likelihood of a woman's giving birth to a Down's Syndrome child increases as the mother gets older. While the likelihood of a 30-year-old woman giving birth to a Down's Syndrome child is 1 in 1,000, at age 40 the risk increases tenfold, to 1 in 100; at 45, it is still higher—one out of every 50 infants is likely to be a Down's baby. Although the reason for the increased frequency of this birth defect among older mothers is not known with certainty, the prevailing theory is that since each female child is born with all the egg cells she will ever have, these eggs are subject to deterioration with aging or with exposure to toxic substances. The older the woman, the greater the possibility that her egg cells could sustain damage resulting in a mutation. Given the enhanced risk, it is now common practice for pregnant women 35 or older to undergo a prenatal diagnostic procedure such as **amniocentesis** or **chorionic villus sampling**. By removing and culturing fetal cells, medical personnel can determine whether the developing child has Down's Syndrome or any of approximately 100 other genetic diseases. If test results are positive, the parents then have the option of terminating the pregnancy.

Two other human abnormalities resulting from a change in chromosome number are Klinefelter's Syndrome, found only in males, and Turner's Syndrome, restricted to females. Whereas a normal man has an X and a Y sex chromosome, victims of Klinefelter's Syndrome have an extra X, or 47 chromosomes altogether. This condition, one of the most common of all genetic abnormalities, can cause a variety of problems, ranging from learning disabilities, language difficulties, behavioral problems, infertility, and, in about one-third of cases, enlargement of the breasts following puberty. Many of these symptoms respond to therapy, enabling Klinefelter males to lead normal, productive lives even though they will never be able to father children (nevertheless, many marry and are sexually active). The frequency of Klinefelter's births is relatively high—about 2 out of every 1,000 male births—and is only slightly more prevalent among children of older mothers. Turner's Syndrome, by contrast, occurs when one X chromosome is missing; i.e., the victim has only one sex chromosome, for a total of 45 instead of the normal 46. This malady is out-

BOX 6-2

Microbial Killers

Toxic chemical pollutants may be the current "hot button" issue among many environmentalists today, but historically the primary focus of environmental health practitioners has been reducing the incidence of infectious epidemic disease. Fostered by poor living conditions and spread through contaminated food and water, bacterial, viral, and parasitic pathogens have been responsible for the vast majority of human deaths from time immemorial until the early 20th century. Even today, throughout much of the developing world infectious killers such as tuberculosis, malaria, and diarrheal diseases remain leading causes of mortality.

In North America and Europe, however, deaths caused by infectious microbes began to decline noticeably about 100 years ago, thanks in large part to drinking water purification, sewage treatment, and vector control. In the United States, infectious disease mortality rates dropped by approximately 2.8% annually between 1900 and 1937 (with the exception of 1918 when a worldwide outbreak of "Spanish flu" sent death rates soaring everywhere). From 1937 until 1952, mortality rates due to infectious diseases dropped even more precipitously—8.2% per year—as cases of pneumonia, influenza, and tuberculosis plummeted. These years witnessed the introduction of powerful new antibacterial drugs—sulfonamides, penicillin, streptomycin, isoniazid—but it's likely that a number of factors in addition to improved medications account for mortality declines. From the mid-1950s until 1980 infectious disease death rates continued to drop, albeit more slowly than during the preceding 15 years. By this time it had become an

article of faith that humankind (or at least that segment fortunate enough to live in affluent, sanitized, well-fed nations) had forever left behind the "age of pestilence and famine"—characterized by high rates of infectious disease mortality, especially among children and young adults. Like it or not, we had moved, so it was believed, into the modern age of degenerative diseases where most deaths occur among the elderly and are due to chronic ills such as cardiovascular disease or cancer.

Dismissal of microbial threats as a thing of the past has proven premature, however. In 1981 medical recognition of Acquired Immune Deficiency Syndrome (AIDS) reminded the world that pathogens still lurk among human populations. From 1981-1996 the U.S. witnessed a steady rise in mortality rates due to infectious diseases, primarily AIDS and tuberculosis. Unfortunately, AIDS was but the most recent of several frightening diseases to make headlines over the past several decades. Medical researchers now speak of "newly emerging pathogens" to describe outbreaks of previously unknown ailments such as Lassa fever, Legionnaires' Disease, toxic shock syndrome, Ebola virus, hantavirus, and E. coli 0157:H7 food poisoning. In addition, old microbial diseases are now showing up in new places, South America's cholera epidemic of the mid-1990s being a case in point. Other killers of yesteryear are surfacing in new forms; in late 1997, "bird flu"—a strain of influenza previously documented only among avian species—broke out in Hong Kong, killing four of the 16 people infected. Fears that the Hong Kong outbreak might herald a return of the 1918 influenza pandemic that killed over 21 million people worldwide fortunately weren't realized, but medical authorities fully expect more such unwelcome surprises. AIDS may be the first large-scale modern epidemic of infectious disease, but almost certainly it won't be the last. The world today is more vulnerable than ever before to the global spread of infections. As ever more crowded human populations invade previously undisturbed ecosystems, especially in the tropics, opportunities for contact with animal pathogens proliferate. The rapid expansion of global commerce and tourism provide easy access for microbes on one continent to travel quickly to distant locations, either riding along with cargo, harbored by stowaway insects, or incubating in the bodies of travelers. Unfortunately, the Western world's single-minded preoccupation with finding a cure for cancer and other degenerative diseases has caused us largely to ignore the microbial

pathogens which remain an ever-present threat. The nations of the world still lack an "early warning system" to ensure the quick detection of new diseases when they first appear or to identify old diseases when they show up in unexpected places or in clever disguises. Continued delay in confronting this challenge due to a misplaced faith in humanity's supposed conquest of infectious disease is a risky tactic. As Dr. Richard Krause of the U.S. National Institutes of Health commented nearly 20 years ago, "Plagues are as certain as death and taxes."

References

Armstrong, G.L., et al. 1999. "Trends in Infectious Disease Mortality in the United States During the 20th Century." *Journal of the American Medical Association* 281, no. 1 (Jan. 6):61-66.

Garrett, Laurie. 1994. *The Coming Plague*. Farrar, Straus, and Giroux.

wardly expressed by retarded sexual development (no breast development, failure to menstruate or ovulate), unusually short stature (generally under 5 feet), a webbed neck, and broad chest. Treatment methods developed within recent years have made it possible for an increasing number of Turner's Syndrome women to live near-normal lives. Interestingly, the incidence of Turner's Syndrome is far lower than that of Klinefelter's—about 1 in 3,000 female births. This discrepancy appears to be due to a very high rate of intrauterine deaths among fetuses with only one sex chromosome (Klug and Cummings, 1997).

Cause of Mutations

That mutations occur is not in question; their underlying cause is less well understood. A great many mutations occur spontaneously due to natural causes. Some of these spontaneous mutations have been attributed to radiation exposure from cosmic rays and radioactive minerals in the earth's crust. However, it is thought that such relatively low levels of background radiation are insufficient to account for the majority of spontaneous mutations, the cause of which remains a mystery.

Since the early 1900s, a number of substances identified as capable of inducing mutations have been introduced into the human environment and have raised serious concerns within the scientific community regarding their potential for increasing mutation rates. Such substances are known as

mutagens. X-rays were the first mutagens to be recognized, their mutagenic effect on fruit flies being described in 1927 by the great geneticist H. J. Muller at Indiana University. Subsequently a number of chemical compounds have been found to possess mutagenic properties, among them formaldehyde, mustard gas, nitrous acid, colchicine, and vinyl chloride. Many other candidates are now under suspicion as being possible mutagens.

Mutation Rates

Although the probability of any given human gene in an egg or sperm cell undergoing a spontaneous mutation is difficult to estimate accurately, it is generally regarded as low. However, one must keep in mind that each person has millions of genes. The chances of a mutation occurring in at least one of those genes is thus quite large. In fact, the English geneticist Harry Harris asserts that, on the average, every newborn child may be "expected, as the result of a new mutation in either of its parents, to synthesize at least one structurally variant enzyme or protein." Since only those mutations which occur in an egg or sperm have the potential to be passed on to subsequent generations, studies of mutation frequency have focused on these so-called "genetic mutations." Typically mutations occurring in a person's sex cells have no effect upon him or her but present a risk to succeeding generations of offspring. On the other hand, a mutation occurring in any cell other than an egg or sperm (somatic mutation) can adversely affect the person who sustained the mutation, but such injury will not be inherited by his or her children and thus represents no threat to the human gene pool.

In this context it is of interest to note that about 15% of all women who know they are pregnant suffer spontaneous miscarriages, usually within the first four months after conception. Of these fetal losses, about 5–6% are caused by abnormal chromosomes. It is suspected that the impact of chromosomal defects on the viability of developing fetuses is actually much higher than the above numbers suggest, with many conceptuses never reaching the stage of implantation in the uterus. Some researchers estimate that perhaps as few as a third of all human pregnancies reach full term because of genetic abnormalities that preclude survival of the fetus (Sack, 1999).

The great concern among geneticists today is that exposure of populations to the artificial mutagens so common in the modern environment could further increase mutation rates. Since most mutations are harmful to some degree, it is in humanity's long-term interest to keep mutation rates as low as possible.

Birth Defects

As we have seen in the previous section, mutations in parents' sex cells can result in their children being born with structural or functional abnormalities, but by no means are all birth defects due to mutations. Of the roughly 150,000 infants in the United States whom the Centers for Disease Control and Prevention (CDC) estimates are born with birth defects each year, mutations are believed to account for approximately 25% of the total. Since birth defects constitute the leading cause of infant mortality in the United States, efforts to understand why fetal malformation occurs and how to prevent such a tragic course of events assume added urgency.

Living things are far more sensitive to adverse environmental influences during their early stages of development than they are at any other time. Embryos that are perfectly normal genetically can be seriously or fatally damaged if exposed to extraneous hazards. Investigations over the past several decades have revealed the sad truth that the womb is not the safe haven it was once assumed to be.

The likelihood that all abnormal development is triggered by some aspect of the environment (even hereditary disorders were at some point initiated by a mutation) has given rise to the science of **teratology**—the study of abnormal formations in animals or plants—and to the search for **teratogens,** substances that cause birth defects.

Table 6-1   Some Known Human Teratogens

Teratogen	Effect
Ionizing Radiation	
X-rays	central nervous system disorders,
Nuclear fallout	microcephaly, eye problems,
	mental retardation
Pathogenic Infections	
German measles	congenital heart defect, deafness, cataracts
Syphilis and herpes simplex type 2	mental retardation, microcephaly
Cytomegalovirus	kidney and liver disorders, pneumonia, brain damage
Toxoplasmosis	fatal lesions in the central nervous system
Drugs and Chemicals	
Thalidomide	phocomelia
Methyl mercury	mental retardation, sensory and motor problems
DES	vaginal cancer in girls, genital abnormalities in boys
Dioxin	structural deformities, miscarriages
Anesthesia	miscarriages, structural deformities
Alcohol	mental retardation, growth deficiences, microcephaly, facial irregularities
Cigarette smoke	low birth weight, miscarriage, stillbirth
Dilantin	heart malformations, cleft palate, harelip, mental retardation, microcephaly
Valproic acid	spina bifida
Accutane	cardiovascular abnormalities, deformation of the ear, hydrocephaly, microcephaly
Tegison	same effect as for Accutane

Interest in birth abnormalities is undoubtedly as old as humanity itself, although prior to the 20th century most ideas regarding birth defects involved considerably more fantasy than fact. From ancient times until fairly recently, some societies believed that the emotional state and visual impressions of an expectant mother could influence the physical development of her child. For this reason women in ancient Greece were encouraged to gaze at statuary representing the ideal human form, while Norwegian mothers-to-be were cautioned against looking at rabbits, for fear their babies would be born with harelip! The Babylonians and Sumerians regarded certain types of malformations as portents of coming events; medieval Europeans regarded them as evidence that the mother had indulged in intercourse with Satan or other demons and occasionally used this event as an excuse to execute the unfortunate mother and child. The so-called "Theory of Divine Retribution," also prevalent in Europe during the Middle Ages, viewed the birth of a defective child as God's punishment on the parents for past sins. With the rebirth of scientific inquiry in the Western world following the Renaissance, less mythical interpretations of teratogenesis were sought. In the 17th century birth defects were attributed to such factors as the narrowness of the mother's uterus, poor posture of the pregnant woman, or to a fall or blow on the abdomen during pregnancy. Though inaccurate, these explanations at least were an attempt to find a rational explanation for what remained a mysterious phenomenon. Gregor Mendel's discovery of the laws of genetics, followed by an explosion of research into the mechanism of heredity, led in the early 20th century to acceptance of the idea that all developmental errors could be attributed to faulty genes. This view prevailed until the mid-20th century, but a series of significant discoveries and observations since that time has once again altered our perception regarding teratogenesis and has given new impetus and urgency to the field of teratology.

The first key discovery to contradict the prevailing view that heredity is all-important emerged from animal studies investigating the influence of maternal diet on the outcome of pregnancy. In 1940 a report was published showing that specific types of nutritional deficiencies in pregnant rats caused predictable types and percentages of malformations in their offspring (Warkany, 1972). This finding effectively shattered old ideas about the overriding importance of genes and the conviction that the fetus could parasitize the mother if necessary to ensure normal development. Continued research into the influence of maternal diet on fetal development has confirmed and broadened these original findings. It is now known that a wide range of nutrients, from proteins to trace minerals to specific amino acids, are essential for normal development. Conversely, an excess of some of these necessary substances (e.g. phenylalanine, vitamin A) can exert teratogenic effects. Among the birth abnormalities associated with a specific nutritional deficiency are neural tube defects such as spina bifida and anencephaly. Recognition that up to 75% of these devastating birth abnormalities could be prevented simply by increasing a pregnant woman's dietary intake of **folic acid**, one of the B vitamins, led the FDA to mandate the fortification of flour, corn meal, pasta, and rice with this micronutrient. The FDA action, which took effect on January 1, 1998, marks the first time the federal agency has required fortification of a food for the express purpose of preventing a birth defect.

In 1941 an unusually large number of babies in both the United States and Australia were born suffering from congenital cataracts, heart defects, or deafness. Epidemiological studies launched to try to determine the cause for such an outbreak found that the only common thread linking all the victims was the fact that during the first trimester of pregnancy, their mothers had contracted German measles *(Rubella),* which had reached epidemic proportions that year. The fact that a virus could cross the placental barrier and damage the fetus was thus established.

While these two developments demonstrated that mammalian embryos are vulnerable to such commonplace environmental influences as inadequate diet and infections, the most dramatic confirmation that certain environmental factors (in this case an artificially synthesized drug) must be regarded as a potential risk to the unborn came only in the early 1960s with revelation of what has since come to be referred to as the "Thalidomide Tragedy."

Thalidomide was a **drug** first synthesized by a pharmaceutical company in Germany in 1953 and subsequently developed and widely marketed in western Europe as a mild sedative and as a treatment for morning sickness. Preliminary testing on laboratory animals indicated that thalidomide had little injurious effect even when taken in quantity (in fact, humans who attempted to commit suicide using the drug survived extremely large doses). With evidence of its safety regarding overdosing, but with virtually no testing for other side effects, the German manufacturer put thalidomide on the market as a nonprescription sleeping pill and, thanks to an aggressive advertising campaign stressing its safety, thalidomide (sold under the trade name *Cantergan*) became the most widely used sedative in Germany and was extensively sold in the United Kingdom; altogether, the drug was marketed in 48 countries during the early 1960s. Two American **drug** companies initially showed interest in acquiring thalidomide but concluded from their own tests that the drug was less effective than the brands they were already marketing. Somewhat later another American firm, impressed by the growing popularity of thalidomide in Europe, began another series of tests and released the drug for prescription use in Canada. In the United States, however, a doctor with the Food and Drug Administration had nagging doubts about some unexplained neurological results among long-term thalidomide users and restricted use of the drug in this country to a small clinical human trial. At about this time (1960) the European medical community was becoming increasingly puzzled by the sudden increase in what had formerly been an extremely rare type of birth abnormality. In near-epidemic proportions children were being born with a condition known as **phocomelia** ("seal-limb"), in which there is typically a hand or foot attached directly to the torso without an arm or leg. In some cases, however, even the hands and feet were absent, the babies being born with only a head and torso. The presence of large numbers of babies with such an obvious deformity couldn't be overlooked, but intense questioning of the parents regarding their hereditary background, blood type, radiation exposure, or chromosomal aberrations in other children failed to reveal a common link. Finally two alert physicians made the connection between thalidomide use early in pregnancy to the birth of limbless babies. Subsequent studies revealed that 40% of the women who had taken thalidomide during their first trimester of pregnancy delivered babies afflicted with phocomelia.

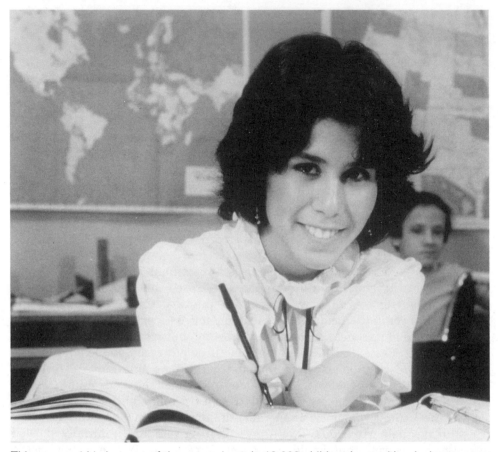

This young girl is but one of the approximately 12,000 children born with missing arms or legs as a result of fetal exposure to thalidomide—a nonprescription sedative widely used in Europe during the early 1960s. *[March of Dimes Birth Defects Foundation]*

As proof of thalidomide's teratogenic properties gained acceptance, use of the drug was gradually discontinued in country after country, but not before nearly 12,000 children had been permanently disabled.

Ironically, thalidomide's unsavory reputation may yet be redeemed. Research demonstrating that thalidomide acts by inhibiting blood vessel growth has suggested its potential for combating a number of serious human ailments, including brain cancer, AIDS, and lupus. The drug also offers hope for treating diabetic retinopathy and macular degeneration, the two leading causes of blindness in the United States. In July 1998, the FDA approved the use of thalidomide for treating a serious inflammatory skin condition in patients with leprosy (*erythema nodosum leprosum*) and by October of that year thalidomide became commercially available in the U.S. for the first time. Produced exclusively by Calgene Corporation under the trade name "Thalidomid," thalidomide is now being prescribed for hundreds of critically ill cancer patients as tests of its safety and efficacy are ongoing (Henderson, 1999; FDA, 1998).

In the early 1970s, not long after the heart-breaking photos of thalidomide babies had receded from media attention, another teratogenic chemical made headline news. Diethylstilbestrol, or **DES**, was first synthesized in 1938 and widely prescribed to pregnant women in the United States and Latin America for several decades thereafter. Because its biological action resembles that of natural estrogen, doctors began administering it to women experiencing problem pregnancies in the mistaken belief that it would prevent miscarriages. In the late 1950s one drug company, touting the miraculous properties of DES, even urged that *all* pregnant women use the drug to produce "bigger and stronger babies!" Eventually it was demonstrated that DES had no beneficial health effects; in fact, when given in high doses before the 20th week of pregnancy, DES actually *increased* the risk of miscarriage. Gradually the popularity of the drug began to wane, but not before an estimated 5 million pregnant women had used it. Little more was heard about DES until the late 1960s when doctors at Massachusetts General Hospital in Boston made the connection between a rare form of vaginal cancer (clear-cell adenocarcinoma) in young female patients and the use of DES by their mothers during pregnancy. The fact that teratogenic effects could lie hidden for years, only to manifest themselves when the affected child became an adult hit the medical world like a bombshell—obviously birth defects don't have to be immediately visible to be important. Over the years that followed, several hundred cases of vaginal cancer were diagnosed among "DES daughters." While DES-related troubles initially focused on the daughters of women who had taken the drug, it gradually became apparent that girls were not the only victims nor was vaginal cancer the only problem. Many DES sons exhibit congenital deformities of the reproductive system and reduced fertility—problems experienced by DES daughters as well. DES daughters are at heightened risk of tubal pregnancies, miscarriages, and premature deliveries—if they are able to become pregnant in the first place. Perhaps most ominous of all are recent research results suggesting that DES exposure *in utero* causes genetic changes in a female embryo's egg cells that may pose a cancer threat to yet a third generation—the DES *granddaughters*. Unfortunately, hopes that the sad saga of DES would be confined to the generation exposed in the womb may prove too optimistic (Colburn et al., 1996; Newbold et al., 1998).

The thalidomide and DES episodes not only emphasized the importance of testing new drugs for their teratogenic effects, but also raised the profoundly disturbing question of what other drugs and medicines widely used by pregnant women might be doing to their unborn babies. That harmful effects could indeed result from medications used by pregnant women was confirmed again in the early 1980s when a French physician linked numerous cases of spina bifida to maternal use of valproic acid to control epileptic seizures (Harris and Wynne, 1994). A very beneficial medication for the mother's health problems, valproic acid proved devastating for unborn children exposed to the medication *in utero*. Valproic acid and thalidomide produced such distinctive types of abnormalities that they could scarcely go unnoticed. Conceivably, however, other teratogens that result in slight impairment of mental abilities, slight physical abnormalities, or diminished vigor might never be suspected as harmful. These tragic episodes stimulated research, still ongoing, into what other substances present a threat to the unborn. Though much remains to be learned, investigations over the past several decades have implicated an increasing number of drugs and chemicals as proven or suspected teratogens.

Among them, in addition to thalidomide and DES: dioxin, organic mercury, lead, cadmium, anesthetic gases, alcohol, and—responsible for by far the largest number of birth abnormalities and miscarriages—cigarette smoke. In spite of the gruesome lessons of past tragedies, pregnant women continue using various drugs (e.g. aspirin, antacids, barbiturates, tranquilizers, cough medicines), drinking, and smoking, even though it is generally accepted that excess use of any of the above substances carries some risk of fetal damage.

Self-administered drugs or medications are not the only source of teratogenic exposure, of course. Hundreds of thousands of American workers currently are employed in occupations that expose them to reproductive hazards—lead, anesthetic gases, ethylene oxide (used as a sterilant for many hospital supplies), and certain pesticides. While few well-documented associations between specific workplace chemicals and reproductive problems (i.e. miscarriage, reduced fertility, neonatal death, birth defects) exist at present, this doesn't mean such a linkage is nonexistent. Very few well-designed clinical or epidemiologic studies on the issue have been conducted, making it impossible to draw definitive conclusions. Nevertheless, a 1985 review of 2,800 chemicals evaluated for their ability to induce birth defects in animals indicated that more than a third exhibited some teratogenic potential (Chivian et al., 1993). Unfortunately, most workplace teratogens are identified only after significant numbers of employees experience personal tragedies. Among the more recent reproductive hazards to make headlines are two glycol ethers, widely used as solvents in the manufacture of computer chips. Studies conducted on female workers exposed to the chemicals during the chip-making process found that the women suffered miscarriages 40% more frequently than did nonexposed women in the industry and experienced 30% fewer pregnancies. As a result of these findings, several of the corporate giants in the semiconductor industry are allowing pregnant female employees to work outside the chip fabrication area of the plant and have announced their intention to phase the hazardous chemicals out of the production process altogether (Markoff, 1992; "Solvents Used," 1992). The widespread assumption that such workplace precautions need apply only to female workers is now being challenged by provocative, though inconclusive, evidence that a *father's* exposure to environmental hazards may also lead to defective offspring. It has long been observed that men working as painters, farmers, or mechanics—jobs involving exposure to certain solvents and pesticides—tend to be at higher risk of fathering children with birth defects than do men in other occupations. These observations have stimulated a new look at the impact which mutagenic or teratogenic substances might have on sperm production or on the chemical composition of semen, and thereby on the development of a fertilized egg (Stone, 1992).

While some progress in elucidating the mechanism of teratogenesis has been made in recent years, much more research is needed. Nevertheless, some broad generalizations about the causation of birth defects can be made. Perhaps most critical is the finding that fetal vulnerability to teratogens depends on the stage of development at the time of exposure. By far the most sensitive period is the time of tissue and organ formation (organogenesis), a period lasting from about the 18th day after conception to approximately the 60th day, with the peak of sensitivity around the 30th day. During this time, interfer-

Maternal consumption of alcohol during pregnancy is now recognized as a serious problem worldwide, its most dramatic consequences manifested here in the birth defect known as Fetal Alcohol Syndrome (FAS). FAS children generally suffer from low IQ, attention deficits, memory problems, and hyperactivity. The majority exhibit abnormalities of the upper lip, teeth problems, and an unusual shape of the head, face, ears, palms, and back/neck/spine. *[From "Fetal Alcohol Syndrome in Adolescents and Adults" by Ann Pytkowicz Streissguth, PhD., et al., JAMA, April 17, 1991, Vol. 265. Courtesy of FAS Research Fund]*

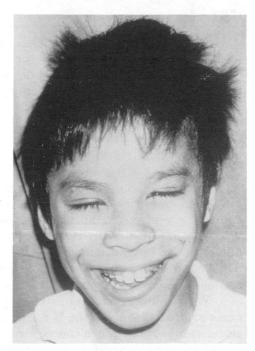

ence with development can result in gross structural defects. In the case of the thalidomide episode, it was found that virtually all of the thalidomide mothers had taken the drug precisely during those few days when the limb buds were forming. Those women who used thalidomide before or after this critical time gave birth to normal babies. Similarly, DES exposure after the 20th week of pregnancy did not result in reproductive tract deformities, while exposure before the tenth week increased the risk of cancer in DES daughters. During the first week after conception, when the embryo is a relatively undifferentiated mass of cells, any damage caused by teratogenic exposure will be lethal to the developing embryo. After the 8th week, though the fetus is barely an inch long, its organs are already basically formed. Exposure to teratogens after this time can cause such harm as mental retardation, blindness, or damage to the external sex organs, but the time for major structural deformation has passed. It must be recognized, however, that individual genetic differences in both mother and child will determine the extent of damage caused by teratogenic exposure. No teratogen causes birth defects in 100% of those exposed; if a group of women, all at the same stage of pregnancy, were exposed to equal concentrations of the same teratogen, some would give birth to babies with serious abnormalities, others with only moderate damage, and some would deliver infants who were perfectly normal (Harris and Wynne, 1994).

A second widely accepted generalization about teratogenesis is that as the dosage of a teratogen increases, the degree of damage increases. Basing their assumptions on the results of animal studies, teratologists thus presume the existence of a threshold below which no injury of any kind can be demonstrated. Determining exactly where that threshold is for any particular substance is, however, uncertain at best, and expectant mothers are well advised to limit their exposure to potential teratogens to the greatest extent possible.

Cancer

Few words arouse such emotions of sheer terror and hopelessness today as does the term "cancer." As the second leading cause of death in the United States at the present time (heart disease ranks first), cancer appears to have assumed epidemic proportions. Throughout the industrialized nations, cancer now accounts for 20–25% of all deaths each year; worldwide, cancer claims an estimated 6.6 million victims annually. In the United States, over 1,500 people die of cancer every day, with a yearly toll exceeding 560,000. Cancer is not an age-specific disease; although incidence rates are highest among the elderly, cancer is the second-leading cause of death, after accidents, among children aged 1–14. In general, cancer death rates are considerably higher in developed countries than in the developing world, but the *types* of cancer which are most prevalent in various parts of the world differ sharply. Malignancies associated with cigarette smoking, asbestos exposure, or high-fat diets are far more common among populations in industrialized countries, while cancers linked to certain food preservatives, viral infections, or fungal toxins in food are more prevalent in the developing world.

While cancer *incidence* rates continue to climb, with over a million new cases being diagnosed in the U.S. each year, the same is no longer true of cancer *mortality* rates. Since cancer record-keeping began in 1930, cancer death rates increased inexorably, year after year, reaching a peak in 1990. In 1991, however, overall U.S. cancer mortality rates began a slow but steady decline that researchers are convinced will continue for at least 20 years. The welcome reversal is attributed to a variety of factors: decades of anti-smoking campaigns and other preventive efforts, earlier detection when malignancies are more likely to respond to treatment, and improvements in medical care (Cole and Rodu, 1996). For some types of cancer, the turn-around in mortality rates was achieved long before the 1990s. For over a half-century, deaths due to cancer of the uterus, cervix, and stomach have fallen by more than 70% in the United States. In the case of uterine and cervical cancers, credit for the decline in death rates is attributed to widespread use of the Pap smear test which provides early diagnosis when the disease is still treatable. Experts estimate that a further 90% reduction in the current annual number of U.S. cervical cancer deaths (est. 4600) could be achieved if all American women would take advantage of this simple procedure. Regarding stomach cancer mortality, which is lower today in the United States than anywhere else in the world (at present the East Asian and eastern European countries have the highest incidence of stomach cancer mortality), favorable trends are probably due to improved methods of transport and to refrigeration which have made fresh produce available year-round. These advantages of modern life are significant in terms of cancer prevention because they have led to increased consumption of fresh fruits and vegetables (known to contain anticarcinogenic compounds), thereby lessening dependence on the salted, pickled, or smoke-preserved foods that are thought to pose a cancer risk.

More recently, colorectal cancers have also begun to decline in both North America and western Europe; liver cancer, bladder cancer, and childhood leukemia mortality rates exhibit similar downward trends. Most encouraging, however, is the long-awaited reversal in the lung cancer death rate.

Although lung cancer continues to kill three times as many Americans as colon cancer, the second-leading cause of U.S. cancer mortality, death rates for this disease are finally beginning to drop, falling by 3.9% between 1991–1995. Other smoking-related cancers declined by 2% during the same period—an indication that anti-smoking education efforts are finally paying off. Unfortunately, death rates for some forms of cancer continue to rise: non-Hodgkins lymphoma (due in part to the increasing incidence of this disease among AIDS patients), malignant melanoma, pancreatic cancer, multiple myeloma, and chronic leukemia among the elderly (Cole and Rodu, 1996).

Cancer, of course, is not a new disease; ancient societies, like their modern counterparts, were familiar with the ravages of cancer. Indeed, all multicellular organisms, plant and animal, are subject to the occasional development of malignancies. However, cancer's rapid rise to prominence as a leading cause of illness and death during the 20th century has imbued the malady with an aura of dread and fatalism. Until recently, progress achieved in the so-called war against cancer remained disappointingly limited after decades of intensive medical research and the expenditure of billions of dollars. Major gains *were* achieved in prolonging a cancer patient's survival time after the initial diagnosis, and notable successes were scored in reducing deaths from childhood leukemia and Hodgkins lymphoma; nevertheless, the "magic bullet" that would provide a cure for cancer was nowhere in sight. Research and observation strongly suggested that a majority of cancers were associated with environmental causes (using the term "environment" in its broadest sense to include diet, smoking, sun exposure, chemical pollutants, and so forth), yet the mechanism for such interaction remained unknown. Within the past decade however, several major breakthroughs in cancer research have revolutionized our understanding of carcinogenesis. While a great deal more remains to be learned, these findings have provided important information on how once-healthy cells become malignant and offer new hope for both prevention and treatment of this formidable killer.

What Causes Cancer?

"Cancer" is a collective term used to describe a number of diseases that differ in origin, prognosis, and treatment. It is essentially a condition in which the regulating forces that govern normal cell processes no longer function correctly, leading to uncontrolled cell proliferation. Cancerous cells, unlike normal ones, continue to divide and spread, invading other tissues where they interfere with vital bodily functions and eventually lead to death of the organism. The search for agents responsible for initiating this chain of events has been ongoing for years and has focused on a number of possibilities including pathogens, hereditary factors, oxidation damage within cells due to normal metabolic processes, and exposure to a wide range of environmental **carcinogens** (substances that can cause cancer) such as toxic chemicals and radiation.

Viruses are definitely known to cause some forms of cancer in animals (e.g. viral leukemia in cats, Rous sarcoma in chickens) and are suspected of being involved in the type of human cancer known as Burkitt's lymphoma. Similarly, there appears to be an association between hepatitis-B infection

Figure 6-2 Cancer Death Rates, by Site, U.S., 1930–1995

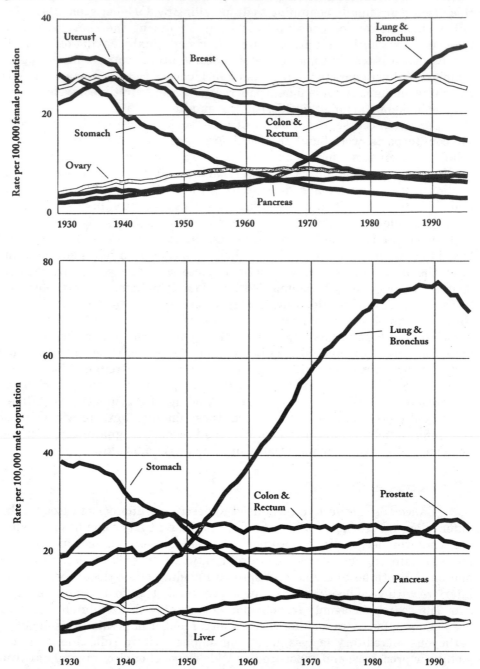

Note: Rates are per 100,000; age-adjusted to the 1970 U.S. standard population. Uterus cancer rates are for uterine cervix and uterine corpus combined. Due to changes in ICD coding, numerator information has changed over time. Rates for cancer of the uterus, ovary, lung and brochus, liver, and colon and rectum are affected by these coding changes.

Source: American Cancer Society's Facts and Figures—1999. Reprinted with permission.

and the development of liver cancer, as well as between a herpes-type virus and some cases of cervical cancer, the latter suspicion based on the fact that cervical cancer is most common among women who have had intercourse with various partners. For decades it had been assumed that **bacteria** had no part to play in the cancer drama, but in 1994 researchers at Stanford University reported that the risk for non-Hodgkins lymphoma of the stomach is markedly higher among people infected with the bacterium *Helicobacter pylori,* the common microbe that was recently recognized as the leading cause of stomach ulcers (three years earlier another research team demonstrated an association between this same bacterium and a different form of stomach cancer, gastric carcinoma). Interestingly, while non-Hodgkins lymphoma of the stomach is extremely rare in the United States, it is relatively common in the Veneto region of Italy where 90% of the population is infected with *H. pylori* (Parsonnet et al., 1994; Isaacson, 1994).

Since the rediscovery of Mendelian principles of genetics in the early 1900s, **heredity** has been a prime suspect for cancer causation, particularly because certain kinds of malignancies are more common in some families than in others. It is well-established that a few types of cancer *are* hereditary; among the best known inherited cancers are retinoblastoma, a cancer of the eye, and familial polyposis, a rare type of colon cancer. For the most part, however, studies carried out decades ago discounted heredity as a significant factor in cancer causation. These studies compared the incidence of specific types of cancer among descendants of immigrants to the United States and members of the same ethnic group remaining in the homeland. For example, a 1944 study of the incidence of liver cancer showed that African-Americans have much lower rates of this disease than do native African populations; similarly, Japanese-Americans exhibit low rates of stomach cancer—comparable to those of the general American population—while stomach cancer remains very common in Japan. By contrast, these Japanese-Americans, like other U.S. residents, experience typically high rates of colon cancer, a disease quite rare in Japan. A subsequent study of immigrants to Australia and Canada found that a woman's risk of breast cancer shifted from the rate prevailing in her country of origin toward the rate observed among native-born women in the country to which she moved. Thus women who emigrated from England, where breast cancer rates are relatively high, experienced a lowering of risk in their new country of destination; conversely, female emigrants from Asian countries, where breast cancer rates are lower than those prevailing in Canada and Australia, were more likely to develop breast cancer in their adopted countries than were women in their homelands. Study results strongly suggest that risk of breast cancer has little to do with heredity, but rather is associated with as-yet unidentified environmental and lifestyle factors. Since most of the women emigrated as adults, it also suggests that one's risk of breast cancer can be altered later in life (Kliewer and Smith, 1995).

Although few types of cancers are directly associated with "cancer genes," a tidal wave of new discoveries during the past decade has demonstrated the existence of an inherited *predisposition* to cancer that explains the prevalence of specific types of malignancies within certain families. These findings not only help to explain why some people exposed to known carcinogens remain hale and hearty while others sicken and die, but also offer promising therapeutic approaches for reducing cancer mortality among those likely to develop the disease. A classic example of genetic predisposition to cancer is that of hereditary non-polyposis colon cancer, a common type of colorectal malignancy. Victims of the disease carry an inherited defective gene which, in its normal state, produces a DNA repair protein that acts as a cellular "spell checker," correcting errors in the order of nucleotide base pairs during DNA replication. In mutated form, the gene is no longer able to produce its key protein, so mistakes occurring after replication rapidly accumulate throughout the genetic material, creating a situation that may eventually result in cancer (Leach et al., 1993; Fishel et al., 1993). For individuals with a predisposition for hereditary non-polyposis colon cancer (about 10% of all colon malignancies), the chances of eventually developing colon cancer range between 70–90%, with many victims developing tumors before the age of 50. The practical significance of these recent findings is therefore immense: if carriers could be identified through genetic screening programs, they could begin having regular colonoscopic examinations at an early age in order to detect precancerous polyps when they can be easily removed. Similarly, identified bearers of the defective gene could be strongly advised to adopt the low-fat, high-fiber diet that is known to reduce the risk of colorectal cancer (Weinberg, 1998; Papadopoulos et al., 1994; Bronner et al., 1994).

A great many **environmental agents** such as cigarette smoke, radon gas, sunlight, heavy metals, X-rays, chemical pesticides, some air pollutants, and high-fat diets are known to be carcinogenic. These environmental factors, acting in conjunction with an individual's inherited predisposition to cancer and with acquired susceptibility, are believed to be responsible for an estimated 80–90% of all human cancers. The exact mechanism by which such agents induce a malignancy is still not completely understood, but recent progress in unraveling cancer's mysteries has brought us tantalizingly closer to that goal (Perera, 1997).

How Does Cancer Develop?

Carcinogenesis is a multistep process that begins when a single cell undergoes a mutation. The mutant cell then slowly proliferates to form a small group of genetically identical precancerous cells. This first step, termed **initiation**, is possibly provoked by a brief interaction between the target cell and a carcinogenic agent. It has been demonstrated that many environmental carcinogens (e.g. ultraviolet light, aflatoxin, vinyl chloride, certain components of tobacco smoke, etc.) bond tightly with DNA to form DNA-carcinogen **adducts**, causing genetic damage that can eventually lead to cancer. Researchers can utilize the unique "biomarkers" left at characteristic locations along certain genes to identify the causative agent of a specific cancer—a development with obvious implications for environmental lawyers representing clients claiming harm from toxic pollutants (Semenza and Weasel, 1997)!

Cells that have undergone initiation do not inevitably give rise to malignancies, however. Tumor progression is dependent on the **promotion** of initiated cells by long-term exposure to nonmutagenic agents that stimulate cell proliferation, thereby expanding the number of initiated cells and increasing the likelihood that additional mutations will occur within this population. It has long been observed that onset of malignant disease almost always occurs many years after initial exposure to a cancer-causing agent. This characteristically long **latency period** can be explained by the fact that **progression** of cancer requires considerable time (10–30 years or more, depending on the type of cancer) for a precancerous tumor to accumulate the 3–7 additional independent, random mutations generally needed to cause malignant growth.

During the 1990s, a number of significant findings by cancer researchers further clarified the nature of the molecular changes within genes that lead to the outward manifestation of cancer. It is now known that two major types of genes are of fundamental importance in cancer causation: **proto-oncogenes** and **tumor-suppressor genes**, both of which play an essential role in regulating the cell cycle. Proto-oncogenes tell the cell when to begin dividing; in so doing, they orchestrate orderly fetal development, the routine replacement of worn-out cells, healing of wounds, and so forth. Mutant versions of these genes, called **oncogenes** (from the Greek word *onkos*, meaning "lump" or "mass"), cause cells to divide endlessly when they should not. By contrast, normal tumor-suppressor genes halt uncontrolled multiplication of cells, acting in a manner analogous to the brakes on an automobile. In mutant form, normal gene function is inactivated, resulting in runaway cell proliferation. A number of mutant tumor-suppressor genes and oncogenes have now been identified as key contributors to the development of many cancers. The *ras* oncogene is known to occur in 50% of colon cancers and 90% of pancreatic cancers. Even more ubiquitous is the tumor-suppressor gene, *p53*, found in altered form in the tumors of more than half of all cancer patients, regardless of the type of cancer involved. Normal functioning of *p53* is especially important because, in addition to preventing uncontrolled cell division, the gene gives instructions for a cell to self-destruct when it detects irreparable damage to DNA during cell division. Because of its role in preventing the dangerous proliferation of mutant cells, *p53* is sometimes referred to as the "guardian of the genome."

Research has shown that the progression of a precancerous tumor to a full-blown malignancy requires a series of mutations that both activate specific oncogenes and inactivate specific tumor-suppressor genes. This sequence of events can be, and usually is, blocked by a number of different bodily defense mechanisms that limit the number of times a cell can divide before dying ("cell mortality") or that cause defective cells to self-destruct ("apoptosis"). Only when all such obstacles are surmounted does cancerous growth commence (Weinberg, 1998).

Undoubtedly, the next few years will witness unprecedented expansion of our knowledge regarding cancer causation—knowledge that will provide an increasing number of weapons for fighting and eventually controlling this dreaded disease. In the meantime, however, society must continue ongoing efforts to prevent exposure to the myriad of environmental agents which are believed responsible for the majority of cancers. While new evidence of inherited predisposition to specific cancers explains why some people are more likely to develop cancer than others, it holds true nevertheless that with most cancers even susceptible individuals are unlikely to develop a malignancy in the absence of adverse environmental exposure. Conversely, even individuals who are not genetically predisposed can experience the DNA damage leading to carcinogenesis if exposure to cancer-causing agents is excessive. By eliminating contact with known carcinogens, one can drastically reduce the incidence of a malignancy—as in so many other realms of life, prevention is the best cure for cancer.

Environmental Carcinogens

The fact that an environmental agent can cause cancer was first reported more than two hundred years ago when, in 1775, an English physician, Sir Percival Pott, recognized an association between cancer of the scrotum and exposure to soot. Every patient he examined with this relatively rare ailment had, as a child, worked as a chimney sweep, being lowered naked into chimneys to clean out the soot that accumulated there. In the process, the boys were covered with soot and grime themselves and with the low standards of personal hygiene that characterized those times, some of this soot remained in the folds of the scrotum for long periods, eventually resulting in the development of scrotal cancer years later (more recently the active ingredient in this soot was identified as benzopyrene, known as a very potent carcinogen). Not until the 20th century, however, was much research directed toward detecting environmental carcinogens. Work during the early 1900s revealed the cancer-causing properties of a number of coal tar products and of X-rays, but not until mid-century as age-adjusted cancer rates began to soar did the search for cancer causation acquire new urgency. Since that time the public has been bombarded with so many dire warnings that the average citizen may be excused for thinking that indeed everything causes cancer. This of course is untrue, but the very large number of new chemicals and products that are introduced each year, many without adequate testing for harmful side effects, justifies concern. Epidemiologic surveys carried out on the "geography of cancer" indicate that the incidence of certain types of cancer is elevated in heavily industrialized areas.

Researchers and environmentalists alike continue to debate the extent to which present cancer rates reflect exposure to chemical pollutants as opposed to personal habits such as smoking or diet. The outcome of this controversy is obviously of political and economic importance, since extensive regulation would be required to control the former, while education and persuasion represent the practical limits to modifying the latter. Several of the most prominent public concerns in relation to cancer causation include the following.

Smoking. Tobacco use, particularly cigarette smoking, is now recognized as far and away the leading contributor to cancer mortality. Rates of lung cancer are most reflective of the impact of smoking on health, and the drastic rise in this disease in the United States neatly parallels the increase in the smoking habit in American society. Today about one-third of all U.S. cancer deaths are due to lung cancer, and of the 170,000 new lung cancer victims diagnosed annually in recent years, 87% are cigarette smokers (most of the others are individuals industrially exposed to carcinogens such as asbestos fibers or those exposed to radon gas inside their homes). Death rates among lung cancer victims, as opposed to victims of some other types of cancer, are quite high largely because lung malignancies are seldom diagnosed before the mass has reached a size of about 1 cm in diameter. By that time it has been growing for about 10 years and has usually spread to other parts of the body.

Lung cancer rates began their steady rise in the mid-1930s, approximately 20 years or so after cigarette smoking became popular. Interestingly, until the mid-1950s it was widely assumed that women were resistant to the disease because the incidence of lung cancer among females was negligible compared to that among men. Since the mid-1950s, however, lung cancer mortality among women has been rising rapidly in a fashion parallel to that of males several decades earlier, reflecting social pressures which inhibited women's smoking prior to the "female emancipation" of the 1920s and 1930s. By the late 1980s, lung cancer had surpassed breast cancer as the leading cause of cancer mortality among women, making it for the first time the number one cancer killer among both sexes. As the advertisement for Virginia Slims puts it, "you've come a long way, Baby"—all the way from virtually no lung cancer prior to the 1950s to the current situation where 43 out of every 100,000 American women are diagnosed with lung cancer each year (American Cancer Society, 1999). Thanks to increasing public awareness of the many adverse health impacts of tobacco use following the 1964 Surgeon General's report, the incidence of cigarette smoking among American adults steadily declined from 42% in 1965 to 25% in 1990, a figure that has held relatively steady since that time (National Center for Health Statistics, 1998). According to the Centers for Disease Control and Prevention (CDC), smoking prevalence within the adult population is slightly higher for men (27%) than for women (22.6%) and is highest among Native Americans (36.2%) as compared with other ethnic groups. Smoking prevalence is inversely associated with educational level, reaching its peak (41.9%) among men who never completed high school (the value of education in reducing smoking incidence is called into question, however, by a study conducted at the Harvard School of Public Health showing that cigarette use on American college campuses rose by 28% between 1993–1997). Health officials are disappointed that the consistent downward smoking trend that prevailed from 1965 until 1990 now seems to have stalled. They are even more concerned that between 1991–1997 tobacco use among high school students increased by 32%. While frequent tobacco use is still significantly higher among white teenagers than other ethnic groups, the *rate* of increase in adolescent smoking has been most dramatic among African-Americans (up 80% between 1991–1997) and young women. The popularity of smoking among teenage girls is particularly disturbing in view of the now well-documented adverse impact of smoking in relation to problem pregnancies and birth defects.

Another unfortunate trend in recent years, ironically motivated at least in part by concerns about the health hazards of *inhaling* cigarette smoke, has been the upsurge in use of smokeless tobacco, particularly by teenage males. A CDC Youth Risk Behavior Survey in 1997 reported that 15.8% of male high school students were using snuff or chewing tobacco (keeping company with five million adults), a practice that exposes the user to amounts of nicotine equivalent to that in cigarettes. While use of smokeless tobacco products circumvents concerns about *lung* cancer, it certainly is not risk-free—the incidence of oral cancer is several times higher among snuff-dippers than among nonusers, while risk of cancer of the cheek and gums is nearly 50 times higher.

BOX 6-3
Lab Tests for Carcinogenicity—Are They Valid?

In 1977 a Canadian study documenting an excess incidence of bladder cancer among male rats fed a 5% diet of saccharin created a furor among an American public unconvinced that the food additive posed a real health threat and dismayed at the possible banning of the only non-caloric sweetener on the market at that time. Intelligent assessment of the implications of the saccharin research was not helped by the statement by a top FDA official that humans would have to drink 800 cans of diet soda daily to consume an amount of saccharin equivalent to that fed the experimental rats. The issue was widely aired in outraged letters to Congress and newspaper opinion pages, laughed about on late-night talk shows, and used as the butt of cartoonist's jokes. The public was given the impression that the tests were meaningless as far as human health was concerned, an attitude aptly expressed by Congressman Andrew Jacobs of Indiana who proposed passage of a bill requiring that products containing saccharin bear the label: "Warning: the Canadians have determined that saccharin is dangerous to your rat's health."

Unfortunately, the Congressman's remarks, echoed by millions of his fellow Americans, reveal a profound lack of understanding regarding the methods routinely used for determining the safety of new chemicals. The objections raised to the Canadian saccharin tests—and to animal testing procedures in general—focus primarily on two points:

1. The question of dosage. Does *everything* cause cancer when present in excess? Contrary to popular belief, only carcinogens cause cancer. A test animal might be fed a mountain of sugar or salt and die of toxemia, but it will not develop a malignancy because neither substance is a carcinogen (some would qualify this statement by pointing out that because hyper-obesity is a risk factor for certain types of cancer, excessive consumption of chocolate fudge sundaes could lead to cancer; nevertheless, it would be difficult to argue that ice cream is an environmental carcinogen in the same sense that aflatoxins or nitrosamines are known to be). Feeding or exposing test animals to extremely high doses of a suspected chemical is a widely accepted procedure necessary for obtaining meaningful results within a reasonable period of time, given the constraints of such experiments. In a typical study, for reasons of expense and space considerations, only 50 to 100 experimental animals are used in each test group. Such animals have a relatively short life span in comparison with humans, so in order to compensate for the long latency period involved in cancer initiation and to increase the chances for a weak carcinogen to be revealed in the small study population, massive doses are used. This method simply facilitates the collection of data within a reasonable time and at considerably less expense than would be possible using larger test populations and lower dosages.

That such tests are valid and that administration of large doses, per se, does not lead to carcinogenesis are supported by the results of past experimentation. A researcher at the National Cancer Institute some years ago reported that of 3,500 suspected carcinogens tested in the routine manner, only 750 proved, in fact, to be carcinogenic—hardly support for the thesis that large doses in themselves are cancer-causing.

2. **Animals aren't humans.** Do the substances that cause cancer in mice, monkeys, or rats predict cancer causation in humans? The prevailing assumption among researchers is that the basic biological processes in all mammals are fundamentally the same. For ethical reasons it is impossible to prove the thesis that any chemical which causes cancer in animals also causes the disease in humans—to do so would require deliberately exposing humans to a known animal carcinogen and waiting to see if cancer develops! However, numerous tests have been successfully carried out to prove the reverse: every substance known to induce human cancer causes cancer in animals as well (with the sole exception of arsenic, a heavy metal that is a human carcinogen, is mutagenic to bacteria and to cells grown in tissue culture, yet has never been shown to have carcinogenic potential in animals). Thus it seems logical to assume that the opposite is true also and that animal testing is a valid method for determining which chemicals are carcinogenic. What animal testing cannot tell us, however, is how strong or weak a given carcinogen will be in humans. This is because different species show varying degrees of sensitivity to the same substance, some developing cancer only at high levels of exposure while others are vulnerable to relatively low doses. Unfortunately it is not possible to calculate the level of human risk based on the risk level in animals. We may be more or less vulnerable; the tests indicate only which substance can be expected to result in a given number of human cancer cases.

Animal models, of course, provide but one of several methods for studying the mechanism of carcinogenesis. Other approaches for advancing our understanding of cancer include: **mutagenesis studies using bacteria** which, due to their very large population size and short generation time, allow rapid screening of numerous potential carcinogens; **tissue culture research**, which permits examination of DNA damage and mutagenesis in eukaryotic cells (as opposed to prokaryotic bacterial cells); and **epidemiologic studies** of cancer incidence among human populations. Each of these lines of investigation has inherent limitations, and results yielded by one type of study may not always correspond with conclusions drawn from an alternative mode of inquiry. For example, nickel compounds are potent carcinogens in both humans and animals but are not mutagenic to bacteria. Conversely, organic mercury compounds damage DNA in bacterial cells and are mutagenic to cells in tissue culture, but have not been shown to induce cancer either in humans or animals. Cadmium and chromium, however, show carcinogenic potential in all four systems.

The disturbing lack of consistency in results among these various test models has led some observers to question the validity of current testing procedures and to challenge government regulations based on the results of carcinogenicity studies on animals. Most investigators would argue, however, that in an admittedly imperfect world, we must continue to use the only tools currently available, always bearing in mind their limitations and exercising due caution when interpreting data or extrapolating results from such experiments. As one cancer researcher remarked in defense of animal tests, "...half a loaf is better than no loaf at all!"

Elsewhere in the world, the number of smokers and the number of cigarettes smoked per person continue to climb. With a few notable exceptions, effective anti-smoking campaigns are rarely encountered outside the United States and Canada. Newly affluent developing countries in particular are witnessing an explosive increase in cigarette sales—South Korea, China, and Brazil have experienced significant increases in per capita cigarette consumption. In China, where 70% of adult males smoke, the number of cigarettes smoked per person has risen from just one per day in 1950 to four in the 1970s to 14 by the mid-1990s. As a result, Chinese health officials are bracing for a literal epidemic of tobacco-related disease in the years ahead. It is expected that by the first decade of the 21st century one million Chinese men will die each year of diseases caused by smoking—a number predicted to rise to 3 million per year by mid-century (Liu et al., 1998; Niu et al., 1998). Fortunately, tobacco use in China remains almost exclusively a male vice; only 1% of Chinese women smoke. Elsewhere, in a number of countries where smoking by females has long been socially unacceptable, increasing numbers of women are now taking up the habit. In Spain, for example, half of all 20-year-old women now smoke, compared with just 3% in their grandmothers' generation. Russia and the eastern European nations constitute several of the most rapidly expanding markets for tobacco sales. In those formerly Communist countries, so voracious is the craving for cigarettes that demand far exceeds supply, and Western companies are rushing in to fill the void (Brown, Kane, and Ayres, 1993). Between 1991–1997, U.S. cigarette exports to the nations of the former Soviet Union rose from 4.6 billion to almost 15 billion; watch for the Russian cancer statistics of 2020!

Such trends cause dismay to those who realize that cigarette smoke contains more than 4,700 chemical compounds, of which at least 43 are known carcinogens, including benzo(a)pyrene, arsenic, cadmium, benzene, and radioactive polonium. Since these substances are inhaled, it is not surprising that the lungs are the tissue most directly affected. However, smoking has also been documented as a major cause of cancer of the mouth, esophagus, larynx and pharynx—and contributes to the development of bladder, kidney, pancreatic, and colon cancer. Whatever their age, smokers who quit live longer than those who continue to smoke. However, they continue to have a higher risk for certain types of cancer than do people who never used tobacco. Most troubling are research findings that smoking during childhood or adolescence, when lung tissue is particularly sensitive, confers a heightened lifelong risk of cancer even when the individual involved subsequently kicked the habit. Such results are especially disturbing in light of the growing numbers of very young smokers. As one cancer researcher remarked, "We have a generation of people who smoked as teen-agers, quit, changed their lifestyles, and now are just walking time bombs for cancer to develop" (Wiencke et al., 1999).

Altogether, it is estimated that smoking is responsible for fully 30% of all cancer-related deaths. In light of these realities, those who look forward to a long and healthy life would do well to consider the categorical advice offered by a former U.S. Surgeon General:

> There is no single action an individual can take to reduce the risk of cancer more effectively than to stop smoking—particularly smoking cigarettes.

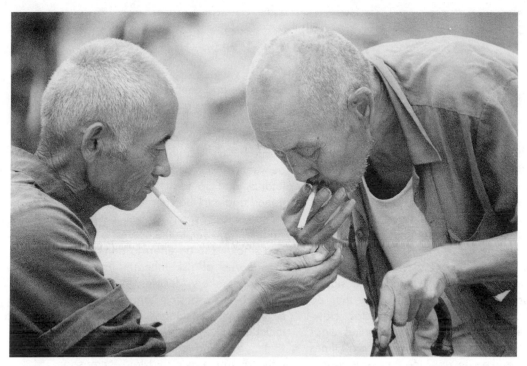

In China, 70% of adult males smoke, and the number of cigarettes smoked per day has been rising steadily, prompting health officials to brace for an epidemic of smoking-related diseases in the years ahead. *[Reuters/Will Burgess/Archive Photos]*

Dietary Factors. Approximately one-third of all U.S. cancer deaths are believed to be due to dietary factors, but judging from media accounts, most of us misidentify the main culprits. Recent scares about everything from coffee to charcoal broiled meat to peanut butter having the potential to cause cancer have prompted consumers to fear that many food additives and contaminants are potential carcinogens—a concern that is reflected in the growing popularity of so-called "natural" or "organic" foods. This topic will be discussed at greater length in the chapter on Food Quality. Suffice it to say here that although some food additives—particularly the coal tar dyes used for artificial coloring and sodium nitrite in hot dogs—are known to be carcinogenic in tests on laboratory animals, no solid evidence yet exists to indicate that human cancer rates are rising because of these substances in food. However, bearing in mind the long latency period of many forms of cancer and the fact that many additives have been widely used for only a few decades, it may yet be too early to state categorically that such chemicals won't cause future problems.

Ironically, while many people worry, perhaps unjustifiably, about synthetic food additives, they pay little attention to findings regarding naturally occurring carcinogens in food. Substances called **aflatoxins,** potent carcinogens produced by the fungus *Aspergillus flavus*, cause liver cancer in both humans and animals and are suspected of being responsible for the high rates of that disease observed in parts of Africa and Southeast Asia. Aflatoxins are known to act synergistically with the hepatitis B virus and with chronic alco-

BOX 6-4

Synergism: 1 + 1 = 5

Virtually all laboratory tests to determine carcinogenicity of suspected substances are based on responses to single-source exposures. Results of such testing methods may significantly underestimate risks in the real world because it is now well known that certain substances in combination are far more hazardous than either one would be if acting independently. For example, people who smoke cigarettes are 10 times more likely to develop lung cancer than are nonsmokers; asbestos workers incur significantly higher risk of lung cancer than do people not exposed to asbestos. However, a person who both smokes cigarettes and works with asbestos is 60 times more likely to get lung cancer than is a person exposed neither to cigarette smoke nor to asbestos—far higher than the risk factor for either type of exposure separately. This phenomenon, where the interaction of two or more substances produces an impact greater than the sum of their independent effects, is known as synergism and can perhaps be most easily thought of as a situation where 1 + 1 = 5.

Synergistic effects are well documented in relation to interactions between various air pollutants, water pollutants, and so forth and will be mentioned again in the chapters dealing with those topics. Synergism has been most studied, however, in the context of cancer and smoking in an effort to demonstrate the degree of risk inherent in various types of smokers' lifestyles. In addition to the smoking-asbestos connection, other synergistic associations with smoking include:

1. Smoking and alcohol consumption—as much as a thirtyfold increase in the risk of mouth and throat cancer.

2. Smoking and living in areas of high air pollution—elevated risk of lung cancer.

3. Smoking and working with chemicals or in uranium mines—high lung cancer risk.

hol consumption (National Research Council, 1996). The toxin-producing mold grows on peanuts, pistachios, corn, rice, and certain other grains and nuts when temperatures and humidity are high. If large quantities of aflatoxin are present in the food, liver damage and death may occur very quickly; in small amounts, consumed over a period of time, aflatoxins are among the strongest carcinogens known. Other natural carcinogens in food include safrole, an extract of sassafras long used to flavor root-beer until banned by the FDA in 1960, and oil of calamus, used until 1968 to flavor vermouth. On a more cheerful note, it also has been demonstrated that many foods contain *anti*carcinogenic compounds whose regular inclusion in one's diet can be protective against certain types of cancer. Most notable in this regard are members of the cabbage family—broccoli, cauliflower, cabbage, kale, and brussels sprouts—whose cells contain **sulforaphane**, one of the most potent anticarcinogens yet discovered. Cooked tomato products rich in **lycopene**—especially tomato sauce, tomato juice, and pizza—have long been associated with a reduced risk of prostate cancer. Other tasty sources of protection against cancer include yellow and green vegetables, citrus fruits, apricots, cantaloupe, brown rice, wheat germ, soy products, onions, and garlic (Giovanucci et al., 1995; Kliewer and Smith, 1995; Davis, 1990).

Perhaps most important of all in reference to food and cancer is the conviction among many researchers that there is a direct correlation between high fat intake and rates of colon and prostate cancer, as well as a relationship between stomach cancer and consumption of smoked, salt-pickled, and salt-cured foods. In addition, being excessively overweight seems to favor development of cancer of the endometrium in women (Willett, 1994; National Research Council, 1982). However, the widespread suspicion among health experts that breast cancer incidence is closely associated with high-fat diets was dispelled by results of a 14-year study of almost 89,000 women, which demonstrated that women who consume large amounts of fat have no higher risk of developing breast cancer than women whose diet is low in fat. Reducing dietary fat intake confers significant benefits in preventing heart disease, but apparently has no impact one way or the other in reducing breast cancer risk (Holmes et al., 1999). Although much remains to be learned concerning the relationship between dietary factors and cancer, current scientific evidence strongly suggests that a diet rich in a wide variety of fruits, vegetables, beans, and grain products and low in meat, dairy products, and other high-fat foods can significantly reduce overall cancer risk.

Air Pollution. It has long been known that urban air contains a number of carcinogenic substances, benzo (a) pyrene among the most potent. Obtaining conclusive proof that breathing polluted air, by itself, induces cancer has been complicated by the fact that many cancer victims living in regions of poor air quality are also smokers. However, a number of well-designed epidemiologic studies, along with research utilizing techniques from molecular genetics, have yielded results demonstrating a clear association between polluted air and increased incidence of lung cancer. In southern California, a study of more than 6,000 nonsmoking Seventh-Day Adventists who had lived in areas with elevated levels of particulate matter, sulfur dioxide, and ozone found an excess rate of lung cancer among both men and women within this population (Beeson et al., 1998). Halfway around the world, in a heavily industrialized region of Poland where coal combustion for industry and home heating has fouled the air for decades, studies have shown a close correlation between lung cancer incidence and residence in highly polluted neighborhoods. Scientists working in Krakow have demonstrated how air contaminants can damage the molecular structure of genes. Examining DNA from white blood cells of Polish central-city residents, researchers found that certain polycyclic aromatic hydrocarbons (PAHs) produced from burning coal bond to the DNA molecule to form PAH-DNA adducts. Since adducts at that location on the gene had previously been linked to elevated lung cancer risk, this finding provides additional evidence that certain air pollutants damage the genetic material and hence play a direct role in cancer causation (Whyatt et al., 1998).

Occupational Exposure. Since the days of Sir Percival Potts' observations on scrotal cancer among chimney sweeps, it has been recognized that certain occupations entail heightened risk of specific diseases. In recent

BOX 6-5

Public Outcast #1

Tobacco is a filthy weed,
That from the devil does proceed;
It drains your purse, it burns your clothes,
And makes a chimney of your nose.

—Dr. Benjamin Warehouse (1754–1846)

Vilification of cigarette smoking is nearly as old as the habit itself, as attested by this bit of doggerel attributed to a disapproving English physician nearly two centuries ago. However, the opprobrium directed against nicotine addicts has never been as widespread nor as intense as it is today. Once the national epitome of success and sophistication, the smoker is rapidly becoming a social outcast. "Nonsmoker's Rights" has become a battle cry, relegating the once-admired Marlboro Man to the status of second-class citizen. Why this sudden evaporation of public tolerance for a habit still prevalent among one out of every four American adults? Why do most states now restrict smoking in public places? Why has the U.S. government banned smoking on all commercial domestic flights? Nonsmokers have always suffered physical discomfort when forced to breathe air polluted with tobacco smoke, yet as long as the belief persisted that smokers were only endangering their own health, nonsmokers felt they had no right to complain. Personal grumbling turned to open militancy only with medical evidence proving that not only are cigarette smokers killing themselves in record numbers (over 430,000 Americans die from tobacco-related diseases each year), but they're damaging the health of family members, friends, and coworkers as well. With growing public awareness of the impact of "pas-

sive smoking" (i.e. exposure of nonsmokers to indoor air pollution from tobacco smoke), the three-fourths of Americans who don't smoke have resolved to remain the silent majority no longer.

Tobacco smoke inhaled by a nonsmoker can originate either from the "mainstream" smoke exhaled by a smoker or from the "sidestream" smoke emanating from the burning end of the cigarette. The latter accounts for approximately 85% of the pollution in the proverbial "smoke-filled room" and contains higher concentrations of carcinogens per unit weight than does mainstream smoke. While the sidestream smoke is significantly diluted by the volume of air in the room, two of its major components—carbon monoxide and nicotine—nevertheless have been measured at concentrations exceeding the ambient air quality standards in public places and meeting rooms. For nonsmokers who frequent these smoky environments, blood levels of carboxyhemoglobin are as high as if they had just smoked five cigarettes; their nicotine levels also are equivalent to those of a light smoker.

Although nonsmokers forced to live or work in smoky surroundings are far more likely to die of heart disease than any other tobacco-related illness, much of the health research on passive smoking has focused on an association with enhanced lung cancer risk. Basing its conclusions on numerous studies conducted in several different countries, EPA estimates an average of 3,000 nonsmoking Americans die annually of lung cancer due to working or living in an atmosphere contaminated with tobacco smoke. Studies in Japan and Greece likewise support a link between passive smoking and lung cancer mortality. EPA's 1993 designation of **environmental tobacco smoke (ETS)** as a Class A carcinogen added further weight to nonsmoker's demands for pollution-free indoor air.

Far more prevalent than nagging worries about lung cancer are the more mundane health complaints by nonsmokers forced to inhale someone else's smoke. Although eye irritations, headaches, nasal symptoms and cough may not be life-threatening problems, they seriously diminish the nonsmoker's sense of well-being, as do the allergic reactions, wheezing, and sore throats reported by numerous sufferers. A 1998 study of California bartenders both before and after the state prohibited smoking in bars and taverns revealed a rapid improvement in the men's respiratory health after the ban took effect. The vast majority of subjects reported a significant reduction in wheezing, coughing, labored breathing, and phlegm production once their work environment became smoke-free.

The most tragic victims of passive smoking are those members of society least able to speak out in their own defense—infants, children, and the unborn. That parental smoking could be considered another form of child abuse has been amply documented in numerous studies. The EPA estimates that a minimum of 150,000 serious respiratory ailments among young children are caused each year by exposure to environmental tobacco smoke, with those under the age of 18 months facing the

greatest risks. Bronchitis, pneumonia, asthma, and wheezing all occur more frequently among children whose parents smoke. Researchers estimate that ETS causes 8,000–26,000 additional cases of asthma each year and aggravates symptoms in many more. Medical researchers have demonstrated that asthmatic children exposed to significant levels of secondhand smoke suffer 70–80% more attacks than children subjected to little or no such exposure. A significantly greater number of children whose mothers smoke are hospitalized for respiratory conditions than are children of nonsmoking mothers. Children suffering from asthma have been shown to experience marked improvement when their parents quit smoking.

Even more vulnerable are children in the womb. When a pregnant woman smokes (and 25% of pregnant Americans do smoke), she is exposing her fetus to nicotine, carbon monoxide, radioactive polonium, and numerous other toxic chemicals. Carbon monoxide appears to be the most fetotoxic of these, causing a rise in carboxyhemoglobin in the blood of both mother and child and resulting in retarded fetal growth rates. Pregnant women who smoke 20 or more cigarettes daily are at heightened risk of bearing an infant with cleft lip and palate; maternal smoking during pregnancy also is associated with a significantly higher chance of giving birth to a mentally retarded child. Medical experts estimate that 20–40% of all low-weight births can be directly attributed to maternal smoking during pregnancy. Infants born to smoking mothers weigh on the average about 10% less at birth than do babies of nonsmokers. Since low birth weight is a major risk factor for infant mortality, it is not surprising that approximately 10% of all U.S. neonatal deaths each year are blamed on maternal smoking. Smoking during pregnancy also is blamed for an estimated 50,000 miscarriages annually and for 11–14% of all premature births, the risk of which rises the more heavily the mother smokes.

Considering the extent to which a smoker's habit can adversely affect those around him or her, it's no wonder that smoking is increasingly viewed as antisocial behavior. The proliferation of clean indoor air regulations across the country are undoubtedly annoying to smokers whose freedom to light up in public has been sharply curtailed. Nevertheless, to health-conscious nonsmokers, aware that ETS is ranked as the third leading preventable cause of death in the U.S., mandated smoke-free zones constitute a quite literal breath of fresh air.

References

Drews, Carolyn D., et al. 1996. "The Relationship Between Idiopathic Mental Retardation and Maternal Smoking During Pregnancy." *Pediatrics* 97, no. 4 (April):547–553.

Eisner, Mark D., et al. 1998. "Bartenders' Respiratory Health After Establishment of Smoke-Free Bars and Taverns." *Journal of the American Medical Association* 280, no. 22 (Dec. 9):1909–1914.

Shaw, Gary, et al. 1996. "Orofacial Clefts, Parental Cigarette Smoking, and Transforming Growth Factor-Alpha Gene Variants." *American Journal of Human Genetics* 58, no. 3 (March):551–561.

decades the proliferation of new synthetic chemicals in industry, as well as the continued use of older substances only recently recognized as hazardous, has been reflected in cancer rates far higher among certain segments of the workforce than among the general public. Estimates of the number of American workers potentially exposed to chemicals considered by the National Institute of Occupational Safety and Health (NIOSH) to be proven or likely carcinogens range from three to nine million; many others work with materials suspected to be carcinogens but on which the necessary testing has not yet been done. Although there has been considerable difference of opinion between industry and labor regarding the health impact of exposure to carcinogens in the workplace, researchers estimate that occupational exposure accounts for 4–38% of U.S. cancer incidence (Chivian et al., 1993). Until passage of the Toxic Substances Control Act in 1976, giving the federal government the power to require testing of potentially hazardous substances before they go on the market, hundreds of new chemicals with unknown side effects came into industrial use each year. Unfortunately, the carcinogenicity of many substances was recognized only after exposed workers, like human "guinea pigs," fell sick or died. Some of the most significant industrial carcinogens thus discovered include:

- **Asbestos,** one of the best known occupational hazards, which is expected to cause the death of 30–40% of all asbestos workers
- **vinyl chloride,** a basic ingredient in the manufacture of plastics, found in 1974 to induce a rare form of liver cancer among exposed workers
- **anesthetic gases** used in operating rooms have been identified as the

reason nurse anesthetists develop leukemia and lymphoma at three times the normal rate and also experience higher rates of miscarriage and birth defects among their children

- **benzene,** long known to be a powerful bone marrow poison capable of causing aplastic anemia, has now been shown to cause leukemia as well
- **coke oven emissions** have been linked with cancers of the lung, trachea, bronchus, and kidneys and are now regulated as hazardous air pollutants when vented to the outdoor air
- **benzidine, naphythylamine,** and several other chemicals associated with rubber and dye manufacturing pose an excess risk of bladder cancer to exposed workers in those industries
- **hardwood dust** inhaled by cabinet and furniture makers can lead to malignant nasal tumors
- **radioactive mine dusts** have been a particular problem in uranium mines, resulting in lung cancer rates among miners four times higher than the national average

Although pressure from labor unions and adoption of protective government legislation have resulted in some improvements in reducing occupational hazards, standards set for protecting workers are far less stringent than those set for protecting society at large. In addition, until a few years ago workers often lacked basic information about the nature of the materials with which they worked and were thus unable to take precautionary action even if they desired to do so. A major step forward in this regard was promulgation by the Occupational Safety and Health Administration (OSHA) in 1983 of its Hazard Communication Standard, intended to provide employees in manufacturing industries access to information concerning the hazards of chemicals which they encounter in the workplace. Essentially a federal "Employee Right-to-Know" law, this ruling requires that manufacturers inform their employees of any workplace hazards and how they can minimize risk of harm. Manufacturers must also ensure that all chemicals are properly labeled and that Material Safety Data Sheets for each chemical are available for any employee who requests them.

Reproductive/Sexual Behavior. The National Cancer Institute estimates that 7% of all cancer deaths can be linked with reproductive factors or sexual practices. For reasons thought to relate to hormone levels, breast cancer incidence is significantly higher among women who experienced early onset of menstruation, childless women or women who first gave birth at a late age, and women who were older than average at the time of menopause. Conversely, research suggests that mothers who breast-feed, especially *teenage mothers* who nurse their babies for at least six months, cut their risk of developing breast cancer before menopause nearly in half. For women in their 20s and 30s, prolonged breast-feeding reduces cancer risk by approximately 22%. Although such risk factors are largely beyond the control of the women involved, those who fall into one or more of these categories should be especially conscientious about having regular mammograms once they reach age 40.

Risk factors for cervical cancer are more subject to self-control: early age at the time of first intercourse and multiple sex partners predispose a woman to subsequent development of this type of cancer. Chances of contracting uterine cancer are enhanced by early onset of menstruation, late menopause, a failure to ovulate, a history of infertility, or by excessive obesity. Estrogen replacement therapy, frequently prescribed for menopausal and post-menopausal women, may also increase the risk of uterine cancer. For this reason, most physicians now advise a hormone replacement regimen consisting of both estrogen and progesterone, a combination believed to offset the risk associated with using estrogen alone (American Cancer Society, 1999).

Preventing Cancer

The preceding discussion should make it apparent that while we still have much to learn about the nature of carcinogenesis, we have already discovered enough to suggest a variety of personal actions that individuals can take to reduce substantially their own risk of developing cancer. Malignancies caused by tobacco use, responsible for more than 170,000 U.S. cancer deaths every year, could be prevented entirely; the same is true for the 20,000 cancer deaths caused by heavy alcohol consumption. Proper nutritional choices, along with regular exercise and maintaining proper body weight, could significantly reduce the estimated one-third of fatal cancers attributed to dietary factors. Avoiding excessive sun exposure and using a high-SPF sunscreen when such exposure is unavoidable could have a major impact on reducing new cases of skin cancer, currently totaling over one million annually in the United States. Although medical science continues its aggressive search for a cancer cure, even the most optimistic researchers affirm that *preventing* cancer from ever developing is the most effective way of combating this dreaded, but certainly not inevitable, disease.

References

American Cancer Society, *Cancer Facts and Figures—1999*.

Beeson, W. Lawrence, David E. Abbey, and S.F. Knutson. 1998. "Long-Term Concentrations of Ambient Air Pollutants and Incident Lung Cancer in California Adults: Results from the AHSMOG Study." *Environmental Health Perspectives* 106, no. 12 (December): 813–828.

Bronner, Eric C., et al. 1994. "Mutation in the DNA Mismatch Repair Gene Homologue hMLH1 Is Associated with Hereditary Non-polyposis Colon Cancer." *Nature* 368 (March 17).

Brown, Lester R., Hal Kane, and Ed Ayres. 1993. *Vital Signs 1993*. Worldwatch Institute, W. W. Norton.

Chivian, Eric, M.D., et al., eds. 1993. *Critical Condition: Human Health and the Environment*. Physicians for Social Responsibility. The M.I.T. Press.

Colburn, Theo, Dianne Dumanoski, and John P. Myers. 1996. *Our Stolen Future*. Dutton, Penguin Books USA.

Cole, Philip, and Brad Rodu. 1996. "Declining Cancer Mortality in the United States." *Cancer* 78, no. 10 (Nov):2045–2048.

Davis, Debra Lee. 1990. "Natural Anticarcinogens: Can Diet Protect Against Cancer?" *Health & Environment Digest* 4, no. 1 (Feb).

Fishel, Richard, et al. 1993. "The Human Mutator Gene Homolog MSH2 and

Its Association with Hereditary Nonpolyposis Colon Cancer." *Cell* 75 (Dec. 3).

Food and Drug Administration (FDA). 1998. "Once-Feared Drug Provides Relief for Leprosy Symptoms." *FDA Consumer* 32, no. 6 (Nov):2.

Giovanucci, E., A. Ascherio, E.G. Rimm, M.J. Stampfer, G.A. Colditz, and Walter Willett. 1995. "Intake of Carotenoids and Retinol in Relation to Risk of Prostate Cancer." *Journal of the National Cancer Institute* 87, no. 23 (Dec. 6):1767–1776.

Harris, John A., M.D., and Jackie W. Wynne. 1994. "Birth Defects Clusters: Evaluating Community Reports." *Health & Environment Digest* 7 (Feb).

Henderson, Charles W. 1999. "Thalidomide Making Comeback to Treat Cancer, AIDS." *Cancer Weekly Plus* (Jan. 25).

Holmes, Michelle D., David J. Hunter, Graham A. Colditz, Meir J. Stampfer, Susan E. Hankinson, Frank E. Speizer, Bernard Rosner and Walter C. Willett. 1999. "Association of Dietary Intake of Fat and Fatty Acids with Risk of Breast Cancer." *Journal of the American Medical Association* 281, no. 10 (March 10):914–920.

Isaacson, Peter G., M.D. 1994. "Gastric Lymphoma and Helicobacter Pylori." *New England Journal of Medicine* 330, no. 18 (May 5).

Kliewer, Erich, and Ken Smith. 1995. "Breast Cancer Mortality Among Immigrants in Australia and Canada." *Journal of the National Cancer Institute* 87, no. 15 (Aug. 2):1154–1161.

Klug, William S., and Michael R. Cummings. 1997. *Concepts of Genetics*. Prentice Hall.

Leach, F. S., et al. 1993. "Mutations of a mutS Homolog in Hereditary Nonpolyposis Colorectal Cancer." *Cell* 75, no. 6 (Dec. 17).

Liu, Bo-Qi, Richard Peto, Zheng-Ming Chen, Jillian Boreham, Ya-Ping Wu, Jun-Yao Li, T. Colin Campbell and Jun-Shi Chen. 1998. "Emerging Tobacco Hazards in China: 1. Retrospective Proportional Mortality Study of One Million Deaths." *British Medical Journal* 317, no. 7170 (Nov):1411–1422.

Markoff, John. 1992. "Danger of Miscarriage Found for Chip Workers." *New York Times*, Dec. 4

National Center for Health Statistics. 1998. *Health: United States, 1998, with Socioeconomic Status and Health Chartbook*. Hyattsville, MD.

National Research Council, National Academy of Sciences. 1982. *Report on Diet, Nutrition, and Cancer*.

National Research Council. 1996. *Carcinogens and Anti-Carcinogens in the Human Diet*. Washington, DC: National Academy Press.

Newbold, Retha R., Rita B. Hanson, Wendy N. Jefferson, Bill C. Bullock, Joseph Haseman, and John A. McLachlan. 1998. "Increased Tumors but Uncompromised Fertility in Female Descendents of Mice Exposed Developmentally to DES." *Carcinogenesis* 19, no. 9 (Sept):1655–1663.

Niu, Shi-Ru, Gong-Huang Yang, Zheng-Ming Chen, Jun-Ling Wany, Gong Hao Wang, Xing-Zhou He, Helen Schoepff, Jillian Boreham, Hong-Chao Pan, and Richard Peto. 1998. "Emerging Tobacco Hazards in China: 2. Early Mortality Results from a Prospective Study." *British Medical Journal* 317, no. 7170:1423–1424.

Papadopoulos, Nickolas, Nicholas C. Nicolaides, et al. 1994. "Mutation of a mutL Homolog in Hereditary Colon Cancer." *Science* 263 (March 18).

Parsonnet, Julie, M.D., et al. 1994. "Helicobacter Pylori Infection and Gastric Lymphoma." *New England Journal of Medicine* 330, no. 18 (May 5).

Perera, Frederica P. 1997. "Environment and Cancer: Who are Susceptible?" *Science* 278, no. 5340 (Nov. 7):1068–1073.

Sack, George H. 1999. *Medical Genetics.* McGraw-Hill.

Semenza, Jan C., and Lisa H. Weasel. 1997. "Molecular Epidemiology in Environmental Health: The Potential of Tumor Suppressor Gene *p53* as a Biomarker." *Environmental Health Perspectives* 105, suppl. 1 (Feb):155–162.

"Solvents Used in Making Computer Chips Linked to Workers' Miscarriages at IBM." 1992. *Environmental Health Letter,* Sept. 16.

Store, Richard. 1992. "Can a Father's Exposure Lead to Illness in his Children?" *Science* 258 (Oct.2)

"Studies Yield Conflicting Findings on Environment's Link to Cancer." 1994. *Environmental Health Letter,* April 27.

Warkany, J. 1972. "Trends in Teratologic Research." *Pathobiology of Development,* edited by E. Perrin and M. Finegold. Williams and Wilkins.

Weinberg, Robert A. 1998. *One Renegade Cell: How Cancer Begins.* Basic Books.

Whyatt, R.M., R.M. Santella, W. Jedrychowski, S.J. Garte, D.A. Bell, R. Ottman, A. Gladek Yarborough, G. Cosma, T.L. Young, T.B. Cooper, M.C. Randall, D.K. Manchester, and F.P. Perera. 1998. "Relationship Between Ambient Air Pollution and DNA Damage in Polish Mothers and Newborns." *Environmental Health Perspectives* 106, suppl. 3 (June):821–826.

Wiencke, John K., Sally W. Thurston, Karl T. Kelsey, Andrea Varkonyi, John C. Wain, Eugene J. Mark, and David C. Christiani. 1999. "Early Age at Smoking Initiation and Tobacco Carcinogen DNA Damage in the Lung." *Journal of the National Cancer Institute* 91, no. 7 (April 7):614–619.

Willett, Walter C. 1994. "Diet and Health: What Should We Eat." *Science* 264 (April 22).

CHAPTER 7

Toxic Substances

What is it that is not poison?
All things are poison and nothing is without poison.
It is the dose only that makes a thing not a poison.

—Paracelsus (16th Century)

Human illness or death due to contact with toxic materials in the environment is certainly not unique to the modern age. Hippocrates described the symptoms of lead poisoning as early as 370 B.C.; mercury fumes in Roman mines in Spain made work there the equivalent of a death sentence to the unfortunate slaves receiving such an assignment; for centuries Turkish peasants living in homes built of asbestos-containing volcanic rock have been dying of lung disease. Yet for the most part, such examples of illness caused by direct contact with toxic substances have been confined to certain occupational groups or to people who, by chance, happened to be living in an area where there was an unnaturally high concentration of some toxic material. By and large, in the past large populations seldom, if ever, were exposed to significant amounts of toxicants on a sustained basis. Today, however, that situation is changing, thanks in part to the tremendous increase in industrial production during the 20th century, as well as to the "chemical revolution" that has witnessed the introduction of thousands of new synthetic compounds into widespread use in recent decades. Some of these substances, several of which were briefly mentioned in the preceding chapter, are largely confined to an occupational setting and pose little threat to the general public, although of course they are a major concern to workers and their families. Others, however, are now virtually omnipresent throughout the human environment and are generating considerable controversy as to the degree of public health threat they present.

In this chapter we will describe the process by which chemicals are tested for toxicity and their health risks assessed. We will then take a closer look at several of these substances—some naturally occurring, others artificially produced—to which human exposure is nearly universal and which are known to cause serious health damage.

Testing for Toxicity

"Toxic" or "toxicant" are terms scientists use to describe a chemical that provokes an adverse systemic effect on living organisms. That is, **toxicants** have the ability to cause harm to organs or biochemical processes away from the site on the body where exposure occurred. In this sense they differ from other harmful chemicals such as corrosives or irritants, which damage only the tissues they contact. For example, spilling concentrated acid on one's hand will result in a painful chemical burn, followed by loss of skin, but damage is localized to that area. By contrast, ingesting small amounts of arsenic over an extended time period can result in cirrhosis of the liver, skin discoloration, and peripheral nerve damage, among other problems. "Poison," a word many people use as a synonym for toxic, actually has a much narrower meaning, referring to a chemical that can cause illness or death at a very low dose of exposure—approximately 3/4 of a teaspoon for an adult or 1/8 of a teaspoon for a toddler. Very few chemicals are capable of causing death in such low amounts, hence the list of true poisons is much shorter than commonly believed. Another term frequently equated with "toxic" is "hazardous," whose actual meaning is more complex. The hazardous nature of a substance is dependent both on its inherent capacity to do harm (e.g. its degree of toxicity, corrosiveness, flammability, etc.) and, equally important, on the likelihood of that substance coming into contact with people. Methyl parathion, one of the most toxic insecticides, presents an extreme hazard to migrant farm workers entering a just-sprayed field without protective clothing; the very same chemical presents virtually no hazard when stored in its original container inside a securely locked storeroom.

The study of toxic substances, or **toxicology**, in an informal sense is probably as old as the human species. Long before written records were kept, ancient peoples learned through trial and error which plants and animals should be avoided because of their toxic properties. Among classical civilizations, knowledge of mineral toxicants was well-established and was extensively applied to the art of poisoning one's enemies! Modern toxicology is a relatively recent offshoot of pharmacological science, its origin as an independent field of inquiry prompted initially by the needs of occupational medicine. Toxicology has gained added importance in recent decades due to the rapid growth of the chemical industry and associated public concerns regarding health effects of toxic chemicals.

Whether a chemical provokes a toxic effect—or any effect at all—is dependent on a number of variables, the most important of which is the **dose-time** relationship, that is, the amount of the chemical in question (dose) and the duration of exposure (time). Depending on the nature of the dose-time relationship, toxicity can be categorized as either acute or chronic. A chemical's **acute toxicity** refers to its ability to cause harm as a result of one-time exposure to a relatively large amount of the substance. Most accidental childhood poisonings (e.g. drinking a liquid pesticide stored in a cola bottle) represent harm caused by acutely toxic chemicals. **Chronic toxicity**, by contrast, refers to a chemical's ability to impair health when repeated low-dose exposure to the chemical occurs over a long time period. Interestingly, the effects of acute vs. chronic toxicity for the same chemical are often quite different in terms of symptoms and bodily organs involved. As an example, with acute exposure lead poisoning manifests itself as severe abdominal pains, while chronic lead toxicity provokes anemia and nervous system damage. Not only is there no correlation between acute and chronic toxicity symptoms, there also is no connection between their relative potency. A chemical that is very toxic in acute exposure situations may be nontoxic chronically. Similarly, a chemical with minimal acute toxicity may present a greater danger when exposure is chronic.

Another parameter influencing toxicity is the chemical's route of exposure. Toxic substances can enter the body through the mouth when a person eats, drinks or smokes (**oral**); through the skin (**dermal**); or via the lungs if the substance is inhaled (**respiratory**). Depending on the chemical in question, toxicity will vary, depending on the route of exposure—very few chemicals are equally toxic by all three routes.

Toxicity is also profoundly affected by species, a fact which troubles those questioning the validity of animal testing procedures. Chemicals that are very toxic to some animal species may be only slightly toxic or nontoxic to others, including humans. Close taxonomic relationship is no predictor of how a particular species will react in a toxicity test. For some chemicals, toxicity in both humans and monkeys is very similar, while for other substances humans may join cats and dogs in being highly sensitive while monkeys suffer no adverse effects. Just as genetic variability *among* species influences toxicity, so do genetic differences *within* a population. Individual susceptibility, based on each person's (or each guinea pig's) biochemical makeup, explains the range of effects among members of a group exposed to exactly the same dose of any substance.

Determining the acute, subchronic, and chronic toxicity of a chemical is necessary in order to establish protective regulations. Acute toxicity is generally described using the technical term LD_{50} (LD=lethal dose), which refers to the amount of the chemical, administered in one dose, that is required to kill 50% of a population of test animals within a 14-day period. LD_{50} is expressed as the number of milligrams of chemical per kilogram of body weight. Thus the lower the LD_{50}, the smaller the dose required to kill; in other words, the lower the LD_{50}, the more acutely toxic the chemical is (substances legally termed "poisons" are those with an LD_{50} of 50 or less). For obvious reasons, acute toxicity testing is restricted to populations of laboratory animals; thus when results are used to estimate lethal doses for humans, considerable judgment must be exercised, recognizing that humans may be more or less sensitive than the test species. For some chemicals, unfortunately, direct human results may supplement animal data. When known quantities of a toxicant are involved in accidental poisonings, suicides, murders, or industrial accidents, these quantities can be related to the severity and type of symptoms and then compared with animal test results. If such data indicate the chemical is more or less toxic to humans than to animals, the human results supersede the animal data.

Testing for subchronic and chronic toxicity is more difficult, time-consuming, and expensive than acute toxicity testing and considerably less is known about the long-term effects of a chemical than about its acute effects. Symptoms of chronic toxicity may take months or years to manifest themselves, and because such symptoms are often similar to other common health complaints they may be misdiagnosed.

Testing for subchronic and chronic toxicity involves animal feeding experiments, most commonly using rats or dogs. After determining the daily dose of chemical the animals are likely to be able to tolerate for long periods (a determination based on the chemical's LD_{50}), the animals are divided into three or more test groups, plus a control group. Each group will have the same number of animals and a balanced male/female ratio. Beginning at the time the animals are weaned, each group of test animals is fed a specified level of the toxicant mixed with its feed. One group receives a dose expected to have significant sublethal chronic effects; one group receives an amount of the toxicant predicted to have no effect; the third group is fed a level of toxicant intermediate between the other two. The control group is treated in exactly the same manner as the other animals except that no toxicant is added to its food. Subchronic toxicity tests typically are run for 90 days, their main intent being to establish levels of exposure at which no adverse effects can be observed and to identify which organ or organs suffer damage after repeated exposure to the toxicant being tested. Daily records are kept detailing the animals' appearance and behavior. At the end of the three-month test period, the animals are killed and autopsied, being carefully examined for evidence of organ damage or other adverse changes. Tests for chronic toxicity are conducted in the same manner as described for subchronic testing, except that the duration of exposure to the chemical is considerably longer. Chronic toxicity tests are usually carried out for a time period equivalent to the average lifespan of the test animals (generally rats or mice). Since determination of a chemical's carcinogenicity is a prime goal of chronic toxicity tests, autopsies performed at the conclusion of the test period are focused specifically on the incidence and location of tumors.

The data collected from these studies are plotted on a **dose-response curve**, which has three parts. The first portion of the curve, on the far left, is horizontal—an indication that low doses of the toxicant produce no ill effects. The middle portion of the curve begins at a point called the **threshold**, where increasing dosage is beginning to provoke adverse symptoms. The curve continues to climb upward as the dose increases until, in its final portion, it again flattens out after reaching its maximum effect (i.e. death). The dose-response curve describes one of the most basic principles of toxicology—the greater the dose of a toxicant, the greater the effect. If all groups of test animals displayed the same symptoms of harm, or if the group fed the lowest level of toxicant suffered more adverse health effects than the group receiving the highest dose, it could be concluded that something other than the toxicant caused the observed problems. Demonstration of the existence of thresholds is also of great importance to an understanding of toxicity. Because the threshold of toxicity for a chemical varies among species, as well as within a population of the same species and even in the same individual, depending on age and health status, it will probably never be possible to determine precisely where the threshold of tolerance is for any particular person. Nevertheless, knowing

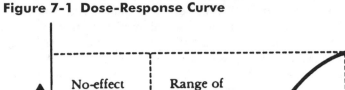

Figure 7-1 Dose-Response Curve

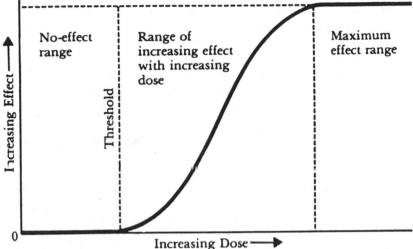

that there *is* a safe level of exposure facilitates regulation by providing a basis for establishing **margins of safety**—a buffer zone between the highest level of a chemical that produces no adverse effect in an animal species and a level of exposure assumed to be safe for humans. In the United States, a hundred-fold margin of safety has traditionally been employed for regulatory control of toxic substances. This number was arbitrarily chosen, based on the assumptions that 1) humans are 10 times more susceptible to the toxic effects of chemicals than are laboratory animals and 2) the more vulnerable members of the population—young children, the elderly, the immunocompromised—are 10 times more sensitive than the average healthy adult. In spite of the uncertainties inherent in such assumptions, the fact that legal exposure limits to toxicants are well below the no-effect level should lend comfort to citizens beset by the chemophobia so widespread in modern society (Ottoboni, 1991).

Assessing Health Risk

As fears of the potentially harmful health effects of chemical exposure have increased in recent decades, a concerned public has demanded that government act to manage such risks. Doing so effectively requires decision makers to determine whether a particular substance presents a greater danger than society is willing to accept, to examine the available options for controlling such hazards, and then to adopt policy measures (i.e. regulatory controls, product bans, market-based incentives, educational efforts) that reduce or eliminate unacceptable risk. **Risk management,** however, is dependent on accurate **risk assessment**—determining whether something suspected of presenting a human health threat is in fact dangerous, estimating how much injury or harm is likely to result from a given level of exposure, and determining if those consequences are serious enough to warrant action.

Health risk assessment began to receive serious professional attention early in the 20th century when adverse effects associated with certain types of occupational exposures were described. Investigations into the relationship between levels of exposure and the observed human health effects led to the identification of **no-observed-effect-levels (NOELs)** and the establishment of adequate margins of safety for exposure. By the early 1970s, creation of the U.S. Environmental Protection Agency and the Occupational Safety and Health Administration—agencies charged with writing regulations and implementing the provisions of a number of far-reaching new environmental, health, and safety laws—gave health risk assessment a major boost. By necessity, risk assessment became a prime component of the regulatory decision-making process, and modern quantitative methods of analysis emerged in response to this need. During the past 30 years, health risk assessments have been employed for a wide range of regulatory issues: food additives, pesticide residues, drinking water contaminants, indoor air pollutants, and so forth. Although hazardous substances can adversely affect human health in various ways—immune system dysfunction, reproductive or teratogenic effects, organ damage, nervous system impairment—the potential carcinogenicity of suspect chemicals has been the main focus of health risk assessments in recent years.

Health risk assessment constitutes a four-step process:

1. *Hazard identification.* Aimed at determining whether or not a particular substance or agent has an adverse effect on human health (e.g. is the substance carcinogenic?). Such a determination is typically made on the basis of animal testing, as described in Box 6-3. If these tests indicate no harm from exposure, there is no need for further investigation; on the other hand, if exposure to the substance causes death or injury to some of the test animals, risk assessment proceeds to the next step.

2. *Dose-response assessment.* Since health effects of the same substance can be either harmful, beneficial, or neutral, depending on the amount of exposure received, determining the dose at or below which no effects are detected is important for establishing safety standards. For noncarcinogenic toxic substances this is a relatively straightforward process; empirical evidence has shown that biological effects of exposure to noncarcinogenic chemicals appear only after a **threshold level** has been exceeded. Exposing laboratory animals to varying doses of the agent in question permits identification of the **lowest-observable-effect-level (LOEL),** the **no-observed-adverse-effect-level (NOAEL)**—the dose at or below which no *harmful* effects are observed, and the **no-observed-effect-level (NOEL).** This dose-response information facilitates the determination of threshold levels of exposure.

For carcinogens, however, the situation is complicated by a working assumption, adopted by regulatory agencies on the premise it's better to be safe than sorry, that there is *no threshold* for cancer-causing substances—even one molecule of a carcinogen can initiate cancer. Evidence has been growing that this assumption is incorrect and that, for some carcinogens at least, a threshold does, in fact, exist. Nevertheless, the no-threshold approach to regulating carcinogens still applies. All parties to the controversy agree, however, that the risk of developing cancer is much greater when the exposure dose is high than when it is low.

3. *Exposure assessment.* Attempting to determine the numbers and types of people (age, sex, health status, etc.) who might be exposed to the substance in question, as well as estimating the duration, magnitude, and geographic extent of exposure, constitute the third step in the risk assessment process. In many real-life situations, some of the necessary information is unavailable—particularly actual exposure data—and those performing the analysis frequently must resort to computer modeling based on generalized assumptions about human behavior and how chemicals move in the environment. Generalizations on behavior include guesses on the kinds and quantities of food individuals in the target population eat each day; how much water they drink; how much time they spend indoors vs. outdoors. Assumptions regarding the environmental mobility of a chemical deal with its chemical stability, whether it dissolves in water or animal fat, how quickly it evaporates, or whether it binds to soil. The validity of assumptions about such parameters, in the absence of actual measurements, is questionable, making exposure assessment one of the weaker links in the information chain.

4. *Risk characterization.* Combining the information obtained from the first three steps of the risk assessment process, analysts produce a comprehensive picture of the types of adverse health effects likely to occur in exposed populations and the frequency with which such effects can be expected to occur. Risk is usually expressed in terms of quantitative probability—for example, one cancer death per 10,000 exposed population or "10^{-4} risk." For noncarcinogens, the risk characterization typically yields **Acceptable Daily Intakes (ADIs)** derived from dividing animal study NOELs by safety factors.

Information gathered through the risk assessment process is of great value to risk managers, but such data are incapable of answering many of the values-based questions with which decision makers wrestle: how safe is "safe enough"? what trade-offs between risks, benefits, and costs of control are justified? will reducing an existing risk merely replace it with a newer, more dangerous one? which among competing risks merits the greatest attention and resource allocation for abatement? Societal values and priorities must inevitably be taken into account in resolving these issues. Trade-offs among competing interests, political considerations, legal obligations, and scientific uncertainties are all factors that risk managers weigh as they decide how best to reduce hazards and protect public health. Risk assessment, while not perfect, provides a valuable tool for making appropriate decisions (American Chemical Society, 1998).

Polychlorinated Biphenyls (PCBs)

In 1964 Dr. Soren Jensen, a Swedish chemist at the University of Stockholm, began a project to determine DDT levels in human fat and wildlife samples; instead he discovered that the tissues he was examining contained large amounts of synthetic organic chemicals called PCBs. His findings, published in 1966, were greeted with widespread surprise and disbelief because PCBs, unlike DDT and other chlorinated hydrocarbon pesticides, were not being deliberately released into the environment but were restricted to use in industrial settings. Despite the initial skepticism, subsequent studies by researchers in many countries confirmed Dr. Jensen's findings. Virtually every tissue sample tested, from fish to birds to polar bears to animals living in deep sea trenches, contained detectable levels of PCBs. Extensive research during the decades that followed revealed that of all the chemical contaminants known, PCBs are the most widespread throughout the global environment.

How Could This Situation Come About?

Polychlorinated biphenyls were first synthesized in 1929, their production being taken over in 1930 by Monsanto, which sold the chemical under the trade name Arochlor. PCBs, which range in consistency from oily liquids to waxy solids, are extremely stable substances with a high boiling point, high solubility in fat but low solubility in water, low electrical conductivity, and high resistance to heat—all qualities which made them valuable for a wide variety of industrial uses. Primarily employed as cooling liquids in electrical transformers and capacitors, PCBs have also been used in hydraulic fluids, in carbonless carbon paper, insulating tapes, adhesives, paints, caulking compounds, sealants, and as road coverings to control dust.

The chemical stability that made PCBs so attractive to industry, however, is the very characteristic that has made them such an environmental and health hazard. Although designed for industrial use, there are many way in which PCBs can inadvertently escape and contaminate the environment: 1) discharge of PCB-laden wastes from factories into waterways have resulted in mammoth pollution problems, the most notorious episodes being Outboard Marine Corporation's dumping of PCBs into Waukegan Harbor (on Lake Michigan) and a similar situation in the Hudson River, traced to two General Electric plants; 2) vaporization from paints or landfills or burning of PCB-containing material can result in the chemical becoming airborne and then reentering the ecosystem with precipitation. EPA estimates that approximately 89% of PCBs now entering Lake Superior are deposited via airborne fallout (EPA, 1994). A classic example of fire causing extensive PCB contamination occurred early in 1981 in Binghamton, New York, where PCB-containing electrical equipment in the basement of the newly built 17-floor State Office Building caught fire. Although the blaze was quickly extinguished, inspectors subsequently discovered that contaminated soot had been carried through the air conditioning system and deposited throughout the entire building. Air sampling indicated that this soot contained 10–20% PCBs, as well as lesser amounts of dioxin and dibenzofurans formed during the combustion process. The ensuing cleanup operation took seven years to complete and cost New York taxpayers $37 million (Fawcett, 1988); 3) leaks in industrial equipment have resulted in numerous instances of PCB contamination, such as the case during the summer of 1979 when 200 gallons of PCBs leaked from an electrical transformer at a feed processing plant in Billings, Montana, contaminating about a million pounds of meal used in chicken feed. Subsequently, $2.7 million worth of chickens and eggs had to be destroyed because the birds had

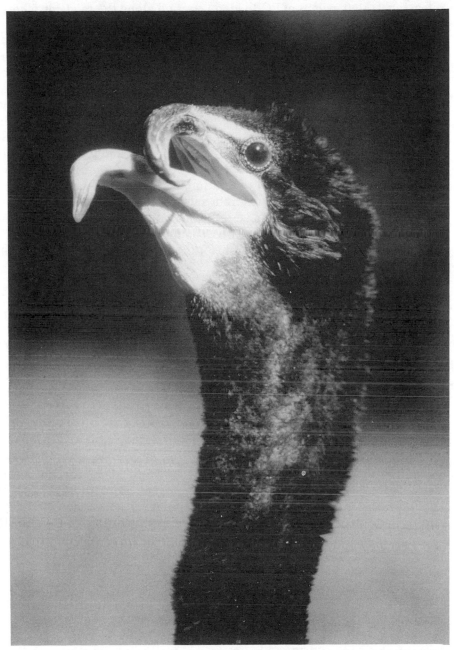

This double-crested cormorant, with its twisted and deformed beak, is a glaring example of the toxic effects of PCBs. *[Thomas A. Schneider]*

eaten the contaminated meal before the leak was discovered (Regenstein, 1982); 4) accidental spills or illegal dumping are a source of concern because the high cost of legally disposing of PCB wastes has tempted some haulers to dump such materials along roadsides, in ditches, or other out-of-the-way places. In August of 1978 such "midnight dumpers" opened the discharge pipe of their truck while driving along 210 miles of back roads in North Carolina, releasing 31,000 gallons of PCB-laden waste oil along the roadside where most of it remains to this day.

Whatever the route, once PCBs enter the environment they persist there for decades, resisting breakdown. Contamination of living organisms with PCBs generally occurs via the food chain, the concentration of the chemical increasing as it moves from lower to higher trophic levels ("biomagnification," see chapter 8). Within an individual organism, especially among higher-level consumers such as carnivorous birds, fish, and humans, PCBs accumulate in fatty tissues such as liver, kidneys, heart, lungs, brain, and breast milk. By 1976, after more than forty years of PCB production and use, 99% of all breast milk sampled in the United States contained PCBs. A quarter of the samples tested exceeded the legal level of contamination, which would have caused a commercial product to be banned from sale (Steingraber, 1997). With continuing exposure, PCB concentrations in the body increase over a period of time, a process known as **bioaccumulation.** Though ingestion of PCBs with food is the primary route of human exposure to these chemicals, PCBs can also be inhaled or absorbed through the skin.

PCB Threat to Health

Widespread human exposure to PCBs has concerned health and regulatory officials because laboratory testing has shown the chemicals to be toxic to several animal species even at very low concentrations. In experiments with rodents, minks, and Rhesus monkeys, PCB exposure has resulted in the development of a number of adverse health effects: liver disorders, miscarriage, low birthweight, abnormal multiplication of cells, and (in rats only) liver cancer. Researchers presumed that chemicals which could produce such effects in some mammalian species were likely to have similar effects on humans, and the knowledge that virtually everyone on the planet has been exposed to at least trace amounts of PCBs was considered cause for alarm. Evidence that many foods, especially freshwater fish, were contaminated with PCBs prompted the U.S. government to take regulatory action. In 1973 the FDA established tolerance levels for PCBs in food; passage of the Toxic Substances Control Act in 1976 specifically banned the production, sale, distribution, and use of PCBs in open systems; and in 1977, Monsanto, the sole U.S. manufacturer of the chemicals, terminated PCB production.

In the meantime, research on the human health impact of PCBs continued and today a wealth of scientific data exists on the chemical's toxicological effects. Contrary to popular perception, the acute toxicity of PCBs is quite low. The most frequent complaint provoked by high levels of PCB exposure is the appearance of an acne-like skin disorder referred to as **chloracne.** Regarded as the most characteristic symptom of PCB poisoning (or poisoning with any of the related group of chemicals known as chlorinated hydrocarbons), chloracne was an occasional occupational health problem among workers during the early years of PCB production and use. Recognition of this hazard led to the establishment in 1942 of recommended maximum allowable concentrations in the workplace. Since then, with the exception of a few cases of chloracne and possibly diminished liver function, scarcely any adverse health effects attributable to PCB exposure have been documented, even among workers who were exposed to PCBs over a period of many years.

The only large-scale episodes of PCB poisoning occurred in 1968 in Japan and in 1978–79 in Taiwan, both involving widespread consumption of PCB-tainted rice oil, contaminated during processing with PCB-containing fluid from a leaky heat-exchanger. In the Japanese incident, 1,300 people developed chloracne, swelling of the upper eyelids, discoloration of skin and fingernails—conditions collectively referred to as "Yusho (rice oil) disease." Over half the pregnant women who fell victim to Yusho disease subsequently gave birth to infants with similar symptoms, suggesting that PCBs cross the placental barrier and can be toxic to the developing fetus. In both Japan and Taiwan, follow-up studies have revealed that, in addition to PCBs, the contaminated rice oil contained a related, more toxic group of chemicals called dibenzofurans, which may have been responsible for some of the health problems initially blamed on PCBs alone. No deaths directly attributable to these chemicals have occurred among the victims of rice oil poisoning, however the Yusho incident appears to have resulted in some cases of chronic illness (Ottoboni, 1991).

Since few members of the general public ever receive the relatively high levels of exposure experienced by Yusho disease victims or by workers in an occupational setting, the main focus of worry about PCBs' possible health impact has focused on chronic toxicity, specifically their potential to cause cancer. Since animal studies indicate that PCBs are carcinogenic in rodents, it was feared that the same would be true in humans—one of the main reasons advanced to justify banning the chemical. However, after decades of research, no link between chronic PCB exposure and human cancer has been found. In 1999, the largest epidemiologic study to date found no increase in cancer deaths among more than 7,000 workers exposed to PCBs from 1946–1976 (Kimbrough et al., 1999). The evidence thus appears convincing that even among those occupationally exposed to the chemical, PCBs do not cause cancer in humans. PCBs have not yet been acquitted of all charges of adverse human health effects, however. Their role as one of a group of so-called "endocrine disruptors" is now being actively investigated (see Box 7-1) and may yet vindicate the legal action taken against them a quarter century ago.

Although PCB production in the United States halted in 1977, the chemicals remain very much a part of the American scene. During the years 1929–1977, 1.4 billion pounds of PCBs were produced in the United States. Decades later, millions of pounds remain in use, mainly in closed systems such as high voltage capacitors (common on ordinary utility poles), electrical transformers, and fluorescent light ballasts. In addition, approximately 500 million pounds of PCBs have been dumped into landfills and waterways where they continue to pose an environmental threat. As existing PCB-containing equipment becomes obsolete and is replaced, safe methods for disposing of this material must be found. While several promising new technologies for treating PCB-contaminated soils have been developed recently and are undergoing feasibility testing, high-temperature (2200°F or above) incineration is the EPA-approved method at present for destroying wastes containing high concentrations of PCBs.

BOX 7-1

Hormonal Havoc

Until recently, PCBs, dioxins, and a host of other persistent organic pollutants were the focus of public fear and scientific scrutiny largely because of their presumed role as major contributors to rising cancer rates. Decades of intensive research have failed to support the widespread conviction that these chemicals are important environmental carcinogens, but a growing body of evidence now suggests they play a more insidious role as **endocrine disruptors**.

At least 50 different chemicals have now been identified as capable of interfering with the normal functioning of the endocrine system in both animals and humans. The culprits include lead and mercury—both naturally occurring heavy metals—but the majority are synthetic compounds, including many long-lasting chemicals which concentrate as they move up the food chain and tend to be dispersed widely throughout the environment. PCBs, dioxin, DDT, chlordane, atrazine, lindane, phthalates, and styrene are but a few of the synthetic organic chemicals known to act as endocrine disruptors. Although several of these compounds, including DDT and chlordane, are no longer being manufactured or used in most developed countries, they are still detectable in trace quantities throughout the environment and, unlike conventional toxicants, can wreak hormonal havoc even when present in extremely minute concentrations. Indeed, in terms of dose-response relationships, endocrine disruptors are unusual in that low levels of exposure tend to elicit a greater adverse response than do high doses.

Endocrine hormones play a pivotal role in regulating such vital processes as fetal development, sexual differentiation, reproduction, brain development, and immune system functioning; anything that prevents the correct chemical messages from being received is bound to cause trouble. Endocrine disruptors are believed to interfere with these processes by acting as "hormone mimics," replacing the natural hormones which bind to the hormone receptor molecules within cells, or as "hormone blockers," preventing natural hormones from attaching to a receptor. Embryonic development is particularly vulnerable to the effects of endocrine disruptors. Exposure that provokes only temporary effects in adults can produce permanent and far-reaching damage to an embryo or fetus if it occurs at a critical developmental stage.

Evidence demonstrating the harmful impact of endocrine-disrupting chemicals has come primarily from wildlife studies. As early as the 1950s and 1960s, researchers noted that animal populations as diverse as eagles in Florida, trout in Lake Ontario, and commercially raised mink in Michigan were experiencing reproductive failure, a problem eventually traced in part to their exposure to synthetic insecticides, dioxins, and PCBs, respectively. In the 1970s, biologists in California reported another strange phenomenon among western gull populations—females nesting with other females. Over the next 20 years, similar same-sex pairings were observed in waterfowl populations in the Great Lakes, Puget Sound, and off the coast of Massachusetts, leaving scientists bewildered as to what could be causing the sexual confusion among these far-flung groups of birds. In the late 1980s, wildlife biologists in Florida, searching the shores of Lake Apopka for alligator eggs, discovered to their dismay that only a small percentage of the eggs collected were viable; and half the baby alligators from the few eggs that did hatch died within ten days. Even more surprising was the fact that when male alligators were captured and examined closely, approximately 60% exhibited abnormally small penises. Alligator populations in other Florida lakes were flourishing, indicating some sort of localized problem. Researchers knew that almost a decade earlier, a spill from a nearby chemical factory had polluted Lake Apopka with the insecticide dicofol, but by the time biologists were scratching their heads over alligator reproductive failures, the lake appeared to be clean again. Whatever was causing the observed problems was obviously potent in very minute quantities.

Reports of abnormal sexual development and behavior, congenital abnormalities, and immune system dysfunction began appearing with increasing frequency in scientific journals during the late 1980s and early 1990s. More and more, researchers attributed the problems they were seeing in the field to substances that acted like the sex hormones estrogen, progesterone, or testosterone to alter normal sexual development, or that interfered with thyroid metabolism, thereby adversely affecting development of the brain or reproductive organs. Knowing that differences between endocrine system functioning in humans and other animal species are negligible, scientists began expressing their concerns that the problems they were observing among wildlife populations might be occurring in humans as well.

Direct evidence for human health damage caused by endocrine disruptors is less compelling than that for wildlife effects, however. Demonstration of a link between fetal exposure to diethylstilbestrol and subsequent abnormalities of the reproductive system in DES-sons and daughters provides the most clear-cut association, but the fact that the exposure dose received by these individuals was much higher than the levels of endocrine disruptors in the general environment makes it problematic to extrapolate findings from long-term DES studies to the wider public. In the 1980s several European studies that documented a dramatic decline in human sperm counts over the past several decades attracted considerable attention and caused some observers to speculate that endocrine disruptors might be responsible. However, subsequent surveys in various parts of the world have yielded conflicting results, some corroborating the earlier research, others indicating no change in sperm counts or even an increased count in some groups studied. To date, investigators have been unable to reach a consensus on whether sperm counts are falling or not and on the extent to which endocrine disruptors are responsible for such a decline if it has, in fact, occurred.

Another source of evidence cited as suggestive of human health damage caused by endocrine disruptors is a study that focused on the children of mothers consuming significant amounts of PCB-tainted Lake Michigan fish during pregnancy. Babies whose mothers had eaten the most fish tested highest for blood PCB levels and were smaller at birth than babies born to mothers who hadn't consumed Lake Michigan fish. Developmental testing of these children continued at intervals during their childhood years; researchers found that the children whose pregnant mothers had eaten the most fish were less cooperative in terms of behavior, had poorer memories, lower

IQ, and had a shorter attention span than did the children of nonfish-eating mothers. These results are particularly worrisome because the PCB levels to which these children were exposed were not a great deal higher than concentrations prevailing among the general population.

Accurately assessing the human impact of endocrine disruptors is fraught with difficulties, not the least of which is the lack of a control population to compare the effects of exposure vs. nonexposure. Even in the most remote spots on the planet, people carry a measurable body burden of PCBs, DDT, and other persistent organic pollutants. Indeed, the Inuit people inhabiting islands in the Canadian Arctic, west of Greenland, exhibit some of the highest PCB levels ever detected in human populations. Another challenge confronting health researchers is accounting for the additive or synergistic effects of exposure to the dozens of different chemicals to which humans are simultaneously exposed every day.

Despite these difficulties, intensive research efforts are currently underway to assess whether and to what extent endocrine disruptors are undermining our biological future as individuals and as a species. In the United States a number of federal agencies and institutes have launched close to 400 research projects dealing with the issue; many state environmental agencies are actively investigating the problem also, as is the chemical industry itself. Overseas, a number of national governments and international organizations, including the U.N.'s World Health Organization, are engaged in research efforts as well. It may be many years before these projects provide definitive answers, but in the meantime there are a number of actions individuals can take to reduce exposure to hormone mimics and hormone blockers.

- Avoid use of chemical pesticides to the greatest extent possible; don't permit children or pets to play on pesticide-treated lawns.
- Heed state-issued fish advisories; don't fish downstream from golf courses due to pesticide runoff from these heavily-treated grasses.
- Limit consumption of fatty meats and dairy products.
- Wash fruits and vegetables thoroughly to remove pesticide residues; better yet, grow your own chemical-free produce.
- When using a microwave oven, don't allow plastic wrap to touch food.

Reference
Colborn, et al. 1996. *Our Stolen Future*. Dutton.

Dioxin (TCDD)

In the wet spring of 1983 public apprehension about the dangers of dioxin soared when the U.S. Environmental Protection Agency announced that inhabitants of the tiny riverside community of Times Beach, Missouri, should abandon their homes and evacuate the town. Soil analyses had revealed high levels of dioxin contamination due to oiling of roads for dust control in the early 1970s; the oil had been scavenged from a trichlorophenol factory by a waste hauler and was heavily laced with the toxic chemical.

Table 7-1   Preliminary List of Chemicals Associated with Endocrine System Effects in Animals and Humans (*) or In Vitro (+)

Known	Probable	Suspect
Atrazine	Alachlor	Aldicarb
Chlordanes	Aldrin	Butyl Benzyl Phthalate
Chlordecone (Kepone)(*)	Amitrole (Aminotriazole)	tert-Butylhydroxyanisole (+)
DDD	Benomyl	p-sec-Butylphenol (+)
DDE	Bisphenol A(+)	p-tert-Butylphenol (+)
DDT	Cadmium (*)	Carbaryl
1,2-Dibromo-3-Chloropropane (*)	2,4-D	Cypermethrin
Dicofol (Kelthane)	Di(2-Ethylhexyl) Phthalate	2,4-Dichlorophenol (+)
Dieldrin	Endrin	Dicyclohexyl Phthalate
Diethylstilbestrol (DES)(*)	Heptachlor	Di(2-Ethylhexyl) Adipate (+)
Dioxins (2,3,7,8-)	Heptachlor Epoxide	Di-n-butyl Phthalate (+)
Endosulfans	Hexachlorobenzene	Di-n-hexyl Phthalate
Furans (2,3,7,8-)	β-Hexachlorocyclohexane	Di-n-pentyl Phthalate
Lindane	Lead (*)	Di-n-propyl Phthalate
Methoxychlor	Mancozeb	Esfenvalerate
p-Nonylphenol	Maneb	Fenvalerate
PCBs	Mercury (*)	Malathion
Toxaphene	Methyl Parathion	Methomyl
Tibutyl Tin	Metiram	Metribuzin
	Mirex	Nitrofen
	p-Octylphenol	Octachlorostyrene
	Parathion	PAHs
	Pentachlorophenol	p-iso-Pentylphenol (+)
	Polybrominated Biphenyls (PBBs)	p-tert-Pentylphenol (+)
	Styrene (*, +)	Permethrin
	2,4,5-T	Ziram
	Trifluralin	
	Vinclozolin	
	Zineb	

Note: Chlordanes includes α- and γ-Chlordane, Oxychlordane, and cis- and trans-Nonachlor; Endosulfans includes α- and β-Endosulfan and technical grade Endosulfan.

Source: Illinois Environmental Protection Agency (IEPA). 1997. *Endocrine Disruptors Strategy.* February.

Times Beach is but one of numerous places around the world where industrial accidents, deliberate dumping, or inadvertent use of dioxin-tainted pesticides have resulted in environmental contamination which has provoked alarm, sometimes panic, among local residents. Public concerns, in turn, have been generated by debatable statements by some researchers that "dioxin is the most toxic substance ever created by humans," and by allegations of a wide range of health problems and genetic disorders among American servicemen exposed to dioxin during their tour of duty in Vietnam. Widespread fears that serious human health damage can be caused by infinitesimally small amounts of the chemical have led to such controversial regulatory actions as the evacuation of Times Beach and the suspension of the selective herbicides 2, 4, 5-T and silvex, yet the results of numerous follow-up studies on exposed populations fail to show a single case where human death has resulted from dioxin exposure. What are the facts about this chemical whose very name seems to generate hysteria?

Chemically related to PCBs and other chlorinated hydrocarbons, dioxins form a large group of chemicals of widely varying levels of toxicity. The most dangerous dioxin is 2, 3, 7, 8-tetrachlorodibenzo-p-dioxin, generally referred to as TCDD or, simply, "dioxin." TCDD, unlike its chemical cousin PCB, has no industrial usefulness and has never been intentionally manufactured; it is formed as an unwanted by-product in the production of certain herbicides and the germ-killer hexachlorophene. Dioxin can escape into the atmosphere when it evaporates from TCDD-contaminated soil and water or when dioxin- or other chlorine-containing compounds are burned (EPA researchers say that municipal and medical waste incinerators currently constitute the leading source of dioxin emissions in the United States). Airborne dioxins can be carried long distances before they eventually are rained out or settle as dry deposits on soil, plant surfaces, or bodies of water. There they bind tightly to soil particles or sediment at the bottom of lakes and streams. Although TCDD undergoes rapid photolysis, if protected from light exposure dioxin breaks down very slowly—experimental evidence suggests that its half-life in soil may exceed 10 years. Thanks to regulatory controls on industrial emissions and the banning of 2,4,5-T, dioxin levels in the environment have fallen by about 50% since the late 1980s. Nevertheless, TCDD in minute quantities is still very widespread, present in soil, dust, chimneys of woodburning stoves and furnaces, eggs, fish tissues, and animal fat. Most humans have accumulated small amounts of dioxin in their fatty tissues largely through consumption of meat, fish, and dairy products, with only 1% or less of the total body burden coming from such sources of exposure as contaminated air or water.

Statements asserting that dioxin is the "most toxic of all synthetic chemicals" are somewhat misleading because they are based on the observation that extremely low doses of TCDD are fatal to guinea pigs, by far the most sensitive species to the chemical's lethal effects. Hamsters, by contrast, can tolerate doses of dioxin up to 1,900 times the amount that would kill a guinea pig. For other test species, dioxin's lethality ranges somewhere between the extremes represented by guinea pigs and hamsters. However, dioxin is capable of producing many adverse effects other than death, and while any given species may exhibit a biological response at the far end of the range for a particular TCDD-induced problem, most species, humans included, respond similarly for most effects. For example, dioxin produces chloracne in rabbits, monkeys, mice, and humans at roughly equivalent levels of exposure. Interference with immune system function, fetal toxicity, and cancer are other adverse effects of dioxin exposure to which humans, rats, guinea pigs, and hamsters exhibit similar sensitivity. On the other hand, some of TCDD's effects are strikingly species-specific. Teratogenic effects of dioxin are apparent only in mice, which develop cleft palates at doses below the lethal level. Similarly, while dioxin acts as a liver toxin in a number of species, no signs of liver damage have yet been observed in highly exposed humans. By contrast, TCDD is carcinogenic in most species, producing malignant tumors at multiple sites—but only at high levels of exposure. Perhaps most significant among dioxin's long-term effects revealed by animal tests (presumed valid for humans as well) is the chemical's ability to disrupt the hormonal systems that control reproduction. Evidence from both wildlife and laboratory studies shows that exposure to dioxin (and to chlorinated organic chemicals in general) may result in reduced fertility, fetal loss, changes in sexual behavior, thyroid dysfunction, and suppression of the immune system. Indeed, some scientists conclude that these effects are far more significant than the carcinogenicity concerns that have been the focus of most toxicological research in relation to dioxin (Colburn et al., 1996; Birnbaum, 1994).

The implications of all this so far as human exposure is concerned remains somewhat problematic. Over the years thousands of people, particularly chemical industry workers, have had extensive exposure to the chemical at relatively high levels (e.g. a 1949 incident in a Monsanto plant in Nitro, WV, exposed more than 200 workers to dioxin; more spectacularly, a 1976 explosion at a trichlorophenol factory near Milan, Italy, released a toxic cloud that settled on the nearby suburb of Seveso, exposing 37,000 people of all ages to considerable amounts of dioxin). It is estimated that additional millions have been exposed to low concentrations (e.g. the farmers and ranchers using dioxin-contaminated herbicides, military personnel exposed to Agent Orange, residents of Times Beach and other communities where dioxin-laced waste oils were sprayed on dirt roads, consumers of TCDD-tainted fish, etc.). With the exception of the chemical industry workers whose dioxin exposure was 500 times greater than that experienced by the general public, the only confirmed human health problems associated with TCDD have been acute symptoms such as chloracne, muscle aches and pains, nervous system disorders, digestive upsets, and some psychiatric effects.

Among the thousands of Seveso residents exposed to dioxin fallout from the 1976 industrial accident, the only health problems reported in the months following the explosion were about 200 cases of chloracne, almost all of them involving children, though over 200 animal deaths in the area were reported (Ottoboni, 1991). Nevertheless, a statistically significant increase in deaths due to soft tissue sarcoma (a type of cancer) and respiratory cancer has been confirmed among a group of men who were highly exposed while working for more than 20 years in chemical manufacturing plants. Among this group, workers who had been exposed to dioxin for the longest period of time had TCDD blood levels of 3600 ppt. By comparison, for adults living in the industrialized world, the average blood level of dioxin is 6 ppt, while members of the U.S. military who handled dioxin-contaminated Agent Orange exhibited peak levels around 400 ppt (Fingerhut et al., 1991). In 1993, publication of a study carried out by a team of Italian researchers reviewing the medical records of thousands of Seveso residents documented an increase in soft tissue sarcomas, cancer of the gall bladder, and multiple myelomas among citizens exposed to the highest levels of dioxin ever recorded among civilian populations. However, the overall cancer rate for the region was lower than expected. Another study of U.S. chemical industry workers whose exposure to TCDD averaged less than one year revealed average blood concentrations of 640 ppt—a level 90 times higher that the national norm—yet the cancer death rate among these men 20 years after exposure was scarcely distinguishable from that of the general public (Dickson and Buzik, 1993). In 1997 the International Agency for Research on Cancer officially classified TCDD as a group 1 human carcinogen, basing its designation on studies showing an excess of all cancers among several groups of highly exposed workers. Results from a follow-up study of one of these groups, involving over 5,000 U.S. chemical workers, confirmed an increased cancer incidence due to dioxin exposure—but only among those who experienced doses 100–1,000 times higher than those encountered by the general public (Steenland et al., 1999). Such findings have led most researchers to the conclusion that while dioxin *does* cause cancer in humans at very high levels of exposure, it poses a minimal threat of malignancies at the low concentrations commonly encountered.

For those charged with protecting the public health and setting regulatory requirements regarding TCDD exposure, the dioxin issue presents some difficult decisions. Without question the chemical is acutely toxic to laboratory animals and produces serious chronic health problems in many animal species as well. However, in spite of extensive human exposure to TCDD, only a handful of transitory acute effects have been confirmed in people. It must be noted that one of the problems in determining the health effects of dioxin is the fact that TCDD virtually never occurs alone; rather, it is but one of many chemicals in a mixture which may include PCBs, dibenzofurans, chlorophenols, and other dioxins. Since the identity of these other chemicals is frequently not known or not reported, it could be risky to attribute a given observed health effect to TCDD alone. While some investigators argue that dioxin presents less of a health threat to humans than to other animal species, others are convinced that the subtle effects observed in laboratory animals are having an impact on people as well. Citing animal data regarding TCDD's adverse impact on reproduction and on immune system function as justification for continued regulatory controls, such authorities are convinced of the necessity to limit human exposure to dioxin as much as possible (Colborn et al., 1996).

Asbestos

Probably no other hazardous substance has resulted in so many deaths and cases of disabling disease as has asbestos, the collective term for a group of six fibrous silicate minerals (amosite, chrysotile, tremolite, actinolite, anthophyllite, and crocidolite) found almost worldwide. Centers of commercial asbestos production are Canada, Russia, and South Africa, though in recent years production has been shifting to developing countries such as Brazil, India, Pakistan, Korea, and Indonesia. Utilized by humans ever since Stone

Age potters employed the substance to reinforce their clay, asbestos was woven into cloth during Greek and Roman times and was regarded as having magical properties because of its invulnerability to fire.

In modern times asbestos has acquired great economic value as an essential component in thousands of commercial products and processes. By the late 1970s, over six million tons of asbestos were being produced worldwide. About two-thirds of the asbestos used in the United States is employed in building materials, brake linings, textiles, and insulation, while the remaining one-third is consumed in such diverse products as paints, plastics, caulking compounds, floor tiles, cement, roofing paper, radiator covers, filters in gas masks, conveyor belts, potholders, ironing board covers, theater curtains, fake fireplace ash, and so on.

Unfortunately, in addition to being very useful, asbestos also represents an occupational hazard of major proportions. It is now estimated that of the 8–11 million current and retired workers exposed to large amounts of asbestos on the job, 30–40% can be expected to die of cancer. Exposure to asbestos is primarily through inhalation of tiny fibers suspended in the air. While airborne fibers may occur naturally in regions characterized by outcroppings of the mineral, they are more commonly associated with the deterioration of manufactured asbestos-containing materials or with the demolition or renovation of buildings containing asbestos. Fiber levels tend to be highest near asbestos mines or factories and are higher in cities than in rural areas, but virtually any air sample, regardless of where it is taken, will contain some asbestos fibers. Once inhaled, asbestos fibers are deposited in the air passages

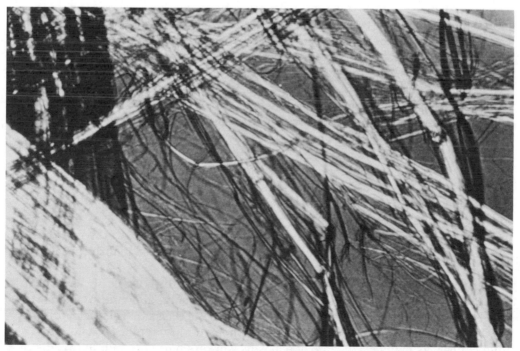

Asbestos fibers magnified to show the needle-like configuration of these hydrated silicate minerals. *[Illinois Department of Public Health]*

and cells within the lungs. Most of these are quickly carried away by the mucus that lines the respiratory tract, being transported up to the throat where they are swallowed, carried to the stomach, and eventually excreted with the feces. Some, however, remain trapped deep in the lungs and may never be removed.

Although inhalation represents the primary route by which asbestos enters the human body, people may also be exposed to the mineral in drinking water. Asbestos fibers can be released into water supplies when cement asbestos pipes corrode or when asbestos-containing wastes piled near mine sites are washed into lakes or rivers. While most municipal drinking water supplies experiencing asbestos contamination have relatively low concentrations, under one million fibers per liter, residents of cities such as San Francisco, Philadelphia, Seattle, New York, Atlanta, and Boston may be consuming water with fiber levels 10 to 100 times this amount. Asbestos that is swallowed, fortunately, presents much less of a health hazard than that which is inhaled. Most fibers are simply carried through the stomach and intestines and are excreted within a few days. A small portion, however, may lodge in the cells lining the gastrointestinal tract, while a few may move through the intestinal lining and enter the blood stream. These may either become trapped in other tissues or be excreted in the urine.

Asbestos-Related Diseases

Several different types of asbestos-related diseases are known, the most significant being the following.

Asbestosis. A chronic disease characterized by a scarring of the lung tissue, asbestosis most commonly occurs among workers who have been exposed to very high levels of asbestos dust. It is an irreversible, progressively worsening disease, the first symptom of which is shortness of breath following exertion. Lung function is adversely affected, the maximum volume of air a victim can inhale being reduced. In most cases, it takes 20 years or more of exposure to asbestos before symptoms of the disease appear; unfortunately, by this time asbestosis has usually reached an advanced state. The severity of asbestosis is influenced not only by the duration of exposure, but also by the type of asbestos fibers inhaled and by the synergistic effects of cigarette smoking. Until about 40 years ago when concerns about workers' health led to regulations regarding dust levels in asbestos factories, asbestosis was the leading cause of death among asbestos workers. Since the 1940s, however, rates of severe asbestosis have been substantially lowered. Yet even today standards for permissible levels of asbestos exposure are based on those amounts deemed low enough to protect workers from asbestosis, in spite of the fact that this disease is no longer the most significant asbestos-related health threat.

Lung Cancer. With the gradual reduction in dust levels in asbestos factories, deaths due to asbestosis have been decreasing, allowing workers to live long enough to develop today's leading cause of asbestos-related mortality, lung cancer. Compared to the 4–5% of the general population who die of lung cancer, as many as 20–25% of asbestos workers now succumb to this disease. The risk is especially great when exposure to asbestos fibers is accompanied by exposure to cigarette smoke. Studies have shown that while asbestos exposure alone increases an individual's risk of lung cancer death by a factor of seven, exposure to both asbestos and cigarette smoke entails a 60 times greater risk of lung cancer than that experienced by persons who are not exposed to asbestos and don't smoke.

Mesothelioma. This previously rare cancer of the lung or stomach lining today kills more than 5% of all asbestos workers. Like many other forms of cancer, mesothelioma is characterized by a long latency period, onset of disease symptoms occurring 25–40 years after initial exposure. Even very low levels of asbestos can result in mesothelioma, as evidenced by cases among young adults whose only contact with the mineral involved childhood exposure to their fathers' asbestos-contaminated work clothes. Mesothelioma is of special interest to researchers because, unlike other forms of cancer, the only known causative agent for this disease is asbestos. Thus mesothelioma is considered a "marker disease" indicating asbestos exposure. Since no effective treatment exists, mesothelioma is an invariably fatal ailment, with death generally occurring within two years of diagnosis.

Gastrointestinal Cancer. Cancer of the GI tract, which includes cancer of the colon, rectum, esophagus, and stomach, strikes asbestos workers with greater frequency than it does the general public, although a direct causative link is still not conclusively established. It is known that inhaled asbestos fibers can pass from the lungs to the stomach, colon, or intestines, and cell culture studies have demonstrated that the epithelial cells of the human intestine are particularly sensitive to damage by asbestos. There is also some evidence to suggest that people whose drinking water contains high concentrations of asbestos fibers may be at slightly elevated risk of gastrointestinal cancer. With the exception of esophageal cancer, the risk of gastrointestinal cancer is not enhanced by smoking.

Although research has not yet been able to establish conclusively the degree of asbestos exposure necessary to initiate cancer, evidence suggests that some individuals who were exposed to high levels of asbestos for only one day developed cancer years later as a result. For this reason the current presumption is that there is *no safe level for asbestos exposure*. Some scientists have argued that the development of asbestos-related disease is dependent on the mineral type of asbestos to which an individual is exposed. However, most researchers believe that fiber *size* is a more important determinant of asbestos' cancer-causing potential than are its chemical or physical properties. Experimental data suggest that long fibers (those exceeding 1/5000 of an inch in length) are more injurious than short fibers (less than 1/10,000 of an inch).

While *any* amount of asbestos exposure entails some degree of hazard, the extent of that risk is determined by a combination of several factors, among the most important of which are:

- level and duration of exposure
- time since exposure occurred
- age at which exposure occurred
- personal history of cigarette smoking
- type and size of asbestos fibers

While asbestos workers constitute by far the largest percentage of victims, others may be affected through indirect exposure. Mesothelioma has claimed casualties among people living in the vicinity of asbestos factories and among children of asbestos workers, whose only exposure to the fibers was from their fathers' work clothes when they returned from the factory. When asbestos is brought into the home, it becomes a permanent part of the domestic environment, embedded in carpets and draperies and suspended in the air where it constitutes a 24-hour/day source of exposure not only to the less vulnerable healthy adults of the household but also to the very young, the sick, and the elderly who are the groups most susceptible to any type of environmental irritant. For this reason, asbestos workers today are cautioned to shower and change clothes at the workplace in order to avoid inadvertent contamination of their homes with asbestos fibers.

Asbestos Problems in Public Buildings

Until the mid-1970s most asbestos-related health concerns were focused on the millions of American workers who had experienced significant levels of occupational exposure to the hazardous fibers. It thus came as an unwelcome surprise when the EPA warned that the general public has been receiving asbestos exposure for years simply by working or living in any of the estimated 700,000 commercial, governmental, or residential buildings which contain friable asbestos ("friable" refers to asbestos material which, when dry, can be crumbled to a powder by hand pressure).

Of greatest concern was the revelation that as many as two to six million schoolchildren and 300,000 teachers in 31,000 primary and secondary schools across the nation might be inhaling asbestos fibers on a daily basis. During the years 1946–1973, asbestos-containing fireproofing materials were extensively used in constructing or renovating schools throughout the country. By 1973 increasing documentation of the health threats posed by asbestos had caused the EPA to ban all spray applications of asbestos in insulating and fireproofing materials and in 1977 new restrictions totally halted the spray application of asbestos. Such regulation had no effect, however, on existing asbestos-containing materials which, by this time, were beginning to deteriorate in many schools, releasing potentially dangerous asbestos fibers into the classroom environment. When asbestos-containing dust is swept up by janitors or disturbed by students' coming and going, it becomes resuspended and can remain in the air—at breathing level—for as long as 80 hours. The high levels of asbestos fibers measured in the indoor air of many schools have prompted concerns for elevated rates of lung cancer and mesothelioma among today's schoolchildren 20–40 years hence. The initial EPA response to this perceived threat was to issue an advisory to school districts throughout the country, informing them of the situation and requiring that they inspect their buildings for the presence of asbestos-containing materials (ACM). If friable asbestos was found, the districts were to notify parents or the PTA of that fact. The federal authorities apparently assumed that if an asbestos hazard was identified, parental concerns about their children's safety would be sufficient to ensure prompt remediation of the problem. Such did not prove to be the case, however, as financially strapped school districts, in the absence of a firm federal mandate, postponed expensive remediation projects. By 1983, 66% of the nation's school districts had not yet even inspected for asbestos or had failed to report doing so to the EPA.

Consequently, in the fall of 1986, President Reagan signed into law the far-reaching Asbestos Hazard Emergency Response Act (AHERA), requiring that all primary and secondary schools be inspected for the presence of asbestos; if such materials are found, the school district must file and carry out an asbestos abatement plan. EPA was charged with promulgating rules detailing correct inspection procedures, establishing asbestos abatement standards, certification programs for contractors, and standards for the transportation and disposal of asbestos.

Asbestos Abatement

When an asbestos hazard is identified, those charged with remedying the situation have several options from which to choose:

1. *Encapsulation.* This is a technique in which exposed asbestos is heavily coated with a polymer sealant to prevent further release of fibers.

2. *Enclosure.* Feasible when the area affected is relatively small, this process involves building a nonpermeable barrier between the source of exposure and surrounding open areas.

3. *Removal.* A labor-intensive process whereby all asbestos containing materials are physically removed from the structure.

Of the various abatement alternatives, complete removal is the most expensive and time consuming. It also entails the risk of worker exposure to asbestos fibers and, if carelessly done, could endanger the public as well. However, since removal absolves a building's owner of future liability and because encapsulated asbestos requires periodic reinspection, removal may, in the long run, be cheaper than encapsulation. In addition, federal laws require that any buildings that are going to be demolished or renovated, other than private homes or apartments with four or less dwelling units, must be inspected for the presence of asbestos-containing material. If any friable asbestos is found it must be removed before work can commence. Essentially this means that if a school district chose encapsulation as its asbestos abatement option and subsequently decided to tear down or substantially renovate that building, it would first have to hire a contractor to remove all encapsulated asbestos materials, thereby paying twice to have the job done. For these reasons, even though encapsulation is an acceptable method of reducing asbestos exposure, most asbestos abatement projects today involve complete removal.

Asbestos removal projects must adhere to strict federal and state regulations to protect both workers and the general public. Under the Clean Air Act provisions for hazardous air pollutants, EPA has set a standard of "no visible emissions" for any asbestos removal activities. Asbestos-containing materials must be wet down before work commences and must be kept damp throughout the course of the project, right up to final disposal. Damp asbestos wastes must be containerized in thick plastic bags or plastic lined containers, tagged with an appropriate warning label, and transported in a covered vehicle to an approved sanitary landfill. Since asbestos is not classified as a hazardous waste, the EPA-approved method of asbestos disposal is to bury the material in an area of the landfill separate from other household wastes, covering the containers with at least six inches of soil or with some other nonasbestos materials before compacting. Final cover of an additional 30 inches of nonasbestos material is required.

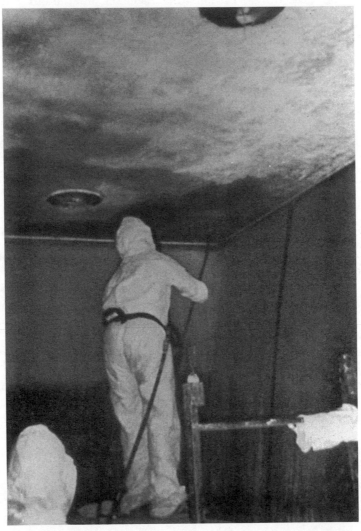

Workers in protective clothing soak an asbestos-containing acoustical ceiling prior to removal of the asbestos. *[Courtesy of Occupational Training & Supply, Inc.]*

Legal Status of Asbestos

The mass of evidence documenting asbestos' adverse health impact has led to passage of legislation in several countries restricting the use of this otherwise valuable material. The United Kingdom, Germany, and Sweden have all banned some uses of asbestos and are searching for acceptable substitutes. Japan is similarly discouraging imports of the material. In Brazil, by contrast, asbestos consumption is growing by about 7% annually.

In the United States, action against asbestos is proceeding on several fronts. Occupational exposure, which in the 1970s was lowered first to 5 and subsequently to 2 fibers/cm^3 of air, has now been reduced to 0.1 fibers/cm^3 over an eight-hour time-weighted average. Employers are required to sample at factory sites every six months and daily at construction sites unless employees are wearing respirators. In situations where fiber levels exceed standards, employers must install exhaust ventilation and dust control systems and air vacuuming methods to reduce worker exposure to asbestos dust. Medical surveillance of workers, provision and laundering of protective clothing, maintenance of respirators, provision of showering and changing facilities—all are employer responsibilities to enhance the health and safety of asbestos workers. For the protection of the general public, the federal government has banned the use of asbestos in a number of consumer products: certain pipe coverings and patching compounds, artificial fireplace logs, sprayed-on decorations, and hair dryers. Since 1997, production of asbestos-containing materials for home construction and use has been banned. In spite of these prohibitions, however, consumers cannot always assume that products they buy are asbestos-free. Items imported from countries without legal restrictions on asbestos (Canada being a notable example) may still contain the mineral. Even in the United States, asbestos-containing products are not legally required to be labeled as such and therefore buyers wishing to know product content are advised to contact the manufacturer or the U.S. Consumer Product Safety Commission.

Lead

Lead poisoning is entirely preventable, yet it is the most common and societally devastating environmental disease of young children.
—Dr. Louis Sullivan, former Secretary of Health and Human Services

Dr. Sullivan's remarks regarding the impact of lead on children's health were prompted by the recognition that three to four million American youngsters at that time had blood lead levels high enough to impair their brain function. By the late 1990s, the Centers for Disease Control and Prevention (CDC) estimated that subclinical (i.e. lacking visible disease symptoms) lead toxicity was affecting about 11% of all urban children in the United States; among inner-city African-American children, the percentage affected was estimated at double that figure—22% (CDC, 1997). Future medical historians may regard it as ironic that as a new century dawns, a substance whose toxicity has been well established for millennia is regarded as the single most important environmental health problem affecting American children.

Human contact with lead, a mineral element naturally occurring throughout the environment, dates back to at least 4000 B.C. when it was first smelted as a by-product of silver processing. Because it is malleable and easy to work, doesn't rust, corrode, or dissolve in water, and binds readily with other metals, lead has been widely used since ancient times as an alloy; as an ingredient in paints, glazes, and cosmetics; and for gutters and piping. Indeed, the word "plumbing" is derived from the Latin word for lead, *plumbum*—hence lead's chemical symbol, Pb.

Among those who worked with the metal, it early became apparent that in addition to being commercially valuable, lead is a potent human poison. Over the centuries, evidence of the multifaceted aspects of lead's toxicity has continued to mount. More than two thousand years ago, Roman doctors were describing patients suffering with symptoms of gout, an ailment associated with chronic lead poisoning; modern commentators theorize such problems may have been caused by the Roman practice of lining wine casks, cooking pots, and aqueducts with lead. Lead poisoning may also have contributed to the low birth rate and high incidence of mental retardation among the Roman aristocracy. A major source of exposure to the metal among wealthy Romans is thought to have been a grape juice syrup, *frumentum*, which was brewed in lead pots and subsequently used to sweeten foods and wine; even one teaspoonful of this syrup would have been more than enough to cause chronic lead poisoning. Unfortunately, later generations learned little from the Roman experience; during medieval times, Europeans in large numbers fell victim to "Saturnine poisoning," a result of using soluble lead acetate to sweeten sour wine, and even in the 16th century widespread outbreaks of lead poisoning were occurring in France as a result of storing wine in lead-lined vessels.

Sources of Lead

Today, as in centuries past, lead is used in a wide range of industrial products. The single largest use of lead, over 70% of total U.S. consumption of the metal, is for lead storage batteries (virtually every car on the road contains 20 pounds of lead in its battery); other lead-containing products include ammunition, brass, coverings for power and communication cables, glass TV tubes, solder, and pigments. With world production estimated at more than three million tons annually, lead is produced in larger amounts than any other nonferrous metal. Not surprisingly, lead is now found throughout the environment—in soils, water, air, and food. Until the mid-1980s, automobile emissions constituted the major source of environmental lead. With the phaseout of leaded gasoline in the United States and a number of other countries, amounts of lead entering the atmosphere have declined sharply. Correspondingly, Americans' blood lead levels have fallen as well, down by more than 80% since the mid-1970s. In the approximately 100 countries where leaded gasoline is still used, however, environmental contamination from this source remains a serious problem. Researchers in India report that over half the children in six large metropolitan areas have elevated blood lead levels, a fact they blame on fallout of lead particles from automobile emissions (Sharma, 1999). In the United States today, airborne lead originates primarily from the burning of lead-contaminated used oil, from the smelting of ores and other industrial processes, and from the incineration of municipal refuse. Currently more lead is released into soil than into the air, primarily as the result of lead-containing solid wastes being dumped in landfills (aware of this hazard, a number of states have passed laws banning landfill disposal of lead batteries). Weathering of lead-based paints, particularly around the foundations of older structures, and fallout of airborne lead further contribute to the buildup of lead in soils.

Route of Entry into Body

In years past, ingestion of lead-tainted food and water constituted the main source of lead intake for most Americans. Canned foods and beverages represented a significant hazard because over 90% of such cans had lead-soldered seams. Leaching of the toxic metal from the solder into the cans' contents was commonplace, especially when the food items were acidic (e.g. tomato products, citrus, or carbonated drinks). Airborne fallout of lead from automobile emissions onto vegetables or fruits growing near busy highways was responsible for lead concentrations as high as 3,000 ppm on such crops. Drinking water, too, has been identified as a source of exposure for as many as 40 million Americans whom EPA estimates live in homes where tap water contains elevated levels of lead due to the presence of lead pipes or lead solder in household plumbing. Other sources of drinking water contamination include brass faucets on kitchen or bathroom sinks and brass pump fittings in private wells, all of which can leach dissolved lead into tap water (see chapter 15). Fortunately, Americans' exposure to lead from all these sources has been declining sharply since the phaseout of leaded gasoline (a process completed in the U.S. by 1995), the substitution of plastic (PVC) for metal piping in new and replacement home plumbing systems, and the 1991 prohibition on the manufacture of lead-soldered food or soft drink cans. However, imported foods continue to pose a hazard since few other countries restrict the use of lead solder.

Ironically, housepaint remains the most important source of lead poisoning problems, even though the use of lead in paints was halted years ago. Lead was used in residential paint in the U.S. from 1884–1978; until 1953 the use of paint containing as much as 50% lead by weight was common in the United States. In that year a consensus was reached within the industry to reduce paint lead levels, resulting in a steady decline in the manufacture and use of interior lead-base paint (most European countries had recognized the problem decades earlier, signing a treaty in 1921 to prohibit the use of *interior* paints containing lead). Exterior lead-base paint continued to be widely available until the mid-1970s, although its lead content by then was considerably less than that of paint produced prior to the 1950s. In 1977 the Consumer Product Safety Commission banned all house paints, interior or exterior, as well as paints on toys or furniture, which contained more than 0.06% lead by weight. Lead-base paint can still be used, even today, for painting bridges, ships, and other steel structures and for a variety of industrial and military applications and sometimes this paint ends up being applied in homes by workers who have access to the material and fail to realize its hazardous nature ("Preventing Lead Poisoning," 1991).

Although the use of leaded paint has been illegal for more than 20 years, it is estimated that three million tons of lead from paint remains in the 57 million U.S. homes and apartment complexes built before 1980. In such structures, deterioration or renovation activities may expose older layers of paint, providing access to toddlers who may inadvertently consume the poison chips or paint dust. While at one time it was believed that chewing on window sills or eating flakes of the sweet-tasting paint was the major lead-poisoning hazard to children, researchers are now convinced that the prime culprit is ordinary household dust, contaminated by tiny particles of lead from the gradually deteriorating paint. Simply by playing in their own homes and doing what children normally do—putting dirty fingers in their mouths—youngsters can swallow enough lead to cause serious health problems. Growing recognition of the extent of lead contamination in the nation's housing supply has prompted action by the federal government, requiring that, as of December 1996, anyone selling or renting a home or apartment must sign a form disclosing any knowledge of lead-based paint in the structure and must agree, if requested by the buyer or renter, to have the building tested for the presence of lead.

Lead presents a hazard outside as well as inside homes. Soil or dust adjacent to housing once painted with lead-base paints may contain lead levels high enough to pose a risk to small children playing in such locations; soil near busy streets or highways frequently features high lead levels also, thanks to airborne fallout of lead emissions from motor vehicles. Once deposited, lead may remain in soils as long as two thousand years. Researchers estimate that in the United States alone, more than 50 years of leaded gasoline use has left an environmental residue of 4–5 million metric tons of lead dust, the bulk of this amount being deposited along busy highways running through cities. This disproportionate concentration of lead in urban areas further increases the lead hazard for poor and minority children in inner-city areas, already at risk due to dilapidated housing conditions. Studies have shown that children living in neighborhoods where soil lead content is high often exhibit elevated blood lead levels (Mielke, 1999).

Interestingly, *ingested* lead poses a much greater hazard for young children than it does for adults. Whereas only 10% of lead swallowed by adults passes from the intestine into the bloodstream, 40% of the lead ingested by preschoolers remains within their bodies, making such youngsters the highest risk group for lead poisoning within our population. The fact that development of the blood-brain barrier isn't complete until a child reaches approximately three years of age means that lead can readily move into the central nervous system, further explaining why lead exposure is more hazardous for infants and toddlers than it is for other age groups. Particularly vulnerable are malnourished children; absorption of lead from the gastrointestinal tract occurs more readily among youngsters suffering from deficiencies of protein, calcium, zinc, or iron. Thus poor nutritional status is considered an additional risk factor for childhood lead poisoning (Chao and Kikano, 1993).

While young children constitute the primary victims of lead poisoning, persons of any age group are susceptible to the metal's toxic effects. The National Institute of Occupational Safety and Health (NIOSH) estimates that over three million Americans work in occupations involving potential lead exposure; of these, tens of thousands are estimated to suffer from lead poisoning each year, primarily through inhalation of airborne lead (30–40% of inhaled lead reaches the bloodstream and is deposited in the lower respiratory tract where it is almost completely absorbed). Occupational exposure to lead

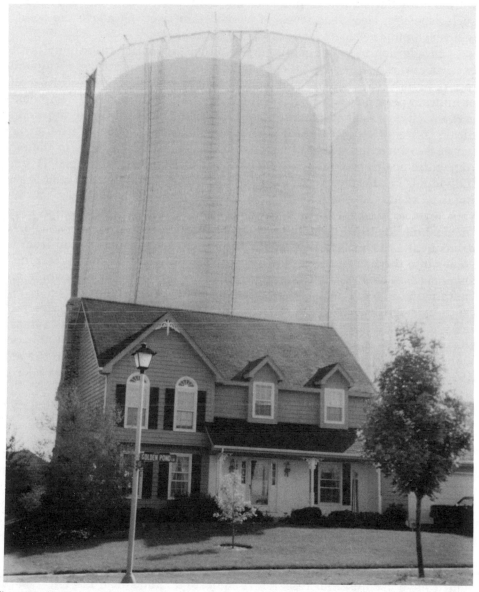

The water tower in Wheaton, Illinois was draped with fabric in order to contain lead dust after the exterior was sandblasted to remove lead-based primer. *[Ray Schnurstein, City of Wheaton]*

has been regulated by OSHA since 1978 through specified **permissible exposure limits (PELs)** to airborne lead concentrations and by standards for allowable blood lead levels. Nevertheless, standards are not sufficiently enforced, with the result that significant worker exposure is an ongoing problem (Stauding and Roth, 1998). Those most at risk are construction workers who renovate or demolish bridges, approximately 90,000 of which in the United States are coated with lead-base paints. Such work is often performed without training or the use of personal protective equipment and may involve the use of acetylene torches or sandblasting, either of which can result in workers' inhalation of lead fumes or dust. After several weeks or months of such exposure, blood lead levels of workers can rise well above the point at which symptoms of acute lead poisoning are apparent.

In addition to bridge maintenance, other occupations that may involve excessive worker exposure to lead include battery manufacturing, shipbuilding, radiator repair, smelter and foundry operations, and certain crafts. Police or military personnel working at firing ranges have also reported symptoms of lead toxicity, a result of inhaling fumes released when lead-containing ammunition is fired (CDC, 1993; Franklin, 1991). Occasionally, some rather bizarre instances of lead poisoning illustrate the challenges facing those in the environmental health profession: over a period of seven months during 1991, eight individuals in Alabama were diagnosed with various symptoms of lead poisoning (e.g. anemia, abdominal pains, weakness in the arms, seizures, and nervous system damage) which developed as a result of drinking illegal "moonshine" distilled in an old automobile radiator containing lead-soldered components! Such a practice, which results in the leaching of lead from the solder into the home-brewed liquor, is a frequent source of lead poisoning in some rural Alabama counties and accounts for the fact that moonshine may contain up to 74 µg/L of lead (CDC, 1992).

Although lead concerns understandably focus on human health problems, it shouldn't be overlooked that environmental lead constitutes a hazard to other species as well. Especially vulnerable are waterfowl, large numbers of which have died after eating lead fishing sinkers lost by anglers. In the mid-1990s, EPA banned the manufacture and distribution of lead sinkers in order to alleviate this problem.

Regardless of whether the route of exposure is ingestion or inhalation, upon entering the body, lead first moves into the bloodstream where its half-life is estimated at 36 days. For this reason, measurements of blood lead levels, calculated as micrograms of lead per deciliter of blood (µg/dL), are considered to give the most accurate indication of short-term lead exposure. Some lead makes its way into soft tissues such as the brain and kidneys; approximately 50–60% of the lead that enters the body is excreted relatively quickly, mainly through the feces but also in urine. Over a period of time the remaining lead is slowly deposited and stored in the bones, particularly in the long arm and leg bones where it can remain for years (the estimated half-life of lead in bones is 27 years). Lead also accumulates in children's baby teeth, which have been used in research to indicate a child's lead burden. Lead in bones can act as a cumulative poison, becoming increasingly concentrated over an extended time period. Although once thought to be inert, it is now known that lead in bones can be suddenly released back into the bloodstream by a number of conditions such as high fever, osteoporosis, or pregnancy, resulting in cases of acute lead poisoning.

Biological Effects

A potent toxin that can adversely affect people in any age group, lead can damage human health in a number of ways. It interferes with blood cell formation, often resulting in anemia; lead can cause kidney damage, sterility, miscarriage, and birth defects. Because lead has a strong affinity for nerve tissue, injury to the central nervous system is perhaps the most serious manifestation of lead poisoning. Depending on the degree of exposure, lead poisoning can be reflected by hyperirritability, poor memory, or sluggishness at lower levels all the way to mental retardation, epileptic convulsions, coma, and death at high levels.

Lead is a poison that exhibits what health experts refer to as a **continuum of toxicity**; any amount of exposure, however small, carries with it some degree of harm. Not surprisingly, as levels of exposure increase, risk of adverse health effects rise correspondingly (as is the case with exposure to any hazardous substance, identical levels of lead may provoke a varying range of responses in different people). Until about the 1960s, it was widely believed that a diagnosis of "lead poisoning" was appropriate only when blood lead levels were high enough to cause such overt symptoms as anemia, kidney disease, brain damage, or death. Such conditions can be manifested when blood lead levels exceed 70 µg/dL (typically, brain damage only occurs at blood lead levels above 100 µg/dL). At that time, levels of blood lead below 60 µg/dL weren't regarded as dangerous enough to warrant monitoring or treatment. By the early 1970s, however, new evidence regarding lead's deleterious effects on biological systems prompted a reevaluation of the U.S. Public Health Service's level of "undue lead absorption"—the blood lead level at which medical intervention is recommended. In 1971 that level was lowered to 40 µg/dL, further lowered to 30 µg/dL in 1975, to 25 µg/dL in 1985, and, most recently, in 1991 was again reduced to an action range of 10–15 µg/dL. Current analytical devices are incapable of measuring blood lead levels below 10 µg/dL (Florini, 1990).

The justification for the steadily declining levels of blood lead that define a case of lead poisoning can be found in the results of numerous studies carried out over the last several decades, which have conclusively shown that even at levels previously considered safe, chronic low-level exposure to lead can inhibit the normal development of children's intellectual abilities. A landmark study launched in 1979 in the Boston suburbs of Somerville and Chelsea among second-grade students revealed that those whose baby teeth (which they had willingly withheld from the Tooth Fairy to contribute to science!) had a relatively higher lead level also exhibited a greater incidence of unruly classroom behavior, a lesser ability to follow instructions, and lower scores on I.Q. tests than did classmates with low lead levels in their teeth (Needleman et al., 1979). Yet none of the children would have been categorized as lead-poisoning victims based on the prevailing view at that time regarding "safe" levels of lead. Eleven years later, in 1990, a follow-up study was carried out to see whether the effects of low-level childhood lead poisoning persist into young adulthood. In light of the millions of children who have experienced some lead exposure, the results of this investigation were depressing: in comparison with classmates whose baby teeth had minimal levels of lead, the higher-lead students, by then 18-year-olds, exhibited a significantly greater school drop-out rate, higher incidence of reading disabilities, lower class rank, and higher absenteeism—all a legacy of childhood lead exposure (Needleman, 1990).

Lead Poisoning: Treatment and Prevention

Children with blood lead levels of 45 µg/dL or higher typically are treated through the use of **chelation**, a process which employs a drug that binds to lead, sequestering the metal and facilitating its excretion from the body. Most commonly, chelating agents are administered in a hospital setting where the patient must remain for a five-day period of treatment and testing (another type of chelating agent that can be given orally at home has been approved for use in less serious cases). Some forms of chelation therapy can be quite painful and the process, while essential in forestalling further impairment to the nervous system, cannot reverse damage that has already occurred. Nor is chelation a one-time solution to lead poisoning problems. Since the chelating agent is generally unable to reach all of the lead stored in bones and teeth, blood lead levels frequently rebound following chelation therapy, the result of additional lead moving from bony tissues into the bloodstream. Many lead poisoning victims are forced to suffer repeated bouts of hospitalization for years after the initial treatment. Children whose lead poisoning symptoms are relieved by chelation therapy frequently require special education and therapy long after cessation of treatment and, in the all-too-common situation where they return to the same lead-contaminated environment responsible for the initial poisoning, their symptoms will promptly recur. For this reason, removal of the child from the source of exposure or, conversely, removal of lead from the child's environment, constitutes the prime strategy in restoring a lead-poisoned child to good health. Unfortunately, evidence suggests that mild brain damage persists in lead-poisoned children even after their blood lead levels were markedly reduced (Tong et al., 1998).

Preventing Childhood Lead Poisoning

Since the health impact of lead, even at very low levels, has been shown to be so devastating and because damage, once it occurs, may never be completely reversed, *prevention* of lead poisoning should be a high-priority societal goal. As mentioned previously, the near-total phaseout of the use of lead in gasoline, paint, food containers, and home plumbing has drastically reduced human exposure to this toxic metal in recent years. Nevertheless, almost 900,000 U.S. preschoolers continue to exhibit elevated lead levels due to lead-contaminated paint and dust still present in millions of homes. Other household items may present a threat as well. Vinyl miniblinds, introduced to the U.S. in the late 1980s, include several brands containing lead. A study of childhood lead poisoning cases in North Carolina revealed that for 9% of the children surveyed, miniblinds were the main source of exposure. While no-lead blinds are now available, a product recall on the lead-containing versions

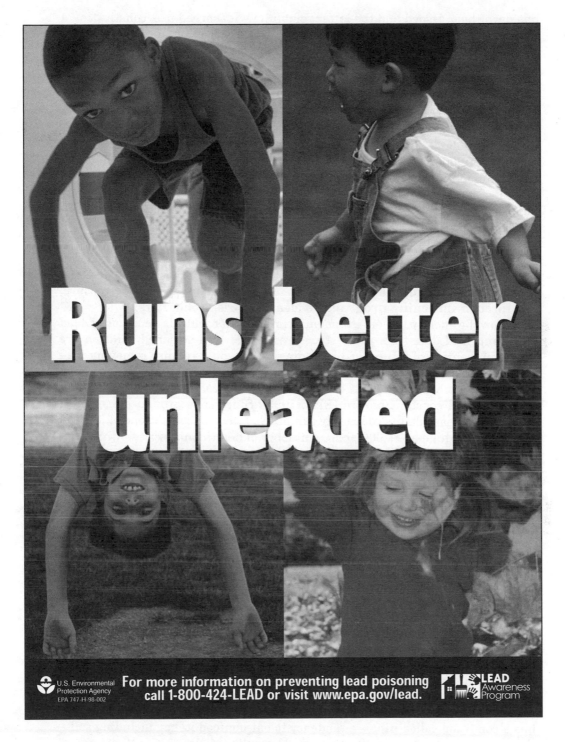

Campaigns to create public awareness, such as this poster developed by the EPA, are an important tool in preventing childhood lead poisoning.

has never been issued and the latter remain in widespread use, constituting a hazard to millions of youngsters (Norman, 1998). Food or juice served from improperly fired pottery or china coated with a lead-containing glaze has caused sporadic cases of lead poisoning, as has consumption of wine or other alcoholic beverages stored in lead-crystal decanters. Lead hazards continue to surface from unexpected sources; in 1994 Arizona state health officials issued an advisory, warning parents about lead-tainted crayons imported from China after a toddler was poisoned by eating a jumbo crayon, ironically labeled "Non-Toxic" (Arreola et al., 1996). More recently, in 1999 Nike, Inc., had to issue a recall of 110,000 pairs of infant Air Jordan shoes after discovering they had been trimmed with red lead-based paint from a Taiwanese supplier. Children may also be inadvertently exposed when a family member engages in such hobbies as making pottery (lead glaze), stained glass, oil painting (some artists' paints contain lead), or furniture refinishing. Parents who work in occupational settings involving lead exposure may unintentionally carry lead dust home on work clothes, thereby exposing children to the toxic metal. A two-pronged national effort has been launched to combat childhood lead poisoning through **environmental intervention** to remove sources of lead exposure, and through **screening programs** to identify at-risk youngsters.

For the most part, environmental intervention entails removal of lead paint and lead dust from those structures where lead-poisoned children are living; prevention of future lead poisoning cases would require removing lead paint from all homes, with special emphasis on the estimated 26 million residential units where such paint is in a deteriorating condition and presents an imminent and constant hazard (EPA, 1995). Since soils around homes with exterior lead-base paints commonly exhibit elevated concentrations of lead (in some cases as high as 11,000 ppm), a number of health authorities also recommend soil abatement programs for neighborhoods where childhood lead poisoning is prevalent. Such efforts would involve removing the top 6–7 inches of soil, replacing this with clean dirt, and then revegetating the area. However, recent epidemiologic studies have shown that in urban areas where children were experiencing low-level lead exposure, blood lead levels declined only slightly when soil abatement activities were carried out. Thus although lead in soils *does* contribute to children's body burden of the metal (studies have shown that blood lead levels rise by 3–7 µg/dL for every 1000 ppm increase in soil or dust concentrations), the considerable expense of contaminated soil removal may not be cost-effective; significantly greater health benefits can be achieved by targeting available funds to interior paint abatement. In many situations where potential exposure to lead in soil is a concern, simply covering bare soil with sod, indoor-outdoor carpeting, or planting foundation shrubs along the base of the structure can eliminate or greatly reduce the opportunity for children to come into contact with contaminated soil—and at a much lower cost than removal activities would entail. However, in situations where soil lead levels are extremely high or where a child suffering from lead poisoning has a condition called **pica**—a tendency to eat nonfood items, including soil—then soil abatement could effect beneficial results (Mielke, 1999; Weitzman et al., 1993; Xintaras, 1992).

In the absence of a strong federal commitment to environmental lead remediation, the focus of prevention efforts on the part of government has

BOX 7-2

Dream Turned Nightmare

The old Victorian farmhouse in upstate New York was a homeowner's dream. Built in the mid-19th century, the two-story wood-and-stone structure featured 10 rooms arranged around a central hallway whose focal point was an elegant center staircase. The solid wood floors, moldings, and doorframes had been painted many times and looked a bit dingy, but the young New York City executive and his wife who moved into the house in late June of 1987 knew the basic woodwork was sound and were convinced that with some energetic stripping and varnishing the place would be as good as new—the ideal location to raise their 5-year-old daughter and 20-month-old son, far from the stress and pollution of big-city life.

In early August, after hiring two workmen to perform the renovations, the family left for vacation, hoping that during their absence the job of sanding layers of old paint off floors, walls, and woodwork would be completed. Upon returning in mid-September, however, they found the work only partially finished and signs of work in progress were all too evident. The workmen had neglected to seal off the area undergoing repairs and a thick layer of dust had spread throughout the house, settling in every nook and cranny. Over the next several weeks, renovation activities shifted into high gear as the workmen used torches, heat guns, and chemical woodstrippers to remove over a century's accumulation of paint from door frames and moldings in the central hallway.

In an effort to keep the children out of the work area, a young woman was hired as a babysitter to come to the house five days a week, accompanied by her own toddlers, aged two and three. Whenever possible, she tried to keep all the children occupied outdoors, while the mistress of the house pursued her career from an office in the home. The two family dogs were less easily persuaded to avoid the work area; one of them, a 10-year-old mongrel, took a special liking for one of the carpenters and spent most of her time sitting at his feet, conscientiously licking the fresh paint dust off her coat as he sanded.

By mid-October, renovations were nearly complete, but some unsettling developments indicated all was not well. The dog, previously healthy, was rushed to a veterinarian with symptoms the owners described as "shaking and twisting." Suspecting poisoning, the veterinarian asked the wife about possible lead exposure; upon hearing that the dog lived in a home where extensive renovations were underway, the vet took a blood sample that immediately confirmed his hunch. Chelation therapy was promptly begun on the animal, but in spite of a brief period of initial improvement, the dog died of kidney failure a few days after returning home.

By this time, the paint removal process was taking its toll on the human members of the household as well. In early November the mother reported feeling tired and weak; her daughter frequently complained of stomach aches in the morning prior to catching the bus for kindergarten. The father experienced severe nausea after spending a weekend at home while workmen used acetylene torches for paint removal. After blood tests revealed that all family members, including the baby, were suffering from lead poisoning, the mother and children were admitted to the hospital for a five-day course of chelation therapy. Shortly after returning home, the mother discovered she was two months pregnant; realizing the devastating teratogenic effects of lead, she decided to undergo a therapeutic abortion. Over the next several weeks, the little girl had to endure chelation therapy five times; her brother was treated twice, and both children continued to receive close medical evaluation. Nor were family members the only victims; the babysitter and her two youngsters were subsequently tested and they, too, had elevated blood lead levels requiring chelation. The workmen, however, who might be expected to have the highest lead levels of all, were never tested and no information on their health status has been reported.

While the menace posed by lead-base paints in deteriorating inner-city structures has been recognized for decades, increasing numbers of "yuppie lead poisoning" incidents such as that just described have only recently begun to attract public attention. Suburban or rural homeowners are generally far less aware of the lead hazards of housing renovation than are their urban counterparts who for years have been deluged with such information by public health activists. Anyone intending to engage in structural restorations involving the potential for lead exposure needs to be aware of the hazard and to take appropriate precautions. Small children and pregnant women in particular should not remain in a dwelling while such activities are underway and should not return until a thorough cleanup has been performed. The example described here also demonstrates how health problems experienced by nonhuman species (in this case, the family dog) can be early warning signs of more widespread environmental exposure and illustrates the importance of good communication between family doctors and veterinarians. Awareness that lead poisoning recognizes no ethnic or socioeconomic boundaries, coupled with greater parental vigilance and caution, is essential if we are to eliminate this devastating, yet entirely preventable, childhood disease.

Reference

Marino, Phyllis E., M.D., et al. 1990. "A Case Report of Lead Paint Poisoning During Renovation of a Victorian Farmhouse." *American Journal of Public Health*, 80, no. 10 (Oct).

shifted to blood lead screening to identify children at risk and to provide prompt treatment to those with elevated blood lead levels before damage becomes irreversible. Since many youngsters live in areas where the risk of lead poisoning is extremely low, screening efforts are being targeted at children living in older homes and children from low-income families. Although the prevalence of lead poisoning and its more severe manifestations have steadily declined since the 1970s, the fact that the disease still affects 5% of the U.S. population (Silbergeld, 1997) means that society must persevere in efforts to eradicate humanity's most ancient toxic hazard.

Mercury

This liquid metal, the "quicksilver" of ancient times, has been used for a wide variety of purposes for at least 2,500 years—and has been contributing to illness and death among those exposed to it for an equal period of time. Although at very low levels of exposure mercury does not appear to be damaging, the margin of safety is small. Mercury is a valuable constituent of many industrial products and processes. It has been used as a catalyst in the manufacture of plastics, as a slime retardant in paper making, in fluorescent light bulbs, as a fungicide in paints, as an alloy in dental fillings, as an ingredient in many medicinal products (mercury's first medicinal use was for the treatment of syphilis when that disease reached epidemic proportions in 16th-century Europe), in the manufacture of scientific instruments, and for many other purposes.

Mercury has always been present in the environment in trace amounts, entering soil or water from vaporization and weathering of mercury compounds in the earth's crust or via volcanic activity. However, concentrations have been increasing in modern times due to coal combustion, mining and smelting of mercury-containing ores, and incineration of mercury wastes. Emissions from medical waste incinerators are a particular concern, since wastes from hospitals and other health care facilities contain up to 50 times more mercury than does ordinary municipal refuse. Industrial processes such as electroplating, paper milling, mining and ore processing, chlorine and caustic soda production, textile manufacturing, and pharmaceutical production produce a mercury-laden effluent that is sometimes discharged into waterways. Evaporation of mercury from paints during the drying process can add significant quantities of this substance to the air; studies have shown that mercury concentrations in indoor air may be one thousand times higher immediately after a room is painted than they were before painting. Several well publicized cases of children developing symptoms of mercury poisoning after mercury-containing latex paints were applied to their homes led to an agreement among U.S. paint manufacturers to stop adding mercury to their products. Nevertheless, although the production of interior paints containing mercury halted in 1990, followed by similar action regarding exterior paint in 1991, the fact that many people keep partly used containers of paint for future use means that paint will remain a potential source of mercury exposure for years to come.

Mercury emissions to the environment are gradually declining due to a decrease in demand for the metal, especially in the paint and chlor-alkali industries and for battery and wire manufacturing. Mercury recycling initiatives to divert mercury wastes from landfills and incinerators are helping to curb environmental releases, as are efforts to substitute mercury-free products for those containing the toxic metal (i.e. digital thermometers in place of mercury thermometers).

Health Effects of Mercury Exposure

The action of mercury on the human system depends primarily on the form of mercury to which the victim is exposed, either inorganic metallic mercury or the far more toxic organic mercury.

Inorganic Metallic Mercury. This form of mercury frequently attacks the liver and kidneys; it also can diffuse through the alveolar membranes of the lungs and travel to the brain where it can cause such neurological problems as lack of coordination. Inorganic mercury can enter the system either by inhalation of mercury vapors or by absorption of mercury compounds through the skin after prolonged contact. Examples of human poisoning with inorganic mercury include the malady prevalent among hatmakers in 17th-century France called the "Mad Hatters' Disease" (immortalized by a character of the same name in Lewis Carroll's *Alice in Wonderland*). This neurological disorder, manifested as tremors and mental aberrations, resulted from the practice at that time of soaking animal hides in a solution of mercuric nitrate for purposes of softening the hairs. Since the hatmakers' bare arms and hands were in frequent contact with the solution as they manipulated the hides, skin absorption of mercury led to development of the disease symptoms.

Poisoning by inhalation is more common than skin absorption, however, and represents the most common form of occupational exposure to mercury. A survey conducted by NIOSH estimated that 70,000 American workers may be exposed to mercury vapors on the job. These include nurses, lab technicians, machine operators, miners, plumbers, dentists and dental hygienists, and many others. Even the families of potentially exposed workers may be at risk if mercury is carried home from the occupational setting on contaminated work clothing. Exposure to mercury vapors from dental fillings (standard amalgams are approximately 50% mercury by weight) has provoked concern about the potential for chronic poisonings, but there is no convincing evidence to support such worries. Most authorities feel the amount of mercury that dental fillings contribute to the average person's daily body burden of the metal is too small to pose any credible health risk.

Many people have become ill and some deaths have been reported among persons exposed to mercury fumes when large quantities of mercury were accidentally spilled within confined, inadequately ventilated areas. If such an accident should occur, the mercury should be cleaned up as quickly as possible, regardless of how small an amount is involved, because vaporization of the metal over time could pose a serious health hazard to anyone in the vicinity, particularly small children and pregnant women. If the spill is on a smooth surface, such as a countertop or uncarpeted floor, a piece of paper can be used to roll the beads of mercury carefully onto another piece of paper and then placed in a zip-lock bag or glass jar with a tight-fitting lid. Never try to blot or wipe up mercury with a rag or paper towel—since the metal is not absorbent, doing so will simply disperse the mercury into smaller droplets and make it even more difficult to collect. If the spill occurs on carpeting, cleanup will be more difficult and usually requires seeking advice and assistance on decontamination from local health authorities. Because of the severe inhalation hazard posed by metallic mercury, a vacuum cleaner should *never* be used to clean up mercury droplets, since this will only exacerbate the problem by hastening vaporization and increasing air concentrations of the metal. Persons cleaning up spilled mercury need not worry about suffering acute inhalation poisoning, but they should either wear gloves or remove any rings, because mercury readily forms an amalgam with gold. Good ventilation with outside air during cleanup operations is important; windows should be opened and a fan used to direct air out of the room for at least an hour. Mercury collected should be kept in a tightly sealed container and disposed of in a manner

BOX 7-3

Quicksilver's Dangerous Allure

The Arkansas teenagers who stole nearly 40 pounds of pure metallic mercury from an abandoned neon-sign factory in Texarkana joined a long line of mercury poisoning victims seduced by the bewitching allure of the silvery liquid. As the mother of one of the boys later remarked to a reporter, "They thought it was cool." Unaware of its dangers, the two 17 year olds shared their prize with friends who coated their hands and arms with "quicksilver," poured it onto their bedroom floors to watch the metallic globs flow and coalesce, and sold it in small vials to classmates similarly fascinated. One young man even dipped a cigarette in mercury and proceeded to smoke it—and soon began coughing up blood.

By early January 1998, officials of Texarkana realized they were confronting a major public health emergency, as symptoms of mercury poisoning began showing up all over town. Several people, including one of the boys who had originally found the substance, were hospitalized with symptoms ranging from vomiting and difficulty with breathing to seizures. Because a number of the teenagers had played with the mercury at home—contaminating carpets, furniture, and clothing—eight houses had to be evacuated temporarily and stripped of most of their furnishings. In one home mercury fumes killed the family dog and caused several small children to be taken to the hospital. Eventually about 175 people were tested for mercury exposure; of those, seven had levels high enough to require treatment. Federal EPA officials, arriving in Texarkana to take charge of decontamination efforts, estimated the cost of cleaning up homes,

testing exposed residents, and removing hazardous chemicals from the abandoned factory at $1 million.

Similar thefts of carelessly stored mercury have resulted in human exposure and illness all too frequently; EPA reports that one out of every five calls received by the agency's emergency response section involves a mercury-related problem. A wider-scale, if less dramatic, misuse of mercury that has public health officials around the country seriously worried is the ritualistic use of the metal by several Hispanic and Caribbean ethnic groups in the United States. Many adherents of religious beliefs such as Santeria (Cuban), Voodoo (Haitian), Espiritismo (Puerto Rican), and Palo Mayomba (Caribbean) regard mercury as conveying good luck because it flows smoothly; conversely, they believe that because of its slippery nature, mercury prevents evil and envy from sticking to the person who possesses it. For this reason, devotees often wear mercury in a small pouch or amulet around the neck or sprinkle it inside their homes or automobiles. Others mix mercury with bath water or perfume or burn the metal in devotional candles. Santeros (those who practice Santeria) incorporate mercury into potions intended to attract a lover or acquire money; they may sprinkle mercury around baby cribs or beds or feed it directly to infants; they add the metal to wine and oil as well as to creams or lotions that are then rubbed onto the skin.

For such a dangerous substance, mercury is amazingly easy to obtain. Surveys conducted by public health authorities in several large U.S. cities indicate that shops called "*botanicas*" in Hispanic and Haitian neighborhoods commonly sell small capsules or glass vials of metallic mercury under the name "*azogue*." All too often, the azogue capsules lack any warning label alerting buyers to the health hazards of mercury.

While public health authorities have only recently initiated efforts to determine whether ritualistic use of mercury is actually causing human illness, they worry that the potential for slow poisoning of entire families certainly exists and may already be occurring. Since in its less severe form mercury poisoning is characterized by vague symptoms easily mistaken for other ailments, the problem may not be identified until after serious damage has been done. The ritualistic practices described earlier are typically performed indoors and as the mercury evaporates into the air, anyone in the room risks inhalation exposure. Mercury embedded in carpets, upholstery fabric, or floor cracks constitutes a long-term source of exposure that could also endanger future residents of the dwelling. The danger is particularly acute for infants and small children who spend considerable time playing on the floor where mercury concentrations tend to be highest and whose still-developing nervous systems make them especially vulnerable. Given the long history of mercury use among the ethnic groups mentioned, health educators face a challenging task in trying to persuade them to abandon dangerous traditions. Nevertheless, if ongoing surveys reveal that health damage is, in fact, occurring, a vigorous effort to raise public awareness of quicksilver's dark side should be promptly undertaken.

References

ATSDR. 1999. *Toxicological Profile for Mercury (Update)*. U.S. Department of Health and Human Services.

Cropper, Carol M. 1998. "Teen-Agers' Vandalism Leads to Mercury Crisis," *New York Times* (Jan. 24), A8.

Gwynne, S.C. 1998. "The Quicksilver Mess," *TIME* (Jan. 26).

recommended by local health or environmental officials (ATSDR, 1999).

In contrast to the serious dangers posed by *inhalation* of mercury, *swallowing* the metal—as could occur if a child bites down on an oral thermometer—poses no health threat. Metallic mercury is poorly absorbed by the gastrointestinal tract and is soon excreted in the feces.

Organic Mercury. Far more toxic than elemental mercury are the organic mercury compounds such as methyl mercury which, being extremely soluble, can readily penetrate living membranes. Organic mercury circulates in the bloodstream bound to red blood cells and gradually diffuses into the brain, destroying the cells that control coordination. Symptoms of organic mercury poisoning generally don't appear until a month or two after exposure, showing up initially as numbness in the lips, tongue, and fingertips. Gradually speech becomes slurred and difficulty in swallowing and walking becomes apparent. As mercury levels rise, deafness and vision problems may develop and the victim tends to lose contact with his or her surroundings. Before the nature of mercury poisoning was understood, such people were often thought to be neurotic or mentally ill and were occasionally placed in insane asylums.

Because consumption of mercury-contaminated fish or shellfish is the most likely route for human exposure to methyl mercury, many states issue **fish advisories**, warning consumers—particularly pregnant women—to limit consumption of fish caught in specified waterways due to potential mercury contamination (*Note:* similar advisories are issued for PCB contamination). The World Health Organization in 1990 also voiced concerns that women could harm their unborn children by a regular diet of mercury-tainted fish. However, evidence from a comprehensive study conducted in the Seychelles Islands among people who rely on fish as the mainstay of their diet indicates concerns may be exaggerated. Women in the Seychelles, who eat fish approximately 12 times weekly, have body burdens of mercury considerably higher than those found in most Americans, yet no resulting developmental damage has been detected in their children. Basing its action on these findings, the Agency for Toxic Substances and Disease Registry (ATSDR) in 1999 amended its minimal risk level (MRL) for methyl mercury in fish, increasing its recommended safe level from 0.1 to 0.3 micrograms per kilogram of body weight per day. It should be noted, however, that ATSDR's standard is only a guideline; the Food and Drug Administration still limits the amount of mercury in fish sold commercially to 1 ppm (ATSDR, 1999).

Several tragic episodes involving methyl mercury poisoning have been documented in past decades. In 1972 more than 6,500 Iraqi villagers became seriously ill and 459 died after eating bread that had been made from seed wheat coated with an organic mercury fungicide. A similar situation, fortunately on a much smaller scale, occurred in the United States three years earlier when several members of a family in Alamagordo, New Mexico, suffered permanent neurological impairment after they butchered and ate a hog that had been fed fungicide-treated seed corn. Undoubtedly the most infamous episode of mass poisoning with methyl mercury occurred during the years 1953–1961 in the coastal town of Minamata on the Japanese island of Kyushu. A plastics factory, Chisso Corporation, had for a number of years been discharging inorganic mercury wastes into the waters of Minamata Bay where many of the local residents earned their livelihood by fishing. In the anaerobic conditions among the sediments at the bottom of the bay, the inorganic mercury was converted into highly toxic methyl mercury by the bacterium *Methanobacterium amelanskis*. Readily soluble, the methyl mercury thus began moving through the aquatic food chain, being passively absorbed by microscopic algae which were subsequently eaten by zooplankton, which were eaten by small fish, etc., the methyl mercury becoming increasingly concentrated at each higher trophic level (mercury concentrations in predator fish at the top of aquatic food chains commonly reach levels 100,000 times higher than those present in the surrounding water).

Trouble first became apparent in Minamata when the town cats developed what residents first thought must be a strange viral disease, yowling continuously and sometimes leaping into the sea to drown. When the townspeople themselves started to complain of vague maladies such as extreme fatigue, headaches, numbness in their extremities, and difficulty in swallowing, it was first suspected that they were contracting some sort of illness from the sick cats. Eventually the true nature of their mutual problem was discovered—methyl mercury poisoning derived from a diet composed primarily of mercury-contaminated fish. By this time more than 100 people had been stricken with such symptoms as mental derangement, inability to walk or use chopsticks, visual disturbances, and convulsions. Forty-four of the Minamata victims died during this period and many others were permanently disabled. As this sad episode unfolded, the teratogenic properties of methyl mercury became apparent. Twenty-two brain-damaged babies were born during this period to mothers who themselves exhibited no outward signs of mercury poisoning, though several mentioned experiencing a slight numbness of the fingers during pregnancy and analysis showed a high level of mercury in their hair. Subsequent studies have revealed that methyl mercury has a special affinity for fetal tissue, easily crossing the placental barrier where it severely damages the developing child while leaving the mother unharmed. The ultimate human toll of Chisso's poisoning of Minamata Bay included 700 deaths and 9,000 individuals left with varying degrees of paralysis and brain damage. Estimates are that as many as 50,000 persons living within 35 miles of the bay who consumed its fish have suffered at least mild symptoms of mercury poisoning (Weisskopf, 1987). After years of legal wrangling over compensation, several thousand plaintiffs reached a settlement with Chisso in 1996, agreeing to drop lawsuits in return for a $24,200 lump sum payment to each Minamata Disease victim, plus additional payments to five national victims' groups. A year later, in 1997, the regional government (Kumamoto Prefecture) declared that Minamata Bay is once again safe for fishing with mercury in the waterway's marine life having fallen below the level the government considers dangerous (Pollack, 1997).

Ironically, as Japan's tragic episode of methyl mercury poisoning draws to a close, Minamata Disease is now claiming new victims along the Amazon. Brazil is in the throes of a modern-day gold rush, with an estimated half-million prospectors roaming the Amazon basin, searching along riverbeds for traces of the precious metal. Employing methods that would have looked entirely familiar to California's "Forty-niners" a century and a half ago, prospectors utilize mercury to separate gold from the muck dredged from the river. In doing so they are releasing an estimated 250 tons of mercury into the Amazon watershed each year. Following the same sequence of events that transpired decades ago in Minamata, mercury has reached high concentrations in Amazonian fish. Villagers who eat the tainted fish are now showing signs of neurological disorders and have detectable body burdens of methyl mercury. A visiting epidemiologist from the Japanese Ministry of Health, surveying the scene, remarked on the suffering still endured by survivors in Minamata and observed, "It should not happen again" (Pearce, 1999).

In addition to the toxic materials discussed in this chapter, there are many other substances capable of causing health damage in humans when present in more than trace amounts or when exposure to even very low levels persists over an extended time period. Cadmium, fluorides, selenium, copper, nickel, chromium, and arsenic are but a few of the naturally occurring toxins that are known, under certain conditions, to affect human health adversely. Unfortunately, because the symptoms of exposure to toxic substances are often so vague or so similar to those of other more common ailments, they are frequently either ignored or misdiagnosed. Thus it would not be surprising to find that health damage due to such toxins is more prevalent than commonly assumed at present.

References

Agency for Toxic Substances and Disease Registry (ATSDR). 1999. *Toxicological Profile for Mercury.* U.S. Dept. of Health and Human Services, Public Health Service.

———. 1990. *Toxicological Profile for Asbestos,* TP-90-04. U.S. Dept. of Health and Human Services (Dec).

American Chemical Society. 1998. *Understanding Risk Analysis.*

Arreola, P., L. Boyer, C. Fowler, C.M. Neumann, K. Schaller, and Z. Weaver. 1996. "Lead-Tainted Crayons from China. Part I: Secondary Prevention in Arizona." *Journal of Environmental Health* 58, no. 7 (March):6–10.

Birnbaum, Linda S. 1994. "The Mechanism of Dioxin Toxicity: Relationship to Risk Assessment." *Environmental Health Perspectives.*

Centers for Disease Control and Prevention (CDC). 1997. "Blood Lead Levels—United States, 1991-1994." *Morbidity & Mortality Weekly Report* 46:141–146.

———. 1993. "Lead Poisoning in Bridge Demolition Workers—Georgia, 1992." *Morbidity & Mortality Weekly Report* 42, no. 20 (May 28).

———. 1992. "Elevated Blood Lead Levels Associated with Illicitly Distilled Alcohol-Alabama, 1990-1991." *Morbidity & Mortality Weekly Report* 41, no. 17 (May 1).

Chao, Jason, M.D., and George D. Kikano, M.D. 1993. "Lead Poisoning in Children." *American Family Physician* (Jan).

Colborn, Theo, Dianne Dumanoski, and John Peterson Myers. 1996. *Our Stolen Future.* Dutton, Penguin Books USA.

Dickson, L. C., and S. C. Buzik. 1993. "Health Risks of Dioxins: A Review of Environmental and Toxicological Considerations." *Veterinary and Human Toxicology* 35, no. 1 (Feb).

Environmental Protection Agency (EPA). 1995. "Report on the National Survey of Lead-Based Paint in Housing: Base Report." EPA A747-R95-003.

———. 1994. "Deposition of Air Pollutants to the Great Waters." EPA-453A/R-93-055, May.

Fawcett, Howard H. 1988. *Hazardous and Toxic Materials: Safe Handling and Disposal.* John Wiley & Sons.

Fingerhut, Marilyn A., et al. 1991. "Cancer Mortality in Workers Exposed to 2,3,7,8-Tetrachlorodibenzo-p-Dioxin." *The New England Journal of Medicine* 324, no. 4 (Jan. 24).

Florini, Karen L. 1990. *Legacy of Lead: America's Continuing Epidemic of Childhood Lead Poisoning.* Environmental Defense Fund.

Franklin, Deborah. 1991. "Lead: Still Poison After All These Years." *Health* 5, no. 5 (Sept-Oct).

Kimbrough, R.D., M.L. Doemland, and M.E. LeVois. 1999. "Mortality in Male and Female Capacitor Workers Exposed to Polychlorinated Biphenyls." *Journal of Occupational and Environmental Medicine* 41, no. 3 (March 10):161–171.

Mielke, Howard W. 1999. "Lead in the Inner Cities." *American Scientist* 86 (Jan-Feb): 62.

Needleman, H. L., et al. 1990. "The Long-Term Effects of Exposure to Low

Doses of Lead in Childhood." *The New England Journal of Medicine* 322:83–88.

Needleman, H. L. et al. 1979. "Deficits in Psychologic and Classroom Performance of Children with Elevated Dentine Lead Levels." *The New England Journal of Medicine* 300:689–95.

Norman, Edward H. 1998. "Childhood Lead Poisoning and Vinyl Miniblind Exposure." *Journal of the American Medical Association* 279, no. 5 (Feb. 4):342.

Ottoboni, M. Alice. 1991. *The Dose Makes the Poison.* Van Nostrand Reinhold.

Pearce, Fred. 1999. "A Nightmare Revisited." *New Scientist* 161, no. 2172 (Feb. 6):4.

Pollack, Andrew. 1997. "Japan Calls Mercury-Tainted Bay Safe Now." *New York Times*, July 30.

Preventing Lead Poisoning in Young Children. 1991. U.S. Dept. of Health and Human Services, Centers for Disease Control.

Regenstein, Lewis. 1982. *The Poisoning of America.* Acropolis Books.

Sharma, Dinesh C. 1999. "Alarming Amounts of Lead Found in Indian Children." *The Lancet* 352, no. 9153 (Feb. 20):647.

Silbergeld, Ellen K. 1997. "Preventing Lead Poisoning in Children." *Annual Review of Public Health* 18:187-210.

Stauding, Kevin C., and Victor S. Roth. 1998. "Occupational Lead Poisoning." *American Family Physician* 57, no. 4 (Feb. 15):719-728.

Steenland, Kyle, Laurie Piacitelli, James Deddens, Marilyn Fingerhut, and Lih Ing Chang. 1999. "Cancer, Heart Disease, and Diabetes in Workers Exposed to 2,3,7,8-Tetrachlorodibenzo-p-dioxin." *Journal of the National Cancer Institute* 91, no. 9 (May 5):779–786.

Steingraber, Sandra. 1997. *Living Downstream: An Ecologist Looks at Cancer and the Environment.* Addison-Wesley.

Tong, Shilu, Peter A. Baghurst, Michael G. Sawyer, Jane Burns, and Anthony J. McMichael. 1998. "Declining Blood Lead Levels and Changes in Cognitive Function During Childhood: The Port Pirie Cohort Study." *Journal of the American Medical Association* 280, no. 22 (Dec. 9):1915.

Weisskopf, Michael. 1987. "Japanese Town Still Staggered by Legacy of Ecological Disaster." *The Washington Post*, April 18.

Weitzman, Michael, et al. 1993. "Lead-Contaminated Soil Abatement and Urban Children's Blood Lead Levels." *Journal of the American Medical Association* 269, no. 13 (April 7).

Xintaras, Charles. 1992. "Impact of Lead-Contaminated Soil on Public Health." Agency for Toxic Substances and Disease Registry, U.S. Dept. of Health and Human Services (May).

CHAPTER 8

Pests and Pesticides

Rats!
They fought the dogs and killed the cats,
And bit the babies in the cradles,
And ate the cheeses out of the vats
And licked the soup from the cooks' own ladles.
                    —Robert Browning, "The Pied Piper of Hamelin" (1845)

The tale of the mythical ratcatcher of Hamelin, who rid that medieval town of its plague of rodents—and subsequently of its children as well—has been told and retold for centuries. Whether based on historical fact or not, the legend accurately conveys the sense of dismay and helplessness experienced by pre-industrial societies when confronted with disastrous pest outbreaks. History records countless incidents of the devastating impact that certain insects, rodents, fungi, and so forth, can have on human health and well-being. Such organisms are typically referred to as "pests," a term derived from the Latin word *pestis* ("plague"), which was applied to a number of deadly epidemic diseases that periodically swept through the ancient world.

What Is a Pest?

Biologically speaking, there is, of course, no such thing as a "pest"; no classification system divides living things into categories labelled "good species" and "bad species." The term "pest," then, is a purely human concept and refers broadly to any organism—animal, plant, or microbe—which adversely affects human interests. Pest species comprise only a small percentage of the total number of organisms on earth, the vast majority being either beneficial or, more commonly, neutral so far as their impact on humans is concerned. Pests are not restricted to any one taxonomic group; representative species can be found among such invertebrates as insects, mites, ticks, and nematodes. Several bird species such as starlings, pigeons, and English sparrows can be considered pests, as can some mammals—rats, mice, moles, rabbits, and, in some situations, deer, coyotes, or even elephants! Many types of microorganisms, such as disease-causing bacteria, viruses, rickettsia, and fungi, are pests, as are weeds—any "plant out of place," growing where it's not wanted.

Problems Caused by Pests

Conflict between people and pests has existed since time immemorial and is generated primarily when such organisms compete with humans for the same resources, cause us discomfort, or are vectors of disease. The need to protect human interests by limiting pest damage has created a demand for better methods of combatting such problems and constitutes the chief justification for the development and use of chemical pesticides. Although the use of such toxic compounds has, for a variety of reasons, come under increasing scrutiny and criticism in recent years, it is important to review the types of problems caused by pests in order to understand why suggestions to limit or abolish the use of chemical pesticides generates such controversy.

Resource Competition

Insects, weeds, and plant pathogens (fungi, nematodes, bacteria and viruses) are responsible for the loss of an estimated 30–35% of the global harvest each year, despite more than 50 years of escalating chemical warfare against agricultural pests. Insect problems are particularly severe on corn and cotton (over 10% of all pesticide use worldwide is directed to cotton production; in the United States, corn, citrus, cotton, and apples account for the largest percentage of insecticide applications). Fungal diseases cause significant losses primarily to fruits and some vegetables, while yield reductions due to weed infestations are most pronounced on acreage devoted to corn and soybean production. In addition to such losses in the field, about 6% of the annual harvest in the United States (and a substantially larger share in developing nations) is lost to pests while in storage or transit.

A reduction in current pesticide use would undoubtedly result in a further increase in crop loss due to pest depredation—a cause for concern both to farmers and to humanitarians worried about feeding a hungry world. The extent of such loss is hotly disputed, however. The U.S. Department of Agriculture estimates that without pesticides, American agricultural production would drop by at least 25% and food prices would rise by 50%. Others, however, calculate that preharvest losses of all crops resulting from a significant reduction in pesticide use would be minimal. A noted entomologist at Cornell University estimates that if American farmers were to adopt a variety of nonchemical control techniques they could cut current levels of agricultural pesticide use by 50% without experiencing any decline in yields. Under this scenario, substituting nonchemical for chemical controls would result in food price increases of less than 1% (Pimental, 1991).

Although loss in farm production is the major example of resource competition between humans and pests, many other instances of conflict can be cited: **termites** cause incalculable damage to structures, especially in the tropics; in the United States alone, property owners spend an estimated $2 billion annually to control these wood-destroying pests. **Cockroaches**, the bread-and-butter of the structural pest control industry, are found worldwide and are universally despised for contaminating food and materials in homes, restaurants, supermarkets, cruise ships, warehouses—literally every place where careless humans provide them with a source of food and water. **Rats and mice** cause enormous economic losses, consuming as much as one-third of the world's harvest and rendering many stored food supplies unusable due to contamination with rodent hairs, droppings, and urine (Mallis, 1997).

Sources of Discomfort

Itching, buzzing, creeping, and crawling may not seem like serious concerns, but the creatures responsible have been driving people to distraction for millennia and have been the targets of a great deal of pesticide use in recent decades. Some of the major villains involved in producing acute human discomfort, if not illness, include the following.

Lice. Head lice, body lice, and crab lice are all human parasites that can cause severe itching, secondary infections, and scarred or hardened skin. Lice are typically associated with people living in crowded conditions where opportunities for bathing and laundering clothes are limited. With the introduction of DDT following World War II, the incidence of lice infestations dropped to low levels. As the use of this insecticide became restricted, however, cases of head lice among schoolchildren have been increasing.

Fleas. Aside from the flea species which transmit the deadly plague bacterium (see next section), fleas commonly found on domestic animals can cause severe irritation, loss of blood, and discomfort. Although most fleas prefer to feed on their animal host, they frequently bite humans if the normal host is absent. Such bites can be extremely painful and may cause swelling and a reddening of the skin.

Mites. These tiny insect relatives are responsible for the serious skin condition known as scabies, as well as a number of other forms of dermatitis such as "grocers' itch," acquired by handling mite-infested grain products, cheese, dried fruits, and so on. Mites that normally live as ectoparasites on birds may become very serious pests of humans when they migrate in large numbers into homes after starlings or sparrows leave their nests. For this reason, householders should discourage birds from nesting on eaves or windowsills or other locations in close proximity to homes. **Chiggers,** a type of mite inhabiting many parts of the southern or midwestern United States, can cause extreme skin irritation lasting for a week or more when they attach themselves to a human host, usually around the waist or armpits.

Bedbugs. Hiding during the day in mattresses, bedsprings, cracks in the wall, and so on, bedbugs cause many a sleepless night and produce large, intensely itchy welts on sensitive victims. Fortunately they are not known to transmit any disease.

Spiders. Although many people harbor an irrational antipathy toward spiders, the vast majority of these eight-legged creatures are quite harmless to humans. Even the fearsome-looking tarantula—the loathsome villain in many a B-grade Hollywood thriller—is actually rather docile. Now widely sold as pets, tarantulas can be handled with ease and rarely bite; even when they do, their venom is of little harm to most people. Only three U.S. species present any real danger: the **black widow** (female only), the **brown recluse** (both sexes), and the **aggressive house spider** (males more venomous and more likely to bite than females). The black widow, though more abundant in warmer regions of the country, can be found throughout the United States; primarily an outdoor spider, the black widow is typically found around piles of wood or other debris where the female spins a nondescript-looking web. Black widow venom acts as a nerve poison, but while bites may be quite painful they are very seldom fatal, even in the absence of medical attention. Contrary to popular myth, the diminutive male black widow is *not* devoured after mating by his much larger bride—unless she is unusually hungry!—but generally spends a parasitic post-nuptial existence in the vicinity of her web, waiting for any leftovers that may come his way. The brown recluse spider, whose range covers much of the south-central and southeastern United States as far north as Missouri, Illinois, and Indiana, is most often encountered within dwellings where it hides in attics, closets, and other dark, seldom-disturbed places. It is a shy, retiring species that bites only when provoked—usually when rolled on at night or when clothes are taken out of storage. The poison injected by the bite of a brown recluse differs from that of a black widow in that it is *cytotoxic*, causing tissue death in the vicinity of the wound. Scarcely noticeable at first, the bite gradually becomes very painful and frequently develops into an open ulceration that persists for weeks and eventually leaves a large ugly scar. The aggressive house spider, a European immigrant whose range in North America is currently limited to British Columbia and five states in the northwestern U.S., has only recently been identified as the source of spider bites long attributed to the brown recluse (which doesn't live in that part of the country). Like brown recluse venom, that of the aggressive house spider is a cytotoxin, causing tissue necrosis very similar to that of a brown recluse bite. *Unlike* the brown recluse, however, aggressive house spiders are true to their name and tend to bite without provocation. Large (40 mm in length) and fast-running, these spiders tend to live in or near houses, often in rock walls, along foundations, or in woodpiles (many bites occur when firewood is being carried inside). Large numbers of males enter basements and ground floor rooms of homes in the autumn and dogs and cats are frequently bitten on the face as they attempt to investigate, occasionally dying as a result. These are *not* nice spiders! (Akre and Myhre, 1994).

In addition to the above, the buzzing of flies, mosquitoes, gnats, cicadas, June bugs, or wasps—even when these insects are not carrying disease organisms—can provoke extreme annoyance. Certain plant species also, particularly poison ivy and its relatives, have been prime targets of chemical herbicides because of the intensely irritating rash which contact with these plants can produce.

Vectors of Disease

Public health practitioners, along with farmers, were among the first to greet the introduction of synthetic chemical pesticides with great enthusiasm. Compounds such as DDT were viewed as perhaps the ultimate weapon in freeing humanity from the threat of a number of insect- or rodent-borne diseases responsible for millions of deaths and illnesses each year. Quite appropriately, the first use to which DDT was put involved the wartime dusting of refugees in Italy to curb an outbreak of typhus fever. The success of this effort led to extensive spraying campaigns in many parts of the world against the vectors of such dreaded killers as malaria, yellow fever, river blindness, bubonic plague, and encephalitis. Although the medical community's high hopes for complete eradication of the carriers of these diseases have proven overly optimistic, pesticide use has played a significant role in lowering death rates and improving public health in many parts of the world. Some pests of particular public health importance include mosquitoes, flies, body lice, rat fleas, and ticks.

Mosquitoes. Mosquitoes have probably been responsible for more human deaths than any other insect, though their role as disease-carriers was not recognized until late in the 19th century. Worldwide, even today millions of people become ill each year due to such mosquito-borne ailments as malaria, yellow fever, dengue, filariasis, and encephalitis. In the past, there have been major outbreaks of all these diseases, particularly malaria and yellow fever, in parts of the United States. In recent years, entry of large numbers of infected immigrants or returning tourists from regions where malaria is still endemic have been responsible for 1,000–1,200 cases of malaria acquired abroad but diagnosed and reported in the United States each year. Since the mosquito vectors responsible for transmitting malaria in the U.S. are common species (*Anopheles quadrimaculatus* and *A. freeborni*), the opportunity still exists for future outbreaks. Such a situation occurred in New Jersey in 1991 when three state residents contracted malaria from local anopheline mosquitoes whose previous meal had been the infected blood of tourists from Mexico and Korea (Mallis, 1997).

Of mosquito-borne disease outbreaks within the United States today, only encephalitis continues to occur with some frequency. During times when mosquito populations are high and when the viral pathogen of the disease has been detected in birds or small mammals (the virus is generally carried to humans by a mosquito which has previously bitten an infected bird), chemical spraying may be carried out by local authorities to prevent the possibility of encephalitis, a disease which in severe cases can permanently damage the central nervous system or even kill its victim. Although the last major U.S. outbreak of a mosquito-borne disease occurred in 1975 (a St. Louis encephalitis epidemic that killed 142 and sickened more than 2,000 throughout the Midwest), vector-control officials had a new cause for worry in the late 1980s when some unwelcome stowaways arrived with a shipment of used tires in the port of Houston. *Aedes albopictus,* the **Asian tiger mosquito**, quickly spread from Texas throughout much of the eastern United States, presumably hitchhiking on the truckloads of used tires which ply the interstate highway system

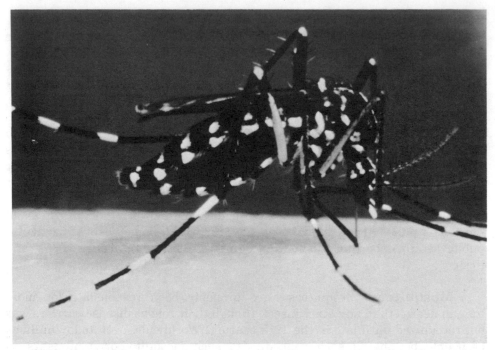

Asian Tiger Mosquito: a vicious biter and potential disease vector, *Aedes albopictus* has spread rapidly through the southern and midwestern states since its accidental introduction to the U.S. in 1985. *[American Mosquito Control Association/L. Munstermann]*

(the insect lays its eggs just above the waterline in treeholes or artificial containers—like tires). Because tiger mosquito eggs can overwinter, *A. albopictus* has already become established as far north as Minnesota (CDC, 1997). Unlike many other mosquitoes, it can also live inside houses year-round, breeding in pet water dishes and in the saucers under flowerpots. The tiger mosquito is a vicious biter and, in its Asian homeland, is an important disease vector. Although as yet no outbreaks have been attributed to the newcomer, researchers have determined that *A. albopictus* has the ability to pick up and transmit the viral pathogens for dengue fever and encephalitis and fear that it has the potential to become the most important carrier of mosquito-borne diseases in the United States. These fears were given added urgency in 1992 when a tiger mosquito captured in Florida, just 12 miles from Disney World, was found to be harboring the virus for Eastern equine encephalitis, the most deadly form of the disease which, until now, has been carried primarily by salt marsh mosquitoes whose preferred habitat is remote from human settlements. The tiger mosquito, by contrast, lives in close proximity to people and thus represents a more serious public health concern.

Flies. Many species of flies, particularly the common housefly, are important carriers of serious gastrointestinal diseases such as typhoid fever, cholera, dysentery, and parasitic worm infections due to their habit of feeding on human and animal wastes. If such wastes contain pathogenic organisms, the fly can pick these up either on the sticky pads of its feet or on its body

Table 8-1 Some Serious Pest-Borne Diseases of Humans

Disease	Causative Agent	Vector	Method of Infection
African sleeping sickness	trypanosome	tsetse fly	bite
Cholera	bacterium, *Vibrio cholerae*	housefly	contamination of foods
Dengue fever	virus	*Aedes* mosquito	bite
Dysentery, amoebic	protozoan	housefly	contamination of foods
Dysentery, bacillary	bacterium, *Shigella sp*	housefly	contamination of foods
Encephalitis	virus	*Culex* mosquito	bite
Lyme Disease	spirochete bacterium *Borrelia burgdorferi*	deer tick	bite
Malaria	protozoan, *Plasmodium vivax*	*Anopheles* mosquito	bite
Onchocerciasis (River blindness)	parasitic worm, *Onchocerca volvulus*	black flies	bite
Plague	bacterium, *Pasteurella pestis*	Oriental rat flea and other fleas	bite or contact with infected rodents
Rocky Mountain spotted fever	rickettsia *Rickettsia rickettsi*	American dog tick	bite
Typhoid fever	bacterium, *Salmonella typhi*	housefly	contamination of food and water
Typhus	rickettsia, *Rickettsia prowazeki*	human body louse	contamination of bite and abrasions
Yellow fever	virus	*Aedes* mosquito	bite

hairs or mouthparts and mechanically transmit them to humans when it alights on food materials. Fly vomitus and feces also frequently contain pathogenic bacteria that can inoculate human food, multiply rapidly in the food medium, and subsequently result in outbreaks of intestinal diseases when the food is consumed by people.

Cockroaches. Contrary to common belief, cockroaches have not been implicated as important vectors of infectious disease, even though laboratory studies have repeatedly shown these insects harbor a wide range of pathogenic microbes on their feet and can mechanically transmit these organisms to food. Some researchers have attributed cases of *Salmonella* food poisoning and other diarrheal illnesses to the presence of large numbers of cockroaches

BOX 8-1
Emerging Pathogens: Hantavirus in the Americas

In the early summer of 1993 a mysterious, often fatal respiratory ailment provoked near-panic in the Four Corners region of the U.S. Southwest. By early June, twelve persons, most of them young and healthy, had suddenly died, gasping for air as fluid filled their lungs; twelve others were critically ill, fighting for their lives. The media promptly dubbed the as-yet unidentified outbreak "Navajo Flu" because those first stricken were predominantly Native Americans on the vast Navajo reservation. As the months passed and new cases were reported from locations thousands of miles apart, it became apparent that the ailment was anything but restrictive in its choice of victims. Five years after the initial outbreak, the Centers for Disease Control and Prevention tallied 183 confirmed cases in 29 states, while the World Health Organization reported 350-400 cases throughout the Americas, ranging from Canada in the north to Argentina and Chile in the south.

The Four Corners outbreak precipitated a crash effort by public health officials to determine what was causing the deadly illness. Investigators quickly eliminated such possibilities as plague or environmental toxins and soon obtained laboratory evidence confirming the culprit as a **hantavirus.** This discovery caused considerable surprise among medical detectives because hantavirus infections, although encountered sporadically over the centuries in other parts of the world, had never before caused acute human illness in the Western Hemisphere—nor had they ever before been manifested primarily as a respiratory disease. In the Americas, hantavirus had assumed a new disguise that initially deceived those who were trying to track it down.

Previous outbreaks of hantavirus-associated illnesses in Asia and elsewhere, usually referred to as "hemorrhagic fever," primarily involved kidney failure. The absence of renal complications among Four Corners victims accounted for much of the early delay in identifying what is now called **Hantavirus Pulmonary Syndrome (HPS).**

Initial manifestations of HPS don't cause particular alarm among those stricken—the fever, chills, headache, cough, muscular aches and pains are similar to the symptoms of many common illnesses. "I thought I was coming down with the flu...so I took a couple of Tylenol and went to bed," remarked one survivor. Very quickly, however, the disease takes a nasty turn as the lungs fill with fluids leaking from the surrounding capillaries, leading to acute respiratory distress. Within days after the onset of symptoms, almost half of those stricken die of respiratory failure. There is as yet no specific treatment for HPS.

Hantaviruses are rodent-borne pathogens, carried by various species of mice, rats, and voles. Most strains of the virus are associated with a specific rodent host. In the Four Corners outbreak the common deer mouse (*Peromyscus maniculatus*) was identified as the carrier, while the cotton rat (*Sigmodon hispidus*) is assumed to be the vector for cases reported in Florida. Generally present in its animal host as a nonsymptomatic chronic infection, the virus is shed in urine, feces, and saliva throughout the animal's lifetime. It can be transmitted to other rodents or to humans either by direct contact or by inhalation of aerosolized rodent excreta containing viral particles. A 1995 outbreak of HPS in Argentina provided evidence for the first time of direct person-to-person spread of the virus, but no other such instances have been reported to date.

The causative agent of hantavirus was first identified as a result of intensive research efforts following an outbreak of "Korean hemorrhagic fever" among U.N. troops during the Korean conflict in the early 1950s. The recent emergence of hantavirus as a dangerous human pathogen in the Americas dramatizes several troubling realities: not only do different strains of the virus exhibit extreme variation in their clinical manifestations, but the geographic areas to which hantaviruses have long been endemic now appear to be expanding. As a result, although the disease is still considered rare, it is important for the public to be aware of its existence and to take precautionary measures. Since the primary risk factor for acquiring hantavirus is **exposure to rodents or rodent excretions**, the main strategy for preventing infection is to avoid contact with these animals and their burrows. There is reason to believe that the 1993 Four Corners outbreak may have resulted, at least in part, from piñon nut-gathering activities by the victims. Thanks to unusually good rains the previous winter, a bumper crop had been produced that spring, supporting a surge in populations of deer mice, which stored large numbers of the nuts in their burrows. Raids on those burrows by human foragers may well have enhanced the opportunity for viral transmission. Similarly, investigations subsequent to the 1998 HPS death of a young man in New Mexico revealed that he spent many hours working on rodent-infested vehicles near his residence and regularly slept on the floor of a rodent-infested mobile home.

Since the rodent vectors of the four different strains of hantavirus known to cause HPS in North America are found in parts of Canada and throughout the lower 48 states, public health departments are issuing advisories to citizens, warning about the new hazard posed by mice. Recommended precautions include the wearing of gloves whenever dead mice are removed from traps and using a household disinfectant (e.g. 1½ cups of chlorine bleach in a gallon of water) to wet-mop areas frequented by mice. Extra efforts should be made to exclude rodents from buildings and from areas adjacent to structures where people live or work. Individuals who work in occupations that might expose them to rodent excretions—farm laborers, electricians, construction workers who demolish or renovate old buildings—should wear respirators or face masks to avoid inhaling virus-laden dust. Campers are advised not to sleep directly on the ground in areas where rodent populations are present, since rodent urine and feces are omnipresent in such environments.

For those who not so long ago blithely assumed that vector-borne diseases are no longer a cause for concern in modern societies, hantavirus has provided a harsh reminder that microbial pathogens are still out there, ready and waiting to strike whenever humanity becomes careless or complacent.

References

Centers for Disease Control and Prevention. 1998. "Hantavirus Pulmonary Syndrome—Colorado and New Mexico, 1998." *Morbidity & Mortality Weekly Report* 47, no. 22 (June 12):449–52.

Sinnott, John T. et al. 1993. "Hantavirus: An Old Bug Learns New Tricks." *Infection Control and Hospital Epidemiology* 14, no. 11 (Nov).

World Health Organization. 1997. "Hantavirus Pulmonary Syndrome in the Americas." *Weekly Epidemiological Record* 72, no. 41 (Oct. 10):305-6.

Figure 8-1   Total Number of Confirmed Cases of HPS Ever Identified, and Location of Cases Identified Jan.-May, 1999

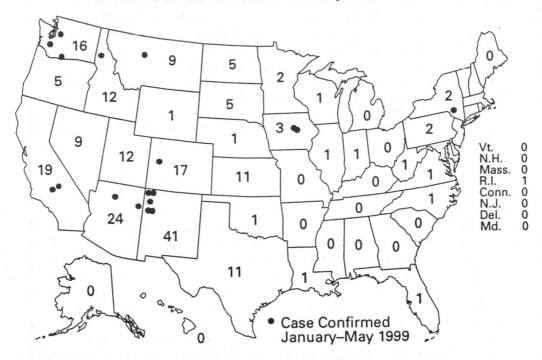

Source: *Morbidity & Mortality Weekly Report*, June 25, 1999.

in or near food preparation areas, but the evidence for a cause-and-effect relationship is inconclusive. Undisputed, however, is the fact that heavy cockroach infestations can cause severe allergic reactions and precipitate asthma attacks. Secretions produced by roaches can induce symptoms ranging from skin irritations and runny nose to difficulty in breathing. Acute reaction to cockroach allergens has recently been recognized as the leading cause for the high incidence of asthma among inner-city children in the U.S. These findings suggest that vigorous cockroach control programs should be an integral part of public health efforts to combat asthma, the incidence rates of which have been dramatically rising worldwide (Rosenstreich et al., 1997).

Body Lice. As mentioned in the previous section, body lice can be a source of intense discomfort, but they are of special public health concern because they are vectors of several serious epidemic diseases. Typhus fever, characterized by elevated temperature, severe headache, and a rash, has been a major killer in past centuries, particularly during wartime when perhaps as many soldiers died from typhus as from swords or bullets. The rickettsial pathogen responsible for the disease is passed from louse to human by the feces of the insect, not its bite. When a person infested with lice scratches the affected area, minor abrasions on the skin permit entry to the rickettsia.

Other lice subsequently feeding on a person infected with typhus ingest the pathogen and spread it as they move from person to person. This method of transmission explains why typhus outbreaks are most prevalent when people are living together in crowded, unsanitary conditions. Insecticidal dusting of louse-infested persons has proven to be an effective method for controlling the spread of typhus fever. Two other louse-borne diseases, also most common during wartime but with much lower fatality rates than typhus, are trench fever and relapsing fever.

Rat Fleas. Aside from the enormous economic damage caused by rats, these pests are of great public health concern because they are vectors of a number of diseases, the most deadly of which is plague (the "Black Death" of medieval times). In September 1994 the first major plague outbreak in half a century terrorized residents of the Indian city of Surat, killing more than 50 people. Even before the Surat incident, plague rates had been steadily rising worldwide since the early 1980s. The vast majority of recent plague victims (90% of total cases reported) have been in Africa, predominantly in the nations of Madagascar and Tanzania, while Brazil, Peru, Myanmar, and Vietnam account for most of the remainder (WHO, 1997).

The plague bacterium actually is carried by fleas on rats, not by the rats themselves. When infected fleas feed on their rat hosts, the rats too sicken and die. If rats are living in close proximity to humans, a flea whose host has died may then hop onto a person for a blood meal and thus spread the plague organism to human populations. Because of the tendency of fleas to substitute hosts when necessary, rat poisoning campaigns should always be preceded by insecticidal spraying of rat-infested areas to kill the fleas first. If this precautionary measure is not taken, one runs the risk of transferring rodent diseases to humans.

While most Americans tend to think of plague as a "long-ago and far-away" type of disease, rat fleas infected with the plague bacterium were introduced into California early in the 20th century and quickly became endemic among wild rodent populations in the region. Since that time the focus of plague infection has expanded steadily eastward; today plague-infected rodent populations have been identified in 13 western states and during the past 50 years approximately 370 cases of human plague have been reported from this region. The incidence of plague outbreaks in the United States seem to be increasing, as rapid suburbanization results in growing numbers of people living in close proximity to wild rodent habitat. A worrisome trend noted in recent years is a rise in the number of human cases in which domestic cats were the source of infection. Because cats typically are allowed to roam freely, those living in areas where plague-infected rodents are common have ample opportunity to contract the disease and subsequently transmit the ailment to their human companions (CDC, 1994). People living, camping, hiking, or hunting in areas where plague is endemic should take precautions to avoid contact with wild rodents and rodent burrows (where infected fleas may be present) and should never approach or handle obviously sick or dying wild animals. Even recently dead rodents can present a disease hazard: one plague death in the Southwest involved a housewife who picked up a dead ground squirrel which her cat had proudly deposited on the doorstep. She presumably

Table 8-2   Reported Cases of Human Plague, by Country, 1980–1994

Continent	Country	No. of cases	No. of deaths
Africa	Angola	27	4
	Botswana	173	12
	Kenya	49	10
	Libya	8	0
	Madagascar	1,390	302
	Malawi	9	0
	Mozambique	216	3
	South Africa	19	1
	Tanzania	4,964	419
	Uganda	660	48
	Zaire	2,242	513
	Zambia	1	1
	Zimbabwe	397	1
America	Bolivia	189	27
	Brazil	700	9
	Ecuador	83	3
	Peru	1,722	112
	United States	229	33
Asia	China	252	76
	India	876	54
	Kazakhstan	10	4
	Mongolia	59	19
	Myanmar	1,160	14
	Vietnam	3,304	158
World Total		18,739	1,853

Source: World Health Organization. 1996. *Weekly Epidemilogical Record* 22:165–172.

was bitten by a hungry flea who found her an acceptable alternative host and subsequently contracted a fatal case of bubonic plague.

Ticks. Among our most common parasites, ticks are a source of profound annoyance to campers, hunters, dog owners, and livestock raisers who frequently discover themselves or their pets providing a blood meal to these tiny pests. Ticks are far more than a nuisance, however. They are vectors of several serious human diseases such as Rocky Mountain spotted fever, a condition that frequently results in death within two weeks and which, contrary to its name, is not restricted to mountainous areas but is found throughout the continental United States, with the largest number of cases being reported from North and South Carolina. Lyme disease, an ailment scarcely heard of by most Americans until a decade or two ago, has now been reported from 48 states (it also occurs throughout Europe and in parts of Africa, Asia, and Australia) and is currently by far the most commonly diagnosed vector-borne disease in the nation (see Box 8–2). The same tick species that carries the Lyme Disease pathogen can also transmit a sometimes fatal bacterial ailment known as ehrlichiosis. Approximately 500 cases of ehrlichiosis, most of them in the northeastern U.S., have been confirmed by medical authorities since the disease was first described in 1985 (CDC, 1998). Q-fever, relapsing fever, tularemia, and tick paralysis are just a few of many ailments which can be transmitted by ticks. Species which most commonly feed on humans generally are found in areas of wild vegetation such as woods, high grass, parks, and along paths frequented by wild animals. Here they lie in wait for a potential human or animal host, clinging to bushes or tall weeds, ready to latch onto an unwary passer-by (contrary to popular belief, they don't drop onto victims from trees). People planning outdoor activities in tick-infested areas should take such precautions as applying tick repellent to exposed areas of skin, wearing socks and long trousers, and avoiding sitting on the ground or on logs. They should also be diligent about checking their bodies for the presence of ticks at least twice a day and immediately removing them, since most tick-borne diseases are transmitted only after the creature has been feeding for several hours.

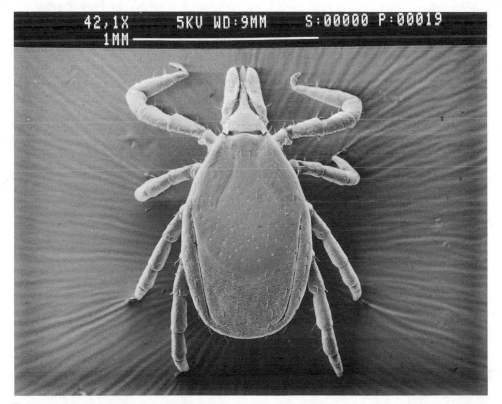

The diminutive deer tick *(Ixodes scapularis)* carries the bacterium that causes Lyme Disease. *[Mathew Nadakavukaren]*

BOX 8-2

"The Woods are Lovely, Dark, and Deep . . ." but Beware of Lyme Disease!

It was late in the fall of 1975 when the small town of Lyme in southeastern Connecticut became the unlikely setting for the opening chapter of a modern-day medical mystery and ultimately bestowed its name on the vector-borne scourge of the late 20th century, **Lyme Disease.** In November of that year, the Connecticut State Health Department was notified of an abnormally high incidence of juvenile rheumatoid arthritis, normally a very rare ailment, in Lyme and several neighboring communities. Suspecting that something was amiss, department officials summoned a team of epidemiologists from Yale to investigate the situation. The geographic distribution and timing of disease outbreaks (most of the victims lived in wooded areas and developed disease symptoms between June and late September) suggested that some sort of vector-borne pathogen was involved, but it took several years of extensive investigation to solve the baffling puzzles posed by this new ailment.

It is now known that the villain responsible for the wide array of unpleasant symptoms which make life miserable for Lyme Disease victims is a spirochete bacterium, *Borrelia burgdorferi,* transmitted to humans (as well as to dogs and horses which are also susceptible) by the bite of an infected deer tick, *Ixodes scapularis* (on the West Coast the main vector is the closely related species, *I. pacificus*).

That the tiny arthropod should first surface as a troublemaker in the well-to-do residential developments spreading into New England woodlands is, in retrospect, not surprising; deer ticks are most abundant in the transitional vegetation characteristic of woody suburban areas where clearings have been cut in the forest or lawns established amidst woods— the type of habitat attractive to deer and a variety of small mammals and birds which provide the main source of sustenance for *I. scapularis.* Similarly, conservation efforts that have resulted in a population explosion among deer herds have also contributed to a corresponding increase in the prevalence of deer ticks.

The tick's life cycle extends over a two-year period; after hatching from eggs laid early in the spring, deer ticks spend their first year as tiny six-legged larvae which feed just once on the blood of a small mammal or bird, then overwinter and molt the following spring into a slightly larger eight-legged nymph. Nymphs also must take a blood meal before molting to the adult stage at the end of their second summer. Although the white-footed mouse is the most frequent host for tick nymphs, an unwary human is also fair game, and it is at this stage of the tick's life cycle that people are most likely to be bitten. Adult deer ticks, about the size of a match-head, climb onto shrubs or vegetation about three feet off the ground and lie in wait for a deer, human, or other large animal upon which they climb, feed once, drop to the ground, and then mate. Because the tick is so small and inconspicuous, a human victim may not even realize he or she has been bitten until disease symptoms appear, generally several days to a month later.

Three distinct phases of the disease have been described, though not all victims experience each stage. The first and most characteristic feature of Lyme Disease, observed in 60–80% of patients, is a spreading red rash (erythema chronica migrans) which begins as a small red bump but expands outward in a circular pattern, 4–20 inches in diameter, resembling a rosy "bull's eye" because of the pale area of skin in the center. Most often occurring on the back, buttocks, chest, or stomach, though not necessarily at the location of the tick bite, this rash is frequently accompanied by a splitting headache, fever, chills, backache, and a feeling of extreme fatigue. The second stage manifests itself primarily as nervous system dysfunction and muscular pains. Some sufferers experience heart problems which may require temporary use of cardiac pacemakers, while others occasionally develop such serious neurological disorders as meningitis or Bell's palsy. The onset of arthritis, usually in the knees or other large joints, typifies the third stage of the disease; attacks generally persist for a few days to several weeks at a time and can be extremely painful. Luckily, since the pathogen causing Lyme Disease is a bacterium, once diagnosed the ailment can be treated by oral administration of an antibiotic such as amoxicillin or deoxycycline. When given early during the rash stage of the disease, such medication generally leads to a quick and complete cure. When used to treat later stages of the disease, antibiotics may or may not be effective—perhaps as many as 50% of patients who have developed chronic symptoms don't respond.

Since surveillance for Lyme Disease was initiated in 1982, the number of cases reported to CDC has escalated dramatically. During the decade of the 1990s, between 9,000–14,000 cases have been diagnosed annually, but the true number of cases is assumed to be much higher (49 states and the District of Columbia require that diagnosed cases of Lyme Disease be reported to the appropriate authorities). As of 1995, Lyme Disease cases had been reported from 48 states and the geographic range of the disease continues to expand. Researchers hypothesize that birds are carrying I. scapularis from one region of the country to another, since tick larvae frequently feed on avian hosts. Three distinct geographical areas are most affected, both in terms of percentage of ticks infected with the pathogen and numbers of human cases reported: the northeastern states, from Massachusetts south to Maryland; Minnesota and Wisconsin in the upper Midwest; and northern California and Oregon, especially along the humid coastal areas and along the western slopes of the northern Sierra Nevada mountains. In the endemic areas of the northeast and north-central U.S., approximately 25–35% of tick nymphs now harbor the Lyme Disease bacterium, while 50–70% of adult ticks are infected. The number of reported human cases in these areas has been increasing in frequency in recent years and now averages between 10–30 per 100,000 population; by contrast, in nonendemic U.S. counties, reported cases are well below 10 per 100,000.

LYMErix, the first vaccine for preventing Lyme Disease, received FDA approval in 1998; a second vaccine is undergoing clinical testing. Although initial results indicate LYMErix is both effective (95% efficacy rate after 3 doses) and safe, at least in the short term, some medical authorities caution that vaccine use needs to be monitored closely for 5–10 years to guard against unanticipated problems in the future.

Welcome though it is, LYMErix is not a panacea against tick-borne disease. Several doses of the vaccine over a period of months are required to confer partial resistance to *B. burgdorferi* and the vaccine gives no protection at all against other serious tick-borne ailments such as ehrlichiosis and Rocky Mountain spotted fever. For these reasons, public health officials continue to advise hikers, campers, or suburbanites living in tick-infested areas to be wary, wear protective clothing, promptly remove any ticks discovered on the body, and contact a physician immediately if mysterious problems arise after a walk in the woods.

References

Habicht, Gail, Gregory Beck, and Jorge L. Benach. 1987. "Lyme Disease." *Scientific American* 257 (July).

Marwich, Charles. 1998. "Guarded Endorsement for Lyme Disease Vaccine." *Journal of the American Medical Association* 279, no. 24 (June 24):1937-38.

Ostfeld, Richard S. 1997. "The Ecology of Lyme-Disease Risk." *The American Scientist* 85, no. 4 (July/Aug):338-46.

Although the previous discussion is by no means a complete listing of the human health problems caused by various pest species, it should convey some realization of the need for pest control and an understanding of why many public health officials feel that abandoning chemical pesticides would entail the risk of increased mortality and morbidity rates due to vector-borne disease.

Pest Control

Early Attempts at Pest Control

Human efforts to control pest outbreaks date back to the development of agriculture approximately 10,000 years ago, when relatively large expanses of a single crop and sizeable numbers of people living close together in none-too-sanitary conditions favored an increase in pest populations which wouldn't have been possible among small, scattered societies living a nomadic, hunter-gatherer type of lifestyle. Early attempts to reduce pest damage included purely physical efforts—stomping, flailing, burning—as well as the offering of prayers, sacrifices, and ritual dances to the local gods. A few effective measures were discovered even at such early dates, however. The Sumerians, in what now is Iraq, successfully employed sulfur compounds against insects and mites more than 5,000 years ago; over 3,000 years ago the Chinese were treating seeds with insecticides derived from plant extracts, using wood ashes and chalk to ward off insect pests in the home, and applying mercury and arsenic compounds to their bodies to control lice. Among the Chinese is found the earliest example of using a pest's natural enemies to control it: by A.D. 300 the Chinese were introducing colonies of predatory ants into their citrus groves to control caterpillars and certain beetles.

During the peak of Greek civilization, records indicate that some of the wealthier citizens used mosquito nets and built high sleeping towers to evade mosquitoes. They also used oil sprays and sulfur bitumen ointments to deter insects. The Romans designed rat-proof granaries, but relied largely on superstitious practices such as nailing up crayfish in different parts of the garden to keep away caterpillars. In medieval Europe people increasingly relied on religious faith to protect them from pest depredations; as late as 1476, during an outbreak of cutworms in Switzerland, several of the offending insects were hauled into court, proclaimed guilty, excommunicated by the archbishop, and banished from the land!

Not until the 18th and 19th centuries did efforts at pest control make any meaningful progress. This was a time when European farming practices were becoming more productive and scientific, and help in combatting agricultural pests was eagerly sought. Botanical insecticides such as pyrethrum, derris (rotenone), and nicotine were introduced at this time. Heightened interest in improved pest control methods was generated during the mid-19th century by several of the worst agricultural disasters ever recorded—the potato blight in Ireland, England, and Belgium in 1848, caused by a fungal disease; the fungus leaf spot disease of coffee in Ceylon which completely wiped out coffee cultivation on the island; and the outbreak of both powdery mildew and an insect pest, grape phylloxera, which nearly destroyed the wine industry in Europe. Such problems led to the development of new chemical pesticides and ushered in a whole new era of pest control. Two of the first such compounds, Bordeaux mixture (copper sulfate and lime) and Paris Green (copper acetoarsenite), were originally employed as fungicides but were subsequently found to be effective insecticides as well. Paris Green became one of the most widely used insecticides in the late 19th century and Bordeaux mixture even today is the most widely used fungicide in the world. Early in the 1900s arsenic-containing compounds such as lead arsenate, highly toxic to both insects and humans, became the most widely sold insecticides in the United States and retained their leading position until the advent of DDT after World War II (Flint and VandenBosch, 1981).

In 1939, Paul Müller, a Swiss chemist working for the Geigy Corporation, discovered that the synthetic compound dichlorodiphenyltrichloroethane (referred to as DDT for obvious reasons!) was extremely effective in killing insects on contact and retained its lethal character for a long time after application. Müller had simply been looking for a better product to be used against clothes moths, but the outbreak of war in Europe gave far wider significance to the new chemical. Military authorities, recognizing that extensive campaigns would be carried out in the tropics where insect-borne disease threatened high troop losses, made the search for better insecticides a top priority. DDT, highly lethal to every kind of insect yet harmless to humans when applied as a powder, was just what the military needed. Initially, production of DDT was exclusively for use in the armed forces where it was employed first as a louse powder and later for mosquito control. At the end of the war DDT was released for civilian use, both in agriculture and for public health purposes. Its use quickly spread worldwide, amidst high expectations of complete eradication of many diseases and greatly reduced crop losses due to insects. Müller was awarded the 1948 Nobel Prize in Physiology and Medicine in recognition of his contribution. The enthusiastic reception given to DDT encouraged chemical companies in their search for new and even more effective synthetic pesticides. By the mid-1950s at least 25 new products which would revolutionize insect control practices were put on the market, among

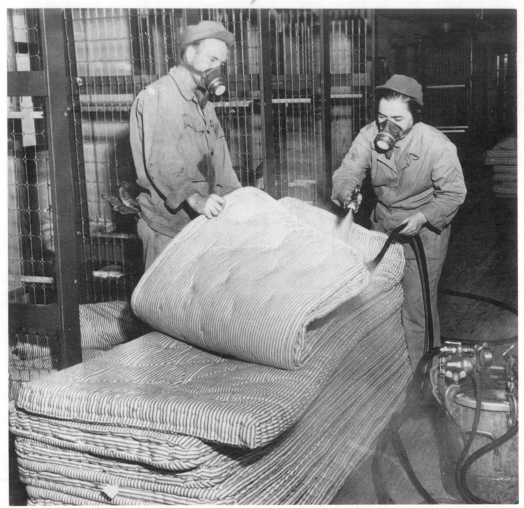

U.S. Army personnel spray mattresses with a DDT solution to combat bedbugs, circa 1944. *[UPI/ Corbis-Bettman]*

the more important of which were chlordane, heptachlor, toxaphene, aldrin, endrin, dieldrin, and parathion (Perkins, 1982). The age of chemical warfare against pests had begun.

Types of Pesticides

Pesticides, substances which kill pests, are subdivided into groups according to target organism. For example, insecticides kill insects, herbicides kill weeds, rodenticides kill rats and mice, nematicides kill nematodes, and so forth. Within each of these groups there may be further subdivisions based on such characteristics as route of intake of the poison or physiological effect on the target organism. A brief survey of some of the most common groups of pesticides currently in use would include the following.

Insecticides. The largest number of pesticides are employed against a wide variety of insects and include **stomach poisons** (taken into the body through the mouth; effective against insects with biting or chewing mouthparts, such as caterpillars); **contact poisons** (penetrate through the body wall); and **fumigants** (enter insect through its respiratory system). Representative types include:

Inorganic insecticides. Most of these compounds, such as lead arsenate, Paris Green, and a number of other products containing copper, zinc, mercury, chlorine, or sulfur, act as stomach poisons and were the most commonly used insecticides until after World War II. Many of these products are quite toxic to humans as well as to insects and their heavy use left significant concentrations of toxic metals in some fields and orchards. Boric acid, widely used in the 1930s and 1940s for cockroach control, is a venerable inorganic insecticide that has enjoyed a resurgence in popularity in recent years because of its low human toxicity. Silica aerogel—a white, fluffy silicate powder which kills insects by absorbing wax from the insect cuticle, resulting in excess water loss and death by dehydration—is another inorganic compound used for household insect control. In addition to these compounds, some petroleum derivatives such as kerosene, diesel oil, and #2 fuel oil have been sprayed on water surfaces to suffocate mosquito larvae.

Chlorinated hydrocarbons. DDT and its chemical relatives (chlordane, heptachlor, lindane, BHC, endrin, aldrin, mirex, kepone, toxaphene, etc.) are all contact poisons. They act primarily on the central nervous system, causing the insect to go through a series of convulsions prior to death. Members of this group are **broad-spectrum** insecticides, meaning that they kill a wide range of insects and other arthropods, and are also **persistent** in the environment, breaking down very slowly and therefore retaining their effectiveness for a relatively long period after application. Because the chlorinated hydrocarbons are not water-soluble, they tend to accumulate in fatty tissues when taken up by living organisms and may remain in the body indefinitely. Since the 1970s, many of the chlorinated hydrocarbons have been banned for most uses in the United States, and more recently in many European countries and Japan, because animal testing has shown them to be carcinogenic.

Organophosphates. Developed first by the Germans for possible wartime use as nerve gases, this group includes some of the most deadly insecticides such as methyl parathion, ranked in the "super toxic" category of pesticides. Organophosphates, like chlorinated hydrocarbons, are broad-spectrum contact poisons, but unlike the chlorinated hydrocarbons they are not persistent, usually breaking down two weeks or less after application. Thus they present far less danger to nontarget organisms. Organophosphates are nerve poisons which act to inhibit the enzyme cholinesterase, causing the insect to lose coordination and go into convulsions. Members of this group range in terms of human toxicity from the extremely deadly parathion and phosdrin (one drop of these in the eye is fatal to an adult) to the moderately toxic diazinon and dichlorvos (the volatile compound used in some pet flea collars), to the slightly toxic malathion, commonly sold for home garden use.

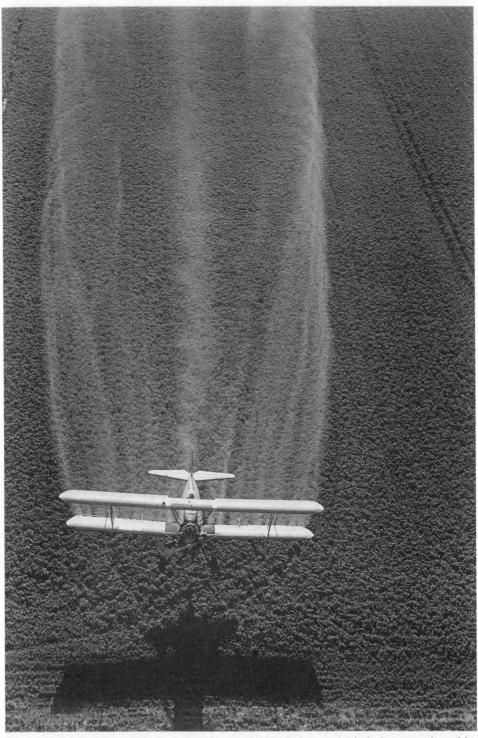

The dusting of agricultural products with pesticides is increasingly being questioned by those concerned with the long-term effects of pesticide exposure on human health and the environment. *[U.S. Department of Agriculture]*

Carbamates. Widely used today in public health work and agriculture because of their rapid knock-down of insects and low toxicity to mammals (a few, however, are quite toxic and their use is restricted to certified applicators), carbamates too are contact poisons which act in a manner similar to the organophosphates. One of the most common of the carbamates, *Sevin*, is widely used as a garden dust and for mosquito control.

Synthetic pyrethroids and other botanicals. Chemical analogs of the natural insecticide, pyrethrum (an extract of chrysanthemum flowers), synthetic pyrethroids such as allethrin, cyfluthrin, resmethrin, permethrin, and fenvalerate are broad spectrum contact poisons widely used in structural pest control, with a growing number of agricultural applications as well. Providing quick knock-down of insects, the pyrethroids are probably the best choice for home or garden use because of their very low toxicity to humans and domestic animals. For this reason, they are among the few insecticides that can be safely used indoors, even in the kitchen. While these products are generally somewhat more expensive than other insecticides, they can be used effectively at much lower rates of application. If it is necessary to use an insecticidal dust, shampoo, or flea collar on young puppies or kittens, a product containing one of the pyrethroids is recommended.

Natural pyrethrum *(Pyrocide)* is still available, as is rotenone *(Chem-Fish),* a poison derived from a tropical legume. **Neem**, an extract of a South Asian tree of the same name, is another botanical insecticide registered for use on ornamental plants and vegetables. Valued in India since ancient times for both insecticidal and medicinal properties, neem seeds and leaves contain nine or more different liminoid compounds that exhibit potent repellent and pesticidal properties effective against at least 200 different species of insects. Like the other botanicals, neem is quite safe for humans—in fact, for centuries South Asians have used neem extensively for dental hygiene and a variety of other medical purposes (National Research Council, 1992).

Herbicides. Weeds in a field may not appear as threatening as hordes of insects, yet the economic losses caused by these unwanted species can be very high. Weeds compete with crop plants for vital mineral nutrients and water, thus reducing crop yields; they make harvesting more difficult and some species, when consumed, poison livestock.

Widescale application of chemicals for weed control is a relatively new phenomenon. Although a few inorganic compounds such as iron sulfate were used against broad-leaf weeds as long ago as 1896, hand-weeding, mechanical cultivation, tillage, crop rotation, and the use of weed-free seeds were the most common methods of reducing crop losses due to weed infestations. After World War II, the first synthetic herbicide (2,4-D) was introduced and has been followed by a succession of more than a hundred different chemical weed killers. Today herbicide use has considerably surpassed insecticide use in American agriculture, both in terms of quantities applied, pounds of active ingredients, and in pesticide expenditures by farmers, who currently spend three times as much for weed killers as they do for insecticides (Aspelin, 1994). Reliance on chemical herbicides for weed control has also risen steadily. For corn and soybeans, the two most herbicide-dependent crops, the percent of crop acres treated has risen from 50% and 27%, respectively, in the mid-1960s to 96% and 97%, respectively, in the 1990s (Lin et al., 1995).

Although herbicides are used most extensively for agricultural purposes, they are also used by public health workers to control weeds that harbor insects and rodents, and to eradicate nuisance plants such as ragweed or poison ivy.

Herbicides may be either selective or nonselective, the former group being by far the more common. Most selective herbicides kill only broad-leafed dicotyledonous plants, a group to which many of the common weed species belong, without harming members of the grass family. Thus they can be used for effective weed control on cereal crops or on home lawns. Examples of some selective herbicides include 2,4-D (the active ingredient in 1,500 over-the-counter weed killers), alachlor, and atrazine. Nonselective herbicides kill any plant with which they come into contact and thus have more limited use, such as spraying railroad and highway right-of-ways. Sulfuric acid and glyphosate *(Roundup, Kleenup)* are examples of nonselective herbicides.

Although most herbicides are thought to be only slightly toxic to humans, in recent years there have been several studies suggesting that herbicide exposure can cause genetic mutations, cancer, and birth defects. Farm workers occasionally blame health problems such as weight loss, nausea, vomiting, and loss of appetite to contact with herbicides. In 1986 researchers reported that Kansas farmers who used 2,4-D for more than 20 days per year had a six times greater risk of non-Hodgkins lymphoma than did a control group with no exposure to herbicides (Blair et al., 1987). In 1991 the *Journal of the National Cancer Institute* reported that dogs, too, are at risk from 2,4-D. If their owners apply the weed killer four times or more each summer, canines are twice as likely to develop malignant lymphoma as are dogs whose owners abstain from herbicide use. Recognition that some of the most widely used herbicides are known or suspected carcinogens has prompted concerns among some federal regulators that residues of these chemicals on food or in well water may be exposing the American consumer to long-term health risks.

During the late 1970s and early 1980s a great deal of public controversy surrounded the use of 2,4,5-T and silvex, selective herbicides that contained traces of dioxin formed as an unavoidable contaminant during the manufacturing process. Notorious as a component of **Agent Orange,** the chemical defoliant used by U.S. military forces during the Vietnam War, 2,4,5-T (actually, the dioxin contaminating 2,4,5-T) was blamed for a wide range of physical and emotional problems among South Vietnamese living in the target areas, as well as among American servicemen who had come into contact with the herbicide during their tour of duty. Although independent studies of veterans' complaints have never been able to confirm an association between the alleged health effects and Agent Orange exposure, production of 2,4,5-T and silvex was terminated in the early 1980s and in 1984 seven chemical companies agreed to an out-of-court settlement for $180 million with a veterans' group claiming health damage. Rapid growth in the commercial lawn care industry, which currently serves an approximate eight million American households (Benbrook, 1996), has provoked a vociferous response in many communities by anti-pesticide activists who warn of the dangers posed to people, pets, and wildlife by toxic lawn chemicals (*"Dandelions won't kill you—*

BOX 8-3

Black-market Poison:
"The Mississippi Stuff" in Chicago

Folks around Ruben Brown's neighborhood in Bellwood, a western suburb of Chicago, described the retired butcher-turned bug exterminator as a friendly fellow—"the guy with the Mississippi stuff"—who traveled door-to-door with his hand sprayer, promising to solve their cockroach problems for a bargain-basement price. Kill roaches he certainly did, but in the process he created an environmental health nightmare that cost millions of dollars to resolve.

Unbeknownst to his satisfied customers, the potent insecticide Brown liberally applied inside their homes was methyl parathion, one of the deadliest of all organophosphate pesticides. Commonly known as "cotton poison" in the South where this chemical is registered for use on cotton and soybeans, methyl parathion is expressly prohibited for use indoors (in Illinois the insecticide is illegal for any use whatsoever). Methyl parathion poisoning can result in death or serious neurological damage; even low levels of exposure may lead to immune system damage, severe headaches, nausea, vomiting, or muscle spasms.

When Brown was arrested in April 1997, investigators were dismayed to discover that his was no small operation. Stored in his home were spraying equipment and 25 gallons of methyl parathion —properly labeled with warnings that the chemical should never be stored or used in residences! Also seized at this time were approximately 40 notebooks meticulously listing names and addresses of all Brown's customers. From these records investigators learned that between 1991–1997 Brown had treated more than 900 homes and apartments in Chicago and 20 sub-urban communities. Not only did he use excessively generous amounts when applying the pesticide, he also frequently left his customers small juice bottles containing methyl parathion concentrate so they could administer follow-up treatments themselves. Given the fact that the undiluted chemical resembles iced tea (or milk, if water is added), the fact that no thirsty child drank the poison is nothing short of miraculous. Ruben Brown subsequently pleaded guilty to misdemeanor charges of illegal pesticide spraying and was sentenced to two years in prison.

In May 1997, soon after Brown's arrest, state and local health authorities, along with EPA officials, launched a massive sampling effort to ascertain the scope of the problem. Using addresses provided by Brown's ledgers, 901 Chicago area homes were tested for methyl parathion residues. Where initial environmental sampling indicated pesticide concentrations high enough to warrant concern for residents' health, biological sampling (i.e. urine assays) of those living in the affected dwellings was carried out to determine the extent of residents' exposure. While not all persons eligible for biological sampling agreed to cooperate, residents at 492 homes supplied samples for analysis. In the majority of cases, results indicated that pesticide residues were either absent or low enough to justify no further action; in some cases, levels were elevated just enough to require additional precautionary testing. However, in those situations where urine samples revealed that at least one resident had absorbed significant levels of parathion, the home in question was targeted for decontamination. During the following twelve months, more than 90 families were temporarily relocated while their homes underwent extensive renovations. A special chemical was employed to seal pesticide residues into walls to prevent release of vapors; old carpeting was removed and replaced, new flooring installed, kitchen and bathroom tiles and fixtures replaced. By the time of project completion, Chicago's decontamination effort had cost over $10 million, an average of about $115,000 per home.

Unfortunately, Chicago's "cotton poison" drama was not an isolated event but rather represents one more example of a growing black-market trade in illicit pesticides. The increasing misuse of dangerous pesticides in urban areas, particularly in low-income minority communities, has resulted from lax controls over pesticides in a few states, primarily in the South, and illegal purchases on the part of uncertified and unlicensed pest control operators who take advantage of casual regulatory practices. Sometimes the chemicals are purchased legally from agrochemical dealers, on other occasions illegally at flea markets or via "tail-gate" dealers at strip malls. In the Chicago case, Mr. Brown admitted he had driven to Mississippi several times to purchase methyl parathion, using pesticide certification cards that belonged to two other men. EPA investigators have documented misuse and illegal sales of methyl parathion, similar to the Chicago incident, in Ohio,

Michigan, New York, Mississippi, Louisiana, Arkansas, Alabama, Tennessee, and Texas.

In an effort to forestall future "cotton poison" episodes, EPA has launched a vigorous program to curb such black-market dealing. Increased enforcement monitoring, particularly within low- income urban areas, to detect and prosecute illegal applicators is part of EPA's "Urban Initiative," conducted in cooperation with state and regional EPA authorities. Of equal, if not greater, importance is a broad-based educational effort to inform the public about safe, effective approaches to cockroach control—including the importance of hiring only reputable, licensed exterminators. The task is immense and will require the help of professional pest control organizations, businesses, health care organizations, and community groups. However, once people are aware of the facts, they generally respond positively. Stressing that she would do whatever was necessary to protect the health of her family, a Chicago grandmother whose apartment was one of those slated for decontamination remarked, "I have a little grandbaby and I didn't want him getting sick or dying. I didn't want to die."

Reference
EPA. 1998. "Methyl Parathion: Cleaning Up Cotton Poison in the Chicago Area." Fact Sheet (May).

pesticides do!"). The increasingly common use by lawn care firms of post-application warning signs, accompanied by recommended safety precautions, has been a positive, if limited, industry response to citizen concerns.

Rodenticides. Although good sanitation and rat-proofing of buildings and food storage facilities provides the only effective long-term control of domestic rodents, use of poisons is an important additional tool in keeping rat populations low. Because some rodenticides used in public health work are extremely toxic to humans as well as to rodents, their use is restricted to certified applicators. General-use rodenticides, chemicals which should not present a serious hazard either to the user or to the environment when used in accordance with instructions, can be purchased by the general public. The rodenticides most commonly recommended for use by householders act as anticoagulants.

Such poisons as warfarin, fumarin, PMP, pival, diphacinone, and chlorophacinone are all multiple-dose poisons which must be consumed over a period of several consecutive days before the rat dies. Thus a child or pet would not be seriously endangered by eating a single portion of bait. Anticoagulants cause internal hemorrhaging, causing the rodents to bleed to death painlessly. These poisons provide excellent control of both rats and mice, although up to two weeks may be required to get an effective kill.

Environmental Impact of Pesticide Use

In the early 1950s, bird-watchers in both the United States and Western Europe were confronted with a baffling mystery—a sudden, inexplicable decline in the populations of bald eagles, pelicans, and peregrine falcons appeared to threaten the very survival of these well-loved species. Investigations into the reasons behind such an unanticipated population "crash" ultimately revealed that the villain was not a disease, nor overkilling, nor a scarcity of food, but rather was the presence in the tissues of these birds of startlingly high concentrations of the new insecticide DDT. Although DDT did not appear to have a direct lethal effect on the adult birds, it interfered with their ability to metabolize calcium, thereby resulting in the production of eggs with shells so thin they broke when the nesting parents sat on them. Thus pesticide-induced reproductive failure—the inability of the birds to produce viable offspring—was ultimately shown to be the factor responsible for the population decline.

This episode represented one of the first glimmerings of awareness on the part of the scientific community at least, that the advent of the new wonder chemicals was not an unmitigated blessing. The public at large, however, remained largely unaware and unconcerned about such matters until the publication in 1962 of Rachel Carson's literary bombshell, *Silent Spring*. This best-seller represented a scathing indictment of pesticide misuse and for the first time made the average American aware of the havoc which indiscriminate reliance on chemicals could wreak on the environment and on human well-being. In retrospect, the publication of *Silent Spring* made "ecology" a household word and was probably the most important single event in launching what became the environmental movement of the 1970s. Carson and many subsequent researchers clearly demonstrated that extensive use and near-total reliance on chemicals for pest control have been accompanied by unanticipated and undesired side effects, many of which have raised problems serious enough to threaten the continued usefulness of these products.

Development of Resistance

Those who dreamed that the new pesticides held promise of complete eradication of certain insect or other pest species were obviously ignorant of the principles that govern how the forces of natural selection act upon chance variations occurring within any population—particularly insect populations whose long evolutionary history demonstrates the remarkable ability of these organisms to evolve and adapt rapidly to changing environmental conditions. The widespread, frequent, and intensive application of chemicals such as DDT in the years following the war was initially successful in drastically reducing pest populations, but eventually was responsible for providing the selective forces that would produce new strains of "super bugs," rendering the original poisons worthless. The mechanism by which this occurs can be visualized by considering a hypothetical population of, say, boll weevils ravaging a field of cotton. Aerial insecticide spraying may kill perhaps 99% of the weevils, but a few will survive, either by chance (perhaps an overhanging leaf shielded them from the spray) or because something in the genetic make-up of a particular individual somehow made it less vulnerable to the poison. Such a hereditary trait might be the production of a particular enzyme capable of detoxifying the pesticide, a less permeable type of epidermis which prevented penetration of the contact poison, a behavioral characteristic that allowed the individual to avoid fatal exposure, or some other factor of this nature. In a pesticide-free environment (the type of situation prevailing prior to the introduction of DDT) such a genetic trait would confer no special advantage to the individual carrying it, so the frequency of such a gene within that population would remain low. Once DDT came into widespread use, however, the boll weevils' environment was radically altered and those few individuals possessing the gene for immunity suddenly enjoyed a tremendous selective advantage. As the accompanying diagram indicates, successive sprayings largely eliminated boll weevils susceptible to the insecticide, but promoted the build-up of a population in which the vast majority of individuals now carry the gene (or genes) conferring resistance to the chemical. In order to combat this new situation, those seeking to control pest outbreaks turn to newer and more powerful chemicals, only to witness the same cycle of events repeat itself.

Since pesticide resistance had appeared as a localized problem even with the old-fashioned insecticides, it shouldn't have come as a total surprise when insects resistant to DDT began to appear in the late 1940s and early 1950s. Among the first species to display immunity were certain populations of houseflies and mosquitoes which, as early as 1946, could no longer be controlled with DDT. In 1951, during the Korean War, military officials were alarmed to discover that human body lice, vectors of typhus, had become resistant to DDT. Among agricultural pests, spider mites, cabbage loopers, codling moths, and tomato hornworms developed resistance to several of the common insecticides; by the mid-1950s when the boll weevil became resistant to many of the chlorinated hydrocarbons, the need for alternative control methods became obvious (Perkins, 1982). At present, more than 500 species of insects and mites are resistant to common pesticides—more than double the number that were resistant just a few decades ago. Largely due to problems of pesticide resistance, crop losses due to insects are nearly twice as high now as they were when DDT was first brought onto the market, in spite of a quantum increase in pesticidal applications by farmers over the past half century. In the public health field, as in agriculture, growing pesticide resistance is causing serious concern. Worldwide, incidence of malaria is now on a sharp upswing as approximately 64 species of mosquitoes have become resistant to

Figure 8-2   Cycle of Pesticide Resistance

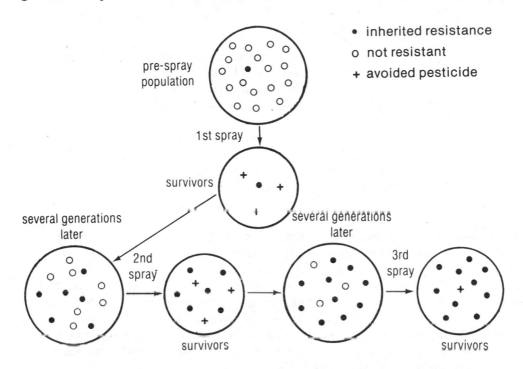

- • inherited resistance
- o not resistant
- + avoided pesticide

insecticides, according to World Health Organization officials.

Problems of pesticide resistance are not restricted to species of arthropods. Some rat populations, particularly those in cities which have long-established rodent control programs, no longer respond to warfarin, the most extensively used rodenticide in the world. More than 150 species of plant pathogens (fungi and bacteria) are now resistant to at least one pesticide, as are 270 weed species (USEPA, 1996). Although herbicide resistance is a relatively recent development and has received considerably less attention among agricultural experts than has the problem of chemically immune insects, weed scientists warn that the phenomenon is already widespread. In Australia wheat growers by the early 1980s were reporting the emergence of new weed biotypes resistant to every selective herbicide which can be used on wheat. Even more ominous was the recent discovery that Australian ryegrass has developed resistance to glyphosate (*Roundup*), the world's best-selling herbicide. This news is particularly worrisome to farmers because new commercial varieties of wheat, cotton, potatoes, sugar beets, canola, and soybeans have now been genetically engineered to survive direct field applications of glyphosate intended for weed control (since glyphosate is a nonselective herbicide, it would ordinarily kill all plants in the area sprayed, crop plants and weeds alike). If glyphosate-resistance becomes widespread among weed species, commercial use of glyphosate-tolerant crop plants will no longer confer any advantage to growers, and agriculture's arsenal of chemical weapons to combat weeds will be further reduced (Fahnestock, 1996).

Killing of Beneficial Species

Only a small percentage of insect species are considered pests, yet the most widely used synthetic insecticides are broad-spectrum poisons, killing both friend and foe alike. The destruction of many beneficial predator insect species as well as the target pest has led to two related types of problems. The first of these, referred to as **target pest resurgence,** occurs when an insecticide application which initially resulted in a drastic reduction in the pest population is quickly followed by a sudden increase in pest numbers to a level higher than that which existed prior to the spraying. This occurs because the natural enemies of the pest, which formerly kept its numbers under control, were also heavily decimated by the spraying. Since any predators which survived the pesticide would subsequently starve or migrate, the pests would then confront ideal conditions—no natural enemies and an abundance of their favorite food (i.e. the crop that had been sprayed). As a result, their populations can increase in size very rapidly, above and beyond the original level.

A second situation, known as **secondary pest outbreak,** involves the rise to prominence of certain plant-eating species which, prior to the spraying, were unimportant as pests because natural enemies kept their populations below the level at which they could cause significant economic damage. After pesticides eliminated most of their predators, such insects suddenly experience a population explosion and become major pests in their own right. In 1995 Texas cotton growers in the lower Rio Grande Valley experienced a devastating outbreak of several secondary pests after some 200,000 acres were targeted for aerial spraying with the organophosphate insecticide, malathion, to control boll weevils. Predictably, the spraying decimated beneficial insects along with the target pest, resulting in an unanticipated outbreak of cotton aphids which spread rapidly through the fields. Shortly afterwards, a beet armyworm infestation mushroomed as well, causing severe losses to the cotton crop. The armyworms were followed by whiteflies, which further reduced yields. In spite of as many as 25 insecticidal sprayings on some farms, many growers lost their entire crop and cotton yields in the area that year plunged 80%, from an average harvest of 300,000 bales to just 54,000 (Meister, 1996).

Environmental Contamination

Liberal use of pesticides on a worldwide basis has resulted in a more thorough contamination of the biosphere than anyone in 1945 would have dreamed possible. Today pesticide residues, especially those of the chlorinated hydrocarbons, are found virtually everywhere in the tissues of creatures as diverse as Antarctic penguins, fish in deep ocean trenches, decomposer bacteria, and every human being. Since no one deliberately sprayed pesticides in Antarctica or in the middle of the Pacific, how could this have happened? Because the chlorinated hydrocarbons are persistent pesticides (meaning that they break down very slowly), they can circulate through the ecosystem for a long time, often traveling long distances from their point of origin. When such chemicals are aerially sprayed on forest, field, or pastureland, less than 10% of the pesticide actually hits the target; the remainder is carried off by air currents and is subsequently deposited miles away where it will eventually be washed into waterways or taken up by living organisms in the food they eat. Even when carefully applied according to label directions, pesticides can vaporize into the air, be washed off the land into lakes and streams during heavy rains, or percolate downward through the soil. The results of this unintended contamination include the following.

Direct Killing of Organisms Exposed to Chemicals. Many species of fish, some birds and small mammals, and a number of plants, including phytoplankton, as well as beneficial insect species, are extremely sensitive to chemical pesticides and die immediately after coming into contact with such substances. A dramatic example of this occurred a few years ago when 700 Brant geese died after walking and feeding on a New York golf course which had been treated with the widely used organophosphate insecticide, diazinon. As a result of this and numerous other bird kills linked to the insecticide, EPA cancelled the use of diazinon on golf courses and sod farms, but the insecticide is still widely applied to lawns and gardens throughout the United States. Another insecticide that has caused high mortality among nontarget species is carbofuran, a carbamate pesticide estimated to kill one to two million birds in the United States each year, including bald eagles. Several years ago, in response to a flood of protests from bird lovers, the state of Virginia banned use of carbofuran. The manufacturer agreed to terminate U.S. sales of the granular form of the poison by the fall of 1994 (birds are particularly attracted to the granules which they swallow, presumably mistaking them for grit); *exports* of granular carbofuran have continued, however, and carbofuran sprays—also a cause of wildlife mortality—have remained on the market both here and abroad. Accidents involving pesticides have frequently wrought havoc on wildlife populations. Several massive fish kills made headline news in 1991; a train derailment along the Upper Sacramento River in California spilled 19,000 gallons of metam-sodium into the water, killing virtually every living creature—fish, crustaceans, insect larvae, algae, and plankton—along a 45-mile stretch of the river. That same year an estimated one million fish, along with uncounted numbers of crabs, crawfish, turtles, and alligators, were killed by canefield runoff of the organophosphate insecticide azinphosmethyl *(Guthion)* in southern Louisiana. The following year a similar incident occurred, again due to pesticide runoff from sugarcane fields, this time causing 25,000 fish to go belly-up (Curtis, Profeta, and Mott, 1993; Williams, 1993).

Indirect Killing Via Depletion of Food or Habitat. When pesticides are targeted against insects, plants, or rodents that serve as a major food source for another group of organisms, the long-term effect can be just as devastating as direct poisoning would be. In New Jersey, populations of certain forest bird species declined by 45–55% after carbaryl spraying for gypsy moth control deprived the birds of their supper. Herbicide use similarly reduces both forage and habitat for many plant-eating insects and can have a "domino effect" when plummeting populations of arthropods adversely impact the food supply of insectivorous birds. On the high plains of Wyoming, a population of native sparrows crashed after herbicidal spraying of sagebrush to enlarge pasturelands for grazing. Unfortunately for the sparrows, the sagebrush supplied essential cover and nesting sites without which the birds couldn't survive (Parker, 1994).

Groundwater Contamination. The discovery in 1979 that 96 wells on Long Island were contaminated with a highly toxic carbamate insecticide, aldicarb, came as unwelcome news to a public which assumed that however polluted our rivers and lakes might be, groundwater supplies were safe from chemical contamination. Any hopes that the New York situation might be an isolated aberration were shattered by the revelation that 3,000 miles to the west, more than 2,000 wells in the fertile San Joaquin Valley were tainted with the nematicide DBCP, a chlorinated hydrocarbon that had earlier made headlines for causing sterility among male pesticide workers exposed to the chemical. In the late 1980s the EPA launched a nationwide survey to determine the extent of pesticide contamination of groundwater supplies. In 1990 the agency released a report showing that 14% of all public and private drinking water wells sampled had measurable levels of at least one pesticide. Two years later the agency reported new results indicating that nearly one-third of rural wells sampled showed unsafe levels of pesticide contamination, with aldicarb and the herbicides atrazine (*Aatrex*) and alachlor (*Lasso*), both suspected human carcinogens, posing the most widespread problems. Agency surveyors reported finding nearly 100 different pesticides in groundwater supplies and concluded that heavy agricultural pesticide use was the main cause of the problem. While the levels of farm chemicals found in well water are too low to cause *acute* pesticide poisoning, they raise concerns about *chronic* health effects among those dependent on such supplies. Since most of the data on groundwater quality has been derived from shallow wells which are presumably more subject to contamination, the full extent of pesticide pollution of groundwater cannot yet be adequately assessed. In addition, because plumes of contamination move so slowly in aquifers, concentrations measured today indicate the impact of agricultural practices years or even decades ago. In the developing nations, where the rate of pesticide use is increasing even faster than in the industrialized world, virtually no groundwater monitoring is being carried out at present; it is quite likely that current agricultural activities may be seriously degrading underground water supplies over vast areas without anyone recognizing the potential threat to future generations (Nash, 1993; "EPA Study," 1992; Curtis et al., 1993).

Indirect Contamination Via Food Chains. Since the chlorinated hydrocarbons are not water-soluble they are not excreted from the body when ingested but instead are stored in fatty tissues such as liver, kidneys, and fat around the intestines. Toxic substances present in minute amounts in the general environment can thus become quite concentrated as they move along a food chain, sometimes reaching lethal doses in organisms at the highest trophic levels. This process, known as **biomagnification**, was the phenomenon responsible for the reproductive failure in the various birds of prey referred to earlier in this chapter. Eagles, pelicans, and falcons are all top carnivores, fish-eaters, at the end of relatively long food chains. As such, they had accumulated amounts of DDT sufficiently high to interfere with important bodily processes, with the results already described.

The classic example of biomagnification can be seen in the case of Clear Lake, California—a favorite fishing spot about 90 miles north of San Francisco. Recreational anglers had long been annoyed by the swarms of nonbiting gnats which were frequently present at Clear Lake. The new synthetic pesticides seemingly offered an easy way of getting rid of a nuisance, so in 1949 it was decided to spray Clear Lake with a dilute solution of DDD (a chemical cousin of DDT which is less toxic to fish). After the first spraying, gnat populations dropped to barely detectable levels, but by 1951 the pesky insects were back in bothersome numbers, so the spraying was repeated. Several more sprayings followed in succeeding years as the gnat populations displayed increasing resistance to the poison. Then some strange side effects became apparent. By 1954 visitors to Clear Lake began reporting significant numbers of carcasses of the Western grebe, a type of water fowl, around the lake. By the early 1960s, the grebe population at Clear Lake had plummeted from 1,000 nesting pairs to almost none. Suspecting that the repeated pesticide applications might somehow be related to the birds' demise, biologists began to measure DDD concentrations in various components of the lake ecosystem. Although the lake water itself contained traces of DDD in barely detectable amounts (0.02 ppm), concentrations of the pesticide increased dramatically when the tissues of living organisms were examined. The facts they uncovered are entirely consistent with the basic principles of a food chain:

Organism	DDD Concentration in Tissues (ppm)
Phytoplankton (producers)	5
Herbivorous fish (primary consumers)	40-300
Carnivorous fish (secondary consumers)	up to 2500
Western grebes (secondary consumers)	1600

The pesticide that had been sprayed on the lake, in what everybody at the time assumed was a safely dilute amount, was absorbed and concentrated by the plankton which were the producer organisms of Clear Lake. When these were consumed by the herbivorous fish (primary consumers), the DDD became more concentrated. By the time these fish were eaten by grebes or by bullheads, the DDD had become sufficiently concentrated to cause the death of the birds.

By the late 1960s the futility of spraying to control the now-resistant gnats became obvious and a gnat-eating fish was introduced into the lake in what subsequently proved to be a very successful method of biological control. As pesticide levels gradually dropped, the grebes returned to Clear Lake and today are once again thriving at approximately their pre-1954 population levels. Numerous other examples of biomagnification involving other chlorinated hydrocarbons and heavy metals (methyl mercury at Minamata, for example) have since been described and illustrate the unanticipated effects which toxic substances can have as they move through ecosystems.

Hazards to Human Health

Although pesticides are used specifically to kill pests, many of them are quite toxic to humans as well. **Acute pesticide poisoning** may account for as many as 300,000 illnesses among American farm workers every year, most of them due to contact with organophosphate insecticides. Poison control centers in the U.S. report over 100,000 pesticide poisonings each year, with 23,000 victims sick enough to visit hospital emergency rooms. Approximately 20 Americans, mostly children, die annually from accidental pesticide poisoning (Benbrook, 1996). On a global basis, pesticides take a much higher toll: the World Health Organization estimates that in the Third World alone, acute poisonings among agricultural workers may be as high as 25 million annually (3% of the work force), with 1% dying as a result of their exposure (Jeyaratnam, 1990). Even these figures may be overly conservative, since field laborers in developing countries seldom seek medical treatment when they feel ill on the job and thus many cases of pesticide poisoning go unreported. While increased emphasis on pesticide safety and improved application equipment has contributed to a marked decline in acute pesticide-related deaths and serious illness in the industrialized nations, such is not the case in most developing countries. Few Third World farm workers receive any training in proper use of farm chemicals, which are commonly misused and overapplied. Adequate protective gear is seldom worn or even provided. Most pesticides in developing countries are applied manually (sometimes by reaching barehanded into a container of pesticidal dust and broadcasting it onto the target area) or by tractor, affording ample opportunity for dusts, mists, or vapors to be inhaled or absorbed through the exposed skin of the applicator. Since field workers seldom have access to running water while working, quick removal of pesticides spilled on garments or on the skin is not possible and workers frequently wear contaminated clothing home, exposing their children, pregnant wives, or elderly parents who are particularly susceptible to health damage from these poisons. Additional exposure to family members may occur when workers, unaware of the danger, bring home empty pesticide containers to use for storing food or water. Although strict adherence to label directions could prevent some of the problems associated with improper handling, storage, and application practices, in fact Third World farm workers seldom read the label instructions, either because they are illiterate or because labels are printed in a language they don't understand (the latter situation poses a safety concern even in the United States where many agricultural laborers read only Spanish and are thus unable to heed warnings printed in English). Even worse, in many developing countries pesticides are often transferred from the original container to another unlabeled receptacle so that the user, even if literate and multilingual, has no way of knowing what hazards the material might present—or even its identity. Finally, a future threat that hasn't received the attention it deserves is the question of what to do with sizeable stocks of outdated or unusable pesticides—many of them persistent chlorinated hydrocarbons such as dieldrin and DDT—more than 15 million pounds (7 million kg.) of which have accumulated in 35 developing countries. In many cases the containers in which these are stored are unlabeled, corroded, and leaking, posing serious problems of environmental pollution and future health problems. Yet,

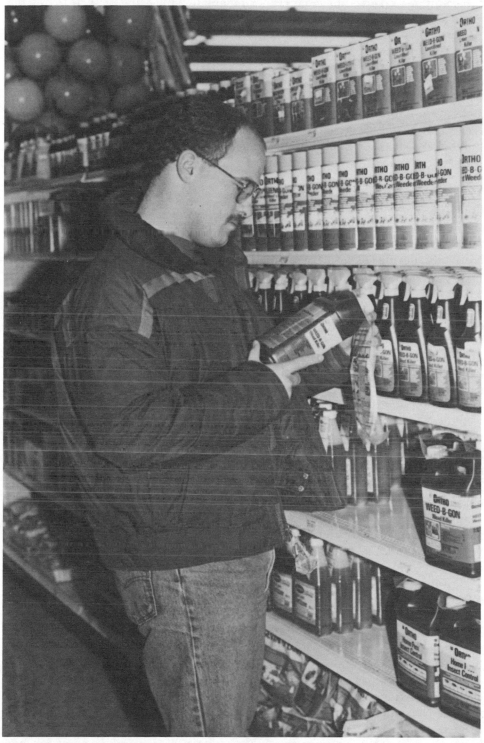

Consumers purchasing pesticides should read label information carefully before using the product. Many human health and environmental problems have been caused by overuse or misuse of these toxic chemicals. *[Author's photo]*

the countries involved have no proper means for disposing of such toxins nor the resources for cleaning up contamination that has already occurred (World Resources Institute, 1994).

To cause harm, a pesticide must be taken internally through the mouth, skin, or respiratory system. Most oral exposure is due to carelessness; for example, leaving poisons within reach of young children, smoking or eating without washing hands after handling pesticides, using the mouth to start siphoning liquid pesticide concentrates, eating unwashed fruit that was recently sprayed, or accidentally drinking pesticides that were poured into an unlabeled container. Exposure through the skin can occur when pesticides are spilled on the body or when wind-blown sprays or dusts come into contact with skin.

Reentering a field too soon after pesticide application or careless handling of discarded containers can also result in absorption of pesticides through the skin. The larger the skin area contaminated and the longer the duration of contact, the more serious the results of such exposure will be. Theoretically, dermal exposure could be reduced significantly through the use of protective clothing and equipment. In practice, however, such precautions are frequently ignored. Such gear is often expensive, cumbersome, and uncomfortable, especially during hot weather. All too often, applicators who know better fail to comply with safety recommendations and have been observed, in some instances, to ply their trade wearing little more than bathing suits! Poisoning due to inhalation is most common in enclosed areas such as greenhouses but can also occur outside when pesticide mists or fumes are inhaled during application or if the applicator is smoking.

Symptoms of acute exposure (i.e. "one-time" cases) include headache, weakness, fatigue, or dizziness. If poisoning is due to one of the organophosphate insecticides, the victim may experience severe abdominal pain, vomiting, diarrhea, difficulty in breathing, excessive sweating, and sometimes convulsions, coma, and death.

In contrast, **chronic pesticide poisoning** (low-level exposure over an extended time period) is characterized by vague symptoms that are difficult to pinpoint as having been caused by pesticide exposure (Bever et al., 1975). The greatest concern regarding chronic pesticide exposure, particularly to chlorinated hydrocarbons, is their potential for causing cancer or reproductive problems.

For many years **cancer** was the prime focus of concern regarding chronic effects of pesticide exposure. Beginning with its prohibition on the use of DDT in 1972, the EPA has gradually banned or restricted most of the chlorinated hydrocarbon pesticides, including endrin, aldrin, dieldrin, mirex, heptachlor, chlordane, and so on, largely because tests showed them to be carcinogenic to laboratory animals (however, these chemicals are still legal in many other countries and continue to be used extensively in developing nations because they are considerably less expensive than alternative products). The environmental consequences of this phaseout have been dramatic. In the United States, concentrations of these persistent pesticides in animal tissues have been steadily declining since the 1970s; certain bird populations which had nearly vanished by the late 1960s due to bioaccumulation of chlorinated pesticides have now largely rebounded. DDT levels in human breast milk also have plummeted by 90% since the EPA ban took effect (Schneider, 1994).

While the impact of pesticide exposure on cancer incidence is still provoking debate among the experts (in California, the largest case-control study to date, published in April 1994, contradicted results of previous research by finding no association between breast cancer and DDT exposure), a growing body of evidence supports the contention that **disruption of the endocrine and immune systems**, not cancer, constitutes the most serious long-term pesticide-related health concern. Since the endocrine hormones regulate a wide spectrum of bodily functions, including fertility and fetal development, compounds which interfere with such hormones have the potential for serious reproductive effects even at low levels of exposure. Scientists have now identified a number of pesticides, including many of the chlorinated hydrocarbons, as well as some synthetic pyrethroids and triazine herbicides, as potent hormone disruptors. Studies of wildlife populations have shown that exposure to these compounds can lead to abnormal sexual behavior (especially feminization of males), birth defects, and impaired fertility among the offspring of pes-

---

Figure 8-3   Dermal Absorption Rates As Compared with the Forearm

The seriousness of absorbing pesticide through the skin depends on the dermal toxicity of the chemical, the size of the contaminated skin area, the length of time the material is in contact with the skin, and the rate of absorption through the skin. As the diagram indicates, different parts of the body have very different rates of skin absorption.

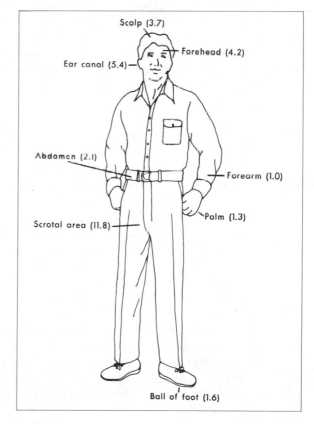

Source: *Illinois Pesticide Applicator Study Guide*, University of Illinois Cooperative Extension Service.

ticide-exposed parents (Curtis et al., 1993). Several of the more notorious pesticide-related tragedies have involved problems caused by the reproductive effects of chronic pesticide exposure. The nematicide DBCP (1,2-dibromo-3-chloropropane), for example, is known to have caused sterility among men in the California factory where it was manufactured, as well as among 1,500 male banana plantation workers in Costa Rica occupationally exposed to the chemical.

Immune system dysfunction can be provoked by either acute or sub-chronic exposure to many commonly used pesticides, including the herbicide 2,4-D and the insecticides malathion, parathion, aldicarb, carbofuran, and most of the chlorinated hydrocarbons (though most of these are no longer used in the United States, their residues persist in the environment). Young children, especially when malnourished, as well as elderly adults appear most vulnerable to pesticides' immuno-suppressive effects and tend to contract infectious diseases more frequently than individuals not exposed to pesticidal compounds. Pesticide-induced immunotoxicity may also be manifested as allergic contact dermatitis, a skin inflammation caused by immune system response to a foreign substance—in this case to pesticide exposure. Allergic reactions to contact with even minute amounts of pesticides can become chronic and in some cases have resulted in farm workers becoming permanently disabled due to chemical intolerance.

The adverse health and reproductive effects induced by endocrine-disrupting pesticides are further compounded when exposure to two or more such chemicals occurs simultaneously. The insecticides endosulfan and DDT, for example, interact synergistically to produce estrogenic effects 160–1,600 times greater than those of either pesticide alone. Inasmuch as humans are constantly exposed to numerous endocrine-disrupting chemicals (including PCBs and dioxins as well as pesticides) in air, food, and water, levels of exposure until now regarded as "safe" may need to be reassessed (Arnold et al., 1996).

The human health impact of **dietary exposure** to pesticides via residues on food has attracted intense public scrutiny since the 1987 publication of a study by the National Academy of Sciences, estimating that traces of carcinogenic fungicides, insecticides, and herbicides on the nation's fruits, vegetables, and meat could result in an additional 20,000 cancer deaths per year in the United States. These findings were hotly disputed by agrichemical interests but generated intense public concern over how pesticides are regulated. Demands for reform received added impetus following publication in June 1993, of a long-awaited study by the National Academy of Sciences on pesticides in the diets of infants and small children. Critical of the EPA's outmoded approach for setting pesticide tolerance levels on agricultural produce (a system based on the estimated amount of any given pesticide the "average person"—i.e. an adult—is likely to consume as part of a typical American diet), NAS scientists concluded that the youngest members of society are at enhanced risk because they consume more calories per unit of body weight and because their diet is less varied than that of adults. Immediately after publication of the NAS report, a second study dealing with the same issue was released by the Environmental Working Group, a nonprofit research organization, stating that up to 35% of an individual's lifetime dose of dietary pesti-

BOX 8-4

"EPA-Registered"—Synonymous with "Safe"?

The war against insects, rodents, and weeds is waged as vigorously on the home front as it is on the farm. An estimated 85% of American households harbor· pesticidal products—three to five different chemicals, on average—which are used in prodigious amounts. Unfortunately, unlike farmers and structural pest control operators who are required to pass competency examinations, the average householder purchasing roach poison at the neighborhood supermarket or weed killer at the local hardware store has little or no idea of the health and environmental hazards such chemicals pose. After all, the reasoning goes, the label says "EPA-Registered"—if the government permits them to be sold, they must be safe! This conviction reflects a dangerous ignorance of how pesticides are regulated and leads to a degree of complacency on the part of the general public that isn't warranted by the facts.

Early laws regulating pesticides focused almost exclusively on protecting farmers from untested, ineffective products, requiring truthful labeling but ignoring issues pertaining to human health or environmental impacts. By the late 1940s, as pesticide use began to grow rapidly, Congress enacted legislation requiring that chemical companies register their pesticide labels with the designated federal agency (originally with the U.S. Department of Agriculture; in 1970 that role was transferred to the newly created Environmental Protection Agency). Thus the fact that a particular product is government-registered simply means that it is legal to sell and use in the United States—nothing more.

By 1972, mounting evidence of human poisonings and environmental damage convinced policymakers that a shift in regulatory focus was needed. In that year, the old Federal Insecticide, Fungicide, and Rodenticide Act (FIFRA) was amended to incorporate health and environmental considerations into the regulatory process for the first time. These amendments mandated that henceforth chemical manufacturers must submit health and safety test results for new pesticides when they seek EPA registration for those products. Basic risk-benefit standards were developed for evaluating data submitted, the intention being to exclude high-risk pesticides from the market while maintaining a plentiful supply of effective chemical products. Also in 1972, EPA canceled the registration of DDT, thus ending its legal use in the U.S., and shortly thereafter the agency took similar action with eight additional chlorinated hydrocarbon insecticides.

With this seemingly protective regulatory framework in place for over 25 years and with most of the notorious cancer-causing insecticides banned from the U.S. marketplace, why shouldn't average citizens assume that pesticides currently in use pose negligible health risks? Several reasons:

1. The requirement for safety testing prior to registration was not retroactive; hundreds of our most acutely hazardous pesticides were already registered for use at the time the new law was enacted. The vast majority of these remain on the market, since only through a lengthy process of collecting scientific data and proving that these "grandfathered" chemicals pose "unreasonable adverse effects" can EPA end their legal use.

2. Safety testing data is required only

for the active ingredients in a given pesticidal product, yet the largest part, by volume, of many pesticides is made up of so-called "inert" ingredients, for which no safety testing is required. Some of these inerts are themselves known to be toxic, yet label requirements don't even require that they be identified by name. Pesticide legislative reform efforts regularly target the issue of inert ingredients, so far to no avail.

3. Many pesticides introduced since 1972 obtained EPA approval on the basis of fraudulent testing data. A scandal that made headlines in the early 1980s revealed that the largest independent laboratory in the nation, Industrial Bio-Test (IBT), had contracts with a number of chemical companies to supply the toxicological test data required for EPA registration. Only after more than 200 pesticides had been registered on the basis of falsified test results did it become known that the company had perpetrated the most massive scientific fraud ever committed in the United States. The IBT executives involved in the deception eventually received prison sentences, convicted of conducting and distributing fake scientific research and then attempting to cover-up their crimes. Nevertheless, many of the products registered during this period remain on the market today. A 1988 amendment to FIFRA requires EPA to speed up the re-registration process for pre-1972 pesticides and for those originally tested by IBT, but that project is far behind schedule and isn't expected to be completed until sometime after 2010.

4. Pesticides like DDT and chlordane, which were removed from commercial use due to concern for their chronic health effects, particularly cancer, were replaced largely by organophosphate or carbamate products that were often more acutely toxic than the chemicals they replaced, and are thus more dangerous to use. A number of these compounds are still commonly purchased for home or garden use, largely because they are cheaper than the less toxic pyrethrins.

In spite of many decades of pesticide regulation, overall use of chemical poisons continues to increase and the health and environmental risks they pose are as great as ever. Following common-sense safety precautions certainly can reduce the chance of injury or illness; follow label directions when using pesticides; keep pesticides in their original containers; keep them out of reach of children and pets; always wear protective clothing when applying chemicals; and avoid spraying when conditions are windy. Nevertheless, the decision to use chemical poisons always entails some degree of risk. Undeniably, pest problems need to be managed, but where nonchemical IPM approaches are equally effective, they represent the wiser, safer choice.

References
Benbrook, Charles M. 1996. *Pest Management at the Crossroads*. Consumers Union.

Schneider, Keith. 1983. "Faking It." *Amicus Journal* no. 4 (Spring).

cides occurs before the age of 5, largely because young children consume proportionately far more residue-laden fruits and vegetables than do adults. Preschoolers, for example, eat 6 times the amount of fruit consumed by their parents and drink 31 times more apple juice in relation to their body weight than do adults. Thus pesticide residue safety levels based on presumed "average" diets may greatly underestimate the actual amount of exposure received by a young child. These reports also emphasized the fact that most foods contain residues of several different pesticides (a laboratory analysis performed on one pear identified 11 different pesticidal compounds), not just one, and that the sources of pesticide exposure are not restricted to food, but frequently include drinking water, lawn chemicals, and household insecticides as well.

All of these factors suggested that the existing regulatory framework for ensuring food safety was inadequate to protect society's most vulnerable members—infants and children (National Research Council, 1993; Curtis et al., 1993). In response to these concerns, the U.S. Congress in 1996 enacted comprehensive legislation to reform and modernize the nation's laws dealing with food safety and the setting of pesticide tolerance levels. The **Food Quality Protection Act of 1996** now requires that when the EPA sets tolerance levels for pesticide residues on food, it must take into account available information on consumption habits of infants and children, as well as the neurological differences between adults and children that make the latter uniquely sensitive to the harmful effects of pesticide exposure. The law also requires EPA to take into account the cumulative effect of multiple residues when establishing pesticide tolerance levels in food, incorporating an additional tenfold margin of safety to protect children, infants, and babies *in utero* (Benbrook, 1996). Unfortunately, heightened awareness on the part of regulatory agencies and the public has not yet been translated into reduced exposure. The Environmental Working Group (EWG), in a follow-up to its 1993 study, reports that foods heavily consumed by youngsters are just as contaminated with pesticides today as they were in 1993. Citing U.S. Department of Agriculture data for 1996, EWG deplores the fact that residues of 67 pesticides were found on twelve of children's favorite fruits and vegetables, up from the 58 reported by USDA in 1993. Even more alarming is the fact that levels of residues known to be carcinogenic increased significantly between 1993 and 1996, while those identified as hormone-disrupting or neurotoxic had remained unchanged. With no concerted federal effort underway to reduce total pesticide use, concerned parents themselves may have to assume responsibility for limiting their children's exposure to pesticide residues in food (EWG, 1998).

Alternatives to Chemical Pest Control

As increasing numbers of pest species become resistant to available chemicals and as concerns over the long-range effects of pesticide exposure on human health and the environment continue to grow, the advisability of continuing to rely exclusively on chemicals for pest control is increasingly being questioned. In recent years a different philosophy of pest control has gained support, a strategy known as **Integrated Pest Management (IPM),** also referred to as "Low Impact Pest Control" or "Low Impact Sustainable Agriculture." After ascertaining that a pest problem does indeed exist, IPM practitioners combine various compatible methods to obtain the best control with the least possible environmental disruption. While the emphasis in IPM is on utilizing natural controls such as predators, food deprivation, or weather to increase pest mortality, it can include pesticide application also, but only after careful monitoring of pest populations indicate a need. Unlike the total chemical control approach, IPM recognizes the extraordinary adaptability of insects and does not attempt to eradicate a particular pest entirely, but rather is aimed at keeping pest populations below the threshold level at which they can cause significant economic loss. Among the methods which could be included in an IPM strategy are the following.

Natural Enemies

Many of our most serious insect and weed pests (such as Japanese beetle, gypsy moth, fire ant, kudzu, water hyacinth, and so on) are foreign imports which rapidly multiplied here in the absence of their natural enemies. Other native pests have caused serious problems only after their predators were eliminated by indiscriminate use of pesticides. Over the past several decades the government has imported more than 500 insect predators in an attempt to control alien species; about 20 of these are now providing significant control of several important pests. Laboratory breeding of large populations of insect predators in hopes of overwhelming certain pests is also being attempted. Great success in controlling scale insects and mealybugs in citrus orchards was obtained by mass-rearing and release of vedalia beetles and certain parasitic wasps. Home gardeners and organic farmers are urged to purchase praying mantis egg cases or containers full of ladybird beetles to achieve effective nonchemical insect control.

Pathogens and Parasites

A further step in biological warfare against insects involves introducing various disease agents into a pest population. About a dozen such microbial pathogens are now being commercially developed or produced in various parts of the world. Two kinds of bacteria have been approved for commercial pest-control in the United States—*Bacillus popilliae*, which causes the milky spore disease of Japanese beetles, and the widely used *Bacillus thuringiensis (Bt)*, which can be used effectively against more than 100 species of caterpillars, including gypsy moth larvae, currently the target of widescale *Bt* applications (Dotto, 1979). Unfortunately, recent observations indicate that some pests are now developing resistance to the toxin released by *Bt*. Among the more promising new approaches to enlisting pathogens in the war against pests is the use of certain fungi whose spores can penetrate an insect's exoskeleton, growing inside the host and digesting its tissues, resulting in death within a few days. One such fungus, *Metarhizium flavoviride* (referred to simply as "*Mf*"), is being tested for control of grasshoppers and migratory locusts; another, under the trade name *Biopath*, has been formulated as a bait and is now commercially available for cockroach control.

Pathogenic viruses are also being viewed as offering a promising method of pest control, since viral diseases in nature are frequently devastating to pest populations. A commercial preparation of polyhedrosis virus that kills the cotton bollworm is being tried on a limited scale and field experiments on control of corn earworm by one of the baculoviruses have been so encouraging that commercial preparations are now available.

A protozoan, *Nosema locustae,* has been successfully employed to control grasshopper infestations. *Nosema* spores sprayed on a wheat-bran bait are consumed by the grasshoppers, germinate inside the insect's stomach, multiply rapidly, and devour the grasshopper from inside.

Sex Attractants

Certain chemical stimulants (pheromones) control many aspects of insect behavior, including mating. Sex pheromones may be excreted by the female to attract the male, or vice-versa. Some of these female pheromones have been synthesized in the lab and used to bait traps which can attract males from miles around. When the males enter the trap, expecting to encounter a receptive female, they are caught by a sticky substance on the bottom or sides of the trap. A variation on this method has yielded encouraging results in efforts to manage the codling moth, an insect whose larvae cause serious economic losses to pear and apple growers. To disrupt mating of adult moths, farmers place 10-inch-long twist-ties impregnated with female moth pheromone high in the branches of their orchard trees. When approximately 400 of these devices are used per acre, the "come hither" scent so pervades the area that male moths are thoroughly confused, not knowing in which direction to fly to find a mate. In this situation, most females remain unmated, lay infertile eggs, and over time the pest populations decline (Benbrook, 1996).

Because the use of sex attractants as just described is effective only against adult insects interested in finding a mate, the technique is of limited effectiveness, since much crop damage is caused by insect larvae. In addition, because most pest species concentrate on a single crop, the market demand for any particular pheromone is relatively small. If the prospects for sales profits are not sufficiently attractive, manufacturers have no interest in producing them! Therefore, in recent years the prime strategy regarding sex attractants has shifted from using them to capture or confuse pest insects to one of employing pheromones to lure "good bugs" (i.e. predator species) into problem areas where they will then encounter—and eat—the "bad bugs." Since most predators eat a wide variety of pests, the same predator species could be a useful control agent in many different situations, a fact which significantly enhances the market demand for its pheromone. Conversely, pheromones could be used to entice the beneficial insects to leave a field prior to chemical spraying against crop pests, thereby avoiding such problems as target pest resurgence or secondary pest outbreaks.

Insect Growth Regulators (IGRs)

Sometimes referred to as "biorational" insecticides, IGRs are chemicals that are identical to or closely mimic growth substances produced by the target pest. IGRs act either as **chitin inhibitors,** preventing proper development of the exoskeleton after molting, or, more commonly, as **juvenoids.**

Table 8-3 Contrasts Between Traditional Pest Control and IPM for Structures

Element	Traditional Approach	IPM Approach
Program strategy	Reactive pest control	Preventive pest control
Program tactics	Routine pesticide application	Applied facilities management
Coordination with sanitation programs	Minimal	Extensive
Inspection & monitoring	Minimal	Extensive
Public education	Minimal	Extensive
Pesticide application	By schedule	By need
Insecticidal formulations	Sprays & aerosols	Baits
Method of applying sprays	Often on exposed surfaces	Mostly crack & crevice treatment
Use of space sprays & fogging	Extensive	Minimal
Approach to rodent control	Emphasis on poisons	Emphasis on trapping, sanitation, exclusion
Approach to bird control	Emphasis on poisons	Emphasis on exclusion
Toxic liability risk	High	Low

Source: Adapted from "Integrated Pest Management (IPM): Desk Guide for Facilities Managers." Prepared by A. Greene, U.S. General Services Administration July 20, 1992 Revision.

When the larvae of insects with a complete metamorphosis (fleas or mosquitoes, for example) contact or ingest juvenoids, these synthetic analogs of natural insect hormones prevent them from emerging as adults after pupating, thus effectively disrupting their life cycle. For insects characterized by a gradual metamorphosis (such as cockroaches) in which there is no pupal stage, nymphs may progress to adulthood but are abnormal in appearance and incapable of reproducing.

Several IGRs are now widely used in structural and public health pest control operations (usually in combination with standard insecticidal formulations to provide a "double whammy"), offering long-term control of such troublesome pests as cockroaches, fleas, ants, and floodwater mosquitoes. An obvious limitation to the use of insect growth regulators is that they are only useful against insects which cause damage as adults; many of the worst agricultural pests are larvae (such as caterpillars and grubs) against which IGRs are ineffective.

Sterile Insect Technique

This method relies on the mass-rearing and release of huge numbers of male insects that have been sterilized by chemicals or radiation, usually gamma rays or X-rays. Subsequent mating of a normal female with a sterile male thus results in the production of infertile eggs. If the ratio of sterilized males to normal males is sufficiently large, most matings will be unsuccessful and over several generations pest populations will die out (the technique is most effective against target pest species in which the females mate only once). This technique was employed with great success on Zanzibar's Unguja Island to eradicate a tsetse fly population that for decades had caused devastating losses to livestock herds. Over a two-year period, from 1995–1997, an average of 50,000 male flies, mass-reared in laboratories and sterilized with a 28-second dose of gamma radiation, were released from airplanes across the island. With sterile males outnumbering the natural population of normal males by 50 to 1, induced sterility among females increased rapidly and the density of fly populations steadily dropped. The ultimate result was the total elimination of tsetse flies from the island (Kinley, 1998). Earlier SIT programs had been similarly successful in eradicating the screw-worm fly from Curacao, Florida, and parts of Central America, as well as the Mediterranean fruit fly from Chile, Mexico, and California. Not applicable in every setting, SIT is most effective when the pest population is geographically isolated, making re-invasion of the area with normal males unlikely.

Host Plant Resistance

Selective use of crop plant species that exhibit genetic resistance to pests is probably the most ecologically sound method for reducing losses due to plant diseases and nematodes. Practical applications of this IPM technique are numerous. For example, savvy home gardeners, as well as commercial growers, insist that the tomato seeds or plants they purchase be varieties bearing code letters that indicate resistance to several important tomato pathogens (e.g. the designation "**VFNT**" informs a prospective buyer that the plant in question is resistant to **V**erticillium wilt, **F**usarium wilt, **N**ematodes, and **T**obacco mosaic virus—and thus is unlikely to require chemical pesticide applications to keep the plant disease-free). Host resistance also has been successfully employed against insect pests such as the Hessian fly, grape phylloxera, spotted alfalfa aphid, rice stem borer, and corn earworm.

More recently, genetic engineering has provided new and faster techniques for introducing desired characteristics from one species into another. In 1995, EPA approved the first **transgenic** corn variety engineered for resistance to the European corn borer (ECB), a moth whose larvae cause significant yield reductions throughout the Corn Belt each year. Scientists spliced a gene for toxin production from the bacterium *Bt* into the DNA of corn, creating a hybrid plant that can poison an invading corn borer larva on the first bite. Theoretically, a crop plant that "fights back," killing its enemy before sustaining damage itself, offers big benefits in terms of increased yields to farmers and a sharp decline in the use of chemical pesticides. In practice, however, widescale planting of *Bt* transgenic varieties seems to be accelerating the

BOX 8-5

Toxic Toys

One of the cardinal rules of pesticide safety is to store containers of these dangerous poisons out of the reach of inquisitive children. Nevertheless, recent research findings suggest that such common-sense measures alone are not sufficient to protect youngsters from pesticide exposure in the home and point to other steps concerned parents can take to reduce the risk of chronic pesticide poisonings.

Surveys have demonstrated that approximately 90% of all U.S. households use pesticides at one time or another—to kill ants marching across the kitchen floor, treat flea-infested pets, eradicate roaches, or to rid the pantry of rodents. Licensed pest control professionals called to a residence to deal with a pest problem typically utilize application methods which leave minimal residues or opportunity for chemical exposure. However, in the all-too-frequent instances when well-meaning but untrained householders or apartment janitors attempt to do the job themselves, pesticides are often carelessly applied and can constitute a serious chemical exposure risk to the small children and full-time homemakers who, on average, spend 21 hours or more each day indoors. During this time, a significant amount of direct contact with pesticides can occur.

The risk is most acute when pesticides are applied inside the home using foggers or pump sprayers that distribute chemicals over broad surfaces such as baseboards, floors, and carpets. In such situations, the finely dispersed liquid particles quickly settle out onto horizontal surfaces. Until recently it was widely assumed that so long as residents avoided contact with still-wet objects,

minimal human health risk was involved. Indeed, the standard warning not to re-enter a treated room for one to three hours following a pesticidal application is based on measurements of pesticide concentrations in the air and the assumption that conditions are safe once droplets have settled and thus are unlikely to be inhaled.

These assumptions have been shattered by a recent study in which residues of the organophosphate insecticide chlorpyrifos (Dursban®, Lorsban®), one of the most widely purchased products for indoor insect control use, were monitored in a treated home over a period of several weeks. Although particles of chlorpyrifos did, indeed, settle out of the air within a few hours after spraying, exposure risk to residents was only beginning at that point. As is true with many pesticides, chlorpyrifos particles gradually volatilize and are carried throughout the room by air currents, moving far beyond the surfaces at which they were directed. This volatilization process continues for more than a week, well beyond the few hours for which product labels suggest caution. Once in the vapor phase, pesticides like chlorpyrifos can diffuse into objects possessing adsorptive properties, including plastic toys, foam-filled pillows, bedding, and especially soft stuffed animals and dolls. Concentrations of pesticides on these items continue to increase over time, generally peaking a week or two after spraying. Toys thus can become important "sinks" and reservoirs for pesticide exposure inside the home; particularly at risk are youngsters between the ages of 6 months and 5 years whose close contact with these objects can lead to absorption of pesticides through the skin or via mouth contact (inhalation of vapors is considered a negligible risk). Because washing contaminated items with soap and water doesn't completely remove adsorbed pesticides, efforts to protect little ones from chemical exposure must focus on prevention rather than after-the-fact actions.

Reconsideration of the need to spray hazardous chemicals indoors, particularly when safer, equally effective formulations (e.g. baits) are readily available, should be the first line of defense. If a decision is made to proceed with spraying, researchers recommend that toys or other objects likely to adsorb chemical vapors not be stored in an open room for at least one week after the pesticidal application, longer if more than one application is made.

While there is no documented clinical evidence demonstrating a cause-and-effect link between pesticide-contaminated toys and childhood illness, public health officials are concerned that toxic toys, added to known dietary intake via pesticide residues on fruits and vegetables, as well as in drinking water, represent but one more source of chronic exposure to health-threatening chemicals—but one that can easily be avoided.

Reference

Gurunathan, Somia et al. 1998. "Accumulation of Chlorpyrifos on Residential Surfaces and Toys Accessible to Children." *Environmental Health Perspectives* 106, no. 1 (Jan):9–16.

development of resistance to *Bt* toxin among insect populations. Although several *Bt*-transgenic crop varieties (corn, cotton, sorghum, potatoes) are now being grown commercially, some plant scientists predict that the usefulness of these products of biotechnology will be short-lived, as pest populations inevitably respond to selective forces by developing genetic resistance to the *Bt* toxin much more rapidly than they would if exposure were not so widespread. If such warnings prove accurate, the usefulness of this valuable and safe biopesticide will be undermined in as little as three to nine years and a much-heralded new technology will be rendered obsolete (Harris, 1991; Kaiser, 1990).

Sanitation

For control of insect and rodent pests in residential areas or business establishments, the most effective way to reduce pest numbers and keep them low is to apply the basic principles of sanitation. To survive and multiply, pests need a source of food, water, and harborage. If these are in short supply, large pest populations cannot be maintained. Strict observance of the rules of good housekeeping—promptly cleaning up spilled food, storing foods in tightly sealed containers, keeping garbage cans covered, avoiding use of mulch immediately adjacent to building foundations, mowing tall grass or weeds near structures, locating woodpiles at some distance from dwellings, regularly collecting and disposing of animal feces—will be far more effective in eliminating flies, rodents, and roaches over the long term than is the temporary palliative

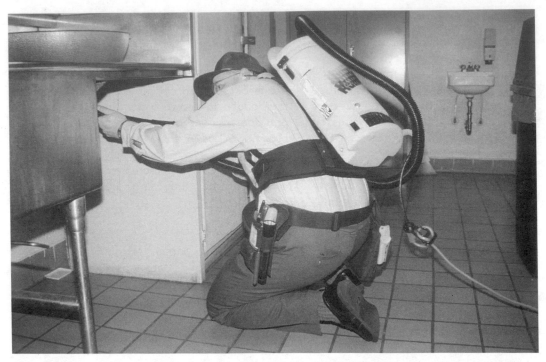

Nonchemical pest control: use of a vacuum equipped with a HEPA filter will remove cockroach allergens in addition to cockroach bodies, feces, and egg capsules. *[Courtesy of Pest Control Technology]*

of pesticidal spraying. Similarly, structural alterations such as screens, metal or cement barriers, and caulk applied to cracks and crevices can assist in "building out" certain household pests. Habitat modification such as changing water in birdbaths frequently, keeping roof gutters free of twigs and leaves to permit complete drainage of rainwater, and maintaining premises free of discarded articles which could collect water can be very effective in reducing mosquito breeding. Pesticide use can provide a "quick fix," but without adherence to good sanitary practices, control will be temporary at best.

None of the above methods alone is the total answer to effective pest management. However, in the proper combination after an accurate assessment of a specific pest situation, IPM techniques promise a safer, more ecologically sound, and ultimately more successful approach to limiting pest damage than does total reliance on chemicals.

References

Akre, Roger D., and Elizabeth A. Myhre. 1994. "The Great Spider Whodunit." *Pest Control Technology* 22, no. 4 (April).

Arnold, S. F., D. M. Klotz, B. M. Collins, P. M. Vonier, L. J. Guillette, Jr., and J. A. McLachlan. 1996. "Synergistic Activation of Estrogen Receptor with Combinations of Environmental Chemicals." *Science* 272 (June 7):1489–92.

Aspelin, A. L. 1994. *Pesticides Industry Sales and Usage: 1992 and 1993 Mar-*

ket Estimates. U.S. Environmental Protection Agency, Washington, DC (June).

Benbrook, Charles M. 1996. *Pest Management at the Crossroads.* Consumers Union.

Bever, Wayne, et al. 1975. *Illinois Pesticide Applicator Study Guide.* Cooperative Extension Service, University of Illinois College of Agriculture, Special Publication 39.

Blair, Aaron, et al. 1987. "Cancer and Pesticides Among Farmers." *Pesticides and Groundwater: A Health Concern for the Midwest.* The Freshwater Foundation.

Centers for Disease Control and Prevention (CDC). 1998. "Statewide Surveillance for Ehrlichiosis, Connecticut and New York, 1994–1997." *Morbidity & Mortality Weekly Report* 47, no. 23 (June 19).

———. 1997. *New Map of the U.S. Distribution of Aedes albopictus—1997.* National Center for Infectious Diseases, Division of Vector-Borne Infectious Diseases, Fort Collins, CO.

———. 1994. "Human Plague—United States, 1993–1994." *Morbidity & Mortality Weekly Report* 43, no. 13 (April 8).

Curtis, Jennifer, Tim Profeta, and Laurie Mott. 1993. *After Silent Spring: The Unresolved Problems of Pesticide Use in the United States.* Natural Resources Defense Council.

Dotto, Sydia. 1979. "Battling the Bugs." *Science Forum* (March/April).

Environmental Working Group (EWG). 1998. "Same As It Ever Was." Press Release, May 21, 1998.

"EPA Study Links Pesticide Use with Ground Water Contamination." 1992. *Environmental Health Letter*, Jan. 28.

Fahnestock, A. L. 1996. "Revitalizing Roundup." *Farm Chemicals Magazine*, (July):16-17.

Flint, M. L., and R. vanden Bosch. 1981. *Introduction to Integrated Pest Management.* Plenum Press.

Harris, M. K. 1991. "Bacillus Thuringiensis and Pest Control," Letter to the Editor, *Science* 253 (Sept. 6):1075.

Jeyaratnam, J. 1990. "Acute Pesticide Poisoning: A Major Global Health Problem." *World Health Statistics Quarterly* 43.

Kaiser, J. 1996. "Pests Overwhelm *Bt* Cotton Crop." *Science* 273 (July):423.

Kinley, David H. 1998. "Aerial Assault on the Tsetse Fly." *Environment* 40, no. 7 (Sept).

Lin, B. H., M. Padgitt, H. Delvo, D. Shank, and H. Taylor. 1995. *Pesticide and Fertilizer Use and Trends in U.S. Agriculture.* Agricultural Economic Report No. 717, Economic Research Service, U.S. Department of Agriculture, Washington, DC.

Mallis, Arnold. 1997. *Handbook of Pest Control.* 8th ed. Mallis Handbook and Technical Training Company.

Mansur, Mike. 1994. "The Food Chain." In *The 1994 Information Please Environmental Almanac.* World Resources Institute, Houghton Mifflin Co.

Meister Publishing Co. 1996. *Ag Consultant Magazine* (March).

Nash, Linda. 1993. "Water Quality and Health." In *Water in Crisis: A Guide to the World's Fresh Water Resources,* edited by Peter H. Gleick. Oxford University Press.

National Research Council. 1993. *Pesticides in the Diets of Infants and Children*. National Academy Press, Washington, DC.

———. 1992. *Neem: A Tree for Solving World Problems*. National Academy Press, Washington, DC.

Parker, Tracey. 1994. "Recent Studies Document the Complex Ways Pesticides Affect Birds." *Journal of Pesticide Reform* 14, no. 1 (Spring).

Perkins, John H. 1982. *Insects, Experts, and the Insecticide Crisis*. Plenum Press.

Pimental, David, et al. 1991. "Environmental and Economic Impacts of Reducing U.S. Agricultural Pesticide Use." *Handbook of Pest Management in Agriculture*. CRC Press.

Rosenstreich, David L., Peyton Eggleston, Meyer Kattan, Dean Baker, Raymond G. Slavin, Peter Gergen, Herman Mitchell, Kathleen McNiff-Mortimer, Henry Lynn, Dennis Ownby, and Floyd Malveaux. 1997. "The Role of Cockroach Allergy and Exposure to Cockroach Allergen in Causing Morbidity Among Inner-City Children with Asthma." *New England Journal of Medicine* 336, no. 19:1356-1363.

Schneider, Keith. 1994. "Progress, Not Victory, on Great Lakes Pollution." *New York Times,* May 7.

U.S. Environmental Protection Agency (USEPA). 1996. *Pesticide Resistance Management: Issue Paper for Pesticide Dialogue Committee Meeting*. Office of Pesticide Programs (June 25).

"Warning About Pesticide Spraying Looms for International Flyers." 1994. *Environmental Health Letter,* Feb. 2.

Williams, Ted. 1993. "Hard News on 'Soft' Pesticides." *Audubon* (March/April).

World Health Organization (WHO). 1997. "Human Plague in 1995." *Weekly Epidemiological Record* 46 (Nov. 14):289.

World Resources Institute. 1994. *World Resources 1994–1995*. Oxford University Press.

CHAPTER 9

Food Quality

It was no uncommon occurrence for a man to find the surface of his
pot of coffee swarming with weevils after breaking up hardtack in it,
which had come out of the fragments only to drown; but they were easily
skimmed off and left no distinctive flavor behind. If a soldier cared to do
so, he could expel the weevils by heating the bread at the fire.
The maggots did not budge in that way.

—John Billings ("Hardtack and Coffee," 1887)

A Civil War veteran's reflections on the insect-infested fare common to
both Yankee and Confederate armies during that historic conflict give evidence that concerns about food contamination and food quality in general are
nothing new. From time immemorial, humans have grappled with such problems as protecting stored food supplies from insects, molds, and rodent infestations; they learned through sad experience about natural toxins in certain
foods and found they could minimize risk of food poisoning through proper
processing and cooking practices. Until the mid-1800s however, problems
related to food quality were relatively limited and localized because most people raised their food at home or purchased it from local producers. Consumers
carefully inspected purchased items for signs of insect infestation, sniffed
meat and fish to detect spoilage, and in general served as their own food
inspectors. Government regulation of food quality prior to the 20th century
was extremely limited, focusing primarily on commercially baked bread. Early
bread laws were designed to standardize the weight of loaves in relation to the
price of wheat; i.e. they were essentially price-fixing laws. Other regulations
prohibited adding foreign substances such as ground chalk or powdered beans
to flour. Subsequent laws provided for inspection of weights and flour quality
(Janssen, 1975).

In the United States, prior to the 1900s the federal government had no
role in regulating food safety, that issue being regarded as solely a prerogative
of state or local authorities (NRC, 1998). However, in the decades following

317

the Civil War, the close-to-home food production, distribution, and marketing systems that had prevailed virtually everywhere in the world up to that time began experiencing revolutionary change. The explosive growth of cities and the expansion of transportation networks—especially the railroad—during these years gave birth to an organized food industry that became national, and eventually global, in scope. The subsequent introduction of refrigerated railcars (and later refrigerated trucks and air freight) made possible the shipment of hitherto unavailable fresh meat and produce to markets thousands of miles distant from their place of origin. This rapid development, in the absence of regulation, was marred by deplorably unhygienic conditions and frequently unethical practices.

The biggest scandal of 19th century food establishments involved the widespread practice of **adulteration**—the deliberate addition of inferior or cheaper material to a supposedly pure food product in order to stretch out supplies and increase profits. Adulteration has undoubtedly been practiced on a small scale for millennia by unscrupulous merchants when they thought they could get away with it, but the anonymity of large, unregulated corporations selling foodstuffs to faceless consumers hundreds of miles away gave great impetus to the proliferation of this age-old practice. Substances used as adulterants in some cases were harmless ingredients, cheating consumers only in a financial sense; in other instances, the adulterants consisted of toxic substances that posed a serious health threat to those consuming the adulterated products. Some foods commonly adulterated during the 18th and 19th centuries included: 1) black pepper commonly mixed with such materials as mustard seed husks, pea flour, juniper berries, or floor sweepings; 2) tea, adulterated on a large scale with leaves of the ash tree which were dried, curled, and sold to tea merchants for a few cents per pound. Green China tea was often adulterated with dried thorn leaves, tinted green with a toxic dye; black Indian tea was more easily adulterated by collecting used tea leaves from restaurants, drying and stiffening them with gum and then tinting them with black lead, also toxic, to make them look fresh; 3) cocoa powder "enriched" with brick dust; 4) milk supplies extended with water; 5) coffee blended with ground acorns or chicory.

Perhaps even more alarming were revelations in the late 19th century that many of the food colors and flavorings in widespread use were poisonous, e.g. pickles colored bright green with copper, candies and sweets brightly tinted with lead and copper salts, commercially baked bread whitened with alum, beer froth produced by iron sulfate. By the turn of the century, over 80 synthetic agents were being used to color foods as diverse as mustard, jellies, and wine. Many had never been tested for adverse health effects and all were being used without any monitoring or regulatory controls; amazingly, some of these chemical additives had been developed as textile dyes and were never intended to be used in food products! Not surprisingly, contemporary accounts document a number of human illnesses and a few deaths attributable to consumption of toxic food colorants in those years (Tannahill, 1973; Henkel, 1993).

A growing awareness of such problems led to congressional passage in 1906 of the **Pure Food and Drugs Act**, one of the first federal laws intended to protect consumers against adulteration, mislabeling of foods, and harmful

ingredients in food. As a result of this act and of subsequent food quality legislation, instances of adulteration in the United States are now much rarer than
they were in former years, though regulations have had to be instituted from
time to time to prevent the gradual degradation of foods, such as the increase
in fat or ground bone content of hot dogs or the decrease in fruit content of
jams or fruit pies. However, occasionally flagrant abuses still do occur. In the
fall of 1993 the Flavor Fresh Foods Corporation of Chicago, as well as 11 of its
corporate officials, pled guilty to charges of defrauding consumers of more
than $40 million through sales of adulterated orange juice. For 12 years Fla-
vor Fresh had been marketing a product labeled as "100% pure orange juice
from concentrate," selling it widely throughout the Midwest. In reality, the
juice contained 55–75% beet sugar, along with other adulterants added to con-
ceal the substitution. The two-year investigation, which culminated in the
convictions of those responsible, demonstrated that unscrupulous attempts to
make a quick dollar at the public's expense are still a threat more than a century after the adulteration scandals of the late 1800s (Ropp, 1994).

Within recent years the focus of public attention regarding food quality
has shifted from adulteration to a concern over the presence of contaminants
and additives in our food supply. The fact that few people today produce their
own foods at home means that almost all of us, to a greater or lesser degree,
have no choice but to rely on foodstuffs produced by a massive food industry—
foods that contain many kinds of additives and, in some cases, contaminants
over which we have very little control. The widespread interest in "health
foods" is due, in no small measure, to the feeling of many people that industrially produced food is somehow less safe and less nutritious than the "natural"
foods of yesteryear. Representatives of the food industry and, indeed, many
scientists, counter that chemical additives are both safe and essential to
ensure an abundant supply of food at affordable prices to a still-growing population. In an attempt to understand the nature of the debate and the rationale
behind existing or proposed regulations, it is helpful to distinguish between
those substances accidentally introduced into foods and those deliberately
added to prevent deterioration or to enhance taste or attractiveness.

Food Contaminants

Substances accidentally incorporated into foods are called **contaminants.** Such contaminants include dirt, hairs, animal feces, fungal growths,
insect fragments, pesticide residues, traces of growth hormones or antibiotics,
and so on, that are introduced into food during the harvesting, processing, or
packaging stage. They serve no useful purpose in the finished product and are
presumed to be harmful unless proven otherwise. (In many cases, however,
common food contaminants constitute an aesthetic affront to consumers
rather than an actual health threat; for example, the thought of eating a fly
wing hidden among the oregano leaves on a frozen pizza may be repugnant,
but it won't make you sick—at least not if you don't see it!) Certainly every
effort should be made to keep our foods as free from contamination as possible;
however, it has never been, and probably never will be, possible to grow, harvest, and process crops that are totally free of natural defects. In order to
ensure that foods are never contaminated by even a few insects, rodent hairs

or droppings, etc., we would have to use much larger amounts of chemical pesticides and would thus risk exposing consumers to the potentially greater hazard of increased levels of toxic residues. Current philosophy holds that it is wiser to permit aesthetically unpleasant but harmless natural defects rather than pouring on more synthetic chemicals. For this reason, the Food and Drug Administration (FDA) has established what it terms **defect action levels**, specifying the maximum limit of contamination at or above which the agency will take legal action to remove the product from the market. It is important to understand that such defect action levels are not average levels of contamination—the averages are considerably lower—but represent the upper limit of allowable contamination. Defect action levels are set at that point where it is assumed there is no danger to human health. Some examples of existing defect action levels are shown in Table 9-1.

Several groups of food contaminants that are less visible but more worrisome are the traces of antibiotics (see Box 9-1) and growth hormones in meat products and toxic pesticide residues on fruits and vegetables. The issue of hormone-treated meat has been rankling relations between the European Union (EU) and major meat-exporting countries (primarily the U.S., Canada, Australia, and New Zealand) since 1989, when the EU banned imports of meat from animals treated with growth hormones. Such hormones, illegal in Europe, are widely used by American beef producers, administered in the form of slow-release pelleted implants inserted under the skin on the back side of the ear flap. Approximately 90% of feedlot cattle in the U.S. are implanted, as are a smaller percentage of sheep (neither hogs nor chickens receive hormone implants). Beef producers have used hormones for decades to hasten weight gain of their animals while using less feed and to produce meat with a lower fat content. The EU justifies its prohibition of hormone-treated meat as a consumer safety measure, fearing that lingering traces of hormones in meat at the time of slaughter could pose human health risks. However, scientific studies in both the United States and Europe conclude there is no evidence of such a threat from the five hormones the FDA has approved for use in U.S. livestock (estradiol, testosterone, progesterone, trenbolone acetate, and zeranol). Because humans daily produce several thousand times larger quantities of these hormones through their own metabolic activities than they are exposed to via meat consumption, health authorities conclude hormones in meat present negligible risk. The Codex Alimentarius Commission, an international group that makes recommendations on food safety questions, has given its support to the use of natural hormones in meat production; similarly, a group of 15 European scientists presented findings to the British Veterinary Association concluding that use of growth-promoting hormones in cattle presents no human health threat. Nevertheless, for reasons U.S. negotiators suspect are due to domestic economic and political considerations, the 15 nations comprising the EU continue to defy a ruling by the World Trade Organization stating that their ban on imports of hormone-treated meat is a violation of free trade rules. Since European public opinion is strongly supportive of the ban, resolution of this dispute appears unlikely in the near future (Hanrahan, 1996).

Early in 1994 a genetically engineered growth hormone intended to boost milk production was introduced onto the market by Monsanto, a move which

Table 9-1   Examples of Food Defect Action Levels

Product	Defect	Action Level
Apricots, canned	Insect filth	Average of 2% or more by count insect-infested or insect-damaged
Beets, canned	Rot	Exceeds average of 5% by weight of pieces with dry rot
Broccoli, frozen	Insects and mites	Average of 60 aphids, thrips, and/or mites per 100 grams
Cherries, maraschino	Insect filth	Average of over 5% rejects due to maggots
Corn, canned	Insect larvae (corn ear worms, corn borers)	Two or more 3 mm or longer larvae, cast skins or cast skin fragments of corn ear worm or corn borer, the aggregate length exceeding 12 mm in 24 pounds
Curry powder	Insect filth	Average of more than 100 insect fragments per 25 grams
	Rodent filth	Average of more than 4 rodent hairs per 25 grams
Olives, pitted	Pits	Average of more than 1.3% by count of olives with whole pits and/or pit fragments 2mm or longer measured in the longest dimension
Peanut butter	Insect filth	Average of 30 or more insect fragments per 100 grams
	Rodent filth	Average of 1 or more rodent hairs per 100 grams
	Grit	Gritty taste and water insoluble inorganic residue is more than 25 mg per 100 grams
Tomatoes, canned	Drosophila fly	Average of 10 fly eggs per 500 grams; or 5 fly eggs and 1 maggot per 500 grams; or 2 maggots per 500 grams

BOX 9-1

Abusing a Valuable Resource

Antibiotics represent one of the great medical advances of the 20th century, relegating once-dreaded bacterial killers to the status of easily curable diseases. Unfortunately, overuse and misuse of these valuable pharmaceutical resources are contributing to the build-up of antibiotic resistance in an ever-increasing number of bacterial populations. Blame for this current state of affairs is widely shared by physicians and patients alike. For years microbiologists have criticized the overuse of antibiotics to treat conditions that would soon be resolved without medication, as well as the misuse of these drugs against viral infections or other health problems that don't respond to antibiotic treatment. The need for more judicious medical use of antibiotics in the face of increasing bacterial resistance is gradually being accepted by doctors and by the general public, but few people are aware that another source of microbial exposure to these drugs is posing a major human health threat.

For decades the widespread use of antibiotics in the livestock and poultry industries has sparked bitter controversy between agro-pharmaceutical interests and food safety experts. Of the 50 million pounds of antibiotics produced in the United States each year, over 40% are used for food animals. Of this amount, about one-fifth is administered for veterinary purposes, to treat animal diseases, while the remainder is incorporated in subtherapeutic amounts into animal feed and trough water to enhance growth and weight gain. Both of these uses have the potential for fostering development of antibiotic resistance among bacterial populations, yet livestock producers have vigorously—and successfully—lobbied against

regulatory controls. Claiming that antibiotic use is necessary to produce affordable meat and poultry, industry spokespersons long argued that no scientific evidence exists to show the practice has adversely affected human health. That argument can no longer be made; by the late 1990s, irrefutable proof of humans infected with antibiotic-resistant foodborne microbes had been traced to drug-resistant bacterial strains in animals.

In 1998, CDC researchers reported that one strain of *Salmonella* (DT104) has rapidly acquired resistance to five of the antibiotics commonly used against it: ampicillin, chloramphenicol, streptomycin, tetracycline, and the sulfonamides. In just seven years—from 1989 to 1996—the percentage of DT104 samples testing positive for multi-drug resistance climbed from 0.6 to 34%, even though the number of human *Salmonella* infections remained relatively constant during the same time period. Although the majority of *Salmonella* infections run their course without need for medication, a small percentage (3–10%) result in dangerous bacteremia (i.e. bacteria invading the bloodstream), requiring antibiotic treatment. If the causative pathogens fail to respond to such treatment, the situation could become life-threatening.

Further evidence of a cause-and-effect relationship between human disease and antibiotic use in meat production made news in 1999 when resistant bacterial isolates from people stricken with *Campylobacter* food poisoning were shown to have the same "DNA fingerprint" as *Campylobacter* strains found on chicken products. Currently, the most common form of bacterial food poisoning in the U.S., *Campylobacter* infections are generally treated, when necessary, with fluoroquinolone antibiotics such as ciprofloxacin. In the early 1990s, fluoroquinolone-resistant *Campylobacter* was quite rare—slightly over 1% of all reported cases—and virtually all of these were acquired during foreign travel. In 1995, the use of fluoroquinolones to treat respiratory infections in poultry flocks was approved by the FDA over the vigorous objections of CDC scientists concerned about the widescale exposure of chickens to a relatively new human drug that the medical community hoped would remain effective for many years. Their worries appeared well-founded, since similar approval of fluoroquinolones for veterinary use in Spain in 1990 had resulted in resistant human *Campylobacter* isolates soaring from almost 0% in 1989 to 30–50% in 1991. As the CDC had feared, within a year after licensure of fluoroquinolone for use on poultry farms, cases of domestically acquired ciprofloxacin-resistant human *Campylobacter* infections began to climb in the U.S., reaching 14% by 1998. Since pharmaceutical companies have no new wonder drugs currently in the pipeline, health authorities are increasingly worried that the livestock industry's profligate use of the same antibiotics needed to treat human disease represents the reckless squandering of a vital resource (of the 17 classes of antibiotics used as growth promoters in food animals, 6 are also used to treat human diseases).

In response to these developments, the Food and Drug Administration has belatedly launched a revision of its guidelines for approval of new animal antibiotics and for monitoring the effects of old ones. FDA is proposing that drug companies do additional tests on new products to determine whether they have the ability to foster the development of antibiotic resistance. Health and consumer advocates argue that the FDA initiative doesn't go far enough, insisting that no drug used to treat human disease should be licensed as an animal growth promoter. Such a prohibition has already been widely adopted in Europe, where increasing numbers of human illnesses due to use of antibiotics for meat production led to a ban on this practice by the European Union (something the FDA says it lacks the authority to do). Nevertheless, although the World Health Organization has recommended a phase-out of the practice, political pressures and seeming public indifference have stymied efforts in the United States to take meaningful action before it's too late.

References

Glynn, M.K. et al. 1998. "Emergence of Multidrug-Resistant Salmonella Enterica Serotype Typhimurium DT104 Infections in the United States." *New England Journal of Medicine* 338, no. 19 (May 7):1333-1338.

Smith, K.E. et al. 1999. "Quinolone-Resistant Campylobacter jejuni Infections in Minnesota, 1992–1998." *New England Journal of Medicine* 340, no. 20 (May 20):1525–1532.

provoked an outpouring of concern from some consumer groups (as well as from some dairy farmers worried about milk surpluses and falling prices). The hormone, alternatively known as **rBGH** (recombinant Bovine Growth Hormone) or **BST** (Bovine Somatotropin), is injected into dairy cows every 14 days, resulting in a 10–15% increase in milk production. After extensive studies evaluating its safety and efficacy, the Food and Drug Administration approved sale of the hormone, making rBGH the first commercially important product of agricultural biotechnology to be incorporated into the nation's food supply. In spite of FDA assurances that there is no human health risk associated with rBGH, many consumer groups remain wary. Critics charge that, by raising milk output per cow, the hormone puts additional stress on the animals, increasing the likelihood of udder infections and thereby necessitating more use of antibiotics and other drugs—thus resulting in more chemical residues in milk. The FDA insists the government has safeguards in place to monitor milk supplies for traces of antibiotics and bacteria and will destroy any milk that is tainted. In 1998, after examining new evidence, the Joint Expert Committee on Food Additives, comprised of representatives of the United Nations' Food and Agriculture Organization (FAO) and World Health Organization (WHO), reconfirmed its position that use of rBGH is safe. Nevertheless, the United States remains the only major country to permit use of the hormone and many American consumers, still unconvinced, are paying premium prices for organically produced milk rather than relying on government assurances of safety (FAO, 1998).

Pesticide residues in food can result from direct spraying of crops or from the consumption by livestock of pesticide-contaminated fodder, traces of which can then be translocated into meat, eggs, or milk. EPA has established **tolerance levels** for all pesticides used on food crops representing the maximum quantity of a pesticide residue allowable on a raw agricultural commodity. Such tolerances constitute the federal government's principle means of regulating pesticide residues in food. These levels are based on results of field trials performed by pesticide manufacturers and reflect the maximum residue concentrations likely when farm chemicals are applied properly. In essence, tolerance levels are set on the basis of good agricultural practices and not on considerations of human health. In 1987 the National Research Council (NRC) of the National Academy of Sciences published an alarming report estimating a significant increase in cancer mortality among American consumers due to ingestion of certain pesticide residues on food, even when the amounts of such chemicals are within the established tolerance levels. A subsequent NRC report issued in 1993 questioned whether existing tolerance levels, established on the basis of estimated adult food consumption patterns, were sufficiently protective of children's health. The report pointed out that youngsters consume more chemically tainted fruit in relation to their body size than do adults and, because of their rapid rate of growth and development, they are more vulnerable than older people to toxic chemicals in food (NRC, 1993; 1987). These concerns led Congress to include a provision in the 1996 **Food Quality Protection Act** that EPA consider the consumption habits and unique vulnerability of children when setting tolerance levels and must be able to guarantee that any tolerance level approved by the agency is safe for children (Merrill, 1997).

While the findings contained in the 1987 and 1993 NRC reports demonstrate the need for strict controls, the National Academy of Sciences contends that under the current U.S. regulatory system, pesticide residues on food pose a negligible health threat to the general population. In a 1996 report, the National Research Council pointed out that although traces of pesticide residues are detectable in food and water virtually everywhere, the amounts present on U.S.-grown crops are typically very low and do not present a significant risk of cancer or other health problems (NRC, 1996).

On rare occasions chemicals may contaminate foods through sheer carelessness or criminal neglect by processors. One of the largest and most costly incidents of chemical food contamination in recent years created havoc in Belgium in 1999 when dioxin-contaminated oil was mixed with animal fat added to livestock feed. The tainted fodder was subsequently distributed to more than a thousand farms throughout Belgium and fed to poultry, hogs, and cattle. The problem was only discovered when chickens stopped laying eggs and subsequently died. Laboratory analysis of the feed revealed the presence of dioxin, but Belgian government officials failed to notify the public or the European Union of this fact and took no immediate action. When the news finally broke more than a month later, pandemonium erupted and virtually every food that might possibly have been contaminated was stripped from grocery shelves. Throughout Europe a ban on Belgian pork, beef, poultry, and eggs was imposed; even the U.S. and some Asian countries refused to accept certain Belgian farm products. Losses to the Belgian agricultural sector, heavily dependent on exports, were estimated at more than $850 million. Although no human illnesses appear to have occurred among unknowing consumers who ate tainted meat or eggs, the incident prompted demands throughout the 15-member European Union for stronger food safety measures (the EU has no equivalent to the United States' Food and Drug Administration) to prevent such problems in the future.

Food Additives

More controversial than the accidental, often unavoidable, food contaminants are the approximately 2,800 food **additives,** substances intentionally added to food to modify its taste, color, texture, nutritive value, appearance, resistance to deterioration, and so forth. The years since the end of World War II witnessed explosive growth of the food chemical industry, as food processors responded to public demand (or occasionally created public demand) by promoting a host of new products—convenience foods, frozen foods, dehydrated foods, ethnic foods, low-calorie foods. Many of these products could not exist in a world free of additives. Nevertheless, a great many people are automatically suspicious of additives with long, unfamiliar, often unpronounceable names; reading the list of ingredients on virtually any supermarket package, can, or bottle seems a bit like a quick tour of a chemical factory. However, there's nothing inherently evil about using additives, provided that the chemical in question has no adverse effect on human health and performs a useful function. Many substances that can technically be termed "additives" have been in use for thousands of years—sugar, salt, and spices constitute just a few examples. Some additives come from natural sources; lecithin, derived from soybeans or corn, is used as an emulsifier to achieve the desired consistency in products such as cake mixes, non-dairy creamers, salad dressings, ice cream, and chocolate milk. Other food additives are factory made but are chemically the same as their natural analogs. The synthetic vitamins and minerals added to foods to improve nutritive value are examples of these; identical in chemical composition to natural vitamins and minerals found in food, they are preferentially used because they are less expensive and more readily available. Such synthetic additives frequently are more concentrated, more pure, and of a

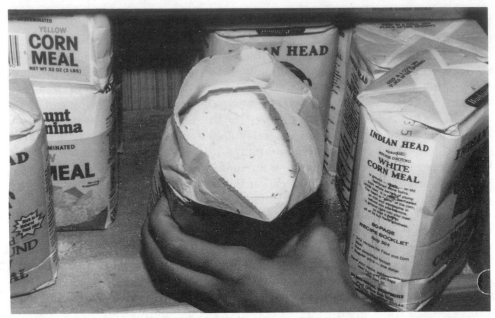

What consumer wouldn't be repulsed by the sight of rodent feces in a package of corn meal? *[NYS Department of Agriculture and Markets, Division of Food Safety and Inspection]*

more consistent quality than some of their counterparts in the natural world. The use of synthetic vitamins and minerals in food over the past half century has had a profound impact on public health in the United States, virtually eliminating certain deficiency diseases that in former years afflicted large numbers of Americans. The addition of vitamin D to milk, iodine to table salt, and niacin to bread has relegated rickets, goiter, and pellagra, respectively, to nearly nonexistent status in this country. Other additives perform such useful functions as retarding spoilage, preventing fats from turning rancid, retaining moisture in some foods and keeping it out of others.

Most people don't quarrel about additives used for these purposes. What does concern many scientists and laypersons alike is that a not-insignificant number of chemicals are used as food additives for purely cosmetic purposes— and many of these have been shown to be toxic, carcinogenic, or both.

Until 1958, food processors wishing to use a new additive were free to do so unless the FDA could prove that the additive in question was harmful to human health. With the passage of the Food Additives Amendment to the Food, Drug, and Cosmetic Act in that year, the situation was reversed: the manufacturer of any proposed food additive or new food-contact chemical (e.g. packaging materials, equipment liners) now has to satisfy the FDA that the product is safe before it can be approved for use. Proof of safety must include such considerations as: 1) the amount of the additive that is likely to be consumed along with the food product; 2) the cumulative effect of ingesting small amounts of the additive over a long period of time; and 3) the potential for the additive to act as a toxin or a carcinogen when consumed by humans or animals (Foulke, 1993). Approval can be rescinded by the FDA at any time if new information indicates that the additive in question is unsafe.

While protection of public health is the main intent of the Food Additives Amendment, the law is also designed to prevent consumer fraud by prohibiting the use of preservatives that make foods look fresher than they really are. A case in point is the regulation forbidding the use of sulfites on meats, since these restore the red color, deceptively lending a just slaughtered appearance to a variety of meat products. On the other hand, sodium nitrite, another additive recognized for its ability to "fix" the red color of fresh meats, can legally be added to meat, fish, and poultry because its primary purpose is to act as a preservative, deterring both spoilage and botulism, a deadly disease caused by the presence of a bacterial toxin. Because it is now known that nitrites can react with other compounds in food to produce **nitrosamines,** substances known to be carcinogenic, food processors wishing to use the additive must take precautionary measures to severely limit nitrosamine formation (Foulke, 1993).

Undoubtedly the section of the Food Additives Amendment that has generated the most heated controversy in recent years is the **Delaney Clause,**

Table 9-2 Common Types of Food Additives

Group	Purpose	Examples
Antioxidants	prevent fats from turning rancid and fresh fruits from darkening during processing; minimize damage to some amino acids and loss of some vitamins	BHA, BHT, propylgallate
Bleaching Agents	whiten and age flour	benzoyl peroxide, chlorine, nitrosyl chloride
Emulsifiers	to disperse one liquid in another; to improve quality and uniformity of texture	lecithin, mono- and diglycerides, sorbitan monostearate, polysorbates
Acidulants	maintain acid-alkali balance in jams, soft drinks, vegetables, etc., to keep them from being too sour	sodium bicarbonate, citric acid, lactic acid, phosphoric acid
Humectants	maintain moisture in foods such as shredded coconut, marshmallows, and candies	sorbitol, glycerol, propylene glycol
Anti-caking compounds	keep salts and powdered foods free-flowing	calcium or magnesium silicate, magnesium carbonate, tricalcium phosphate, sodium aluminosilicate
Preservatives	control growth of spoilage organisms	sodium propionate, sodium benzoate, propionic acid
Stabilizers	provide proper texture and consistency to ice cream, cheese spreads, salad dressings, syrups	gum arabic, guar gum, carrageenan, methyl cellulose, agar-agar

which flatly prohibits the use in food of any ingredient shown to cause cancer in animals or humans (people who question why the FDA bans certain moderately carcinogenic food dyes yet takes no action against cigarettes have to be reminded that the Delaney Clause pertains solely to carcinogenic food additives, not to carcinogens in general; if a food processor should propose to add cigarette smoke as a flavoring to, say, cured meats, this would undoubtedly be prohibited under the Delaney Clause). While many environmental groups feel that the Delaney Clause constitutes the public's sole line of defense against the deliberate addition of carcinogens to the nation's food supply, critics charge that the "zero tolerance" standard implicit in this mandate is unrealistic and an example of regulatory overkill which fails to recognize enormous advances in analytical techniques since the Delaney Clause was enacted in 1958. Whereas the best efforts at chemical analysis during the 1950s yielded results in the parts per million range, today's monitoring devices routinely detect the presence of chemical residues in the parts per trillion. New evidence for the existence of threshold levels of exposure for at least some carcinogens has added fuel to the debate as well (when the Delaney Clause was enacted it was presumed that *any* amount of exposure to a carcinogen, no matter how small, could result in cancer). The Food Quality Protection Act attempted to address these concerns to a limited extent when it amended the Delaney Clause in 1996 by excluding pesticide residues in processed food from regulation as food additives. The revised mandate now permits EPA to approve a tolerance level for residues of a carcinogenic pesticide so long as the agency determines that doing so presents a "negligible risk" (defined as no more than one cancer death per one million population) to consumers. For all other food additives, the "zero tolerance" standard explicit in the Delaney Clause remains intact and continues to generate heated debate (Merrill, 1997).

Since many hundreds of food additives were already in widespread use at the time the 1958 amendment was passed, a portion of this legislation exempted such substances from the rigorous safety testing demanded for new additives. Instead, additives already in common usage were designated "generally regarded as safe" and placed on what is referred to as the **GRAS list.** In order to remove a food additive from the GRAS list, the FDA must demonstrate that the substance in question is harmful. Original screening of existing food additives to determine whether they should be placed on the GRAS list was done rather haphazardly, and by the 1970s it was recognized that long-time usage is no firm guarantee of safety. More thorough studies of certain substances included on the GRAS list have resulted in withdrawal of approval for the use of such once-common food additives as cyclamates (artificial sweeteners suspected of being carcinogenic); safrole (mutagenic and carcinogenic extract of sassafras root, formerly used to give root beer its characteristic flavor); and a number of coal-tar dyes (long used as food colorings but delisted because they were shown to be carcinogenic or to cause organ damage).

Numerous other additives still on the GRAS list are considered of dubious safety by many researchers, yet remain in use due to lack of conclusive evidence or because of industry pressure on FDA regulators. Critics of current policy insist that food additives require a higher standard of care than other environmental chemicals and shouldn't be used if they present a health risk. They base this judgment on the fact that everyone is exposed to chemicals in food, not only those who voluntarily assume the risk. Varying levels of susceptibility among individuals and the effects of simultaneous exposure to other chemicals, including synergistic effects, have to be taken into consideration. Both MSG (monosodium glutamate), a flavor enhancer that can cause the headache, dizziness, nausea, and facial flushing sometimes referred to as "Chinese Restaurant Syndrome," and a group of sulfur-containing compounds known collectively as "sulfites" or "sulfiting agents," added to certain foods, drugs, and wine to prevent discoloration and spoilage, are examples of food additives that serve a useful purpose and pose no danger to the majority of consumers but which can provoke severe allergic reactions among a sizeable minority of sensitive individuals. Because of the vast processed food market, any miscalculation of risk can have far-reaching implications on a public which assumes and expects that special care is being taken with the nation's food supply. Nevertheless, although some health authorities recommend avoiding foods containing nonessential additives (such as artificial colors and flavorings) wherever possible, little evidence exists at present to indicate that the health of Americans is suffering due to the chemical food additives currently in use.

Foodborne Disease

Ironically, while questions dealing with the safety of chemical additives generate most of the public's concern regarding food quality these days, most cases of illness or death due to food involve a number of old-fashioned foodborne diseases commonly referred to as "food poisoning." Food poisoning can result from a variety of causes, including the following.

Natural Toxins in Food

The widely prevalent notion that all "natural" foods are safe and nutritious is a dangerous misconception. The faddish trend toward "living off the land" by collecting and eating various types of wild plants has led to a surge in food poisoning cases, according to some local public health officials. The fact is that there are many common plants, both wild and cultivated, that are poisonous, capable of causing ailments ranging from mild stomach disorders to a quick and painful death if consumed by the unwary. In addition, certain marine fish and shellfish species may contain toxins that induce severe illness or death. Some examples of plants or animals capable of causing a toxic reaction if eaten include the following.

Mushrooms. Mushrooms constitute a gourmet's delight, provided, of course, that the item in question is a nonpoisonous variety. The problem is that there is no simple rule of thumb for distinguishing between those wild forms which are safe and those which are not. Although only a relatively few of the thousands of species found in North America are poisonous, they may look very much like nonpoisonous species and frequently even grow together. One of the most poisonous types, the amanitas (one species of which is called the "Death Angel"), grow commonly in "fairy rings" in woods and on lawns. Just one or two bites of these alkaloid-containing amanitas can be fatal to an adult and, in fact, the vast majority of deaths due to mushroom poisoning are caused by these.

Water Hemlock (*Cicuta maculata*). Sweet-tasting but deadly, this relative of carrots, parsley, celery, and parsnips (to which it bears a strong resemblance) is the most toxic of all native North American plants. Because it is found throughout the continent, since it is quite similar in appearance to edible plants for which it is commonly mistaken, and because it is lethal even in small amounts, water hemlock is responsible for more deaths due to misidentification than is any other plant species. **Cicutoxin,** the poisonous substance in water hemlock, is a neurotoxin present in all parts of the plant and at every stage of development. Concentrations of the toxin are at peak levels in springtime and are highest in the root. In the fall of 1992, a 23-year-old Maine resident died three hours after taking just three bites from the root of a water hemlock plant he had collected in the woods (Centers for Disease Control, 1994). Children have occasionally suffered fatal poisonings after playing with toy whistles made from the hollow stems of water hemlock. Since there is no antidote for cicutoxin, about 30% of reported poisonings have resulted in the death of the victim.

Castor Bean (*Ricinus communis*). This attractive shrub-like plant is commonly grown as an ornamental foundation planting as well as commercially for its oil. The leaves of the plant are only slightly toxic, but the colorful mottled seeds can be deadly, containing a toxin called **ricin.** Children who chew on the seeds experience intense irritation of the mouth and throat, gastroenteritis, extreme thirst, dullness of vision, convulsions, uremia, and death. Only one to three seeds can kill a child; four to eight are generally required to cause fatality in adults.

Jimsonweed (*Datura stramonium*). This common weed contains toxic alkaloids in all parts of the plant. The seeds and leaves are especially dangerous; children have been poisoned by sucking nectar from the flowers, eating the seeds, or drinking liquid in which the leaves have been soaked. A very small amount can be fatal to a child.

Ergot (*Claviceps purpurea*). This fungus, which frequently infects cereal grains, especially rye, produces a toxic alkaloid, ergotamine, responsible for the serious type of food poisoning known as ergotism or "St. Anthony's Fire." When the fungal sclerotia growing on the rye grain are ground up with flour and subsequently consumed in bread, violent muscle contractions, excruciating pain, vomiting, deafness, blindness, and hallucinations can follow. One type of ergotism is characterized by severe constriction of the blood vessels, development of gangrene, and a painful death. Outbreaks of ergotism resulting in thousands of deaths were common until the 20th century, when the decrease in home milling and institution of quality control in commercial mills reduced the level of flour contamination. Even so, small outbreaks of ergotism are still reported from time to time. Interestingly, federal controls do not apply to rye grown for the organic foods market (Klein, 1979).

Aflatoxin. Another mycotoxin (fungal poison) already discussed in chapter 6, aflatoxins are produced by the mold *Aspergillus flavus* which grows on a wide variety of nuts, grains, and peanuts. When consumed, they can cause serious liver damage and are some of the most potent carcinogens known.

Certain Fish and Shellfish. Several different types of food poisoning are associated with eating various marine organisms. **Ciguatoxin,** a poison associated with certain fish living near reefs or rocky bottoms, has accounted for many food poisoning outbreaks in Florida and Hawaii (see Box 9-3). **Scombroid poisoning**, generally associated with deep-sea fish such as tuna and mackerel, is caused by ingestion of a toxin produced by certain bacteria acting on the flesh of fish which aren't handled properly after catching. Onset of symptoms such as a flushing of the skin, headache, dizziness, a burning sensation in the mouth, hives, and the usual gastrointestinal discomfort, generally occurs very quickly, averaging 1/2 hour after eating. **Paralytic Shellfish Poisoning (PSP)** results from eating shellfish such as oysters, clams, or scallops contaminated with saxitoxin, a nerve poison produced by microscopic dinoflagellates (algae). PSP is characterized by numbness in the mouth and extremities, gastroenteritis, and in severe cases, difficulty in speaking and walking; such symptoms occur within 30 minutes to 3 hours after eating. In a small percentage of cases death may result. Protection of the public against PSP depends on effective shellfish sanitation and inspection programs in the states where harvesting occurs.

Microbial Contamination

Microbial pathogens are responsible for the vast majority of food poisoning incidents; in the United States alone, estimates on the frequency of foodborne illness are as high as 81 million cases and 9,000 deaths annually (CAST, 1994), with an economic impact ranging from $6.6 to $37.1 billion in medical costs and lost productivity (Buzby and Roberts, 1997). Since U.S. surveillance and reporting systems for foodborne disease are woefully deficient, such estimates represent, at best, an educated guess and make it difficult to say with certainty whether or not the incidence of foodborne disease is increasing. However, authorities agree the problem is a serious one, as evidenced by numerous well-publicized food poisoning outbreaks and food recalls in recent years. Although the toll in human suffering is immense, food poisoning cases are often misdiagnosed by victims ("I just had a touch of 24-hour flu"), stoically endured (". . . it'll pass in a day or two"), and, due to the nature of symptoms, often not reported (who wants to discuss the details of a bout with diarrhea!). As a result, this entirely preventable malady fails to arouse the public attention it deserves and is perpetuated by widespread carelessness and ignorance of safe food-handling principles. Although food poisoning can, and frequently does, occur with foods prepared and consumed at home, public health officials are most concerned with the potential for large-scale poisoning inherent in the current trend towards more frequent eating outside the home and with the rapid growth and sheer size of the food service industry in the United States today. Institutions such as day care centers and nursing homes, as well as congregate feeding centers for the indigent or homeless also serve meals to large numbers of people on a daily basis. Diners at these facilities comprise many of those most vulnerable to foodborne disease: the very young,

BOX 9-2

Global Supermarket

Within a generation, America's food system has become international in scope. Food imports to the United States, totalling over 30 billion tons annually, have doubled since the 1980s. This booming trade is spurred in part by lower costs of production in many developing countries, but primarily is due to an ever-growing demand by health-conscious consumers for a year-round supply of fresh fruits and vegetables. Since home-grown strawberries, cantaloupes, peaches, or raspberries are virtually nonexistent during a northern mid-winter, such items on supermarket shelves in January obviously originated beyond our shores. Federal officials estimate that since 1995, at least one-third of all the fresh fruit eaten by Americans is imported. Mexico alone supplies as much as 79% of particular off-season crops and the percentage of fresh produce from other developing countries has been rapidly increasing as well.

This burgeoning international food trade has brought many nutritional and gustatory benefits to American consumers, but it has brought some unexpected problems as well. Whereas most foodborne disease outbreaks in the past were associated with contaminated meat or dairy products, recent years have witnessed a sharp increase in food poisoning incidents linked to fresh produce, much of it imported from countries where standards of health and hygiene are less rigorous than those in the U.S. Since fresh fruits are seldom cooked and many fresh vegetables likewise are eaten raw, consumers have little defense against invisible microbial hazards. While most foodborne disease problems, regardless of their place of origin, go unreported, several outbreaks during the late 1990s were large enough to prompt major investigations: in both 1996 and 1997, imported Guatemalan raspberries were linked with over 2300 cases of foodborne diarrhea caused by a previously little-known protozoan parasite, cyclospora, that inhabits Guatemalan waterways. Those same years also witnessed outbreaks of salmonellosis, affecting hundreds of people in 24 states, and ultimately traced to alfalfa sprouts whose seeds originated in Uganda and Pakistan; a food poisoning outbreak at a 1991 convention in Minneapolis was caused by Peruvian carrots contaminated with a new pathogenic strain of *E. coli* bacteria; and a 1991 cholera outbreak was blamed on tainted frozen coconut milk from an unlicensed processing plant in Thailand. In 1997 Japan experienced a food poisoning outbreak caused by contaminated radish sprouts from Oregon-supplied seeds.

Microbial hazards are not the only food quality concern associated with imported foods. The presence of toxic pesticide residues on produce entering the U.S. has been a long-standing issue among consumer advocacy groups. Since the mid-1970s, when EPA prohibited U.S. farmers from using a number of persistent pesticides on American agricultural crops, many consumers assumed their exposure to these chemicals had ceased. Unfortunately, many of the chemicals now banned in North America, Europe, and Japan are still being produced and are sold to developing nations, whose growers use them in prodigious amounts to produce crops for export to U.S. markets. The same tolerance levels set to regulate pesticide residues on domestic produce apply to imported fruits and vegetables, but since less than 1% of all food shipments are ever sampled, violations are seldom detected. On the rare occasion when a sample is taken and sent for laboratory analysis (a process that may require several weeks), the shipment in question isn't detained at the port of entry; therefore even when illegal residues are detected, it is usually too late to prevent marketing and consumption of the product. Also, negative test results don't necessarily mean the product is free of chemical residues, since many of the pesticides used by farmers in developing countries can't be detected by the analytical methods currently available to FDA personnel.

At the same time that safety concerns about imported foods have been mounting, federal efforts to detect problems have sharply declined; according to researchers at the Center for Science in the Public Interest, FDA inspectors at ports of entry are coping with workoads that have doubled since the mid 1990s and are able to check only one or two out of every 100 entering shipments. Authority for regulating food imports is split between USDA, which exercises jurisdiction over incoming meat and poultry, and FDA, which enforces standards on all other food products. Although both agencies maintain the position that imported food should meet the same standards of safety, composition, and labeling as U.S.-produced foods, their ability to ensure that such standards are met are sharply limited. While FDA inspectors can impound suspect imports, they cannot automatically block importation of food shipments from countries whose food safety system is known to be sub-standard. FDA officials are not permitted to inspect foreign processing facilities and are not allowed to travel abroad to investigate an on-going food poisoning outbreak unless invited to do so by the host government.

International efforts to remove trade barriers, thereby creating a "global economy," have further complicated food safety initiatives. Just as American farmers and ranchers charge that European bans on genetically altered seed or hormone-treated beef are efforts to limit competition rather than true safety issues, so growers in developing countries view U.S. scrutiny of their products as a thinly veiled form of protectionism. As one federal food safety official remarked, "Where we see a safety issue, they see a trade issue."

In the long term, safeguarding the quality of food imports can only be achieved through international efforts to develop uniformly high food safety standards in every country and to assist developing nations in improving methods of food production and drinking water quality. Until then, consumers are well-advised to wash fruits and vegetables well, or to peel them, before eating.

References

Gerth, J., and T. Weiner. 1997. "Imports Swamp U.S. Food Safety Efforts." New York Times (Sept. 29), A1.

National Research Council. 1998. Ensuring Safe Food From Production to Consumption. National Academy Press.

the very old, the ill, the immunocompromised. As the number of meals eaten away from home increases, the task of preventing foodborne disease grows more challenging.

It should be noted in passing that food *spoilage* is not the same thing as food poisoning. Spoilage involves the decomposition of foods due to the action of natural enzymes within food, to chemical reactions between food and containers, or to the activities of certain types of bacteria, fungi, or insects, resulting in unpleasant odors, taste, or appearance of the food. However, spoilage organisms do not produce toxins that would cause human illness if they were consumed, nor does eating food containing such live organisms induce sickness. The same cannot be said of food poisoning bacteria, whose presence is not betrayed by the appearance, smell, or taste of the food. The old term "ptomaine poisoning" often used in reference to food poisoning is a misnomer—there is no such thing. Ptomaines are foul-smelling chemical compounds produced by bacterial decomposition of proteins. Eating food containing ptomaines will not produce any illness.

The microbial culprits responsible for food poisoning can be grouped into three general categories: bacteria, viruses, and parasites.

Bacteria. Of the various foodborne diseases, the greatest number of outbreaks can be traced to ingestion of food containing certain pathogenic bacteria or bacterial toxins preformed in the food before it was eaten. Bacterial foodborne diseases are classified either as **infections** or **intoxications,** depending on whether illness is caused by consumption of large numbers of live organisms or by ingestion of preformed bacterial toxins, respectively. The more common types of bacterial food poisoning have rather similar symptom—symptoms which almost everyone has experienced at one time or another: diarrhea, abdominal pain, vomiting, dehydration, prostration, and often fever and chills in the case of bacterial infections (not, however, with intoxications). Onset of such symptoms usually occurs within 1-24 hours after eating the contaminated food, depending on the type of bacteria involved and the amount of food ingested. Examples of foodborne bacterial infections include the following.

Salmonellosis. Often referred to by more descriptive appellations such as "Delhi Belly" or "The Tropical Trots," salmonellosis is one of the most common bacterial foodborne disease in the United States, estimated in recent years to afflict about four million Americans annually. Caused by a number of species of the genus *Salmonella*, the disease is typically associated with eating poultry, meat, or eggs harboring large numbers of the rod-shaped bacterium. Nevertheless, numerous outbreaks have been traced to foods not generally associated with the disease: the largest salmonellosis outbreak in U.S. history, affecting an estimated 200,000 persons (16,000 laboratory-confirmed cases, many more unreported) in Illinois and several other Midwest states in the spring of 1985, was traced to milk. Although potentially an excellent medium for the growth of *Salmonella* and other foodborne pathogens, milk today is considered one of our safest foods due to pasteurization and high standards of sanitation in the dairy industry; less than 1% of all foodborne disease outbreaks in recent years have been traced to contaminated milk. Another unpleasant surprise has been the emergence since the mid-1980s of *Salmonella enteritidis* infections associated with whole, uncracked eggs. Contamination occurs when the bacteria are transmitted from infected hens via their ovaries into the developing egg; short of laboratory testing, neither egg producers or home cooks have any way of identifying which eggs are tainted. It is estimated that one out of every 10,000 eggs (approximately 4.5 million/year) is contaminated. Although the problem was originally confined to the northeastern U.S., it is now nationwide. As a result, today eggs are at or near the top of the list as prime contributors to food poisoning outbreaks in the United States. For this reason, much to the dismay of Caesar salad and homemade eggnog lovers, health agencies now strongly advise against the consumption of raw or undercooked eggs—hard-boiled is the only guarantee of safety!

Inside the small intestine, colonies of *Salmonella* continue to grow and invade the host tissue, irritating the mucosal lining. Sudden onset of disease symptoms most commonly occurs within 12–24 hours after eating the contaminated food, with 18 hours being the most common time interval; discomfort may persist for several days and some victims may remain carriers for months after all outward symptoms have disappeared, shedding bacteria in their feces and remaining capable of infecting others. Severity of the disease ranges from very mild to very severe, with young children, the elderly, and travelers often the most adversely affected. Among otherwise healthy adults, fatalities due to salmonellosis are rare (victims only *wish* they were dead!). However, salmonellosis can be life-threatening to the elderly, to patients in hospitals and nursing homes, and to people whose immune systems are compromised. As many as 2,000 Americans, most of them from one of these highly vulnerable groups, die of salmonellosis each year.

In addition to the obvious short-term effects of the ailment, salmonellosis sufferers may also develop serious chronic disorders as a result of their infection. About 2–3% of victims later contract chronic arthritis, while a much smaller percentage develop painful septic arthritis when the *Salmonella* bacteria invade the joints.

Campylobacter jejuni. One of several ailments often referred to as "Traveler's Diarrhea" because cases used to be most common among vacationers returning home from abroad, foodborne infections caused by *Campylobacter jejuni* have become the most common form of food poisoning in the United States. Estimates indicate the annual incidence of *Campylobacter* infections may be as high as 7 million, resulting in 100–1000 deaths. *C. jejuni* infections are characterized by high fever and bloody diarrhea, along with the nausea and abdominal pain typical of most foodborne ailments; symptoms generally persist for about a week but may last much longer. Most worrisome is the fact that as many as 10% of sufferers develop serious, long-term complications such as Guillain-Barre syndrome, arthritis, or meningitis. Consumption of undercooked chicken or turkey is by far the leading source of *C. jejuni* infections, since the organism is almost always present on poultry carcasses. The marked shift from beef to chicken consumption in the U.S. over the past 30 years has been accompanied by a rapid increase in *Campylobacter* foodborne disease. Other sources of infection include raw clams and other shellfish, inadequately cooked pork, and unpasteurized milk.

E. coli 0157:H7. Among the most dangerous foodborne pathogens, this nasty relative of the harmless *E. coli* strains that are normal inhabitants of the human gut was first recognized as a newly emerging public health problem in 1982. Several sporadic outbreaks occurred during the 1980s, but it was only in 1993 that the disease hit the headlines when four children died and hundreds of people became ill after eating hamburgers at several Jack-in-the-Box restaurants in the Pacific Northwest. Since then, numerous outbreaks have occurred throughout the U.S. as well as in Canada, Australia, Africa,

BOX 9-3

Barracuda Blues

Winter-weary tourists bound for the beaches of Florida or Hawaii seldom expect to encounter any health problems more serious than the occasional painful sunburn. Nevertheless, with growing frequency those living in or traveling to the tropics or subtropics have been falling victim to a bizarre foodborne ailment called **ciguatera fish poisoning**. This affliction, which experts claim is now the most common of all seafood-related illnesses in the United States, accounts for over half the cases of foodborne disease traced to fish consumption.

The active agent in ciguatera poisoning is *ciguatoxin*, produced by a marine dinoflagellate, the free-swimming unicellular alga *Gambiendiscus toxicus*, which lives in association with other algae growing on coral reefs in warm ocean waters. As small herbivorous fish browse on the algae and are, in turn, eaten by larger carnivorous fish, the fat-soluble dinoflagellate toxin is transferred up the food chain, becoming more concentrated at each higher trophic level. Biomagnification of ciguatoxin explains why most cases of ciguatera poisoning are linked to consumption of large reef-dwelling fish. In waters off the Florida coast, red snapper, grouper, and especially barracuda have been identified as the chief culprits; in Hawaii, amberjack is the fish most frequently implicated, while throughout the Pacific region red snapper is the leading cause of reported cases.

Since few physicians are familiar with ciguatera poisoning, it is often misidentified—not surprising since there is no diagnostic test for the ailment and symptoms can be confused with those indicating brain tumors, multiple sclerosis, or chronic fatigue syndrome. Just as there is no definitive test for diagnosis, similarly there is no cure at present (a recently developed treatment utilizing large intravenous doses of mannitol can significantly reduce the severity and duration of symptoms *if* it is administered within 48 hours after the toxin is consumed).

The best safeguard against ciguatera poisoning is prevention—something more easily said than done, since currently there is no commercially available test for determining whether fish are contaminated prior to sale. Nor can one rely on thorough cooking or other food processing methods as an assurance of safety, since ciguatoxin is not broken down by high temperatures, freezing, smoking, drying, or marinating. Therefore, about the only precaution a wary diner can take is to avoid eating large red snappers, groupers, or dishes containing unspecified ocean fish species (ciguatera is *not* associated with freshwater fish). Experts advise consumers *never* to eat barracuda; Dade County, Florida, has banned commercial sales of this fish, since more than a third contain dangerous levels of ciguatoxin (notwithstanding this prohibition, authorities worry that unwary customers may still be purchasing barracuda at dockside from independent fishermen). Fish *livers* should be uniformly avoided as well, since the poison accumulates in that organ. Because illness occurs only when concentrations of the toxin exceed a certain level, authorities concede that red snappers or groupers under five pounds are probably safe to eat; nevertheless, they recommend that other species such as mahi-mahi or yellowtail snapper might be a less risky choice.

In this era of rapidly expanding travel

for both business and pleasure, it's no longer unusual for a person to dine in Tampa, Honolulu, or Tahiti one day and be back home in Seattle, Chicago, or Pittsburgh the next. Consumers (and their physicians) must recognize that their culinary choices can have unexpected consequences and, should they choose to indulge in high-risk foods, be prepared to recognize the symptoms of once-exotic ailments and to seek prompt treatment.

Reference
Brody, Jane E. 1993. "Insidious Poison Lurks in Some Fish." *New York Times*, Sept. 8.

and Europe. In the summer of 1996, the largest outbreak to date killed three and sickened over 12,000 Japanese, mostly schoolchildren, in Sakai City near Osaka (Task Force, 1997). Estimates for the number of pathogenic *E. coli* infections occurring annually range from 10,000–20,000, resulting in approximately 50–100 deaths.

E. coli 0157:H7 normally inhabits the intestinal tract of healthy cattle and is excreted with fecal material. It frequently is found on the udders of cows and thus can be readily transferred to raw milk or to milking equipment. Although the number of bacteria that must be ingested to cause illness isn't known with certainty, most researchers suspect it is quite low—certainly lower than the dose required to cause salmonellosis. Once ingested, *E. coli 0157:H7* multiplies within the human digestive tract, producing a potent toxin that damages cells of the intestinal lining. These lesions permit blood to leak into the intestines, giving rise to the bloody diarrhea which generally develops within several days of eating contaminated food and is one of the characteristic symptoms of infection with this pathogen. Sufferers may also experience abdominal pains, vomiting, and nausea; only rarely will fever be present, however. In most cases the disease runs its course in 5–10 days and the victim recovers completely without treatment. Administration of antibiotics does nothing to improve a patient's condition and may cause kidney problems. Similarly, the use of antidiarrheal medicine is not advisable. For 2–7% of victims the consequences of infection are much more dangerous. If bacterial toxins pass through the damaged intestinal wall and enter the bloodstream, they travel to the kidneys where they can cause **hemolytic uremic syndrome (HUS)**, a serious ailment in which red blood cells are destroyed, leading to kidney failure and possible death. Such patients often require blood transfusions and kidney dialysis. Even with intensive care, 3–5% of patients who develop HUS die.

In the U.S., undercooked hamburgers were initially identified as the food most often implicated in *E. coli 0157:H7* outbreaks. Accordingly, public health agencies renewed their warnings to commercial food establishments and home cooks to cook beef to 160 °F until no traces of pink remain in the center and juices run clear. By the late 1990s, however, an even larger number of *E. coli* food poisonings had been traced to such seemingly harmless foods as alfalfa sprouts, lettuce, and unpasteurized fruit juices (in Japan as well, the Sakai City outbreak was ultimately linked to tainted radish sprouts). In all these cases, poor sanitation at some stage of production or processing allowed food to become contaminated with *E. coli*-contaminated cow manure. Since the

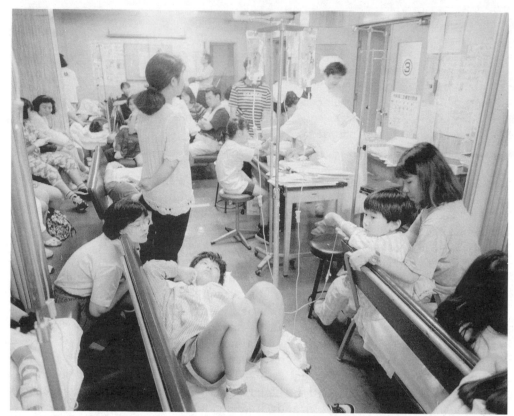

Victims of the 1996 food-poisoning outbreak in Sakai City, Japan crowd the local hospital to receive treatment. The outbreak, which sickened more than 12,000 people, was traced to *E. coli* *0157:H7*. [AP Photo/Yomiuri Shimbun]

foods mentioned above are seldom cooked prior to consumption, live pathogens were present on the food when it was eaten. As a result of these incidents, people at high risk of serious consequences if they contract food poisoning (e.g. young children, the ill or elderly, AIDS patients) are being advised simply to avoid eating sprouts and unpasteurized juice.

Listeriosis. Caused by *Listeria monocytogenes*, a pathogen associated with an extremely wide range of hosts (mammals, birds, fish, ticks, crustaceans) and commonly found in food-processing environments, this disease, once considered rare in human populations, has become a subject of increasing concern in recent years. Listeriosis outbreaks have most frequently been associated with contaminated cold cuts, hot dogs, milk, soft cheeses, and other refrigerated products generally eaten without further cooking. Listeriosis is particularly dangerous in pregnant women, where infection often results in septicemia, miscarriage, or stillbirth. Apparently healthy babies born to infected mothers may develop meningitis within a few days or weeks after birth. Newborns infected with *Listeria* have high fatality rates, as do older victims suffering from diabetes or compromised immune systems (AIDS victims or persons receiving corticosteroids, chemotherapy, radiation therapy, etc.).

Figure 9-1 Foodborne Illness Outbreaks Linked to FDA-Regulated Foods, 1990–1999

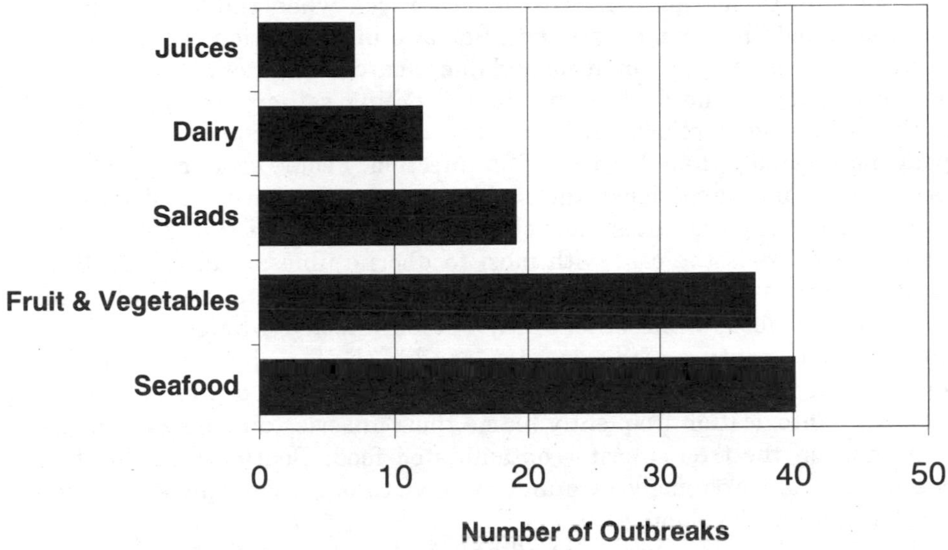

Number of Outbreaks

Source: Center for Science in the Public Interest.

Listeriosis, fortunately, is much less common than salmonellosis or *C. jejuni* diarrhea; on average, less than 2,000 people in the U.S. fall victim to listeriosis each year; fatality rates are high, however—of those stricken, approximately 20% die. Recognition that *Listeria,* unlike other microbial pathogens, grows vigorously at low temperatures, makes this organism a subject of serious concern to regulatory agencies and to the food industry in general, since refrigeration provides no assurance against bacterial multiplication. The FDA has set a "zero tolerance" requirement for presence of *Listeria* in foods.

Vibrio vulnificus. First described as a cause of human illness only in 1979, this free-living marine bacterium lives in unpolluted warm ocean waters. It is commonly found along the Gulf Coast in the southeastern U.S. where it may contaminate oysters and other shellfish. Most human illnesses result from consuming raw oysters, since the bacteria are readily killed by cooking. *V. vulnificus* infections are especially dangerous for individuals with preexisting liver disease resulting from alcoholism, viral hepatitis, or other causes, and for those with compromised immune systems (CDC, 1993).

Among bacterial foodborne intoxications the most important are:

Staphylococcus aureus. Sometimes known as "Roto-Rooter Disease" because of its violent onset, *Staphylococcus* intoxication is estimated to account for between 20–40% of all food poisoning cases. The causative bacteria are present in pimples, boils, hang-nails, wound infections, sputum, and sneeze droplets. People thus constitute the prime source of these organisms, which flourish in such proteinaceous foods as cooked ham, sauces and gravies, chicken salad, egg salad, cream pies and pastries, and so on. Growth of the bacteria within the food medium results in production of an enterotoxin (poison of the intestinal tract) which is not destroyed when the food is cooked. When consumed, the toxin causes irritation and inflammation of the stomach and intestine, resulting in vomiting and diarrhea. Since illness is produced by a poison already in the food at the time of eating rather than by bacterial growth within the victim's intestine, the effects of bacterial intoxication appear more rapidly than do those of an infection. People consuming *Staphylococcus* toxin may experience the sudden onset of vomiting and diarrhea within as little as 30 minutes after eating, although a period of 2–4 hours is more common. As is the case with most foodborne illness, individual differences in susceptibility will result in some people becoming quite ill after eating the tainted food, while others may not be affected whatsoever (Koren, 1980). Due to the nature of the symptoms and to the fact that duration of the illness is relatively brief, seldom persisting for more than a day or two, sufferers of staph intoxication frequently blame their miseries on "the 24-hour flu" rather than on the true culprit—contaminated food. Deaths from this foodborne disease are extremely rare and most victims recover quickly without any complications developing.

Botulism. The most serious of all bacterial foodborne diseases, botulism is caused by the spore-forming soil bacterium *Clostridium botulinum,* which, growing under anaerobic conditions, produces a deadly neurotoxin, the most poisonous substance known. Outbreaks of botulism have been most frequently associated with home-canned, low-acid foods such as beans, corn, beets, spinach, and mushrooms. This is because many home canners fail to realize that a long processing time (or a shorter time at high pressure in a pressure cooker) is necessary in order to kill the heat-resistant bacterial spores. If the spores survive, they can germinate and, in the absence of oxygen, multiply within the food medium, producing the deadly poison. If food contaminated with the botulism toxin is boiled for 15–20 minutes, the poison will be destroyed, but all too frequently such food is eaten uncooked or only briefly warmed, with disastrous results.

Commercially processed foods, mostly smoked fish or vacuum-packed items, occasionally have been identified as the cause of botulism outbreaks, as have some highly atypical sources. In the fall of 1983, one of the worst botulism outbreaks in U.S. history resulted in the hospitalization of 28 victims (one of whom subsequently died) who had eaten "patty melt" sandwiches at a restaurant in Peoria, Illinois. Surprised investigators ultimately identified sauteed onions as the cause of the problem. Contaminated with *C. botulinum* spores from the soil in which they grew, the onions were fried in margarine which provided a protective air-free shield for germinating bacteria. The bacteria proceeded to multiply in the incubating temperatures provided by the warming tray in the restaurant kitchen. By the time the onions were consumed many hours later, enough of the deadly botulinum toxin had been formed to cause the disease outbreak. In an unrelated incident in Baton Rouge, Louisiana, the following year, a restaurant patron was stricken with botulism after eating a foil-wrapped baked potato, warmed up from the previous day. The foil wrapping had provided the anaerobic conditions that permit-

BOX 9-4
Food Irradiation: New Solution for an Old Problem

Reason and scientific facts have finally triumphed over fear-mongering and misinformation as evidenced by the USDA's 1999 decision to approve regulations for the irradiation of raw meat to control foodborne pathogens. This action, qualified by the requirement that packages of irradiated meat must display the easily recognizable radura logo, followed FDA's determination in 1997 that meat irradiation is safe, does not change the taste or smell of meat, and does not significantly alter the nutritional value of the product. USDA had already granted approval of regulations governing irradiation of pork and poultry several years earlier, but the action on raw meat marked a major milestone in gaining acceptance of the new technology. It should be noted that USDA's action does not *require* that meat be irradiated but merely permits it for producers or marketers who desire to utilize this form of food preservation. Groups such as the Food Safety Consortium, most public health officials, and food industry representatives alike hailed the actions of the two federal agencies as important steps toward reducing the incidence of foodborne disease in the U.S. Some experts go so far as to liken approval of food irradiation to the advent of pasteurized milk in terms of its potential benefits to public health, and voice hopes that USDA will expand approval of irradiation to cover ready-to-eat meat products as well.

USDA'S action came after many years of controversy over the pros and cons of utilizing ionizing radiation to kill insect pests and microbial pathogens in food products and to extend the shelf life of fresh produce, meat, and fish. Although irradiation has been used since the mid-1960s to control pests in wheat and flour, as well as to prevent sprout development in potatoes, its broader use has been vociferously opposed by a handful of consumer groups fearful of the possible health or environmental implications. Although the supposedly dangerous "unidentified radiolytic products" these activists claim are present in irradiated food have never been found by independent researchers, anti-irradiation forces remain zealous to their cause. By threatening to boycott any food processor considering irradiation as a food safety measure, activists have had a disproportionate influence in forestalling policy initiatives. Past legislative decisions also have deterred wider adoption of food irradiation. Some observers suggest that commercial use of irradiation might have become common by the 1970s had Congress not amended the 1958 Food, Drug, and Cosmetic Act to designate irradiation as a "food additive" requiring FDA approval, rather than a "process" free of such restrictions. By the 1980s, FDA had given the go-ahead to use irradiation to kill trichina worms in fresh pork, to control insects and to slow ripening in fruits and vegetables, and to kill pests in dry herbs, spices, and tea.

Food irradiation has been approved in 40 other countries, including Japan and most European nations—all with a long history of high standards on food safety issues. Moreover, the process has been endorsed by the World Health Organization, the American Medical Association, and a number of public health organizations. Yet action in the U.S. was noticeably lacking until the early 1990s. The event that galvanized supporters of food irradiation and sparked new interest in the issue was the 1993 *E. coli 0157:H7* outbreak. Food scientists are convinced that, other than thorough cooking, irradiation is the only method known that can completely eliminate pathogenic *E. coli* in raw meat. Numerous food poisoning outbreaks and meat recalls due to contamination with *E. coli* and *Listeria* in the late 1990s reinforced the conviction among food safety experts that food irradiation's time had come.

Government approval doesn't guarantee that irradiated foods will be widely accepted in the U.S., however. Widespread public ignorance and misinformation about the technology has resulted in negligible market demand for irradiated foods; by the end of the 1990s, only a few retail stores were selling irradiated fruits and vegetables and the small amount of irradiated poultry produced was being purchased mainly by hospitals and one restaurant chain. Some consumers avoid irradiated food products due to erroneous ideas about what the process entails. The most common irradiation methods employ gamma rays (generally from a cobalt-60 source), X-rays, or electron beams which, unlike pesticides, accomplish the task for which they were intended without leaving any residue and without rendering the food itself radioactive (just as people receiving dental X-rays or luggage passing through an airport metal detector don't become radioactive themselves as a result). Ideally, the product is irradiated after it is packaged and sealed, thus preventing any opportunity for recontamination. Consumers handling or eating irradiated food are exposed to no radiation whatsoever. To ensure safe operations, food irradiation facilities must adhere to strict regulations promulgated by the Nuclear Regulatory Commission and the

Occupational Safety and Health Administration. Forty years of experience using irradiation to sterilize medical devices, a process very similar to food irradiation, have demonstrated that the technology has performed extremely well in terms of safeguarding employee health and transporting radioactive material. Public opinion surveys have revealed that if consumers are provided with objective, science-based information about food irradiation and about the risks of bacterial foodborne disease, most would purchase irradiated products so long as they are cost-competitive with non-irradiated food; up to 30% of consumers surveyed indicated a willingness to pay 10% more for the irradiated product as extra protection against bacterial contamination.

One consumer advocacy group, the Center for Science in the Public Interest, worries that widespread adoption of irradiation to control foodborne pathogens might tempt meat producers to become lax in maintaining high sanitary standards in processing facilities. Proponents, however, insist that irradiation will never be a substitute for hygienic processing and handling of food but is simply one additional tool—along with production of healthy animals, sanitary processing plants, and proper cooking—to ensure wholesome, pathogen-free food.

In a world where foodborne disease continues to sicken millions of people annually, where pests and spoilage continue to claim a hefty share of each year's harvest, and with increasing concerns about toxic chemical residues on food, the use of irradiation to ensure food safety deserves consumer acceptance.

Reference
Food Safety Consortium, 1999. News release (April 22), Washington, DC.

ted growth of bacterial spores on the potato skin, while remaining at room temperature overnight allowed multiplication of the organism and production of the toxin (Miller, 1984).

Botulism is first evidenced by the usual gastrointestinal distress, which generally appears within 12–36 hours, followed by the onset of such neurological symptoms as double vision, stammering, and difficulty in breathing. If untreated, botulism can result in death due to respiratory paralysis. Another manifestation of the disease that has now become the most common form of human botulism in the United States affects only children under one year of age and is referred to as "infant botulism." This condition can occur when babies are fed honey (or when infant pacifiers are dipped in honey) containing *C.botulinum* spores. When these spores germinate inside the baby's intestinal tract, they release a nerve poison which may cause a weakening of the infant's muscles, resulting in a condition called "floppy baby." Other symptoms of infant botulism include excessive drooling, difficulty in swallowing, droopy eyelids, lack of facial expression, weak cry, constipation, and sometimes respiratory arrest. The condition often requires a lengthy period of hospitalization. Because infant botulism can be provoked by as few as 10–100 *C. botulinum* spores, parents are advised never to feed babies honey (Tarr and Doyle, 1996).

Viruses. Since viruses are unable to multiply outside a living host cell, these pathogens do not increase in number when they are introduced into food materials. Virus-contaminated foods simply serve as a route of transmission— a means by which virus particles can be transported from one host to another. Nevertheless, because the infectious dose needed to cause a viral disease is thought to be quite small, perhaps as low as 10–100 particles, viruses should never be allowed to contaminate food in the first place. Because the viruses associated with foodborne illness are of fecal origin, poor hygienic practices on the part of food handlers or food contact with sewage-polluted water are the most frequent causes of outbreaks. Since viruses are not utilizing the food as a growth medium, *any* type of food is a potential reservoir (i.e. pathogenic foodborne viruses, unlike bacteria, do not have any particular nutritional requirements for survival and hence are not restricted to certain "potentially hazardous foods"). Two of the more prevalent foodborne illnesses of viral origin are:

Hepatitis A (HAV). Most commonly associated with the consumption of raw clams or oysters harvested from sewage-tainted coastal waters, hepatitis A outbreaks have also been traced to foods as diverse as glazed doughnuts, strawberry sauce, sandwiches, orange juice, and salads. Symptoms of the disease, which include jaundice (an indication of liver infection) as well as the usual gastrointestinal distress, generally don't appear until 10–50 days after eating the contaminated food. An infection typically persists for weeks or even months, depending on its severity. An individual suffering from HAV can easily transmit the virus to others if he or she isn't conscientious about good hygienic practices, since the virus is shed in urine and feces. A victim is most contagious 10–14 days before the onset of disease symptoms and remains infectious until about a week after jaundice appears; thus rigorous adherence to routine handwashing practices is of critical importance in preventing the

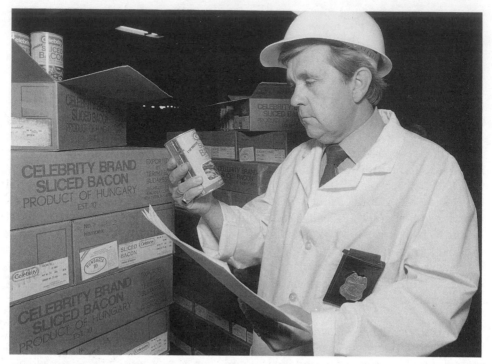

An inspector with the USDA checks a container of Hungarian bacon to verify its eligibility for importation into the United States. *[U.S. Department of Agriculture]*

transmission of HAV. A number of hepatitis A outbreaks have been attributed to direct person-food-person transmission, when an infected food handler failed to wash his/her hands after using the toilet, subsequently touched food which received no further cooking, and then served it to a customer. Since HAV can lead to permanent liver damage, extreme care should be taken to ensure that shellfish are obtained only from safe sources and are thoroughly cooked; similarly, it is essential that food handlers consistently maintain high standards of personal hygiene (Applied Foodservice Sanitation, 1985).

Norwalk virus. A milder affliction than HAV, Norwalk virus causes an infection characterized by nausea, vomiting, abdominal pains, and diarrhea, with headache or slight fever experienced by some victims. The means of transmission (fecal contamination of water or foods) is the same as for HAV. Salads and shellfish are the foods most often implicated in outbreaks, particularly when consumed raw or undercooked (Pierson and Corlett, 1992).

Parasites. Certain parasitic protozoan diseases such as amoebic dysentery or giardiasis are typically associated with ingestion of sewage-contaminated drinking water but have been known to occur when infected food service workers transmitted the microbes to food as a result of faulty handwashing practices. Certain parasitic roundworm infections can occur when untreated sewage ("nightsoil") containing worm eggs is used to fertilize certain vegetable crops. If such produce is consumed raw, the eggs subse-

BOX 9-5
"It Must Have Been Something I Ate—But What?"

Scenario:

Concluding that they deserved a treat after completing mid-term exams, Susan and her roommate Amy decided to indulge in dinner out at an off-campus restaurant Friday evening. After pondering the menu selections, Amy opted for the seafood platter, baked potato, and coleslaw, while Susan chose barbecued chicken, French fries, and a tossed salad with Italian dressing. Both women ordered diet colas and German chocolate cake for dessert, and returned to their room a few hours later well-filled and content. Between 3 and 4 o'clock the next morning, however, Susan woke up feeling miserable, suffering from severe stomach cramps and nausea. She staggered down the hall to the bathroom where she promptly vomited. Shortly afterwards she began to pay repeated return visits to that facility as diarrhea began to take its toll. Susan spent the remainder of the weekend traveling between bedroom and bathroom, but by Monday morning she was beginning to feel human again. Some friends who had heard she was ill inquired as to the nature of her problem, to which she replied, "It must have been something I ate!"

Can You Identify the Cause of Susan's Problem More Precisely?

Theoretically, *any* food could be a route of transmission for foodborne disease. Nevertheless, some foods are implicated in food poisoning outbreaks much more frequently than others and are therefore designated by the U.S. Public Health Service as **potentially hazardous foods**—those which are capable of supporting rapid and progressive growth of infectious or toxigenic microorganisms.

For the most part, potentially hazardous foods are high protein animal products such as poultry, meat, fish, dairy products, and eggs—pathogenic microbes thrive on the same nutritious fare that humans prefer! They also grow well in cooked rice or beans, baked or boiled potatoes, and tofu. Because bacteria must obtain their nutrients in dissolved form, they can only multiply on moist food media, explaining why cooked rice, for example, is designated as "potentially hazardous" while raw rice is not. This inability of bacteria to grow in foods with very low water content is the basis for preservation of such food products as beef jerky or dried apricots. Drying foods does not *kill* microbes, however—it merely prevents their multiplication. If these foods become wet, bacterial growth will resume and their consumption could result in foodborne disease. Certain types of moist foods, peanut butter for example, are not considered potentially hazardous because the sugar and salt they contain tie up the water through chemical bonding, making it unavailable to support microbial growth. Food poisoning bacteria also have specific pH requirements. Most species grow best at pH levels ranging from 4.6 to 9; highly acidic foods such as citrus fruits, tomatoes, most fresh fruits, and pickles are seldom implicated in bacterial foodborne disease outbreaks.

Given this information, a sleuth attempting to discover what menu item was the likely cause of Susan's foodborne illness would, in all probability, zero in on the barbecued chicken; the acidic nature of salad ingredients and the fact that the potatoes were fried at high temperature and served immediately make them less suspect. Although chocolate cake could possibly be a vehicle for disease transmission if the eggs used in making it were contaminated, such an eventuality is uncommon (and the fact that Amy also ate the cake yet remained perfectly healthy further discredits the cake as a plausible suspect). Cola drinks are too acidic to support food poisoning bacteria, leaving the chicken as the only likely candidate—not surprising, since chicken and turkey are among the foods most often implicated in foodborne disease outbreaks. To confirm this suspicion it would be necessary to culture both a sample of Susan's stool and some of the leftover chicken from the restaurant and to show that bacterial isolates from the two are identical. Until such positive laboratory confirmation is obtained, the official cause of the illness can only be termed as "suspected." However, knowledge of which foods are potentially hazardous can prompt both food handlers and consumers to take special precautions with such items to avoid the situations which contribute to food poisoning outbreaks.

Reference
Educational Foundation of the National Restaurant Association. 1985. *Applied Foodservice Sanitation*. John Wiley & Sons.

quently hatch inside the human host and perpetuate the cycle of infection. Other sources of helminthic (i.e. worm) foodborne ailments include the consumption of raw or undercooked fish preparations. In recent years the United States has witnessed a small but increasing number of foodborne helminthic ailments traced to the growing popularity of ethnic specialties such as *sushi* or *ceviche*. Tapeworm infections are the most commonly reported problems, occurring predominantly along the West Coast where most victims admit to having eaten raw fish, mainly salmon. Symptoms of tapeworm infections, as well as time of onset, vary greatly from one person to another: some victims report experiencing severe cramps, nausea, and diarrhea almost immediately after eating; others may not develop symptoms for weeks or months. However, the majority of victims have no symptoms at all and only discover their infection when they pass the tapeworm, or segments of it, in their stool. Tapeworm infections can be eradicated with drugs, but roundworm infections (anisakiasis) are much more serious since there is no effective medication available. Such infections are very painful and may require surgery to remove the parasite. Consumers can easily avoid such problems simply by thoroughly cooking fish until it is flaky (internal temperature should be at 145 °F for five minutes) or by freezing it at -4 °F for 3–5 days before eating in order to kill the worms.

Trichinosis, another foodborne illness caused by a parasitic roundworm, results primarily from the consumption of undercooked pork products (occasionally outbreaks are traced to bear meat or other wild game) which may harbor the larvae of the pathogen, *Trichinella spiralis*. Inside the human host, larvae mature into adult worms and burrow into the intestinal wall, producing new larvae which travel via the circulatory system to muscle tissue. There they embed themselves and produce the typical symptoms of foodborne disease. Although the presence of *Trichinella* in pork is considerably lower today than in past decades (thanks, in part, to prohibitions on feeding uncooked garbage to hogs—a practice which in years past perpetuated the cycle of reinfec-

Table 9-3   Microbial Foodborne Ailments

Because many people assume that food poisoning always occurs within a few hours after eating contaminated food, they frequently misdiagnose the cause of their illness or lay the blame on some innocent menu item in the last meal consumed before disease symptoms appear. In fact, most microbial foodborne ailments manifest themselves 24 hours or more after tainted foods are eaten. The time required before a food poisoning victim feels sick varies depending on the pathogen involved and the amount of contaminated food consumed. Listed below are the time periods typically required for signs of illness to appear for a representative group of foodborne ailments:

Pathogen	Time Frame for Onset of Symptoms
Campylobacter	1 to 10 days (usually 3 to 5 days)
Clostridium botulinum	12 to 36 hours
E. coli 0157:H7	1 to 10 days (usually 3 to 5 days)
Hepatitis A	1 to 7 weeks (usually 25 days)
Listeria monocytogenes	4 days to several weeks
Salmonella	6 hours to 3 days (average 18 hours)
Staphylococcus aureus	2 to 7 hours
Vibrio vulnificus	1 to 3 days

tion), a potential for infection remains nevertheless. Because *Trichinella* larvae are killed by high temperatures, the surest way to prevent trichinosis *is always* to cook pork until well done. *Trichinella is* also cold-sensitive and will die if exposed to a temperature of 5 °F (-15 °C) for 30 days.

Preventing Foodborne Disease

> *You won't be surprised that diseases are innumerable—count the cooks.*
>
> —Seneca (1st century A.D.)

Microbial contamination of foods can occur at any time from the production of food in field or feedlot right up to preparation and serving of the meal. Thus strict adherence to principles of food sanitation are essential at every step from production to processing, transportation, storage, preparation, and service if food poisoning outbreaks are to be avoided. The bacterial pathogens that cause foodborne disease are common inhabitants of the intestinal tracts of humans and domestic animals, present in healthy and sick individuals alike; some are naturally present in boils as well. When discharged in fecal material, these organisms can survive for long periods in litter, feces, trough water, and soil. Livestock feed is often contaminated with *Salmonella* organisms introduced when infected animal by-products are rendered and added to the feed mixture. Animals can become infected from any of these sources and thus bring such pathogens into slaughterhouses and poultry processing plants. Just one infected organ or carcass or animal feces can contaminate cutting equipment or workers' hands and thereby can transfer the bacteria to other carcasses or foods, a process referred to as **cross-contamination.** Once in a processing plant or food establishment, pathogenic organisms can survive on the surface of equipment for long periods and thus constitute sources of food contamination over an extended time period. For this reason, cleaning and sanitizing of grinders, choppers, slicers, and other equipment after each use and frequent washing of workers' hands are important measures in preventing cross-contamination.

Foods, particularly those of animal origin, often contain pathogens such as *Salmonella* and *Campylobacter jejuni* when they enter the kitchen. Once in the kitchen, additional opportunity for contamination of food is presented by the food handlers themselves. The primary reservoir of the *Staphylococcus* organism is the human nose; if kitchen workers cough or sneeze near foods, the bacteria are readily transferred to an appropriate growth medium. If food handlers have infected cuts on their hands, boils, bad cases of acne or other skin eruptions, *Staphylococcus* bacteria likewise can be transferred to food. Similarly, since approximately 40% of all healthy people carry *Salmonella* organisms in their gastrointestinal tract and regularly shed the live bacteria when they defecate, failure of kitchen workers to wash their hands thoroughly after using the bathroom can result in contamination of foods with this pathogen. The low pay, lack of health benefits, limited education, and minimal employment opportunities that characterize the average food service worker complicates efforts to instill in such individuals a strong commitment to safe food-handling practices.

Since so many foods contain at least *some* disease-causing bacteria, it is fortunate that the number of bacterial cells or concentration of bacterial toxins within the ingested food must be relatively high to induce the symptoms of most bacterial foodborne diseases (listeriosis and *E. coli 0157:H7* food poisoning are exceptions to this general rule). Thus the approach to preventing foodborne disease outbreaks must be two-pronged: 1) to the greatest extent possible, avoid microbial contamination of food in the first place through rigorous adherence to rules of good sanitation and hygiene; and 2) maintain environmental conditions that inhibit the multiplication of bacteria that may be present in small numbers within the food medium.

Sanitation

High standards of cleanliness and personal hygiene among those who handle or prepare food are of the utmost importance in preventing outbreaks of foodborne disease. Regulations that local and state public health agencies impose on more than a million retail food establishments in the United States highlight the responsibility of food service personnel for observing good sanitary practices—practices equally relevant to food preparation at home. In its model *Food Code,* a compilation of recommendations that state and local health departments can adopt, if they so choose, when developing or updating their own regulatory requirements, the FDA recommends that food service workers be held accountable for lapses in personal hygiene. The *Code* places a special obligation on employees to notify supervisors if they are experiencing any symptoms of gastrointestinal illness or if they are suffering from boils, dermatitis, or other infections on the hands, wrists, exposed portions of the arms, or other parts of the body, unless covered by a proper bandage (such pus-filled infections are prime sources of *Staphylococcus* bacteria). Thus informed, a supervisor is required to restrict sick employees from direct contact with food or to exclude them from the establishment altogether until health problems have been resolved.

Perhaps the most important of all sanitary practices in protecting food quality is frequent and proper handwashing. The FDA cites germ-laden hands as a major vehicle of disease transmission, a situation resulting largely from negligence on the part of food handlers. Emphasizing that *rigorous handwashing practices represent the single most effective means for breaking the chain of infection*, public health authorities recommend that immediately before handling food, food service workers and home cooks alike should engage in a vigorous 20-second scrub using soap and running water, followed by thorough rinsing under clean water. This procedure should be repeated as often as necessary during food preparation to remove soil and to prevent cross-contamination when changing tasks or after handling soiled equipment. Good handwashing procedures, including using a fingernail brush to clean the fingertips and under the nails, are especially important after food handlers use the toilet, cough, sneeze, smoke, eat, or drink.

Good sanitation of course involves attention to more than employee health and hygiene. General cleanliness of the facility, routine sanitization of cutting tools and food preparation equipment, safe food storage practices, effective dishwashing procedures, proper waste disposal and trash storage—all are important for ensuring that dangerous microbes and food never have a chance to meet.

Time-Temperature Control

When certain environmental preconditions such as optimum pH, moisture, essential nutrients, and temperature are met, populations of pathogenic bacteria in food multiply in accordance with the sigmoidal growth pattern described in chapter 2: after an initial lag phase of about one hour, during which there is negligible increase in numbers while the organisms adjust to new conditions, a period of extremely rapid increase in population size continues until the supply of essential nutrients diminishes and toxic by-products accumulate. At this stage, growth levels off and the number of organisms remains relatively constant until eventually a progressive die-off of cells occurs. Perhaps the most crucial element in determining the rate of bacterial multiplication during this sequence of events is *temperature*. The bacteria responsible for the majority of foodborne disease outbreaks multiply most rapidly within a temperature range referred to as the **Danger Zone,** defined under the FDA's *Food Code* as **41°–140 °F (5°–60 °C).** Temperatures above 140 °F will kill most actively growing bacteria, though bacterial spores and a few thermophilic species may survive. At temperatures below 41°F, growth of the bacterial populations associated with common foodborne illnesses either

BOX 9-6
HACCP—Preventive Approach to Food Safety

In confronting the challenge of how best to ensure the safety of food supplies from biological, chemical, or physical hazards, government regulators and food industry quality assurance personnel alike have traditionally relied on an approach that involved periodic inspections of food processing facilities (e.g. mills, slaughterhouses, canneries, bakeries, supermarkets, restaurants, etc.) and random end-product analyses. The mandated inspection system for meat and poultry still relies on visual examination, the inspector touching and sniffing carcasses to detect signs of disease or spoilage. Most food safety experts decry this approach as outdated and completely useless for identifying the presence of the foodborne pathogens that constitute today's most urgent food quality concerns. The ineffectiveness of trying to protect public health in this manner through sole reliance on efforts to detect problems after-the-fact is attested by the continued prevalence of foodborne disease.

In recent years a paradigm shift has been occurring in the way regulatory agencies approach foodborne disease prevention. Moving away from a nearly century-old reactive food safety strategy, regulators are turning instead to a science-based concept called the **Hazard Analysis and Critical Control Point** system, or **HACCP** (pronounced "hassip"). HACCP has been steadily winning converts among government regulators, food industry executives, and scientific organizations alike. Its endorsement by the National Advisory Committee on Microbiological Criteria for Foods, and the 1992 publication by that group of a document defining HACCP terminology and describing HACCP principles gave a further boost to widespread implementation of HACCP programs throughout the United States and abroad.

So what is this radical new approach? Essentially HACCP is a preventive system of quality control which, when properly applied, can be used to control any point in the food system that might contribute to a hazardous situation. The concept, like so many other innovations to late 20th-century American life, originated with the space program. In the late 1950s, NASA asked the Pillsbury Company to produce a food that could be eaten by astronauts in orbit. Such an undertaking presented a number of challenges, none more daunting than the imperative of ensuring that any food developed be 100% free of microbial, chemical, or physical contamination. The potentially disastrous consequences of a food poisoning outbreak inside a space capsule had to be avoided at any cost. Pillsbury scientists realized that only a proactive preventive system could provide the high degree of safety assurance required. Pillsbury spent the following decade developing and refining its concept and in 1971 adopted the HACCP approach in its own facilities. That same year the FDA awarded Pillsbury a contract to conduct classes for its employees on the HACCP system, and in 1973 the company published the first comprehensive document on HACCP principles as a training manual for FDA personnel. By the early 1980s a number of U.S. food companies, following Pillsbury's example, had established their own HACCP programs, but HACCP's wider application in the public sector remained extremely limited. In 1980, several federal agencies requested that the National Academy of Sciences examine the potential applications for microbiological criteria in food. The result was a 1985 NAS publication that strongly recommended the application of HACCP in regulatory programs, stating that HACCP "provides a more specific and critical approach to the control of microbiological hazards in foods than that provided by traditional inspection and quality control approaches."

Following this ringing endorsement by NAS, an increasing number of federal, state, and local agencies have been redesigning their regulatory approach in conformance with HACCP principles. In 1995, the FDA signed on to the HACCP approach for seafood inspections and by 1997 USDA had launched an effort to implement HACCP programs for meat and poultry inspections, due to be in full force by early 2000.

While food producers must develop individualized HACCP systems tailored to their own processing and distribution conditions, each HACCP program consists of seven basic steps:

1. *Analyze hazard*, identifying potential hazards associated with the food in question, based on close observation of how the food is grown, processed, and distributed—right up to the point of consumption; an assessment is then made of the likelihood of those hazards occurring and preventive measures for controlling such hazards are identified.

2. *Determine critical control points (CCPs)* to minimize or eliminate the hazards identified; CCPs comprise operational steps or procedures such as cooking, chilling, sanitizing, employee hygiene, etc.

3. *Establish critical limits or tolerances* which must be met to ensure that the CCP is under control; some of the criteria most often used include temperature, time, pH, humidity, salt concentration, etc.

4. *Establish a monitoring system* through scheduled testing or observation to ensure that CCP is being controlled.

5. *Establish the corrective action* to be taken when monitoring indicates a deviation from appropriate controls; because of the wide range of possible critical control points, a specific corrective action plan must be developed for each one.

6. *Establish effective recordkeeping systems* that document the HACCP plan.

7. *Establish verification procedures* which demonstrate that HACCP is working correctly; such procedures require minimal end-product sampling (due to safeguards built into the system), relying instead on frequent reviews of plan procedure and affirmation that the plan is being followed correctly. Both the food producer and the appropriate regulatory agencies have a role to play in verifying HACCP plan performance.

Implementing a HACCP program in any given setting is neither quick nor easy. HACCP is a technically sophisticated system requiring extensive site-specific research, discussion, and preparation prior to application. Intensive training of both in-plant personnel and regulatory agency inspectors, as well as a high degree of cooperation between government and industry are essential prerequisites to the success of any HACCP plan. Nevertheless, ultimate results are well worth the effort. According to the NAS analysis, effective use of HACCP in food protection systems is the one approach by which meaningful reductions in the incidence of foodborne disease can be achieved.

References

National Research Council. 1998. *Ensuring Safe Food From Production to Consumption*. National Academy Press.

Pierson, Merle D., and Donald A. Corlett, Jr., eds. 1992. *HACCP: Principles and Applications*. Chapman & Hall.

ceases entirely or is extremely slow; however, the organisms are not killed by cold temperatures and can remain viable for long periods of time, resuming multiplication when temperatures rise. Therefore, the most effective way to prevent buildup of bacterial numbers is to keep foods refrigerated, especially those proteinaceous foods that most frequently harbor pathogenic bacteria. Heating such foods thoroughly will kill bacteria that may be present in the food; the higher the temperature above 140°, the shorter the time the bacterial population will be able to survive (normal cooking times and temperatures are not sufficient, however, to break down *Staphylococcus* toxin).

To ensure complete heat penetration throughout the item being cooked, it is advised that internal temperatures reach the following USDA-recommended minimum levels to guarantee that any pathogens present within the food are killed:

Ground Poultry	165 °F	(74 °C)
Ground beef, veal, lamb, pork	160 °F	(71 °C)
Roast beef or lamb	145 °F	(63 °C)
Roast pork	160 °F	(71 °C)
Ham, fresh	160 °F	(71 °C)
Ham, pre-cooked	140 °F	(60 °C)
Roast chicken, turkey	180 °F	(82 °C)
Chicken or turkey breast	170 °F	(77 °C)
Stuffing	165 °F	(74 °C)

It should be noted that the internal temperature of the item being cooked, rather than the temperature of the oven or burner, is the crucial factor. In many instances, large roasts of beef, ham, or turkey still harbor viable pathogens after cooking because they weren't in the oven long enough for temperatures at the center of the roast to reach the recommended level. In the same way, large pieces of cooked meat held in the refrigerator for cooling frequently have internal temperatures well within the growth range, even though the refrigerator thermostat registers at or below 41 °F as advised. To promote rapid cooling, cooked meat should be sliced into thin layers and placed in shallow pans before being refrigerated.

The most effective methods that food handlers can follow to prevent food-borne disease, be it in the home, in restaurants, or at large public gatherings, is to complete the processing of food within an hour or two while the bacteria remain in the lag phase of growth and to cool foods rapidly if they are not to be consumed immediately.

Unfortunately, although good sanitation and proper time-temperature controls are relatively simple preventive concepts, they are all-too-frequently neglected by homemakers and commercial food establishments alike. Thus bacterial food poisoning, which fundamentally is a result of improper food handling practices and should not even exist in affluent modern societies, will undoubtedly remain our most prevalent food-related health problem.

References

Applied Foodservice Sanitation. 1985. John Wiley & Sons in cooperation with the Educational Foundation of the National Restaurant Association.

Buzby, J.C., and T. Roberts. 1997. "Guillain-Barre Syndrome Increases Food-borne Disease Costs." *Food Review* 20, no. 3:36–42.

Centers for Disease Control and Prevention. 1994. "Water Hemlock Poison-ing—Maine, 1992." *Morbidity and Mortality Weekly Report* 43, no. 13 (April 8).

———. 1993. "Vibrio vulnificus Infections Associated with Raw Oyster Con-sumption—Florida, 1981–1992." *Morbidity & Mortality Weekly Report* 42, no. 21 (June 4).

Council for Agricultural Science and Technology (CAST). 1994. "Foodborne Pathogens: Risks and Consequences." Council for Agricultural Science and Technology, Ames, Iowa.

Food and Agriculture Organization of the United Nations (FAO). 1998. "Expert Committee: No Danger to Humans from Milk and Meat from BST-Treated Cows." *News & Highlights* (March 5).

Foulke, Judith E. 1993. "A Fresh Look at Food Preservatives." *FDA Consumer* (Oct).

Hanrahan, Charles E. 1996. "The European Union's Ban on Hormone-Treated Meat." *Congressional Research Service Report for Congress,* 96-122 ENR (February 8).

Henkel, John. 1993. "From Shampoo to Cereal: Seeing to the Safety of Color Additives." *FDA Consumer* (Dec).

Janssen, Wallace F. 1975. "America's First Food and Drug Laws." *FDA Con-sumer* (June).

Klein, Richard M. 1979. *The Green World: An Introduction to Plants and Peo-ple.* Harper & Row.

Koren, Herman. 1980. *Handbook of Environmental Health and Safety.* Vol. 1. Pergamon Press.

"Lines Drawn in a War Over a Milk Hormone." 1994. *New York Times,* March 9.

Merrill, Richard A. 1997. "Food Safety Regulation: Reforming the Delaney Clause." *Annual Review of Public Health* 18:313–340.

Miller, Roger W. 1984. "How Onions and a Baked Potato Became Sources of Botulism Poisoning." *FDA Consumer* (Oct).

National Research Council (NRC). 1998. *Ensuring Safe Food from Production to Consumption.* National Academy Press.

———. 1996. *Carcinogens and Anti-Carcinogens in the Human Diet.* National Academy Press.

———. 1993. *Pesticides in the Diets of Infants and Children.* National Acad-emy Press.

———. 1987. *Regulating Pesticides in Food: The Delaney Paradox.* National Academy Press.

Ropp, Kevin L. 1994. "Juice Maker Cheats Consumers of $40 Million." *FDA Consumer* (Jan/Feb).

Tannahill, Ray. 1973. *Food in History.* Stein and Day.

Tarr, Phillip I., and Michael Doyle. 1996. "Food Safety: Everyone's Responsi-bility." *Pediatric Basics,* no. 78 (Fall):2–13.

Task Force on the Mass Outbreak of Diarrhea in School Children of Sakai City. 1997. *Report on the Outbreak of E. coli 0157:H7 Infection in Sakai City* (December).

CHAPTER 10

Radiation

The human race has today the means for annihilating itself—either in a
fit of complete lunacy, i.e., in a big war, by a brief fit of destruction, or
by careless handling of atomic technology, through a slow process of
poisoning and of deterioration in its genetic structure.

—Max Born
Bulletin of Atomic Scientists (1957)

There is no evil in the atom; only in men's souls.

—Adlai Stevenson (1952)

Late in the autumn of 1895, a German physics professor, Wilhelm
Roentgen, was busily pursuing a line of research which would soon revolutionize medical science and transform our understanding of the nature of matter
and energy. Roentgen was experimenting with a cathode-ray tube, a device
perfected by the English scientist Crookes two decades earlier which consisted
of a glass vacuum tube through which flowed a high voltage electric current.
By chance, Roentgen noticed that emissions from the tube caused a nearby
sheet of paper coated with a fluorescent chemical to glow, and he observed
that these emanations could be blocked to varying degrees by materials of different densities. Calling his wife to place her hand on a photographic plate,
Roentgen turned on the cathode ray tube; when the plate was subsequently
developed, Roentgen amazed the world with a picture of his wife's bones
inside her hand. Realizing that he had stumbled upon a form of radiation
whose existence was hitherto completely unsuspected, Roentgen appropriated
the mathematical symbol for the unknown and called his discovery "X-rays."
Within a few days after publication of his findings, the medical profession put
the fluoroscope and "roentgenogram" to use—the shortest time gap between
announcement of a major medical discovery and its practical application yet
recorded.

The implications of Roentgen's announcement far transcended the field

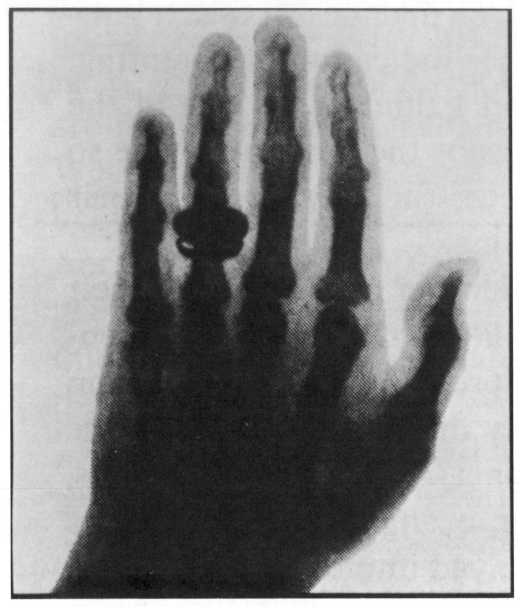

World's first X-ray: this is the "roentgenogram" that Wilhelm Roentgen took of his wife's hand thereby demonstrating the existence of the mysterious emanations that he named "X-rays."

of medicine, however. Upon hearing of Roentgen's findings, the noted French scientist Henri Becquerel became intrigued by the relationship between X-rays and fluorescence and thereupon directed his attention to naturally phosphorescent minerals. In February of 1896, just two months after publication of Roentgen's report, Becquerel placed some crystals of a uranium compound on a photographic plate wrapped in black paper and demonstrated that the emanations from the uranium exhibited the same characteristics as Roentgen's X-rays. Becquerel's work was quickly picked up by Marie and Pierre Curie who termed the mysterious phenomenon "radioactivity" and who soon succeeded in isolating two new radioactive substances, polonium and radium, from uranium ore (Kevles, 1997). Thus the independent discovery of both artificial and natural radioactivity within a three-month time span quickly led to the birth of a whole new field of scientific inquiry with far-reaching implications in physics, biology, medicine, and, unfortunately, warfare.

Ionizing Radiation

Early investigations of radioactivity quickly revealed that the observed emissions were of several different kinds. Some consisted of subatomic particles—protons, neutrons, or electrons—released when atoms spontaneously decay; these came to be known as **particulate radiation**, a group that includes **alpha** and **beta particles**. Other emissions, such as Roentgen's X-rays and naturally occurring **gamma rays,** were shown to consist of highly energetic short wavelengths of electromagnetic radiation, a form of energy which also includes ultraviolet light, visible light, infrared waves, and microwaves. Alpha and beta particles, as well as X-rays and gamma rays, are today referred to as **ionizing radiation** because the particles or rays involved are sufficiently energetic to dislodge electrons from the atoms or molecules they encounter, leaving behind ions, i.e. electrically-charged particles. While certain forms of non-ionizing radiation such as ultraviolet light and microwaves can have an adverse effect on living organisms and will be discussed later in this chapter, ionizing radiation's ability to destroy chemical bonds gives it special significance in relation to both human health and environmental pollution. It is recognized today that when certain particularly vulnerable cells (e.g. fetal cells, sex cells) are exposed to ionizing radiation, birth defects or mutations can result; in any cell, radiation-induced alteration of DNA can lead to cancer. Although discovery of ionizing radiation was immediately hailed as a momentous medical and scientific event, subsequent investigations regarding what is frequently called our "most studied and best understood pollutant" have revealed the importance of extreme caution in dealing with radioactive materials.

Radiation Exposure

Exposure to ionizing radiation is an inescapable circumstance of life on this planet. Every individual, to a greater or lesser extent, comes into contact with ionizing radiation from three general types of sources: naturally occurring, naturally occurring but enhanced by human actions, and human generated.

Natural Sources. Although the fact was not realized until Becquerel's discovery in 1896, earth, air, water, and food all contain traces of radioactive materials which constitute a ubiquitous source of naturally occurring, or "background," radiation. Some of the more significant sources of background radiation include the following:

Cosmic radiation. High energy particles composed primarily of protons and electrons continually stream toward the earth both from outer space and from the sun following episodes of solar flares. An appreciable amount of such cosmic radiation is blocked by the layer of atmosphere surrounding the globe, so that exposure to cosmic radiation is considerably less at sea level than at high altitudes (annual exposure to cosmic radiation approximately doubles with each 2,000-meter increase in altitude above sea level). For this reason, residents of Denver receive about twice as much cosmic radiation as do inhabitants of Los Angeles or Miami, the one million residents of La Paz, Bolivia, receive annual radiation exposures fully 7.5 times higher than do persons living at sea level (Bennett, 1997). While the natural tendency is to assume that something which has always been with us must be harmless, some biologists assert that perhaps 25% of all spontaneous mutations are caused by cosmic radiation.

Radioactive minerals in the earth's crust. Radioactive compounds of uranium, thorium, potassium, and radium are found in soils and rocks in many parts of the world. For example, people living along the Kerala coast in southwestern India, the Morro de Ferro and Meaipe regions of Brazil's Atlantic coast, and in Yangjiang, Guangdong Province in China are all exposed to significantly higher-than-average levels of background radiation due to emissions from thorium-rich monazite sands. Similarly, Floridians living near radioactive phosphate deposits, and residents of New Hampshire, the Rocky Mountain region of the United States, and parts of Sweden—all granite-rich areas—are constantly exposed to external radiation from the soils and rocks around them. In some localities, notably Badgastein in Austria and Mahallat and Ramsar in Iran, high levels of background radiation exposure are received internally due to the ingestion of naturally occurring radioactive minerals in drinking water and to the inhalation of radon gas when bathing in the hot springs for which these regions are famous (Sohrabi, 1998).

Coal deposits frequently contain a number of radioactive elements that are released into the atmosphere when the coal is burned. At a time when many large coal users are contemplating switching to low-sulfur western coal as a means of reducing sulfur emissions, it is interesting to note that western coal contains about 10 times more radionuclides than do eastern or midwestern deposits (Carter, 1977).

Radionuclides in the body. A number of radioactive substances enter the body by ingestion of food, milk, water, or by inhalation and are incorporated into body tissues where their concentration may be maintained at a steady state or gradually increase with age. Plants growing in soil containing radioactive minerals readily take up such isotopes as radium and potassium-40, and in areas where people live on radioactive soils, consuming locally grown foods further increases radiation exposure. In regions where groundwater is in contact with radioactive rock strata, well water used for domestic drinking supplies may constitute a significant source of indoor exposure to radioactive radon gas. Another unavoidable source of radiation exposure is carbon-14, a naturally occurring isotope of carbon, which is inhaled with the air we breathe and is incorporated into the tissues of all living organisms (a fact which has useful implications for scientists who employ C-14 dating techniques to ascertain the age of ancient plant and animal remains).

Enhanced Natural Sources. This category of sources, while not fundamentally different from the group just discussed, is considered separately because of the impact human activities have on levels of exposure which would, under other conditions, be much lower. Examples of enhanced natural sources include uranium mill tailings, phosphate mining, and jet airline travel (due to increased exposure to cosmic radiation at high altitudes). Recently, national attention has focused on what experts consider our single most significant source of radiation exposure—radon gas which, though naturally occurring, can be considered an "enhanced natural source" because it reaches potentially dangerous concentrations only in enclosed environments such as houses and mine shafts ("Ionizing Radiation," 1987). For more information on radon, see the section on "Indoor Air Pollutants" in chapter 12.

Human-Generated Sources. Human beings have evolved and multiplied in an environment where constant exposure to low levels of ionizing radiation was a universal experience. With the exception of indoor radon concerns which are currently the subject of a great deal of attention and remedial action, most naturally occurring radiation is relatively constant and cannot be controlled or reduced in any feasible way. However, human-created sources of ionizing radiation have multiplied at exponential rates during the years since Roentgen first exhibited the X-ray of his wife's hand to an astonished world. It is these artificial sources, which *can* be controlled, that constitute the focus of a growing concern today about the impact of ionizing radiation on human health.

Medical applications. By far the greatest source of exposure to artificial ionizing radiation for the average American comes from the use of medical X-rays and radiopharmaceuticals for both diagnostic and therapeutic purposes. Today approximately 75% of all Americans receive one or more medical or dental X-rays annually. Radioactive isotopes of phosphorus, technicium, iodine, iron, chromium, cobalt, and selenium are widely employed in hospitals for therapy and diagnosis, with as many as one-fourth of all patients in some hospitals receiving applications of some form of nuclear medicine. In addition to X-ray machines and radionuclides, the health professions utilize other such radiation producing devices as teleradioisotope units and accelerators (e.g. cyclotrons, linear accelerators) to generate subatomic particles for radiotherapy. While radiation has provided medical science with an extremely valuable tool, its occasional misuse has been accompanied by some serious health problems; thus a thoughtful weighing of risks versus benefits should precede any decision regarding the application of ionizing radiation for medical purposes.

Nuclear weapons fallout. Since the explosion of the first atomic bomb in 1945 until the signing of the Limited Test-Ban Treaty in 1963, atmospheric testing of nuclear weapons by several of the major powers, primarily the United States and the former Soviet Union, resulted in significant amounts of radioactive fallout worldwide. Such fallout consists of a number of atomic fission products, including strontium-90, iodine-131, cesium-137, and radioactive krypton. Weapons fallout is not always evenly distributed, however. Local fallout close to the test site can be quite intense for about a day following the

BOX 10-1
"See Alice Glow!"—Tragedy of the Radium Dialpainters

The agonizing deaths suffered by scores of young female workers in the radium dialpainting industry in the 1920s and 1930s constitute the most infamous example on record of fatal carelessness in the handling of radioactive materials. The tragedy that befell these first victims of occupational radiation poisoning had its origin in the development, in 1915, of radium-containing luminous paint—a product that promptly found use in the watch-making industry for producing "glow-in-the-dark" wristwatches. To supply the demand for this latest consumer fad, between 1917 and 1925 dialpainting factories were established in Orange, NJ, Waterbury, CN, and Ottawa, IL, cumulatively employing 3,000-4,000 workers over the years they were in operation.

Offering what they touted as "ideal working conditions," firms such as U.S. Radium in New Jersey and Radium Dial Company (later replaced by Luminous Processes) in Illinois selectively recruited a workforce composed of women in their late teens and early twenties, regarding such employees as particularly well-suited for jobs requiring little physical strength but considerable manual dexterity. From moderately prosperous working-class families, these women felt fortunate to find employment in firms offering above-average wages in pleasant surroundings. They also found it exciting to be in daily contact with a substance as magical as radium. In more playful moments they applied the luminous paint to their fingernails, eyelids, and buttons; one particularly vivacious girl in New Jersey laughingly painted her teeth with radium to surprise her boyfriend with a glow-in-the-dark smile! Dialpainters often returned home from work with their hair and clothes liberally speckled with luminous powder and would sometimes amuse friends and family by standing in a dark closet where they cast off a ghostly glow. The dialpainters' most ill-advised practice, however, was lip-pointing. As instructed by supervisors, each worker used her lips to maintain a fine point on the brush as she painted the tiny numbers on the watch dial; in doing so, she inadvertently swallowed small amounts of radium each time the brush touched her mouth. Although most of the ingested radium was subsequently excreted, some was absorbed into the bloodstream and eventually accumulated in the bones where it constituted a chronic source of internal radiation exposure. Knowing little about the properties of radium themselves, the women were reassured by management that the substance with which they were working was quite harmless. In the Ottawa plant one worker interviewed years later recalled a supervisor telling her that radium would "put a glow in our cheeks"! Since radium in those years was also being marketed for medicinal use, such statements were readily believed. Unfortunately, they were untrue.

In 1922, a young New Jersey woman who had worked at U.S. Radium for only three years became the first dialpainter to die of radium poisoning; by then several of her co-workers were gravely ill and within a few years they were dead also. Each of these early deaths involved necrosis of the jawbone, followed by rampant infections that proved uncontrollable in that pre-antibiotic era. Several died of anemia, while other women experienced debilitating weakening of their bones, often resulting in arms or legs breaking from even modest pressure. The largest number of dialpainter fatalities, however, was due to bone cancer or multiple myelomas, which began to appear in the late 1920s. Word of the mysterious ailments plaguing their coworkers began to spread among dialpainters who were increasingly convinced they were confronting a new occupational disease. By 1925, after the death of a 21-year-old employee at the Waterbury plant, managers instituted a ban on lip-pointing, even though the company never officially acknowledged radium as the cause of this tragedy. With definitive scientific proof still lacking, neither industry, government regulators, nor medical researchers were ready to concede that radium was the culprit causing the health problems that were now appearing with increasing frequency.

By 1927, however, the mounting evidence could no longer be ignored; in that year a physiologist hired by industry to refute evidence of radium's harmful effects came to the conclusion that "radium is partially if not the primary cause of the pathological condition described." While the radium industry, much like modern-day tobacco company spokespersons, continued to deny any adverse health effects associated with its product, the medical and scientific community at last recognized radium as a major occupational hazard. With this acknowledgment, the focus of attention shifted to that of winning financial compensation for dying workers and their families. By contemporary standards, such compensation was surprisingly meager. In general, the dialpainters who were affected the worst and the earliest received most of the money awarded; many victims were given nothing at all. While records indicate that altogether 84 dialpainters died of radium-induced cancer and an undetermined but smaller number perished from jaw necrosis or anemia, compensation was awarded to just 13 women in Illinois, 16 in Connecticut, and 10 or 11 in New Jersey. The highest amount received was $5,700; most awards were for considerably lower sums.

The dialpainters' story doesn't have a happy ending for the individuals directly affected. During the 1920s, as the women desperately sought recognition for their plight, they received little support from male-dominated labor organizations; the State Health and Labor Department officials who might logically have been expected to espouse their cause instead supported the politically influential radium industry; scientists and medical researchers likewise tailored their reports to please the corporate sponsors who funded their research or paid their salaries. Nevertheless, publicity surrounding the mounting toll of dying and disabled workers raised general awareness of the problem and eventually resulted in improved worker safety precautions in the dialpainting facilities. The scientific investigations launched in response to an obvious problem gave birth to a new field of study—health physics—and in time yielded the information that formed the basis of health standards for a new generation of industrial workers, scientists, medical personnel, and patients.

Reference
Clark, Claudia. 1997. *Radium Girls: Women and Industrial Health Reform, 1910–1935*. Chapel Hill: University of North Carolina Press.

explosion, a fact which became obvious after the March 1, 1954, detonation of a multimegaton U.S. bomb over Bikini Atoll in the Pacific. Heavy fallout of large radioactive particles and dust contaminated several inhabited islands nearby, as well as a Japanese fishing boat sailing in the vicinity. Many of the Marshall Islanders and the fishermen developed burns, skin lesions, and loss of hair as a result of radiation exposure, and one of the islands, Rongelap, had to be evacuated and remained unoccupied for a number of years following the incident. In some cases air currents or rainstorms can cause radioactive particles and gases to precipitate unevenly. The greatest concern about weapons fallout is focused on those isotopes that enter the human system in food and are incorporated into body tissues. Strontium-90 and iodine-131 enter the food chain when contaminated plant material is consumed by cows and passed on to humans in milk. Strontium tends to displace calcium, being incorporated into bones, while iodine localizes in the thyroid gland; both thereby constitute internal sources of exposure, continuing to emit radioactive particles inside the body over a period of weeks or months in close proximity to vital organs. Radioactive cesium also is ingested in both meat and milk and remains in the body for several months before being metabolized (Hall, 1976). During the peak period of weapons testing, an average individual's radiation exposure due to bomb fallout was 13 millirems annually, a figure which has been steadily falling since 1963 (Eisenbud, 1973). According to a recent report by the National Council on Radiation Protection and Measurements, annual fallout exposure currently averages less than 0.01 mSv (1 mrem) and, barring a resumption of atmospheric testing of nuclear weapons, will continue to decline. Having reached such negligible levels, nuclear weapons fallout need no longer be taken into account in calculating total human radiation exposure.

Nuclear power plant emissions. Public opposition to construction of nuclear power plants often centers around fears concerning radioactive emissions both to the air and in wastewater released from such plants. Radioisotopes such as tritium (H3), iodine-131, cesium-137, strontium-90, krypton, and others are indeed released into the environment during routine operation of a nuclear power generator, but the quantities involved are extremely minute—the average annual dose to individuals living within a 50-mile radius of the plant being less than one millirem, an amount considerably lower than that received from background radiation ("Ionizing Radiation," 1987).

Consumer products. In addition to the sources mentioned above, very small amounts of exposure are received from luminous instrument dials (radium, tritium), home smoke detectors (americium), static eliminators (polonium), airport security checks (X-rays), and tobacco products (polonium). Of these sources, the most significant is tobacco; the radioactive polonium particles in cigarette smoke lodge primarily in the bronchial epithelium of the upper airways—the site of most lung cancers—thereby further contributing to the health risk posed by other carcinogenic and toxic substances in tobacco smoke (NCRP, 1987).

Until recently it was estimated that the average American receives approximately half of his or her annual radiation exposure from naturally occurring background radiation and half from artificial sources, primarily

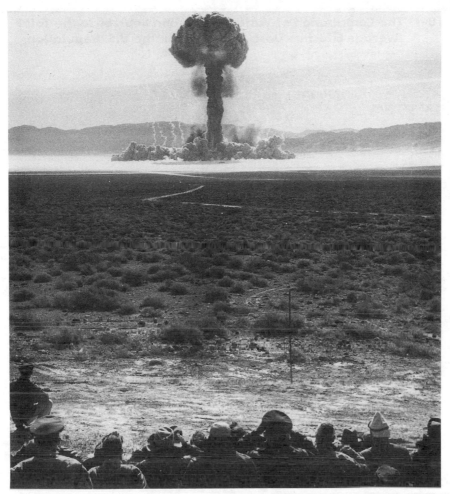

Official military observers watch the mushroom cloud form after an atomic artillery shell was fired in the Nevada desert in 1953. Such tests resulted in significant amounts of radioactive fallout. *[AP/Wide World Photos]*

medical applications. However, a growing realization of the extent to which citizens everywhere are exposed to radon in their homes has prompted a drastic revision in calculations of the contributions of various radiation sources to total average exposures. Due to estimates that as much as 55% of our annual radiation burden results from radon exposure alone, it is now believed that fully 82% of the average American's exposure originates from background (including enhanced) radiation, only 18% from artificial sources (NCRP, 1987). For any one individual, of course, the ratio can vary widely. A person living in an area of unusually high natural radioactivity (e.g. Salt Lake City, Denver) or sleeping in a basement bedroom where radon levels are exceptionally high might receive an even larger portion of his or her total exposure from background sources, while a person undergoing radiation therapy or working inside a nuclear power plant would receive a disproportionate share from artificial sources.

Figure 10-1 The Contribution of Various Radiation Sources to the Total Average Effective Dose Equivalent in the U.S. Population

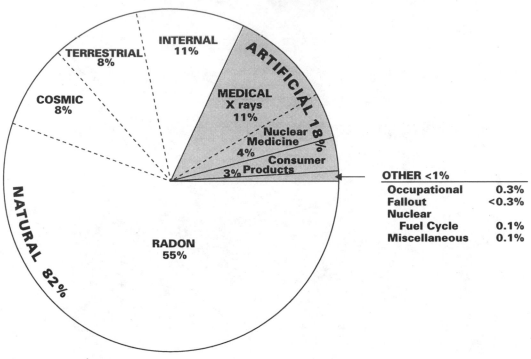

OTHER <1%	
Occupational	0.3%
Fallout	<0.3%
Nuclear	
Fuel Cycle	0.1%
Miscellaneous	0.1%

Source: National Council on Radiation Protection and Measurements, Report No. 93.

Health Impacts of Ionizing Radiation

The advent of X-ray technology for diagnosing and treating human maladies, so eagerly and immediately seized upon by the medical profession, was soon shown to be a double-edged sword so far as its impact on human health was concerned. The first reported case of X-ray induced illness involved an American physician, Grubbe, who began self-experimenting with a homemade cathode ray tube. Within a few weeks he reported acute irritation of the skin on his hand; later cancer developed and eventually his hand had to be amputated. Grubbe's case was not an isolated one. By 1897, scarcely a year after the new technology came into use, 69 cases of X-ray induced injuries had been documented from various clinics and laboratories in different parts of the world (Eisenbud, 1973). One of the most famous early radiation victims was Clarence Dally, Thomas Edison's chief assistant, who "died by inches" after just a few years of working with X-rays. In 1896 Dally had begun experimenting with Roentgen's new device in Edison's West Orange, New Jersey, laboratory, frequently holding his hand in front of the tube to make sure X-rays were being produced. Dally soon noticed slight burns and hair loss, but continued his work. By 1902 he was suffering from oozing ulcers on his hands and eventually had his left hand amputated; cancerous sores then appeared on his right hand and four fingers were amputated, followed by both arms. In such acute pain he couldn't even lie down, Dally died in agony in 1904 (Kevles, 1997). Reports of health damage due to radiation from natural sources were not long in following. Becquerel himself reported a reddening of the skin on his chest as a result of carrying a vial of radium in his vest pocket. He and the Curies subsequently used a radium extract to produce a skin burn on the forearm of a male volunteer, thereby demonstrating that X-rays and natural radioactivity have essentially identical biological effects (Cooper, 1973).

In spite of an increasing awareness of the hazards, as well as the usefulness, of ionizing radiation, the first few decades of the 20th century witnessed numerous cases of radiation-induced illness or death resulting from carelessness, faulty equipment, or simple ignorance. As early as 1903 a dangerous misconception of radiation's curative powers catapulted both X-rays and radium into prominence as the latest medical fads, regarded as modern panaceas for a wide range of ailments. Over a period of approximately 20 years, first in Europe and later in the U.S. as well, radiation treatments were prescribed to hopeful patients both for destroying unwanted external tissue (e.g. warts, birthmarks, excess facial hair) and as an internal medicine. Many researchers during this period were convinced that radiation selectively destroyed diseased cells while actually promoting the growth of healthy ones. Some claimed that the radioactive element radium had germicidal properties, leading one scientist to propose the inhalation of radioactive gas as a treatment for tuberculosis! The discovery during this period that the mineral waters at many health spas were radioactive reinforced the notion that radioactivity must confer health benefits and encouraged promoters of such popular resorts as Saratoga Springs, New York, and Hot Springs, Arkansas, to claim their waters had the power to cure ailments ranging from rheumatism to malaria, alcoholism, chronic skin disease, anemia, and female sterility!

More surprising in retrospect was the medical practice, widespread during the 1910s and 1920s, of administering intravenous injections of radium salts as a treatment for such maladies as high blood pressure, arthritis, leukemia, sexual dysfunction, and senility; rather than curing such ills, the treatment all too often provoked the development of anemia or cancer (Clark, 1997). Outside physicians' offices, a wide variety of radium-based consumer products—candies, liniments, creams, etc.—were being marketed to a gullible public with assurances that the effects of radiation in trace amounts were beneficial to health, perhaps even necessary! One such bogus cure-all, "Radithor," was advertised as a panacea for impotence, high blood pressure, indigestion, and more than 150 other ills. Sold in the United States for over six years, Radithor was taken off the market only after it had induced fatal cancer in a well-known socialite, a Radithor devotee who was reported to have consumed 1,000 to 1,500 bottlefuls of the radium solution between 1927 and 1931. The legal restrictions on sales of radiopharmaceuticals currently prevailing in the United States were a direct result of the outrage provoked by the Radithor scandal almost 70 years ago (Macklis, 1993). To cite another example of a practice that in retrospect seems inconceivably misguided, starting in about 1925, some doctors began irradiating children's scalps to treat ringworm, their heads and throats for enlarged tonsils and adenoids, and their faces to banish acne. Even as late as the 1960s some physicians used low-voltage X-rays to shrink the thymus gland (located in the neck) of infants in the erroneous belief that such treatments would cure colds. Unfortunately, such X-rays could not be precisely focused. As they spread out they irradiated not only the target tissue but the thyroid gland as well. The thyroid is one of the most radiation-sensitive organs in the body, and about 10 or more years following exposure (19 years seemed to be the peak period) significant numbers of these now-teenagers or young adults developed thyroid cancer (Norwood, 1980).

One segment of the population at special risk during the early years of work with radiation was the medical community itself, particularly radiologists whose enthusiastic use of their new machines exposed not only their patients but also themselves to large amounts of radiation on a daily basis. A questionnaire sent to all American radiologists in 1928 revealed that a shockingly high percentage of respondents had been unable to father children and the rate of defective births among those who did have offspring was double that considered normal. Radiologists' mortality rates due to cancer, particularly leukemia, were several times higher than those of their colleagues in other areas of medicine, and the gloved or amputated hand became a macabre symbol of the radiologists' profession. Organizers of a 1920 banquet at a radiologists' convention blundered badly by including chicken on the menu because most of the guests present had lost at least one hand and were unable to cut their meat (Kevles, 1997).

Observations of radiation-induced health problems such as those just described led to extensive research into safer methods of utilizing this valuable but dangerous tool. Since the early 1940s, improvements in equipment design and increasingly stringent standards relating to allowable exposure have significantly reduced the incidence of overt cases of radiation damage. Nevertheless, concerns regarding unnecessary use of X-rays for diagnostic purposes and new understanding regarding long-term effects of low-level exposure require that individuals must be alert to the dangers implicit in any degree of radiation exposure and take an active role in deciding whether such exposure is justified.

Types of Ionizing Radiation

Although any exposure to ionizing radiation is potentially dangerous, the degree and nature of harm varies depending on the type of radiation involved. Early studies of radioactivity revealed that ionizing radiation comprises several different types of emissions, the most biologically significant of which include the following.

Alpha Particles. Basically helium nuclei consisting of 2 protons and 2 neutrons, alpha particles are relatively massive particles which, although the most energetic type of radiation, are the least penetrating. Such flimsy barriers as a sheet of paper, clothing, or even human skin can stop them. The greatest threat to health involving alpha radiation occurs when alpha-emitting particles (e.g. plutonium, radium, radon) are inhaled, ingested with food or water, or taken into the body through a cut or wound. Once in contact with delicate internal tissues, alpha radiation can cause intense damage within a

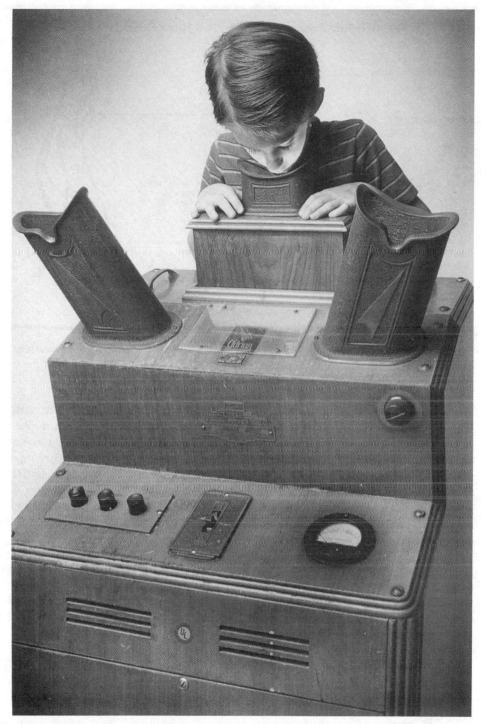

A child looks through a fluoroscopy machine at a shoe store to see if his shoes fit. This and other ill-advised practices were gradually discontinued as the deleterious health effects of radiation exposure became known. *[FDA Consumer]*

Figure 10-2   Penetrating Power of Alpha and Beta Particles and Gamma Rays

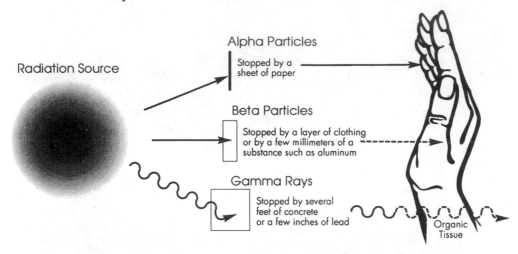

Radiation Source

Alpha Particles
Stopped by a sheet of paper

Beta Particles
Stopped by a layer of clothing or by a few millimeters of a substance such as aluminum

Gamma Rays
Stopped by several feet of concrete or a few inches of lead

Organic Tissue

Source: U.S. Environmental Protection Agency.

localized area. Theoretical projections of large numbers of lung cancer deaths following a nuclear power plant meltdown are based on assumptions of pulmonary damage caused by inhalation of alpha-emitting plutonium dust.

Beta Particles. Consisting of single electrons, beta particles are more penetrating than alphas, capable of passing through the skin to a depth of about a half-inch. Like alphas, however, they are most dangerous when ingested. Since several beta emitters (e.g. strontium-90, iodine-131) are chemically similar to naturally occurring bodily constituents, they may substitute for those elements and concentrate in living tissues (e.g. bones, thyroid), where they continue to emit radiation for an extended period of time, increasing the risk of cancer or mutations. Most fission products in spent fuel rods or in reprocessed nuclear wastes are beta-emitters.

Gamma Rays. These are the most penetrating form of ionizing radiation and generally accompany beta radiation. Shielding with a dense material such as lead is necessary to prevent gamma radiation from penetrating the body and harming vital organs. Short-lived beta emitters such as krypton-85 generally exhibit the highest levels of gamma radiation.

X-rays. Though slightly less penetrating, X-rays have basically the same characteristics as gamma rays.

Dosage

Since ionizing radiation can neither be seen nor felt, human exposure is measured in terms of the amount of tissue damage it causes. Under the International System of Units, the term **gray (Gy)** is the unit of absorbed dose, used to quantify the amount of energy from ionizing radiation absorbed per

BOX 10-2

Half-Life

Not all radioisotopes are dangerous for the same length of time. Each radioactive element is characterized by its own unique half-life (T½)—a period of time during which half of the amount originally present, undergoing radioactive decay, is transformed into something else. The concept of half-life, in essence, is the reverse of exponential growth. Assume, for example, that one has a gram of cesium-137 whose half-life is 30 years. After 30 years there would remain ½ gram of cesium-137 and ½ gram of cesium's nonradioactive daughter product, barium-137; the radiation now being emitted is only half the original value. After 60 years the radioactivity would be only ¼ the original amount; in 90 years ⅛ the original value, and so on.

Obviously the term half-life is not synonymous with safety—½ gram of cesium-137 still presents a hazard. Indeed, highly radioactive substances may have to go through 10 or more half-lives (i.e. 300 years in the case of cesium) before their level of radioactivity is low enough to pose no significant health threat. However, the half-life concept has considerable relevance in assessing relative hazards and in devising waste management strategies.

Isotopes with very short half-lives are intensely radioactive initially; that is, they are experiencing a very high number of disintegrations at any one point in time. However, within a few days or weeks they go through so many half-lives that they no longer present a significant risk. The best management strategy for such wastes is simply to isolate them from human contact during the brief period when they are dangerous. Isotopes with extremely long half-lives will be radioactive virtually forever, but the level of emissions at any one point in time is relatively low; one can briefly handle a piece of long-lived uranium or thorium ore with little concern for radiation injury. The most difficult management problems involve those isotopes with intermediate-length half-lives, elements such as plutonium which, with a half-life of 24,000 years, remains hazardous for hundreds of thousands of years. Human contact with such radioisotopes must be accompanied by stringent safety precautions and ultimate disposal of such material must be carried out in such a way that it remains isolated from the general environment for extremely long periods of time.

Some representative half-lives

Element	Half-life	Element	Half-life
Radon-222	3.8 days	Cesium-137	30 years
Iodine-131	8.1 days	Radium-226	1,600 years
Phosphorus-32	14 days	Carbon-14	5,800 years
Krypton-85	11 years	Plutonium-239	24,000 years
Tritium	12 years	Uranium-235	710,000,000 years

unit mass of material (the gray is replacing the term "rad" which is still in temporary use; a gray is equivalent to 100 rads). The most common unit for measuring effective radiation dose in humans, however, is the **sievert (Sv),** a figure obtained by multiplying the absorbed dose in grays by a factor called the **relative biological effectiveness (RBE).** This measurement reflects the fact that the health impact of radiation depends not only on the amount of energy absorbed, but also on the form of that energy. For example, X-rays and gamma rays which pass through tissue striking only occasional molecules along their path have an RBE of 1; beta particles have RBEs ranging from 1 to 5, depending on their energy level, while the relatively massive alpha particles have an RBE of 10, indicating their greater potential to damage living tissue. For practical purposes, human radiation exposure standards are set in terms of **millisieverts (mSv),** an amount one-thousandth of a sievert, since these represent levels of exposure most commonly encountered by the average individual. Just as the gray is a relatively new term for what formerly was called the rad, sieverts and millisieverts are gradually replacing units, still used in many references, called "rems" and "millirems" (mrem). Under the new system a sievert is equivalent to 100 rems. The average amount of whole-body radiation exposure for a person in the U.S. from all sources is estimated to be 3.6 mSv (360 mrem) a year or 0.01 mSv (1 mrem) per day.

There is little evidence that present average levels of exposure to ionizing radiation are having any adverse effect on the health of the general public. It is well known, however, that higher doses can be extremely injurious to living tissues. Types of radiation-induced biological damage include mutations, birth defects, impairment of fertility, leukemia and other forms of cancer, infections, hemorrhage, cataracts, and reduced lifespan. Humans, and mammals in general, are far more sensitive to ionizing radiation than are lower forms of life. The same degree of damage which a dose of 0.5 Sv (50 rems) can cause in a mammalian cell requires 1,000 Sv (100,000 rems) exposure in an amoeba or 3,000 Sv (300,000 rems) in a paramecium. The frequent reference in horror films to cockroaches inheriting the earth in the aftermath of all-out nuclear war is reflective of the fact that insects also have a very high level of tolerance to ionizing radiation.

Dose **rate,** the quantity of radiation received within a given unit of time, is thought to be very significant in determining the extent of tissue damage incurred, perhaps even more important than total dose. The prevailing view holds that radiation absorbed over an extended period is less harmful than the same amount delivered during a brief time span, due to the existence of bodily repair mechanisms. Furthermore, not only does the risk of damage (e.g. cancer) fall as the dose rate is decreased, but also the latency period becomes longer (Goldman, 1996). A contrary conclusion has been advanced by two noted British epidemiologists who argue that, at least in relation to carcinogenesis, numerous small doses of radiation exposure are *more* likely to induce cancer than is a single large dose. Basing their conclusions on a study of health records of 35,000 nuclear bomb production workers at the federal government's Hanford Reservation in Richland, Washington, these researchers hypothesize that large doses of radiation *kill* cells, while smaller doses simply *damage* the genetic material, giving rise to mutations which increase the likelihood of cancer (Kneale and Stewart, 1993).

High-Level vs. Low-Level Radiation Exposure

Health effects of ionizing radiation can be subdivided into those types of damage caused by high-level and low-level exposure, respectively. **High-level radiation exposure** is defined as a whole-body dose of 1 Sv (100 rems) or more, delivered within a relatively short period of time—minutes or hours. Such exposure will produce obvious symptoms of radiation sickness within a period ranging from a few hours to several weeks, symptoms ranging in severity from temporary nausea to death, depending on the dosage. Levels of ionizing radiation capable of inducing the above-mentioned effects would most likely occur only in such extreme situations as a nuclear bomb explosion, a nuclear power plant meltdown, or in severe industrial accidents involving mishandling of radioactive materials. Such effects are largely reflective of cell death which, if extensive, can be fatal to the organism. Human effects of high-level exposure have been determined from studies of victims of the Hiroshima-Nagasaki atomic bomb explosions, from experience with radiation therapy, and from observations of the results of nuclear accident victims. The 135,000 unfortunate Ukrainians and Byelorussians exposed to large amounts of radioactive debris resulting from the 1986 disaster at Chernobyl constitute a particularly valuable study group for radiation biologists because the radiation doses they received were measured at the time of the accident, unlike the wartime situation in Japan where exposures were estimated after the event. As one British radiation specialist remarked, "The human experiment has now been done. At last we can test our hypotheses" (Hawkes et al., 1987).

Low-level radiation exposure, encompassing dosage levels below 1 Sv (100 rems), seldom results in immediately apparent harmful effects. Nevertheless, because of its potential to cause cell damage rather than cell death, increasing the risk of genetic defects, congenital abnormalities, or cancer—and because almost everyone experiences low-level exposure at one time or another—the human health effects of low doses of radiation have been a prime focus of radiation research for many years.

Radiation-Induced Mutations

Exposure even to very low levels of ionizing radiation can result in gene mutations; indeed, experiments to date indicate that there is no threshold level below which no mutations would be expected (however, at very low levels of exposure the mutation rate will correspondingly be quite low). There is, rather, a direct linear relationship between increasing radiation dosage and an increased number of mutations, either at the gene or chromosomal level. Both diagnostic X-rays and radioactive isotopes used for treating various ailments have been shown to damage chromosomes. Nuclear power plant workers and medical personnel, particularly radiotherapy nurses, who receive small doses of radiation on a daily basis have been shown to exhibit a marked increase in the frequency of mutations in their chromosomes (these can be observed as breaks or changes in chromosome number when chromosome smears are made from a sampling of white blood cells). The number of such abnormalities is generally highest among individuals who have been occupationally exposed to radiation for a number of years, indicating that the damaging effects of radiation exposure are cumulative.

Of greatest concern from a genetic standpoint, of course, are the mutations which accumulate in the gonadal cells which are the precursors of eggs and sperm. The number of new mutations that an individual passes on to his or her children depends on the amount of radiation the sex organs have absorbed from the time of conception up to the moment each of his or her children are conceived. Most radiation-induced mutations are recessive; hence even though most are of a harmful nature, they are likely to persist in the human gene pool, increasing in frequency over several generations before carriers of the recessive gene mate, producing offspring who exhibit the mutant characteristic.

In addition to inducing mutations in sex cells, X-ray exposure has also been shown to be capable of causing chromosomal damage in developing fetuses. Because the majority of such instances involved diagnostic X-rays of women in the very early stages of pregnancy who were not yet aware of their condition, it is now recommended that irradiation of reproductive-age women be limited to the first ten days after the onset of their last menstrual cycle to prevent exposure of an unsuspected embryo. Males and females alike should insist on being provided with a gonadal shield (e.g. lead apron) to reduce the risk of sex-cell mutations whenever X-rays are administered.

Radiation and Birth Defects

Laboratory experiments with animals, as well as direct observations of unintended consequences of humans exposed to ionizing radiation during fetal or embryonic development provide ample evidence of radiation's teratogenic effects. The most tragic and widely studied cases of radiation-induced birth defects involve the Japanese children irradiated *in utero* at the time of the atomic bomb explosions over Hiroshima and Nagasaki and of children who received X-ray exposure while still in the womb. While these sources of fetal/embryonic exposure are now, hopefully, relics of the past, other less acute sources of radiation exposure still pose safety concerns. Among these are natural radionuclides (potassium-40, carbon-14, radon and its daughter products) that can be inhaled or ingested by a pregnant woman with food or water. Radioactive fallout products, such as those released after the nuclear power plant explosion at Chernobyl, constitute another potential source of exposure. Occupational activities of the mother could result in exposure of the unborn child if her work involves production, distribution, or use of radiopharmaceuticals or the treatment and handling of patients undergoing nuclear medicine procedures. Similarly, administration of radiopharmaceuticals to pregnant patients for diagnosing or treating health problems may pose a radiation risk to the embryo/fetus (NCRP, 1998).

Sensitivity to radiation is many times greater during fetal development than at any subsequent period of a person's life, since rapid development and differentiation of tissues is occurring during this time (the more actively cells are dividing, the more vulnerable they are to radiation). In terms of *lethal*, as opposed to *teratogenic* effects, the radiosensitivity of the embryo/fetus steadily decreases during the period before birth. However, the nature and extent of fetal injury (i.e. congenital abnormalities as opposed to death) caused by radi-

BOX 10-3

"Hot" Steel

Public fears regarding radiation exposure typically focus on nuclear power plant emissions or radwaste management facilities. Many observers would argue, however, that careless handling or disposal of an estimated 500,000 radioactive devices—products as seemingly nonthreatening as tritium exit signs in theaters or cesium gauges—pose far likelier exposure risks to the general public. Although companies that produce devices containing radioactive sources must be licensed by the Nuclear Regulatory Commission (NRC) and are required to notify the federal agency (or the appropriate NRC-designated state agency) when these products are transferred or disposed, under present regulations NRC has little routine contact with license holders. As a result, a number of alarming incidents have occurred in which radioactive materials have been sent, either accidentally or illegally, to scrap dealers or metal recyclers where they pose a health threat to workers, the public, and the general environment.

An extreme case involved the theft of several cameras containing cobalt-60 capsules. After tearing off the radioactive warning labels, the thieves sold the cameras to a scrap metal dealer. One camera, containing 35.5 curies of cobalt-60, was later resold to a second dealer and then to a third. That individual, realizing the camera was radioactive, attempted to return it, but in the process the cobalt capsule fell out, landing in the corner of an office building. Subsequently, twelve adults and two children experienced dangerously high levels of radiation exposure, a truck driver developed severe radiation blistering, and five police officers who investigated the incident also suffered low doses of radiation exposure.

Most commonly, it is the workers at scrap metal plants who incur the greatest safety risk. As they bale, cut, shear, and shred metals they may be directly exposed to radioactive sources when the protective shields surrounding these materials are breached. Such incidents represent not only a health and safety issue but also constitute a heavy financial burden to the recycling industry. It is generally the responsibility of the scrap company to arrange for proper disposal of any "ownerless" radioactive device found on company property—an expensive proposition. Scrap dealers who don't discover such materials prior to processing often face far higher costs, however. According to the American Iron and Steel Institute, steel mini-mills pay an average of $8–10 million per incident in decontamination, disposal, and shutdown costs when undetected radioactive devices are inadvertently melted down (fortunately, such events are relatively rare, with 26 known incidents reported in the U.S. since 1983).

Overseas, illegal or inadvertent trafficking in radioactive materials is a growing problem as well, particularly in Europe. Sealed sources, radioactively contaminated metals, and—most worrisome—weapons-grade materials stolen from the former USSR's nuclear arsenal are all the subject of heightened attention by nuclear regulatory authorities. While U.S. officials have been most concerned about the potential for smuggled nuclear materials from poorly guarded Russian weapons sites falling into the hands of terrorists, about 80% of the known incidents to date involve other types of radioactive devices. As in the United States, many radiation sources or contaminated metals are unwittingly sold to scrap dealers, while other transactions are initiated by criminals seeking to sell stolen material for profit. The chaotic state of data-keeping in some countries exacerbates the problem of tracking potentially hazardous materials; Ukrainian officials estimate the existence of perhaps 100,000 radioactive sources whose precise location in that country is unknown. It is assumed that at least some of these materials will end up in scrap yards. In August 1998, a highly radioactive stainless steel plate from a Russian nuclear power reactor was discovered by a British secondary materials dealer in a shipment of scrap metal and had to be sent to British Nuclear Fuels Ltd. for decontamination. Italian authorities recently encountered a strange situation while monitoring shipments of scrap metal entering their country. Routine checks of railcars revealed that when radiation was detected, it was often only around the doors. Further investigation showed that radiation counts were more or less constant over the whole door surface, were almost identical on different doors, and dropped off sharply whenever the monitoring device was moved to another part of the railcar. Intrigued by the mystery, Italian officials used railcar serial numbers to trace the origin of the radioactive doors and discovered they all had been manufactured in Czechoslovakia in 1990, produced with steel that had been contaminated with a cobalt-60 source during the smelting process.

Incidents of this sort, while not frequent, have been worrisome enough to prompt the International Atomic Energy Agency (IAEA) to promote methods for increasing radiation detection efforts worldwide and, working with other organizations, to develop informational materials to assist radiation experts in dealing with this growing problem.

References

"NRC Pushes Staff to Speed Up Proposed Control for Sources." *Nuclear Waste News* 18, no. 5:43-45, Jan. 29, 1998; "International Participants Meet to Discuss Illegal Trafficking." *Nuclear Waste News* 18, no. 37:377-378, Sept. 10, 1998.

ation varies widely, depending not only on the dose absorbed but also on the precise stage of development. Because the fetal tissues are constantly growing and differentiating, the developmental response to radiation exposure on any given day may be quite different from what it would have been the day before or the day after. In addition, there are individual genetic differences in sensitivity to radiation which make it unlikely that any two fetuses would respond in precisely the same manner, even when the doses are identical. In general, radiation exposure during the first 10 days after conception will either kill the fetus or, conversely, have no discernible teratogenic effect at all. Exposure during the following period of organ formation (organogenesis), extending through the eighth week of pregnancy, can result in severe malformations. Both the skeletal system and the central nervous system are especially radiosensitive, thus exposure to X-rays or other sources of ionizing radiation can result in babies being born with abnormally small heads (microcephaly), spinal deformities, eye problems, and permanent growth retardation (the latter effect can be produced by exposure at any time during prenatal development but is most pronounced when exposure occurs during organogenesis). After the second month of pregnancy, radiation does not cause major structural defects but can provoke severe mental retardation, since the third and fourth months of pregnancy mark a period of rapid brain development. Studies of Japanese children irradiated at Hiroshima revealed that the period of highest risk for mental retardation from *in utero* exposure is between the eighth and fifteenth weeks of pregnancy, with another slightly less sensitive period occurring between the sixteenth and twenty-fifth weeks. Late-term radiation exposure has not been linked to structural problems or functional disturbances, but has been shown to increase the risk of developing childhood cancer.

The severity of the effects described increase with increasing radiation dosage; however, the existence of a threshold dose (i.e. a "safe level" of exposure below which no teratogenic effects have been observed) in the range of 0.2 to 0.4 Gy is now generally accepted (Streffer, 1997).

Radiation-Induced Cancer

The potential for health damage as a result of radiation exposure was first recognized in connection with the development of skin cancers among early radiologists, of whom nearly 100 fell victim to this disease within 15 years following the discovery of X-rays. Since then other forms of cancer, most notably leukemia, bone cancer, lung cancer, and thyroid cancer, have also been linked to radiation exposure.

Leukemia is perhaps the classic example of X-ray-induced malignancy. As early as 1911 a report of 11 cases of leukemia among radiation workers suggested a connection between the disease and their occupational exposure. Subsequently, epidemiological studies among radiologists, Japanese survivors of Hiroshima and Nagasaki, patients treated with X-ray therapy, and children who were irradiated in the womb when their mothers received diagnostic X-rays, all confirm the association between exposure to ionizing radiation and the induction of leukemia. Leukemia, like other forms of cancer, is characterized by a latency period following the initial exposure, with development of disease symptoms in this case occurring, on the average, after 5–7 years (some as early as just 2 years after irradiation).

Evidence on the amount of radiation required to induce a malignancy is scarce, particularly at doses less than 0.5 Sv (50 rems). Radiation protection policies since the early 1950s were based on the assumption that *all* radiation exposure, no matter how low, is harmful; low doses were regarded as having the same effects as high doses, though at a lower rate of incidence (a concept known as the **linear no-threshold theory**). The validity of this belief has been challenged in recent years by a growing body of evidence indicating that an exposure threshold for radiation-induced cancer does, in fact, exist and that, more surprisingly, exposure to very low levels of ionizing radiation may actually reduce the risk of cancer and enhance longevity. The scientific rationale for this point of view is that the ability of cells to repair minor genetic damage is stimulated by low-dose radiation, thus increasing the effectiveness of the DNA damage-control biosystem. Proponents of this argument point to the millions of people living in regions of higher-than-normal background radiation (e.g. those areas in India, Brazil, China, Austria, U.S., etc., described in an earlier section of this chapter) whom several epidemiologic studies have shown to have lower rates of cancer than persons living outside

BOX 10-4

Aftermath of Chernobyl

Almost a decade and a half after the name "Chernobyl" became an internationally recognized synonym for nuclear catastrophe, the full impact of that disaster remains a subject of research and controversy. What *is* clear, however, is that the official death tally of 31 persons killed in the explosion, as initially reported by Soviet authorities in the weeks following the accident, grossly understated the accident's true human health and environmental toll.

When reactor #4 of the nuclear power complex near the Ukrainian town of Chernobyl experienced a steam explosion and core meltdown on April 26, 1986, the resulting massive release of radioactive materials contaminated the environment with fallout equivalent to that of several dozen Hiroshima-type bombs. The graphite core of the reactor burned uncontrollably for nine days, in spite of heroic efforts by firefighters to quench the blaze and prevent its spread to the three nearby reactors. Of the 31 fatalities attributed to the accident by Soviet officials, 28 were among these men who knowingly braved lethal doses of radiation, standing their ground even as their boots stuck to the melting tar of the reactor roof. Not until 11 days after the explosion, when liquid nitrogen was pumped under the reactor, did the core cool sufficiently to reduce radiation levels sharply.

By this time the radioactive plume rising from the stricken reactor had spread over much of Europe. Detected first over Sweden, nuclear fallout was carried by shifting winds over most countries of eastern and central Europe, with some radioactive contamination reported from as far away as Scotland. Due to the wind direction at the time of the accident, approximately 70% of the radioactive fallout from Chernobyl was deposited in the neighboring republic of Belarus, where more than 22% of the national territory is now contaminated. Significant contamination also occurred in northern Ukraine in the area surrounding Chernobyl, as well as in nearby regions of Russia.

Evacuation of the population living in the vicinity of Chernobyl was delayed for about 36 hours following the explosion due to administrative confusion and indecision, but eventually resulted in the permanent relocation of about 116,000 people from within a 19-mile (30 km) radius of the plant. The evacuated region, officially designated as the "Scientific Exclusion Zone" (but commonly referred to as the "Dead Zone"), now constitutes a living laboratory where scientists can study the long-term ecological effects of radioactive contamination on biotic communities.

Ukrainians and Belarussians are also subjects of interest to researchers, human "guinea pigs" whose incidence rates of cancer and other radiation-related illnesses will be studied for years to come. Experts are still debating the human health costs of the accident. In 1998, while commemorating the 12th anniversary of the disaster, the Ukrainian and Russian health ministries claimed that 3,600 Ukrainians and more than 10,000 Russian "liquidators" (men who participated in cleanup operations following the explosion) have since died from radiation sickness; thousands of others, the ministries say, are now invalids (other sources, however, cite significantly lower post-accident casualty figures). The government of Ukraine has granted certain financial benefits to about 3.2 million of its citizens—over 6% of the population—as compensation for current health problems, disabilities which curtail their ability to hold a job, or future health risk due to high levels of radiation exposure. Since in Ukraine alone, approximately 2.4 million persons, including some 640,000 children, continue to live in areas regarded as contaminated, the eventual human health toll from radiation exposure could be considerable (amazingly, by the late 1990s, more than 350 people had moved back into their homes in the "Dead Zone," in spite of official prohibitions on doing so). It is known that many of the liquidators, as well as surviving workers at the power plant, received high radiation doses; one machinist in the turbine hall is thought to have received 720 rems exposure—well above the 600 rems generally regarded as lethal—yet his health remains good. Others who suffered such symptoms of radiation sickness as hair loss or skin lesions have since recovered. Nevertheless, although the death rate among those who received high doses of radiation is currently no higher than that of the general population, they tend to get sick almost three times as often and experience the sorts of illnesses usually associated with old age before they reach 45. While the incidence of leukemia and most other cancers has not yet shown a statistically significant increase, this may simply be due to the fact that the 10–30 year latency period characteristic of cancer in general has yet to run its course.

Thyroid cancer, however, constitutes a striking exception to the rule. Of all the documented health problems associated with radiation exposure at Chernobyl, the dramatic upswing in thyroid malignancies, particularly among children, is the most significant. As cattle grazed on pasturelands contaminated by radioactive fallout during the weeks immediately following the accident, iodine-131 traveled via milk to children's thyroid glands where they concentrated to levels 100 times higher than in other tissues. Youthful thyroid glands are 25 times more sensitive to radioactive iodine than are those of adults and within four years of the disaster, cases of childhood thyroid cancer began to be reported with increasing frequency; adult cases attributed to Chernobyl are increasing as well. Given the size of Ukraine's child population, 5–6 cases of thyroid cancer per year would be considered normal. The incidence rate from 1990–1995, however, averaged 37 per year among children aged 0–14, and by 1998 the total number of registered thyroid cancer cases exceeded 1,000. The toll has been even worse in Belarus, especially in the Gomel region which suffered the highest levels of radioactive fallout; there thyroid cancer rates have soared to approximately 200 times their pre-accident level. Since the most significant doses of iodine-131 occurred during the weeks following the accident, children born after October 1986, escaped exposure and are at minimal risk of thyroid problems. However, among young Belarussians, Ukrainians, and Russians who received childhood exposure to radioactive iodine, medical specialists expect to diagnose an additional 3,000 or more cases of thyroid cancer over the next ten years.

While human health problems have, understandably, received the greatest attention by those assessing the long-term damage at Chernobyl, the environmental and economic costs of the tragedy are mounting as well. In Ukraine, about 180,000 hectares (445,000 acres) of radioactively contaminated farmland has been taken out of production and 157,000 hectares (388,000 acres) of forest has similarly been rendered useless. Close to 30% of Ukraine's entire annual budget is spent on problems relating to Chernobyl—significantly more than it spends on health, education, or culture. The financial impact on Belarus has been equally severe—one expert estimates that in the years since the accident, Belarus' economic losses have been ten times greater than the country's annual budget.

Unfortunately, there's no end in sight to Ukraine's Chernobyl-related problems. Perhaps most urgent, the damaged reactor continues to pose serious health and environmental threats. The concrete "sarcophagus" built immediately after the accident to contain further radioactive releases from the molten core was hastily constructed without a structural margin of safety. Experts fear that the sarcophagus, which has already developed hundreds of dangerous cracks, could collapse if overburdened with heavy snow—a disquieting prospect, since engineers have confirmed the presence of some 34 tons of radioactive dust within the sarcophagus. Adding to concerns is the fact that the basement of the sarcophagus is flooded with about 3,000 cubic meters of radioactively contaminated water, due to infiltration of precipitation and routine spraying for dust suppression. There are fears that this water has the potential to contaminate groundwater, the level of which has been rising under the reactor since 1993. Pollution of groundwater in the vicinity is made even more problematic by the existence of large amounts of intensely radioactive wastes buried in shallow trenches on plant grounds and at various locations within the exclusion zone. These burial trenches are situated just 4 meters above the water table and lack waterproof barriers. Inside the sarcophagus, high humidity and standing water are dissolving fission products in the radioactive debris, causing it to crumble and leading to fears that a burst of neutrons (a "criticality incident") could result due to the increasing concentration of fission products.

The international scientific community agrees that the damaged reactor is in desperate need of repairs; in 1997 the Group of Seven (G7) industrialized countries agreed to provide $300 million to make the sarcophagus ecologically safe; the European Union pledged an additional $110 million to the project whose total cost is estimated at $750 million. However, delays in hiring a contractor and an economic crisis in Ukraine have delayed the onset of this project, which is expected to require up to nine years to complete. Unfortunately, Chernobyls lethal legacy of health and environmental threats will continue to bedevil policymakers, scientists, and the medical community for decades to come.

References

Bradley, Don J. 1997. *Behind The Nuclear Curtain: Radioactive Waste Management in the Former Soviet Union.* Columbus, OH: Battelle Press.

Feshbach, Murray. 1995. *Ecological Disaster.* New York: The Twentieth Century Fund Press.

Perera, Judith. 1997. "Ukraine, G7 Countries to Fund Urgent D&D Work." *Nuclear Waste News* 17, no. 42:408 (Oct. 30).

those areas. A study conducted in 1993 on Japanese atomic bomb survivors revealed significantly greater longevity among those exposed to radiation than among unexposed Japanese; a 1991 report on U.S. nuclear shipyard workers showed a statistically significant decrease in mortality rates for deaths from all causes among men occupationally exposed to gamma radiation when compared with unexposed workers. While there is no question that, at doses of 1 Gy or above, cancer risk increases with increasing dosage, intensive investigations conducted over the past 40 years fail to provide convincing data that doses of radiation under 0.2 Gy result in any increased cancer risk. Indeed, the evidence suggests quite the contrary—that very low levels of radiation not only are not harmful but may actually be of health benefit (Pollycove, 1997).

Whatever the case, for purposes of regulation, federal agencies still subscribe to the linear dose-response curve which assumes a directly proportional increase in number of cancer cases with increasing radiation dosage and no threshold level below which cancer incidence would be zero. In the absence of universal agreement, this approach is considered to provide the most prudent way of safeguarding public health. Currently, federal standards set 1.7 mSv/year (170 mR/year), excluding medical exposure, as the maximum permissible radiation dose for members of the general population as a whole, no more than 0.25 mSv (25mR) of which should come from a nuclear power facility. Individuals may receive up to 5 mSv/year (500 mR/year), while workers in radiation-related occupations are allowed average yearly exposures of 50 mSv (5 rems). Persons under the age of 18 are permitted no occupational exposure whatsoever. Such standards have been set for the intended purpose of protecting human health against the long-term radiation effects of cancer and genetic defects. These standards do not reflect levels of absolute safety but rather attempt to strike a balance between possible adverse effects of low-level exposure and the known benefits of nuclear power and other uses of radioactive materials. In the late 1980s the safety of current exposure limits was called into question by new interpretation of data on exposure received by Japanese survivors at Hiroshima and Nagasaki. Post-war estimates of likely radiation levels at varying distances from ground zero, correlated with observed health effects, have formed the basis for radiation standards since the end of World War II. Results from studies conducted during the 1980s suggested that the original data overestimated the radiation dosage received by persons in the affected area. Some researchers now believe that the observable health damage experienced by survivors was caused by approximately one-half the amount of radiation exposure calculated previously. These findings, if correct, imply that current radiation protection standards should be at least twice as stringent as they are now in order to protect public health. More recent studies conducted in the United Kingdom provide additional basis for doubt regarding the adequacy of existing exposure limits. A large-scale survey of British nuclear plant workers who experienced occupational exposure to low levels of ionizing radiation over a period of many years showed a statistically positive association between leukemia death rates and radiation exposure, with risks rising as dosage increased. These results, along with observations that rates of terminal cancer are higher among A-bomb survivors in Japan than among Japanese not exposed to radiation from those atomic blasts, have led Britain's National Radiological Protection Board (NRPB) to urge the adoption of new radiation protection standards. In place of the present 50 mSv yearly exposure limit for occupational exposure, the NRPB is recommending an upper limit of just 20 mSv, while similarly advocating that the annual dose for members of the general public be reduced from 5 mSv to 1 mSv (Perera, 1993; "New Study," 1992; Hawkes et al., 1987).

It should be noted in passing that the above-mentioned consequences of low-level radiation exposure may also be manifested at higher rates among survivors of high-level radiation doses. Mutations, birth defects among offspring, a significantly heightened risk of leukemia and other cancers, as well as cataracts and a general shortening of life span due to premature aging, are realistic possibilities confronting individuals who have recovered from overt symptoms of radiation sickness.

Radiation and Nuclear Power Generation

While medical uses of X-rays and radioisotopes constitute by far the largest amount of non-background radiation exposure, it is not these sources but rather the perceived health threat from nuclear power plants that has received the lion's share of public attention in recent years. Since 1957 when the first commercial nuclear power plant came on line in Shippingsport, Pennsylvania, the percentage of electricity generated by nuclear energy in the United States grew rapidly until the mid-1970s, much more slowly since then—no new commercial nuclear reactors have been ordered by U.S. utility companies since 1978. By late 1999, approximately 20% of the electrical energy in the United States was provided by 103 nuclear power plants. That number could decrease significantly after 2012 when the licenses of currently operating plants begin to expire and the reactors are decommissioned. Economic considerations arising from utility industry deregulation have prompted some observers to suggest that a number of money-losing plants may be closed even before their licenses expire. Alternatively, others predict that many plant owners will request 20-year license extensions and continue to operate the facilities well beyond their originally anticipated lifespan. If the latter forecast proves correct, nuclear power could continue to play an important role in the U.S. energy mix well into the 21st century. Whether or not this situation is desirable has been a subject of controversy for many years.

Even before the serious accident in 1979 at the Three Mile Island power plant near Harrisburg, Pennsylvania, and the catastrophe at Chernobyl in the USSR in 1986, concerns about the safety of nuclear power had given rise to an active and vocal antinuclear movement. Internationally, antinuclear groups have become a powerful political force, echoing the "Hell, no, we won't glow!" sentiments of their American colleagues two decades earlier. Following the 1998 national elections in Germany, the victorious coalition of Social Democrats and the environmental activist Green Party promptly initiated a program to close all 19 German nuclear power plants within 10 years, even though these plants currently produce one-third of Germany's electricity. The only major power now moving resolutely toward increased reliance on nuclear power is Japan where, in spite of public opposition, the government in 1998 approved the first of 20 new light-water reactors that will be constructed over the next several years. Already reliant on nuclear power from 51 operating plants for 37% of its energy demand, Japan views the expansion of nuclear power as vital to efforts to reduce the CO_2 emissions that contribute to global warming. Elsewhere, in spite of the insistence by nuclear power proponents that a new generation of safe, more efficient nuclear generating plants can and should be built to replace facilities being taken off-line, most observers of the current political scene are highly skeptical that a new surge of nuclear power plant construction is likely to occur. Arguments such as those voiced by Japanese leaders that nuclear power is urgently needed to curb greenhouse gas emissions are discounted by a public concerned about the absence of safe methods for permanent radwaste disposal, aware that "accidents can happen," and harboring a visceral fear of anything labeled "radioactive." Given the emotionalism involved, it is important that citizens clearly understand the extent to which nuclear power generation contributes to the overall radiation burden experienced by the general public. Although most attention is focused on the power plants themselves, nuclear power production is dependent upon a number of activities, collectively referred to as the **nuclear fuel cycle**. The three main components of this cycle, along with their environmental health impacts, are described in the following sections.

Front-end. Prior to the generation of power inside a nuclear reactor, the nuclear fuel itself must be mined, processed, and fabricated into fuel rods. Uranium-235 constitutes the fissionable fuel in most nuclear reactors and is mined in a number of locations around the world, including Australia, Canada, parts of eastern Europe, and several western states in the U.S. In the past, when uranium ore was obtained primarily from underground mines, the most significant radiation hazard was the increased risk of lung cancer among uranium miners, caused by the inhalation of alpha-emitting radon gas and radon daughters (radioactive isotopes of polonium and lead) attached to tiny particles of mine dust. Exposure to this occupational hazard contributed to lung cancer mortality rates among U.S. uranium miners (the majority of whom were Navajos recruited by the government to work for the nuclear weapons industry but never warned about the known health risks) four to five times higher than that prevailing among the general population. Similarly, at least 20,000 East German miners, mobilized in the late 1940s and early 1950s to supply uranium for the former Soviet Union's nuclear arsenal, have died or are dying of lung diseases caused by their exposure to radioactive gases and dust (Kahn, 1993). Open-pit uranium mining, while avoiding the occupational health risks entailed by underground mining, is, like strip-mining for coal, environmentally disruptive and often results in soil erosion and contaminated runoff.

The uranium ore extracted from underground or open-pit mines must subsequently be crushed and processed to produce the form of uranium dioxide known as "yellowcake." These milling operations and the enormous piles of sandlike tailings they create (for every ounce of uranium extracted from ore, 99 ounces of waste tailings are generated) constitute by far the most significant source of public exposure to ionizing radiation related to nuclear power production. In the United States, more than 140 million tons of radioactive tailings were left at abandoned mill sites scattered across seven western states, releasing radon into the air and leaching radium into the subsoil. In 1979, the rupture of an earthen dam at a uranium mine and mill site near Churchrock, New Mexico, released 1,100 tons of tailings sludge and 90 million gallons of radioactively contaminated water into a stream running through the Navajo reservation. Considered the worst radwaste spill ever to occur in the United States, this accident resulted in traces of radioactive materials being carried at least 75 miles downstream across the Arizona border. In Grand Junction, Colorado, mine tailings were incorporated into concrete which was used for foundations of homes, churches, and schools. For nearly 20 years until the problem was recognized, approximately 30,000 people living in those dwellings were exposed to levels of radon up to seven times the maximum allowable level for uranium miners; subsequent cleanup efforts at the Grand Junction mill site and over 4,000 nearby properties cost the government close to $700 million. A number of other western communities, including Denver and Salt Lake City, also have used radioactive tailings in constructing roads and the foundations of buildings. Because of the radiation hazards posed by mill tailings (radiation levels 40–400 times above normal background levels), Congress in 1978 passed legislation authorizing the U.S. Department of Energy to clean up 50 uranium-processing sites, as well as nearby contaminated properties. While a number of mills were still active in 1978 when the law was passed, all are now closed and cleanup of surface contamination has been completed. In most cases site remediation involved enclosing the tailings in a containment cell, covering the cell with compacted clay to prevent the release of radon, and, finally, topping the area with vegetation or rocks. Cleanup of contaminated groundwater at these sites is on-going and isn't expected to be finished until at least 2014 (Steinhardt, 1996).

Similar environmental problems associated with uranium milling operations continue to plague a number of European countries. In eastern Germany, Hungary, and the Czech Republic, large areas are today littered with abandoned piles of uranium tailings and other radioactive wastes, confronting the leaders of those countries with massive cleanup challenges.

Today almost all production of uranium in the United States, and in many places elsewhere in the world, utilizes an extraction process called **in-situ leaching (ISL)**. ISL is a closed-loop mining system, whereby uranium is dissolved in place by a leaching agent—usually sulfuric acid—which is injected into the ore deposit, with the liquid subsequently being pumped to the surface where the uranium is recovered out of solution. After processing, the fluid is returned to the well field to continue the leaching cycle. Unlike underground or open-pit mining, ISL methods eliminate worker exposure to radioactive gases, minimize surface disruption, and produce no tailings whatsoever; the only surface wastes associated with the process are small evaporation ponds. Nevertheless, while in-situ leaching is often described by advocates as an "environmentally benign" method of mining uranium, it isn't problem-free. The injection of massive amounts of acid into rock deposits can result in extensive groundwater contamination if proper precautions aren't followed. At an in-situ leaching site that has been operating for more than 25 years in the Czech Republic, highly contaminated liquids have migrated from the leaching zone, seeping along faulty wells to an upper-level aquifer. As a result of this, some 76 million cubic meters of drinking water in northern

Bohemia's largest aquifer are now polluted (Perera, 1997).

Transforming the milled yellowcake into nuclear fuel requires several additional steps. First, the uranium is converted into gaseous uranium hexafluoride, then enriched to increase the concentration of the fissionable U-235 isotope from its original 0.7% (the bulk of uranium ore is U-238, a nonfissionable isotope) to 2–4%, the level necessary to sustain a fission reaction. Finally, at a fuel fabrication facility, the enriched uranium hexafluoride gas is converted into solid uranium dioxide pellets which are then loaded into fuel rods. Cumulatively, these processes have very minimal environmental health impacts, entailing the venting of small, regulated quantities of radioactive emissions into the air and very limited discharges of diluted liquid wastes; occupational exposure among workers in the plants where these activities are carried out likewise is very low.

In summary, the front-end of the nuclear fuel cycle is characterized by relatively low levels of radioactive emissions and minimal public exposure to radiation, the major exception to this being those people living in the vicinity of improperly managed uranium mill tailings and the unfortunate uranium miners whose untimely deaths due to lung cancer can be attributed largely to their workplace exposure to radioactive gases in underground mines.

Power Production. Under normal operating conditions, radiation exposure to the general public emanating from nuclear power plants comes primarily from the deliberate release of controlled amounts of radioactive gases to the atmosphere. Gaseous fission products such as tritium and krypton build up in the fuel rods, leak through the cladding into the reactor building, and must be periodically vented. In addition, small amounts of radioactive materials may be discharged with wastewaters. Overall, the radiation hazard to people living in the vicinity of a normally operating nuclear reactor is minimal, considerably less than that from natural background sources.

The main fear among those opposed to further reliance on nuclear power, of course, is the potential, however remote, of catastrophic release of radioactive materials should a major accident occur. Although most people today realize that it is physically impossible for a nuclear power plant to explode like a bomb (for this to occur the U-235 fuel would have to be enriched to a concentration far above the level necessary to sustain a fission reaction for power production purposes), a **core meltdown,** which represents a worst-type accident scenario, would be nearly as devastating. Overheating of the reactor core, such as might occur if water should cease to circulate among the fuel rods (a "loss-of-coolant" accident), could result in melting of the fuel rods and breaching of the containment vessel. The massive release of highly radioactive isotopes into the atmosphere, such as occurred at Chernobyl, or into groundwater supplies could cause widespread human exposure to lethal doses of radiation, contamination of the general environment with radioactive fallout, and would initiate numerous leukemias and other cancers that would be manifested years later. Although physical destruction of buildings and property would not occur, the biological impact of a core meltdown would be nearly as serious as a bomb blast in terms of human health and environmental degradation. The "defense in depth" concept employed in the construction of nuclear plants, characterized by repeated layers of thick shielding materials and multiple safeguards designed to ensure safety even in the event of partial failure, are intended to prevent this situation from ever becoming a reality.

In spite of such precautions, thousands of mishaps have occurred both here and abroad since the advent of commercial nuclear power. Prior to the Three Mile Island incident, two of the most serious U.S. accidents occurred at the Enrico-Fermi experimental fast breeder reactor near Detroit where part of the fuel in the core melted in early October 1966, and at Browns Ferry, Alabama, where in March 1975, a fire ignited by an electrician's candle raged for seven hours, destroying all the emergency cooling systems in one of the reactors at the complex. In both cases, a core meltdown was only narrowly averted. Each major accident has led to a tightening of safety regulations; a report issued by the Congressional Office of Technology Assessment (OTA) affirmed that safety performance of American commercial nuclear power plants has been generally good. No accidents resulting in damage to the reactor core have occurred since the partial meltdown at Three Mile Island in 1979, nor have any offsite releases of large amounts of radioactivity taken place. Although hundreds of emergency shutdowns occur annually, OTA asserts that the number of such events in recent years has not been abnormal and few of them were serious enough to pose a threat of core damage. OTA also reported that radiation exposure to nuclear plant workers, already well below the limits established by the Nuclear Regulatory Commission (NRC), continues to decline.

The operating record of nuclear power plants in Japan and the countries of western Europe roughly parallels that of the United States. Many concerns have surfaced during the past decade, however, about the deplorable conditions prevailing at a number of nuclear power plants operating in Russia and several of the former Soviet republics. Russian safety experts, nuclear plant workers, and Western scientists have all concluded that the nuclear power industry throughout the former USSR is on the verge of disaster. The tragic accident at Chernobyl in 1986, initially blamed on violations of operating procedures by plant personnel, is now attributed primarily to fundamental design faults in the reactor itself. This conclusion is worrisome because eleven other reactors of similar design are operating in Russia, two more in Lithuania. These plants, in the view of many experts, are "accidents waiting to happen." Neither the Chernobyl-style reactors nor the older Soviet-version pressurized water reactors are enclosed by the concrete and metal radiation containment structures that are a standard feature of reactor design in other industrial countries (Russian reactors built after 1981 do have full containment structures, however). An inventory of nuclear facilities conducted by Russia's State Committee for Nuclear and Radiation Safety Oversight (Gosatomnadzor) in 1993 revealed that many of the nation's older reactors were in dire need of radical reconstruction due to repeated failures of obsolete or worn-out equipment and system components. Some of these older facilities are characterized by such serious design flaws that Committee members concluded they could never be retrofitted to international standards and urged that they be closed. In the Moscow area alone, fifty nuclear reactors were judged to be unsafe and Gosatomnadzor, after concluding its investigation, reported that "Russia's nuclear power plants are incapable of maintaining their equipment in a safe

BOX 10-5

Nuclear Wastelands

There is arguably no country on Earth more radioactively polluted than Russia. Although the Cold War tensions that spurred a nuclear arms race between the former Soviet Union and the United States have now faded, the radioactive remains of four decades of nuclear weapons production continue to threaten human health and environmental quality throughout that vast nation. Extensive contamination caused by negligent rad-waste disposal practices has been reported from locations all across Russia, including numerous sites within the capital city of Moscow itself. Nonmilitary medical, industrial, and scientific research operations generated some of these problems, while others were a result of the ocean dumping of both liquid and solid radwastes from Russian navy vessels, a practice only recently halted. However, by far the worst examples of self-inflicted radiation pollution can be found in the vicinity of three once-secret nuclear cities created by Soviet authorities to produce enriched uranium and plutonium for the USSR's nuclear arsenal. American scientists at Pacific Northwest Laboratory estimate that the current level of radioactive material discharged to the environment at these three sites is about 600 times greater than the combined releases from all remaining nuclear sources in Russia.

Beginning in the late 1940s, the nuclear complexes at Mayak, near the towns of Ozersk and Chelyabinsk in the Ural Mountains of southern Russia, and at Tomsk-7 and Krasnoyarsk-26, both in Siberia, became the centers for spent fuel reprocessing in the former USSR, producing not only bomb-grade material but also enormous volumes of radioactive wastes which were discharged into nearby surface waters, injected into the ground, or buried in shallow trenches. These wastes constitute the largest-ever releases of radioactive materials to the global environment, far exceeding the amounts contributed by nuclear weapons testing.

The Mayak complex was the first Soviet reprocessing facility to commence operations; the plant is still in operation and has been designated as the site for future dismantlement of Russian nuclear warheads. Mayak was built in a low-lying marshy area with a water table just 3–12 feet below ground surface and adjacent to several rivers, a location which greatly enhances the potential for serious water pollution problems. Careful waste management was obviously not a major concern of early Mayak directors; from 1949–1952 large volumes of untreated liquid radioactive wastes, heavily laden with strontium-90 and cesium-137, were dumped directly into the Techa River. In 1951 a radiation survey of the river basin revealed that radionuclides had substantially contaminated the Techa flood plain and bottom sediments, resulting in significant radiation exposure to approximately 124,000 persons living near the river; most seriously affected were the 28,000 villagers who resided close to the river-bank and thus received the largest doses. In 1956, the entire population of the upper Techa basin was evacuated and the contaminated flood plain in other parts of the area fenced off, thereby eliminating further external exposure of the population. Internal exposure, primarily via fish consumption, proved more difficult to control but has measurably decreased over the years. Not surprisingly, a statistically significant increase in leukemia incidence among people living near Mayak was reported over the next 5–20 years.

In the early 1950s, the realization that discharges to the Techa had contaminated about 80% of the river's entire flood plain prompted authorities to construct a series of four dams and reservoirs, both to contain the contamination and to serve as storage basins for liquid low-level wastes, which continued to be discharged to these surface waters. It was assumed at the time that these dams and reservoirs would successfully isolate 98% of the radionuclides which had been deposited on the flood plain. Today the dams are a growing focus of concern among Russian environmentalists who fear that some 200 million curies contained in these reservoirs could be released into the Techa if the dams should break.

An even greater worry in the Mayak region is Lake Karachai, into which high-level liquid wastes from spent fuel reprocessing were discharged after dumping into the Techa River was halted. Russian officials estimate the lake has accumulated a staggering 120 million curies, constituting an acute environmental health hazard today and for centuries to come. In 1990 American observers from the Natural Resources Defense Council reported that radiation levels along the lake shore were so high that a person standing there for an hour would receive a lethal dose. A radioactive plume of contamination has been seeping out of the lake and migrating southward at a rate of about 80 meters per year, resulting in extensive groundwater pollution. In 1997 a member of the Russian Nuclear Society conceded that "we do not see a

solution to radionuclide migration from Karachai in the near future."

Even worse than the radioactive contamination at Mayak are the conditions prevailing at the two Siberian reprocessing facilities. Indeed, the largest discharges of radioactive wastes anywhere in the world have occurred—and continue to occur—at Tomsk-7. Approximately 8 million cubic meters of liquid radwastes, containing 130 million curies, have been dumped into reservoirs and pits that are even more contaminated than Mayak's Lake Karachai. These impoundments are so radioactive that a Moscow photographer wanting to get a shot of the reservoir was allowed by authorities to run up to the edge for only one minute! Still larger volumes of liquid radwastes, estimated by Russian environmentalists to contain from 500 million to 1.2 billion curies, have been pumped directly into sandy geological formations several hundred meters underground via deepwell injection. Citing the fact that these wastes are being injected into aquifers located only a few kilometers from drinking water wells, local environmentalists say the practice invites catastrophe and claim that "we have 22 Chernobyls under our feet."

Although deepwell injection of radioactive wastes at Tomsk-7 has been ongoing since 1963, the Russian government didn't acknowledge the practice until 1992. Officials recently agreed to drill monitoring wells in the area to determine if waste migration is occurring from the injection zone to upper-level aquifers that supply most of the drinking water for the city of Tomsk; some radioactive contamination has already been found in village wells less than five miles from the injection site. Local activists also warn that enough radioactive material could accumulate within the injection zone to cause a criticality event, which could release large amounts of heat and radiation to the environment. Regional administrative officials, economically dependent on the nuclear complex, continue to shrug off such concerns and in 1996 issued a five-year renewal of the facility's permit to continue waste pumping.

At Krasnoyarsk-26 (now renamed Zhelznogorsk) the situation is much the same, though the total volume of radwaste is somewhat less than at Tomsk-7. The three plutonium production reactors that operated during the complex's peak years (only one remains in service) generated huge quantities of radioactive wastes. Today the solid radwastes are simply being stored in special facilities on-site; liquid radioactive wastes are managed either by deepwell injection or by discharge into one of four reservoirs. Although monitoring wells have been placed around the underground repository to detect possible leakage, some observers worry that radionuclides could migrate from the repository into a nearby tributary of the Yenisey River, whose waters eventually flow into the Arctic Ocean.

For Russians demanding improved radwaste management, the current outlook is grim. Most existing and newly generated wastes still are not being treated; radionuclides continue to migrate from open waste impoundments and reservoirs; many engineered storage facilities are no longer considered safe, and inadequate storage capacity is hindering efforts to manage wastes generated by nuclear vessels and radiochemical plants. On-site storage facilities at nuclear power plants are full or nearly so and regional repositories for safe, permanent disposal of these wastes have yet to be developed. Russia still lacks an automated system for accounting and control of its radioactive waste inventory, raising fears of illicit diversion of such materials by organized crime or terrorist groups and, worse yet, financial resources for solving these problems are almost nonexistent. Cumulatively, such deficiencies enhance the risk of future radiation accidents and threaten further radioactive contamination of Russia's air, soil, and water resources.

References

Bradley, Don J. 1997. *Behind the Nuclear Curtain: Radioactive Waste Management in the Former Soviet Union.* Columbus, OH: Battelle Press.

Kryshev, I.I. et al. 1998. "Radioecological Consequences of Radioactive Discharges into the Techa River of the Southern Urals." *Journal of Environmental Radioactivity* 38, no. 2:195-209.

Perera, Judith. 1998. "Opposition Mounts Against Injection of Rad Waste into Tomsk Aquifers." *Nuclear Waste News* 18, no. 28 (July 9):275-6.

state." By the late 1990s, the growing financial crisis in Russia, Ukraine, and elsewhere in the region further compounded the problems facing the nuclear industry. With major customers defaulting on their fuel bills, the cash-strapped nuclear industry found itself unable to pay the salaries of power plant operators, much less finance needed repairs and new equipment. Low staff morale, loss of skilled workers, and growing plant theft increase the risk of serious problems at nuclear power stations throughout the region. Lack of funds also makes closure of troubled plants more problematic, since nuclear plants continue to require costly maintenance and oversight after power production ceases. It has been estimated that shutdown of all the remaining Chernobyl-type reactors alone would take ten years and cost $6–8 billion. As a result, it is likely that for the foreseeable future these plants will remain in operation, posing a constant threat of disaster to all who live downwind (Feshbach, 1995).

Back-end. After a fuel assembly has been in operation for about a year, waste fission products accumulate in the rods to such an extent that the fission reaction can no longer be sustained, necessitating replacement of these "spent" rods with fresh ones. Spent fuel rods, highly radioactive, are initially placed in swimming pool-like cooling tanks where the isotopes with very short half-lives decay within a relatively brief time. The rods are still highly radioactive (and physically hot as well) due to longer-lived fission products still present and also contain appreciable amounts of unused fuel in the form of U-235 and plutonium which formed during the fission process within the fuel rods. To separate these two useful products from the other isotopes that constitute high level radioactive wastes, **reprocessing** of the material in the spent rods was envisioned as a vital part of the nuclear fuel cycle. In this process the fuel is removed from the rods and dissolved in nitric acid, the solution then being treated chemically to separate it into uranium, plutonium, and waste components. This operation represents a potential public hazard, since volatile radioisotopes, particularly krypton, are released into the atmosphere and other radioisotopes are discharged with liquid wastes. Workers inside the reprocessing plant are also exposed to higher levels of radioactivity than are nuclear power plant workers, though conceivably safeguards could be taken to reduce this risk. Although reprocessing was considered an important means to reduce the amount of what would otherwise be considered waste and extend the fuel supply, a moratorium on commercial reprocessing was imposed by President Ford in 1976 and continued by President Carter due to the concern that reprocessing plants would be tempting targets for attack by terrorists attempting to obtain weapons-grade plutonium. Although President Reagan subsequently lifted the ban, financial considerations have deterred private interests from reentering the reprocessing business and at present there is no commercial reprocessing in the United States. Elsewhere, France and the United Kingdom reprocess spent fuel from nuclear reactors, for both their own nuclear power industry and for foreign customers. The Japanese have reprocessing facilities at Tokaimura, about 70 miles northeast of Tokyo, and are building another, larger plant at Rokkasho-mura in northern Honshu, expected to begin operations sometime after 2003. Russia has three formerly secret reprocessing plants, built primarily to obtain plutonium for weapons production during the Cold War years. In 1957 a high-level waste tank at one of these facilities, the Mayak Production Association, near the town of Kyshtym, exploded, releasing about two million curies of radiation over the region. Although the outside world was not told of this event until three decades later, during the year following the accident 11,000 people were evacuated from the area and for many years farming was prohibited on 440 square miles of heavily contaminated land surrounding the site. Today Russia's Mayak reprocessing plant generates badly-needed foreign exchange by reprocessing, for a fee, spent nuclear fuel from other countries. In 1993, one of the plants, Tomsk-

7 in Siberia, experienced an explosion that contaminated 1,500 square meters of land in the vicinity of the plant; radioactive fallout from the accident was detected over a 120-square-kilometer area, with the most heavily contaminated areas registering gamma radiation readings 20 times above background levels (Perera, 1998). Japan's Tokaimura reprocessing facilities have experienced several serious accidents in recent years. A fire and explosion in March 1997 resulted in the exposure of 37 workers to low levels of radiation and released some plutonium into the environment ("Reprocessing Facility," 1997). In the autumn of 1999, improper handling of enriched uranium at a fuel processing plant resulted in a critical reaction that exposed three workers to life-threatening levels of radiation (one of these men subsequently died). Neutrons escaping from the facility irradiated a number of people outside the plant as well; the government's official count of people experiencing radiation exposure was 69, although some environmental groups insisted the actual number was much higher. Regarded as the worst accident to date in Japan's nuclear program, the incident prompted a temporary evacuation order for residents living nearest the plant, while an additional 310,000 people within a six-mile radius were advised to remain indoors until radiation levels subsided (Landers, 1999).

While reprocessing facilities may present radiation hazards both to their workers and to the environment, the most significant source of dangerous radioactive emissions from the back-end of the nuclear fuel cycle is the waste material produced by nuclear reactors. Nuclear power production results in the generation of large quantities of both high- and low-level wastes, the former primarily in the form of spent fuel from reactors, the latter consisting of contaminated clothing, clean-up solutions, wiping rags, hand tools, etc. **High-level wastes** are extremely radioactive, highly penetrating, and generate a great deal of heat, hence must be handled without direct human contact. Currently, most high-level commercial wastes in the U.S. are being stored in cooling ponds at the power plants where they were produced; a relatively small percentage is in storage at facilities in Morris, Illinois, and West Valley, New York, once intended as reprocessing plants.

Responding to criticism that the lack of any clear-cut policy for permanent disposal of high-level radioactive waste could prove the Achilles' heel of the nuclear power industry, Congress in 1982 enacted the **Nuclear Waste Policy Act.** This legislation delegated responsibility for high-level radwaste management to the federal government and designated the U.S. Department of Energy as the lead agency to coordinate the effort to site, construct, and operate the nation's first permanent repository for such wastes. The politically sensitive search for a location for this facility is now focused on Yucca Mountain, Nevada, where extensive characterization studies are underway to determine the site's geologic suitability for deep burial of solidified wastes. Since the fission products in spent fuel rods will be dangerously radioactive for tens of thousands of years, suitability of any site chosen for an underground repository will depend on the ability of surrounding geological formations to absorb heat and to prevent radioactive emissions from escaping into the environment. Issues of special concern at the Yucca Mountain site include the long-term potential for earthquakes or volcanic eruptions in an area of known seismic activity and the possibility of groundwater intrusion into storage caverns in the eventuality of future climatic change. The fact that the area contains numerous mineral deposits raises worries that future generations, ignorant of the hazardous materials entombed on the site, might drill into the repository in search of gas or oil.

In December 1998, the Department of Energy released its long-awaited viability assessment for Yucca Mountain; in its report DOE concluded that although some uncertainties remain, there are no major problems which would disqualify the site from consideration as the nation's high-level rad-waste repository. Department officials stated that scientific and technical work at Yucca Mountain should proceed in order to support a decision by the Secretary of Energy, due in 2001, on whether to recommend the site to the president for development as a geological repository.

If DOE resolves that the site is indeed suitable, it will prepare an environmental impact statement and forward a recommendation to the president that Yucca Mountain be approved as the nation's first permanent repository for high-level radioactive wastes. If the president agrees, Congress must then vote to approve or reject the site. At that point, the State of Nevada has the right to veto the entire project—and will likely do so, given the intense opposition toward the repository being expressed throughout Nevada by the public and by policymakers fearful of their state's image as a "national sacrifice zone." Such an action could be overturned only by a joint resolution by the U.S. Senate and House of Representatives. Only after congressional approval of the site has been obtained can DOE apply to the Nuclear Regulatory Commission for a license to begin construction of the facility. Since approval of the license request can take up to three years and construction of the repository several years more, it is obvious that utility companies have a long time to wait before the spent fuel rods accumulating at reactor sites can be moved to their final resting place (League of Women Voters, 1993). Although the 1982 Nuclear Waste Policy Act mandated that the repository be operational by January 31, 1998, the Department of Energy anticipates that a radwaste facility at Yucca Mountain won't be ready to begin accepting wastes until 2010 at the earliest.

In the meantime, spent fuel rods continue to accumulate at power plants across the country, prompting warnings from utility companies that some reactors may be forced to close prematurely for lack of storage space. Indeed, the Nuclear Energy Institute, a private organization representing industry interests, contends that fully 80 nuclear power plants will have exhausted their on-site storage capacity by 2010. This situation poses a major problem for the federal government as well as for the nuclear power industry. Under terms of the Nuclear Waste Policy Act, Washington has been collecting a one-tenth of a cent fee on every kilowatt hour of electricity generated by nuclear power since 1983, with these revenues being deposited in a special fund ear-marked for development of the permanent repository. In return, Washington made a contractual commitment to the utility companies that it would begin to move spent fuel from reactor sites in 1998. By the time the deadline date arrived, utilities had paid $14 billion into the Nuclear Waste Fund and were furious that the federal government had failed to meet its obligation under the law (a court ruling in November 1997, affirmed DOE's obligation to pick up the spent fuel and stated that the Department could be liable for damages if it did not do so). As a consequence, a coalition of state governments, as well as a number of utility companies, promptly filed suit against DOE. The Department of Energy, while insisting that industry must continue paying into the Fund, is attempting to devise an interim solution in the form of a **Monitored Retrievable Storage (MRS)** facility—a "temporary" away-from-reactor site where spent nuclear fuel could be stored in above-ground dry casks for an indefinite period until a permanent repository is ultimately opened. Already a number of power plants around the U.S. are utilizing dry cask storage, sealing the radioactive wastes inside huge steel containers with 9-inch thick walls and placing them outdoors on a barbed-wire enclosed concrete pad. Legislation has been introduced by congressional supporters of the nuclear industry to develop an MRS facility at Yucca Mountain itself, reasoning that doing so would facilitate transfer of radwastes into a permanent repository if one is eventually built there. Opponents of nuclear power bitterly oppose any away-from-reactor storage, particularly at Yucca Mountain, which they fear would become a *"de facto"* site regardless of its geologic suitability if wastes were already on site as decision-making time approached. They also worry about the potential for accidents involving wastes in transit, but proponents argue that until a permanent disposal site is operational, it is preferable to store mounting stocks of nuclear waste at one carefully maintained location rather than at scores of nuclear power plants across the nation, many of them located in densely populated areas or immediately adjacent to bodies of water.

For a number of years the Department of Energy tried, with very limited success, to attract interest from states, counties, or Native American tribes to host an MRS facility in return for certain financial benefits. In the mid-1990s the Mescalero Apaches in New Mexico seriously considered such an undertaking, but eventually declined. Subsequently, the 124-member Skull Valley Band of the Goshute tribe in Utah entered into a joint venture with eight utility companies to develop a storage facility on 18,000 acres of tribal land 70 miles west of Salt Lake City. Utah state officials are adamantly opposed to the project and are doing all they can to block it. The Goshutes contend that, as a sovereign Indian nation, they are entitled to proceed without state consent if the federal Nuclear Regulatory Commission grants approval. The site, which the consortium hopes to open in 2002, is intended primarily for use by the eight utilities involved, but is large enough to accomodate wastes from other generators as well. To the Goshutes, the proposed development offers a way out of poverty on a reservation described by the tribal chairman, Leon D. Bear, as a place that "doesn't grow much of anything." Arguing that Utah's governor and other antinuclear opponents of the project are guilty of "economic paternalism," Mr. Bear defends the initiative as both safe and of great potential benefit to his people. "My ancestors ate grasshoppers," Mr. Bear commented; "I don't want to live like that" (Fialka, 1998).

While controversy over a monitored retrievable storage facility continues to inflame passions in Utah, elsewhere in the Southwest New Mexico is witness to a radioactive waste management success story. In March 1999, the **Waste Isolation Pilot Plant (WIPP)** opened its gates and in so doing became the world's first certified deep radwaste facility. Designed as a permanent repository for lower-level **transuranic wastes**—plutonium-contaminated rags, tools, and protective clothing from nuclear weapons production facilities—WIPP is a subterranean complex of shafts, tunnels, and rooms excavated more than 2,000 feet (655 meters) underground in a salt formation 25 miles east of Carlsbad, New Mexico. Site selection was driven by a search for the most secure salt bed in the country, salt considered most desirable because of its solid, impermeable nature and because of its tendency under pressure to flow, sealing up any excavated cavities. Although its development was repeatedly delayed by legal challenges related to technical and safety issues, WIPP has won the approval of scientists, regulators, and citizens of Carlsbad as a safe repository. WIPP's opening was welcome news for the ten national weapons laboratories where nearly 60,000 cubic meters of transuranic wastes have been in "interim" storage for years. While no radwastes from commercial nuclear power plants can be sent to WIPP (by law, the facility is reserved exclusively for defense radwastes), the opening of a final resting place for transuranic wastes marks an important milestone in the federal government's efforts to implement a responsible radioactive waste management program (Kerr, 1999).

Low-level wastes, produced not only by nuclear power plants but also by hospitals, research labs, universities, and industries, exhibit low but sometimes potentially hazardous concentrations of radioisotopes. They differ from high-level wastes in having significantly lower levels of radioactive emissions; they are not physically hot, generally require no shielding, and, unlike high-level wastes which remain dangerous for millennia, most decay to harmless levels within 100–300 years. In the United States during the 1950s, many

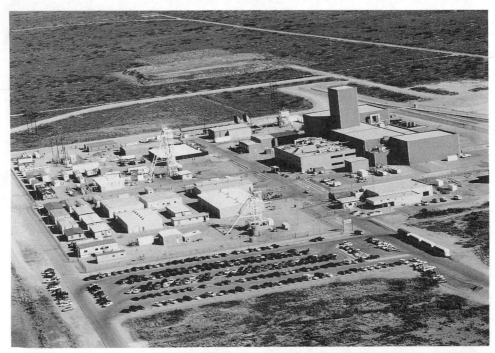

The Waste Isolation Pilot Plant (WIPP) near Carlsbad, New Mexico was built as a permanent disposal site for plutonium-contaminated debris from nuclear weapons production. *[Courtesy of U.S. Department of Energy]*

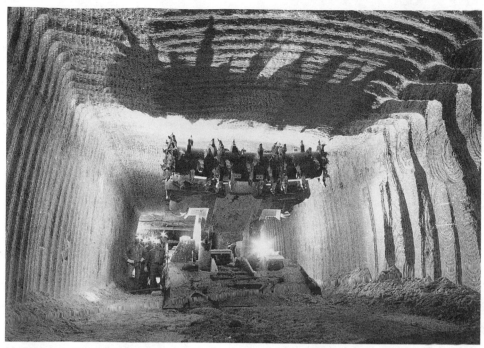

A portion of an underground tunnel at the WIPP facility is shown here, along with a machine used for excavation. *[Courtesy of U.S. Department of Energy]*

low-level commercial radwastes were buried on military reservations along with defense wastes or were simply dumped into the ocean—a practice that didn't cease entirely until 1970 (as recently as the fall of 1993, Russia defied world public opinion and infuriated the Japanese by brazenly dumping more than 900 tons of low-level radwastes into a prime squid fishing area in the Sea of Japan). From 1947–1970 at least 47,500 barrels of radwastes, primarily low-level wastes but also including plutonium wastes from atomic research labs, were dumped at three different sites near the Gulf of Farallones National Marine Sanctuary, an ocean wildlife preserve about 25 miles offshore from San Francisco. While the 55-gallon drums containing the wastes had a 10-year life expectancy in sea water and the concrete encasing the wastes was calculated to remain intact for 30 years, the radionuclides themselves have half-lives ranging from 30–24,000 years. By now virtually all of the barrels have reached their functional life span, but it isn't known for certain whether the radionuclides they contained remain deposited in or on nearby sediments or whether they have already been widely dispersed by ocean currents (Suchanek et al., 1996).

By the 1960s, the commercial nuclear industry was relying on shallow land burial for disposal of low-level wastes, utilizing six privately owned facilities specifically licensed for this purpose. By the late 1970s, three of these sites had closed due to migration of radioactive materials from the trenches, though no radioactive contamination was detected outside site boundaries. Because the states in which the three remaining sites were located (South Carolina, Nevada, and Washington) vigorously objected to being the "nuclear dumping ground" of the nation, Congress was persuaded to enact the **1980 Low-Level Radioactive Waste Policy Act.** This legislation placed responsibility for low-level radwaste management on *state* governments (as opposed to *federal* jurisdiction over high-level wastes), which were required to provide a means of safe disposal for all low-level wastes generated within their borders. Any states failing to do so could find their radwastes barred from disposal at existing sites in other states. However, recognizing that construction of 50 separate disposal facilities was neither necessary nor economically feasible, Congress permitted states to negotiate regional **"compact"** agreements among themselves to provide for the establishment, operation, and regulation of low-level radioactive waste facilities within each compact area.

By 1998 the last of ten regional compacts was approved by Congress; six states and the District of Columbia remained unaffiliated. Each regional compact is required to designate one of its members as the **"host state"**—i.e. the state in which the disposal facility is to be located—and to make numerous decisions regarding operational procedures, disposal fees, and type of facility to be constructed. Since shallow land burial has been deemed unacceptable by most host state legislatures, various designs for engineered structures are being considered, all of which offer much greater assurance of environmental safety than trench burial.

The original 1986 deadline date for completion of regional facilities was extended to January 1, 1993, but in every compact area, intense public opposition to siting has stymied efforts to carry out the requirements of the law. At the end of December 1992, the small facility at Beatty, Nevada, closed its gates and the Hanford, Washington, landfill restricted access to all but 11 northwestern and Rocky Mountain states. In 1988 a new facility owned and operated by Envirocare of Utah, Inc., opened on a site 80 miles west of Salt Lake City. Located within a 100-square mile hazardous waste zone (neighbors include an Army nerve gas storage site and Dugway Proving Grounds), the Envirocare landfill is licensed to manage naturally occurring radioactive materials such as slightly contaminated soil and certain types of low-activity, high-volume wastes. However, at the end of the 1990s the landfill at Barnwell, South Carolina, constituted the only facility willing and able to accommodate the full range of radwaste disposal needs for the nation's nuclear power plants, industries, and other users of radioactive materials. The existence of the Barnwell option has resulted in a virtual halt to facility siting efforts elsewhere around the country. As long as Barnwell remains open to waste generators nationwide, there is little incentive for other states to proceed with programs guaranteed to incur the wrath of voters opposed to living anywhere near a radioactive waste disposal site. As this book goes to press, however, an abrupt change in this situation appears likely. In 1999 South Carolina Governor Jim Hodges, whose campaign platform included a pledge to discontinue his state's role as the nation's nuclear dumping ground, appointed a task force to recommend how this goal could be achieved, while simultaneously providing for the radwaste disposal needs of South Carolina generators. Concerns in the Palmetto State focus on the fact that fully 95% of the incoming radwastes at Barnwell originate out-of-state. In the late 1990s it was estimated that the facility had approximately ten years of remaining capacity, with room for an additional 3.2 million cubic feet of wastes. State officials worry that unless

Figure 10-3   States' Memberships in Compacts

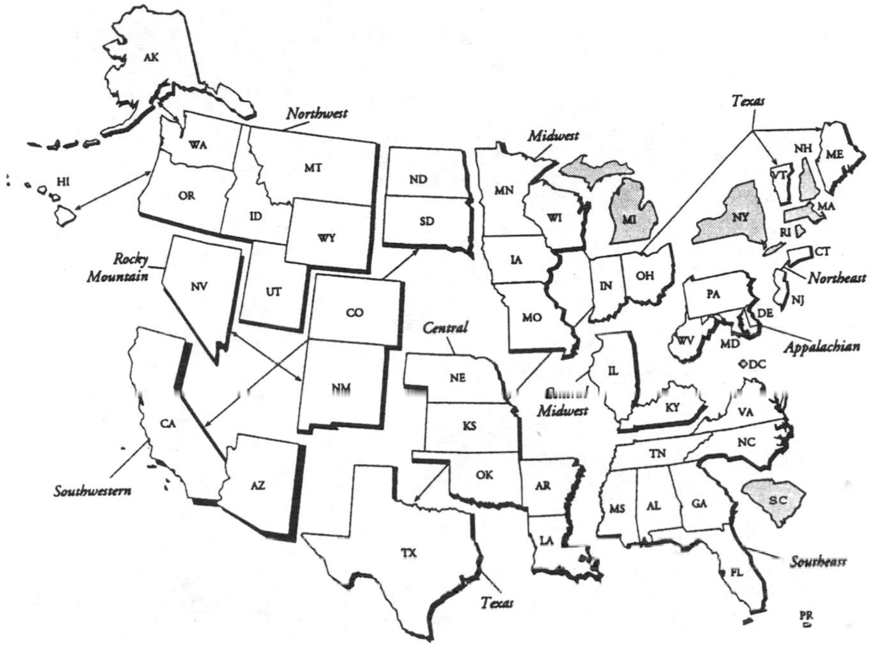

Note: Shaded areas are not affiliated with a compact.
Source: General Accounting Office, RCED-99-238.

access to Barnwell is sharply restricted, South Carolina utilities could be left without disposal options when their plants undergo decommissioning several decades hence. The closure of Barnwell to outside wastes, an event that appears likely to occur within the next few years, will pose major challenges to low-level waste generators. Such an action could revive efforts of states to site regional disposal facilities. Conversely, it could prompt new attempts by private interests to develop new facilities outside the compact agreement framework (in November 1999, Envirocare applied to the state of Utah for a license to manage a full range of low-level radwastes). Some critics, convinced that the present compact system is broken beyond repair, advocate that Congress repeal the 1980 Low-Level Radioactive Waste Policy Act and once again assign to the federal government responsibility for the management of all categories of radioactive waste (GAO, 1999). Nevertheless, whatever option is pursued in the years immediately ahead, the contentious issue of where to locate needed facilities will continue to bedevil efforts to manage low-level radwastes in a responsible manner. While many observers contend that low-level radioactive wastes, properly managed, pose minimal health or environmental hazards, the public's inability to distinguish between the vastly different risks presented by high-level vs. low-level radwastes contributes to the hysteria surrounding the siting issue and makes it difficult to predict how the disposal dilemma will ever be resolved.

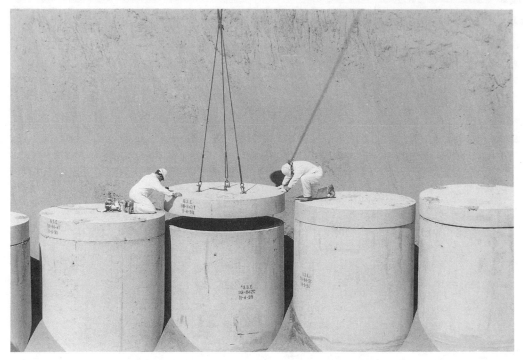

At the Hanford facility in Washington State, low-level wastes are placed in concrete engineered barriers and then placed in a disposal trench. *[Courtesy U.S. General Accounting Office]*

Ultraviolet Radiation

Wavelengths of the electromagnetic spectrum ranging between 40–400 nanometers in length are categorized as ultraviolet (UV) light. Although UV waves longer than 124 nanometers are not of sufficiently high energy to ionize atoms and molecules, certain portions within this range are strongly absorbed by living tissues, particularly by DNA which constitutes the major target of UV damage. Injury to the hereditary material of cells is the reason for the lethal or mutational effects which excess UV exposure can provoke in living organisms. Research has shown that the most detrimental effects to biological systems occur when UV radiation is in the 230–320 nanometer range (referred to as UVB, as opposed to longer-wavelength UVA), peak absorption by DNA occurring at 260 nm. Much of the ultraviolet light naturally present in incoming solar radiation is filtered out by the layer of atmospheric ozone located about 20 miles above the earth's surface (see chapter 11). Living organisms have developed various defense mechanisms to protect themselves against the amounts that do penetrate—shielding devices such as fur, feathers, shells, or darkly-pigmented skin, as well as light-avoidance behavior patterns among a variety of species. Of equal importance has been the evolution of enzymatic mechanisms for repairing UV-induced damage to DNA when levels of injury are not excessive. Without this cellular repair ability it is doubtful whether many organisms could survive existing levels of UV exposure. The importance of such mechanisms can be seen in the example of individuals suffering from

BOX 10-6

Can Sunscreens Prevent Skin Cancer?

Health educators' efforts to promote sunscreen use among a sun-loving public have met with considerable success in recent years. It is now well recognized that sunscreens with an SPF (sun protection factor) of 15, when used properly, are very effective in preventing sunburn as well as protecting the skin against premature aging and wrinkling. However, their role in preventing skin cancer—the primary concern among most users—has been questioned by some researchers who point to the simultaneous rise in sunscreen sales and skin cancer rates.

The problem with assessing the efficacy of sunscreen in protecting against skin cancer is that no studies on people who have used effective sunscreens (those with high SPFs came onto the market only in 1984) for several decades have yet been completed. A number of epidemiological surveys of skin cancer carried out during the 1970s and 1980s on subjects then in their 50s yielded contradictory results—not surprising, considering the fact that skin cancer has a 10–20 year latency period and the individuals studied had not used sunscreen until they were middle-aged, well past the childhood and adolescent period thought to be most critical in determining skin cancer risk later in life.

Dermatologists surmise that one explanation for the rise in skin cancer incidence even among sunscreen users could be due to improper application of these products. For greatest effectiveness, sunscreen should be applied 30 minutes prior to sun exposure so that protective ingredients have time to be absorbed; it should then be re-applied every two hours or whenever perspiration or contact with water removes the original protective layer. Sunscreens should be liberally applied to parts of the body especially prone to sunburn—lips, nose, ears—and should be used on cloudy or hazy days as conscientiously as when the sun is shining brightly. Similarly, sunscreen should be worn when one is out in the snow, particularly at high altitudes. Use of products with an SPF value lower than 15 provides insufficient protection, regardless of skin type (experts are unsure whether *higher* SPF sunscreens offer any additional protection). The best sunscreens are those which are most resistant to being washed off by sweating or swimming—a feature that is largely determined by the product's base material. In general, the most water-resistant sunscreens are those that feel the greasiest (i.e. Vaseline-type ointments); clear lotions and gels are the most easily washed off, while creamy lotions rank midway between.

Although the vast majority of dermatologists are ardent advocates of sunscreen use, some worry that users of these products may assume they can safely remain in the sun for long periods of time, unaware that sunscreens absorb most, though not all, UVB rays (those that cause sunburn), but are ineffective against UVA radiation which, like UVB, has been linked with both skin cancer and immune system damage. For this reason, most experts agree that while sunscreen use is both desirable and recommended to reduce soaring rates of skin cancer, it is not enough. Even more important are common-sense strategies such as staying indoors or in the shade during mid-day hours (10 A.M. to 3 P.M.) when the sun is most intense and wearing tightly-woven long-sleeved shirt and trousers with a broad-brimmed hat when exposure is unavoidable.

Such precautions are particularly important for youngsters, who generally spend much more time outdoors than do adults; indeed, it is estimated that fully 80% of a person's lifetime exposure to UV radiation occurs before age 20. Parents should be especially careful not to allow infants or children to become badly sunburned, since childhood sunburns are widely considered to be a triggering factor for subsequent development of malignant melanoma. Extreme care should be taken to minimize sun exposure of infants; babies under 6 months of age have very sensitive skin and should be kept in the shade when outdoors. Conscientious parents will ensure that strollers are fitted with hoods and babies protected with wide-brimmed hats. Baby oil should never be applied to an infant's skin before going outdoors, since it makes the skin more translucent to harmful solar radiation. Toddlers and older children are somewhat less vulnerable than infants, but dermatologists advise that they, too, should wear protective clothing and hats while playing outdoors. Unfortunately, the inconvenience of these precautions makes it unlikely that such advice will be heeded; accordingly, parents need to do the next best thing and insist that their children regularly use sunscreen.

While not a panacea for reversing the steady rise in skin cancer incidence, sunscreens have an important role to play in alleviating the irreparable skin damage caused both by chronic and acute skin exposure.

References

Epstein, John H. 1998. "Sunscreens and Skin Cancer." *Southern Medical Journal* 91, no. 6 (June).

Fackelmann, Kathleen. 1998. "Do Sunscreens Protect Against Cancer?" *Consumers' Research* 81, no. 8 (Aug):23-26.

Napoli, Maryanne. 1998. "Sunscreens—Not the Protection We Thought." *Health Facts* 23, no. 6:1-3.

the genetic disease xeroderma pigmentosum. Lacking the enzyme needed for repair of radiation-damaged DNA, victims of this ailment have to remain indoors throughout daylight hours or risk the development of multiple fatal skin cancers. There appears to be a tenuous balance between continual UV assault on the hereditary material and its biochemical repair. If the cell's capacity to deal with such damage is overwhelmed, the cell will die.

Since ultraviolet light cannot penetrate very deeply into living tissues, the major concern in reference to UV injury to humans involves the induction of skin cancers, particularly in lighter-skinned individuals who lack protective melanin granules in their epidermal skin layers.

After World War II, when the tyranny of fashion decreed that pale skin was "out" and the bronzed look "in," the apparently irresistible urge among fair-complexioned citizens to spend hours broiling themselves under the sun or at rapidly proliferating tanning parlors has resulted in an alarming increase in the incidence of skin cancer in Western countries. Whereas a child born in the United States in 1930 had about a 1 in 1500 risk of developing skin cancer within his or her lifetime, for a white child born today that risk has soared to 1 in 100 (for blacks the danger is much lower—less than 1 in 1000). The main villain behind these grim statistics is increased exposure to UV radiation, a known carcinogen and mutagen. According to the American

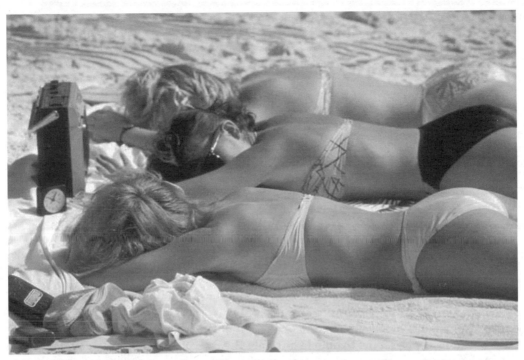

The much sought-after "bronzed" look can come at a high price: skin cancer, premature wrinkling, and immune system dysfunction.

Cancer Society, three major types of skin cancer account for over one million new cases of the disease diagnosed in the United States each year. **Basal cell carcinoma** and **squamous cell carcinoma** represent the vast majority of skin cancers, accounting for fully one-third of all cancers occurring in the United States today. Chronic exposure to sunlight is recognized as the cause of over 90% of these two cancers. They appear, predictably, on portions of the body receiving the greatest sun exposure—face, neck, ears, back of the hands—and until recently were unusual in people under the age of 50. Now, however, numerous cases have been diagnosed among people in their 20s and 30s and occasionally even in teenagers. Not surprisingly, they are also being found on the legs, chest, and back of victims as the sunbathing mania takes its toll.

Fortunately, the majority of such cancers can be treated if detected early, but each year several thousand cases prove fatal when their neglect leads to invasion of underlying tissues. **Malignant melanoma** is much less common than basal cell or squamous cell carcinomas, but far more deadly. By the late 1990s, over 40,000 new victims were being diagnosed with malignant melanoma each year and more than 7,000 annually die of the disease. The incidence of malignant melanoma has been increasing by approximately 4% annually since 1973 and is now the most common form of cancer to strike women under the age of 30. Americans born during the 1990s are at 12 times the risk of eventually developing malignant melanoma as are those born 50 years ago and twice as likely as those born just 10 years ago (DeLeo, 1992).

Figure 10-4   Hazards of UV Radiation

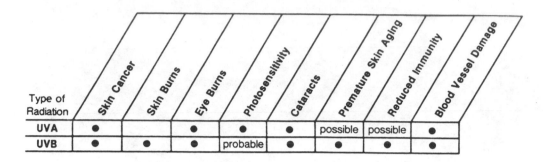

Type of Radiation	Skin Cancer	Skin Burns	Eye Burns	Photosensitivity	Cataracts	Premature Skin Aging	Reduced Immunity	Blood Vessel Damage
UVA	●		●	●	●	possible	possible	●
UVB	●	●	●	probable	●	●	●	●

The American Cancer Institute now estimates an American's lifetime risk of developing melanoma is 1 in 75; in Australia, where melanoma rates are the highest in the world, the chances are 1 in 70.

Unlike the nonmelanoma skin cancers, malignant melanoma appears to develop as a result of occasional severe sunburn, rather than by prolonged, low-dose exposure to sunlight. A blistering sunburn experienced during childhood or adolescence seems to double or triple the risk of subsequently developing malignant melanoma. Interestingly, while basal cell and squamous cell carcinomas develop only on sun-exposed portions of the body, malignant melanomas frequently occur on areas normally covered. They also tend to occur at a younger age than do the other two forms of skin cancer; although the risk of melanoma increases with age, half of all cases occur among those under 50, with incidence rates rising most rapidly among people below 40 years of age. Because of the suspected link between childhood sunburn and melanoma, groups such as The Skin Cancer Foundation are urging parents to be particularly careful in protecting youngsters from excessive sun exposure.

Ill effects of UV-light exposure are not limited to cancer and sunburn. Premature wrinkling, drying, and mottling of the skin are among the less desirable consequences of UV exposure. In recent years the growing popularity of tanning parlors has been accompanied by claims from the owners of such establishments that they provide a safe alternative to sunbathing because they utilize UVA radiation rather than UVB and hence cannot result in burning. Nevertheless, tanning parlor patrons are exposing themselves to several other serious risks. Not only can UVA, like UVB, induce skin cancer, it also causes premature aging of the skin and development of cataracts. In addition, UVA enhances the effect of sunlight: individuals who sunbathe outdoors shortly after a stint in a tanning parlor frequently suffer extremely severe sunburns. Photosensitive reactions to either tanning parlors or outdoor sunbathing can occur when unwary sun-worshippers expose themselves to UV light while taking antibiotics (especially tetracycline), antihistamines, birth control pills, even certain cosmetics. Such a toxic reaction is generally manifested as an unusually severe sunburn immediately following exposure to UV light.

Exposure to even moderate amounts of ultraviolet radiation can be dangerous for individuals suffering from *lupus erythematosus,* an autoimmune ailment. Between 40–60% of lupus patients experience aggravation of skin disease or systemic symptoms when exposed to either UVA or UVB light. Many researchers contend that the threat of UV damage to the body's immune system should be regarded just as seriously as its ability to induce skin cancer. Studies have shown that ultraviolet radiation from both natural and artificial sources can alter the proportions of various types of white blood cells and depress the activity of natural killer-T cells in the bloodstream. Immune system dysfunction caused by UV exposure is not related to the amount of pigmentation in a person's skin, as is the case with skin cancer. Individuals with black or brown skin are just as likely to suffer immune system damage if they spend too much time in the sun as are fair-skinned people. Unfortunately, most sunscreens do *not* appear to be effective in preventing the type of immune system damage provoked by UVB exposure (Sontheimer, 1992; "Sunscreens," 1992). Weighing serious long-term health risks against short-term fashion benefits, dermatologists are unanimous in their recommendation that all UV exposure, whether on the beach or at a tanning salon, be avoided to the greatest extent possible.

Ultraviolet light has some beneficial as well as harmful effects. A certain amount of skin exposure is necessary to promote the bodily synthesis of vitamin D, a deficiency of which can result in the development of rickets, a bone deformity. The germicidal properties of UV light have recommended its use in operating rooms to reduce the danger of bacterial or viral infections. Ultraviolet light applications have also been successfully employed to treat such bacterial skin diseases as acne and boils (Schreiber, 1986).

Microwaves

Electromagnetic radiation comprising wavelengths ranging from approximately one millimeter to one meter (intermediate between infrared and short-wave radio wavelengths) is termed microwave radiation. Since microwave energies are so low, such radiations are typically characterized by their frequencies which, in the case of microwaves of biological interest, generally fall between 100 and 30,000 megahertz (MHZ).

Humans today are continuously bombarded with microwaves from such diverse sources as military radar installations, radio and television transmitters, communications and surveillance satellites, radar and radio frequency transmitters at airports and on planes and ships, microwave ovens, telephone and TV-signal relay towers, walkie-talkies, video display terminals, automatic garage door openers, and so on. Whether or not microwave radiation, particularly at lower levels of exposure, presents a public health threat remains a matter of controversy among researchers. Unlike X-rays, microwaves are nonionizing; instead, when absorbed they cause an increased rate of vibration in the molecules of the absorbing material, resulting in the production of heat. Depending on frequency, microwaves are differentially absorbed by bodily tissues. Those of very low energy (below 150 MHZ) simply pass through the body without being absorbed; those of intermediate frequency (150–1200 MHZ) are absorbed by the deeper tissues without any noticeable heating of the skin. This poses a danger of serious bodily harm, since internal organs can receive highly damaging doses of microwave radiation without the victim realizing that anything is wrong. As microwave frequency increases, tissue penetration decreases and at 3500 MHZ warming of the skin can be felt; above 10,000 MHZ only the surface of the skin is heated and no penetration of the body occurs.

Differential absorption of microwave energy by bodily tissues is to a large degree a function of their water content. Moist tissues such as skin, muscle, and the intestines absorb more microwaves than do bones and fatty tissues. Sensitivity of specific organs to microwaves depends not only on how readily such radiation is absorbed, but also on how effectively blood circulating through the organ can dissipate the excess heat. Experiments have shown that body parts with poor circulation—the eyes, gastrointestinal tract, testes, urinary bladder, and gall bladder—are the areas most susceptible to injury from microwaves (Dalrymple, 1973).

Electromagnetic Fields (EMF)

In 1979 a team of researchers at the University of Colorado Medical Center in Denver reported that children who are exposed to stronger than average magnetic fields, such as those living in the vicinity of power transmission lines, have a two to three times greater risk of developing leukemia than do children living at a distance from such sources. While this study was subsequently discredited because of methodological flaws (e.g. small size of group studied, lack of direct measurements of exposure received), the report sparked intense public alarm about an inescapable component of everyday life. The extremely-low-frequency (ELF) wavelengths produced by the transmission and distribution of electric power, as well as by the plethora of electrical appliances that fill virtually every modern household, are impossible to avoid, so the suggestion that subtle but significant adverse health effects could be caused by electromagnetic fields prompted numerous scientific studies during the 1980s and 1990s. The primary concern of researchers focused on whether exposure to the levels of ELF radiation typical of residential environments could, as some investigators claimed, increase the risk of childhood leukemia; the impact of EMFs in provoking birth defects, miscarriages, learning disabilities, or behavioral modifications also received attention. From the beginning, many scientists were skeptical of any cancer-EMF association, simply because the amounts of radiation emanating from power lines and appliances are so minute in comparison with the earth's own magnetic field. Numerous research efforts to verify a possible EMF-cancer connection yielded inconclusive results; some epidemiologic studies showed a slight risk of cancer with EMF exposure, while others revealed no such association. Significantly, experiments using animal models failed to demonstrate any correlation between laboratory exposure to low frequency radiation and the induction or promotion of cancer. Several major studies in the early 1990s found evidence for an association between EMF and cancer inconsistent and inconclusive; in 1995 the American Physical Society, the world's largest group of physicists, entered the fray, saying its members could find no evidence that electromagnetic fields radiating from power lines have any impact on cancer rates. The Society deplored the fact that public fears about an EMF-cancer connection were responsible for the unnecessary diversion of billions of dollars (estimated at $1–3 billion annually in the U.S.) for moving power lines and installing shielding. The scientific debate was effectively resolved when the National Academy of Sciences issued a major report stating that its review of more than 500 scientific papers failed to provide any evidence that electromagnetic fields adversely affect human health (NRC, 1997) and when scientists at the National Cancer Institute convincingly demonstrated no association between electric power lines and leukemia in children (Linet et al., 1997). Although the public fears raised by two decades of controversy have not been altogether vanquished, the scientific community regards further investigation into the health impacts of EMF as unnecessary—sleeping under an electric blanket or living near a power line doesn't cause cancer!

References

Basso-Ricci, S. 1985. "Cancer Following Medical Irradiation: The Validity of Gray's Hypothesis." *Panminerva Medica* 27.

Bennett, B.G. 1997. "Exposure to Natural Radiation Sources Worldwide." In *Proceedings of 4th International Conference on High Levels of Natural Radiation: Radiation Doses And Health Effects,* edited by L. Wei, T. Sugahara, and Z. Tao. Beijing, China, October 1996.

Carter, L. J. 1978. "Uranium Mill Tailings: Congress Addresses a Long-Neglected Problem." *Science* 202: 191.

_____. 1977. "More Burning of Coal Offsets Gains in Air Pollution Control." *Science* 198.

Clark, Claudia. 1997. "Radium Girls: Women and Industrial Health Reform, 1910–1935." University of North Carolina Press.

Cooper, George, Jr. 1973. "The Development of Radiation Science." In *Medical Radiation Biology,* edited by Glenn V. Dalrymple, M. E. Gaulden, G. M. Kollmorgen, and H. H. Vogel, Jr. W. B. Saunders.

Cushman, John H. 1993. "U.S. Drops Test Plan at Bomb Waste Site." *New York Times*, Oct. 22.

Dalrymple, Glenn V. 1973. "Microwaves." In *Medical Radiation Biology*, edited by Glenn V. Dalrymple et al. W. B. Saunders.

DeLeo, Vincent, M.D. 1992. Testimony before the Senate Committee on Governmental Affairs, June 5.

Eisenbud, M. 1973. *Environmental Radioactivity.* Academic Press.

Feshbach, Murray. 1995. *Ecological Disaster: Cleaning Up the Hidden Legacy of the Soviet Regime.* New York: The Twentieth Century Fund Press.

Fialka, John J. 1998. "Goshute Indians' Plan to Store Nuclear Waste For Eight Utilities Is Opposed by Utah Governor." *Wall Street Journal* (August 26).

Goldman, Marvin. 1996. "Cancer Risk of Low-Level Exposure." *Science* 271 (March 29):1821-1822.

Hall, E. J. 1976. *Radiation and Life.* Pergamon Press.

Hawkes, Nigel, Geoffrey Lean, David Leigh, Robin McVie, P. Pringle, and A. Wilson. 1987. *Chernobyl: The End of the Nuclear Dream.* Vintage Books.

Kahn, Patricia. 1993. "A Grisly Archive of Key Cancer Data." *Science* 259 (Jan. 22).

Kerr, Richard A. 1999. "For Radioactive Waste From Weapons, A Home at Last." *Science* 283, no. 5408 (March 12):1626-1628.

Kevles, Bettyann Holtzmann. 1997. *Naked to the Bone.* New Brunswick, NJ: Rutgers University Press.

Kneale, George W., and Alice M. Stewart. 1993. "Reanalysis of Hanford Data: 1944–1986 Deaths." *American Journal of Industrial Medicine* 23 (March).

Landers, Peter. 1999. "Uranium Leak Feeds Antinuclear Sentiment in Japan." *Wall Street Journal,* Oct. 4.

League of Women Voters Education Fund. 1993. *The Nuclear Waste Primer.* Lyons & Burford.

Linet, M.S., E.E. Hatch, R.A. Kleinerman, L.L. Robison, W.T. Kaune, D.K. Friedman, R.K. Severson, C.M. Haines, C.T. Hartscok, S. Niwa, S. Wachodler, and R.E. Tarone. 1997. "Residential Exposure to Magnetic Fields and Acute Lymphoblastic Leukemia in Children." *New England Journal of Medicine* 337, no. 1 (July 3):1-7.

Macklis, Roger M. 1993. "The Great Radium Scandal." *Scientific American* (Aug).

National Council on Radiation Protection and Measurements (NCRP). 1998. "Radionuclide Exposure of the Embryo/Fetus." NCRP Report No. 128, Bethesda, MD.

———. 1987. "Ionizing Radiation Exposure of the Population of the United States." NCRP Report No. 93, Bethesda, MD.

National Research Council (NRC). 1997. *Possible Health Effects of Exposure to Residential Electric and Magnetic Fields.* Washington, DC: National Academy Press.

"New Study Suggests Recommended Radiation Dose Limit Is Too High." 1992. *Environmental Health Letter,* Feb. 11.

Perera, Judith. 1998. "Officials Charged with Misuse of Funds for Tomsk Cleanup." *Nuclear Waste News* 18, no. 14 (April 2):132.

———. 1997. "EU Offers Some Aid for Massive Eastern Europe Uranium Cleanup." *Nuclear Waste News* 17, no. 35, (Sept. 11):335.

———. 1993. "New Radiation Standards Urged for British Workers." *Environmental Health Letter,* June 11.

Pollycove, Myron. 1997. "The Rise and Fall of the Linear No-Threshold Theory of Radiation Carcinogenesis." *Nuclear Waste News* (June):34-37.

"Reprocessing Facility Blast Leads to Review of Japan's Nuclear Plans." 1997. *Nuclear Waste News* 17, no. 12 (March 20):115.

Schreiber, Michael M. 1986. "Exposure to Sunlight: Effects on the Skin." *Comprehensive Therapy* 12, no. 5.

Sohrabi, Mehdi. 1998. "The State-of-the-art on Worldwide Studies in some Environments with Elevated Naturally Occurring Radioactive Materials (NORM)." *Applied Radiation Isotopes* 49, no. 3:169-188.

Sontheimer, Richard D., M.D. 1992. "Photosensitivity in Lupus Erythematosus." *Lupus News* 12, no. 2.

Steinhardt, Bernice. 1996. *Uranium Mill Tailings: Status and Future Costs of Cleanup.* United States General Accounting Office, GAO/T-RCED-96-85.

Streffer, Christian. 1997. "Biological Effects of Prenatal Irradiation." In *Health Impacts of Large Releases of Radionuclides.* Wiley, Chichester

(Ciba Foundation Symposium 203):155–166.

Suchanek, Thomas H., Manuel C. Lagunas-Solar, Otto G. Raabe, Roger C. Helm, Fiorella Gielow, Neal Peek, and Omar Carvacho. 1996. "Radionuclides in Fishes and Mussels from the Farallon Islands Nuclear Waste Dump Site, California." *Health Physics* 71, no. 2 (August):167-178.

"Sunscreens May Not Afford Protection." 1992. *Environmental Health Letter,* June 12.

United States General Accounting Office (GAO). 1999. "Low-Level Radioactive Wastes: States Are Not Developing Disposal Facilities." GAO/RCED-99-238 (September).

PART 3

Environmental Degradation

How We Foul Our Own Nest

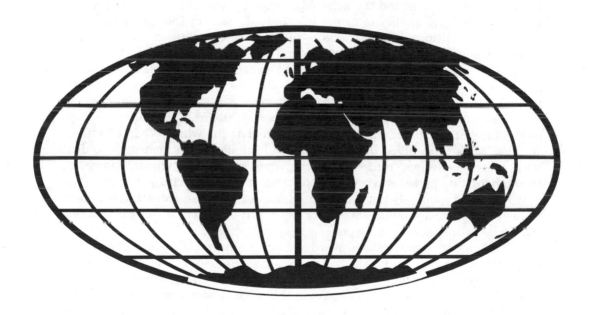

The fouling of the nest which has been typical of man's activity in the past on a local scale now seems to be extending to the whole system.

—Kenneth Boulding

Air pollution, water pollution, excessive levels of noise, and the accumulation of disease-breeding refuse are not phenomena unique to the modern age. Wherever humans have congregated in appreciable numbers, the burning of fuel, the thoughtless disposal of excreta and material wastes, and the din arising from a multitude of human activities have created conditions which adversely affected the health and well-being of the very people responsible for those conditions. For most of human history, environmental degradation was primarily local in scope, concentrated in the relatively few places where humans established urban centers. The extent of pollution in these cities, however, often far exceeded the levels of filth plaguing our environmentally conscious society of today. Streets and gutters clogged with human body wastes, animal excrement, and garbage were a result of both overcrowding and a transference to the city of more casual rural practices. By the time of the Industrial Revolution in the late 18th and early 19th centuries, belching smokestacks from thousands of factories and the noise of machinery and transport vehicles further degraded the quality of urban life. Indeed, back in the "good old days" health and sanitary conditions due to air and water pollution and to inadequate (or nonexistent) refuse collection and disposal were far worse than anything with which we are familiar today. When repeated epidemic outbreaks of waterborne disease killed thousands of citizens or when smog-laden air caused millions to wheeze, cough, and occasionally die, the more enlightened civic leaders began to question society's shortsightedness in fouling its own nest. Many of the most important reforms in civic life which occurred late in the last century involved implementation of public health measures to deal with water pollution, refuse collection, and smoke abatement. However, throughout this period when urban pollution levels were rising, the countryside remained relatively uncontaminated, except for those areas where a local industry—perhaps a metal smelter or pulp mill—created noxious conditions within its own sphere of influence.

The changes that transformed local pollution problems into global concerns have occurred largely in the years since the end of the Second World War. Reverse migration from urban centers into sprawling suburbia was made possible by a quantum increase in the number of automobiles ("infernal combustion engines") whose exhaust fumes guaranteed that air pollution would no longer be restricted to areas of heavy industry. The escalating energy demands of a growing, affluent population were accompanied by construction of massive new power plants, most of them coal-burning and many located in regions previously noted for pristinely clean air. Perhaps most significant was the vast outpouring of new, synthetic chemical products, many of them toxic compounds, which do not break down readily and can be transported immense distances by air currents, water, or in the tissues of living organisms to wreak their havoc far from their place of origin. In spite of the warnings of a few farsighted individuals, several decades of experience were required before society as a whole became aware of the insidious nature and now-massive scope of environmental degradation.

During the decade of the 1970s, a national awakening in the United States regarding issues of ecology and environmental health produced a flood of federal and state legislation aimed at pollution abatement. The battle has been joined and some successes have already been achieved, but it has become increasingly evident that the problem of environmental pollution is far more complex than originally perceived. Issues not even considered until fairly recently—issues such as acid precipitation, carbon dioxide accumulation, ozone layer depletion, contamination of groundwater with toxic organic chemicals, and the fearsome dilemma of what to do about abandoned chemical waste dumps—present policymakers, scientists, and citizens with thorny technical and political problems. Solutions to older questions pertaining to community waste disposal practices, air pollution abatement measures, or stormwater runoff control are well understood but often fail to be implemented due to fiscal constraints.

The concluding chapters of this book attempt to delineate the nature of the pollution problems confronting society as we enter the 21st century. They also describe the legislative tools with which we are now attempting to combat the contamination of our nation's air and water resources in order to prevent future generations from perpetuating the "fouling of the nest" which so endangers our health and well-being.

CHAPTER **11**

The Atmosphere

... this most excellent canopy, the air, look you, this brave o'er hanging firmament, this majestical roof fretted with golden fire...

—William Shakespeare (Hamlet)

The airy canopy above Earth which so inspires poets and painters is a physical characteristic of our planet unique in the solar system. Its existence makes possible the rich diversity of life forms found on Earth, making this globe a veritable oasis in space.

Questions regarding the origin of Earth's atmosphere have intrigued scientists for decades. It is generally assumed that Earth formed almost five billion years ago when particles in a gigantic whirling cloud of dust and gases were pulled together into an aggregate body by enormous gravitational forces. This infant planet had an atmosphere consisting primarily of light gases such as hydrogen and helium, very similar to the present-day atmosphere on the larger planets of Jupiter and Saturn. However, due to Earth's smaller size, gravitational forces were insufficient to retain these elements and they subsequently dissipated into space. This original atmosphere was gradually replaced by a secondary atmosphere produced through the outgassing of volatile materials from the interior of the Earth as the once-molten orb began to cool. Modern phenomena such as volcanic eruptions provide vivid evidence that such outgassing continues right up to the present day.

While there is widespread agreement among scientists that the primitive Earth's atmosphere was significantly different in chemical composition from that of the present, opinions vary as to precisely which compounds were the major constituents of the early atmosphere. For many years it was widely accepted that a mixture of hydrogen, methane, ammonia, and water vapor would have provided the most congenial environment for the origin of life; these must have been the predominant gases in prebiotic times. More recently, however, this assumption has been challenged by observations that gases ejected by volcanoes consist largely of carbon dioxide and water vapor,

411

leading to the conclusion that, unless volcanoes operated very differently in the past than they do today, the main component of Earth's early atmosphere was carbon dioxide, just as it is today on our neighboring planets of Mars and Venus. This concept of a carbon dioxide-rich primitive atmosphere, with mere traces of ammonia and notably devoid of free oxygen, constitutes the prevailing view at present. The origin of our modern oxygen-rich atmosphere is traced to the evolution of green plants, about two billion years ago, whose photosynthetic activities resulted in the uptake of considerable quantities of atmospheric carbon dioxide and the subsequent release of free oxygen—a necessary precursor for the evolution of higher forms of life (Budyko, 1986; Gribbin, 1982).

Although the chemical constituents of the atmosphere have existed in roughly their present proportions for at least several hundred million years, these constituents are in a constant state of flux, reacting with the continents and oceans to form our weather patterns, constantly being removed and recycled (see chapter 1 on "Geochemical Cycles") as a part of great natural processes. The intimate interrelationships between the atmosphere and land, water, and living things make it relevant to refer to such interactions as the **earth-atmosphere system.** This system is essentially a closed one—every material that goes into the air, though it may circulate and change in form, nevertheless remains within the earth-atmosphere system. This fact has disquieting implications for humans who have always viewed the skies as a convenient garbage dump for their volatile wastes—unfortunately, the concept of a pollutant or any other substance "vanishing into thin air" is a physical impossibility.

Composition of the Atmosphere

The modern atmosphere consists of a mixture of gases so perfectly and consistently diffused among each other that pure dry air exhibits as distinct a set of physical properties as is possessed by any single gas. By volume, the composition of dry air can be broken down as follows:

78% Nitrogen (N_2)
21% Oxygen (O_2)
0.9% Argon (Ar)
0.03% Carbon Dioxide (CO_2)
trace amounts—neon, helium, krypton, xenon, hydrogen, methane, and nitrous oxide

Of the four major atmospheric components, only two, oxygen and carbon dioxide, directly enter into biological processes. Oxygen is required by most living organisms for the production of energy, a process known as aerobic respiration; carbon dioxide constitutes the carbon source for photosynthesis—a series of photochemical reactions whereby chlorophyll molecules in green plants absorb sunlight and use its energy to synthesize simple sugars from carbon dioxide and water. Atmospheric nitrogen, on the other hand, can be utilized only by a few species of nitrogen-fixing bacteria and cyanobacteria, while argon is chemically and biologically inert and thus plays no significant role in the biosphere.

Regions of the Atmosphere

Although the composition of its component gases is uniform throughout the atmosphere from sea level to an altitude approximately 50 miles (80 km) above the earth's surface, scientists subdivide this extent into three distinct regions based on temperature zones.

Troposphere. Extending from sea level to an altitude about 8–9 miles above the earth (slightly less above the poles, more above the equator) is the region known as the troposphere. Virtually all life activities occur within this region and most weather and climatic phenomena occur here. In addition to the usual gases, the troposphere also contains varying amounts of water vapor and dust particles. Within the troposphere temperature steadily falls with increasing altitude, a decrease of 5.4 °F per 1000 feet (10 °C/km). The upper limit of the troposphere is known as the **tropopause**.

Stratosphere. Above the troposphere lies the stratosphere, a region distinguished by a temperature gradient reversal. Here the temperature slowly rises with increasing altitude until it reaches 32 °F (0 °C) at a height of about 30 miles (50 km), the upper boundary of the stratosphere known as the **stratopause.** Unlike the troposphere, the stratosphere contains almost no water vapor or dust. It is the site, however, of the **ozone layer,** a region characterized by higher-than-usual concentrations of the rare gas ozone (O_3), an isotope of oxygen (O_2). The ozone layer extends from about 10–30 miles above the earth's surface, being most concentrated between 11–15 miles. Amounts of ozone vary depending on location and season of the year. Ozone concentrations are lowest above the equator, increasing toward the poles; they also increase markedly between autumn and spring.

Mesosphere. Above the stratopause is the region known as the mesosphere, where temperature once again begins to fall with increasing altitude. Since the air becomes progressively more diffuse as the altitude above the earth increases, it is difficult to say precisely where the atmosphere ends. In terms of mass, 99% of our atmosphere lies within 18 miles of the earth's surface—an astonishingly thin blanket nurturing beneath it all the life known to exist in the universe (Strahler and Strahler, 1973).

Radiation Balance

In addition to providing the major source of certain chemical elements necessary for life, the atmosphere performs a vital role in controlling the earth's surface environment by regulating both the quality and quantity of solar radiation that enters and leaves the biosphere.

The source of all energy on earth, of course, is the sun. However, solar energy can be subdivided into several categories, depending on wavelength of the various forms of radiation involved. These categories and their wavelengths are as follows:

Figure 11-1   Regions of the Atmosphere

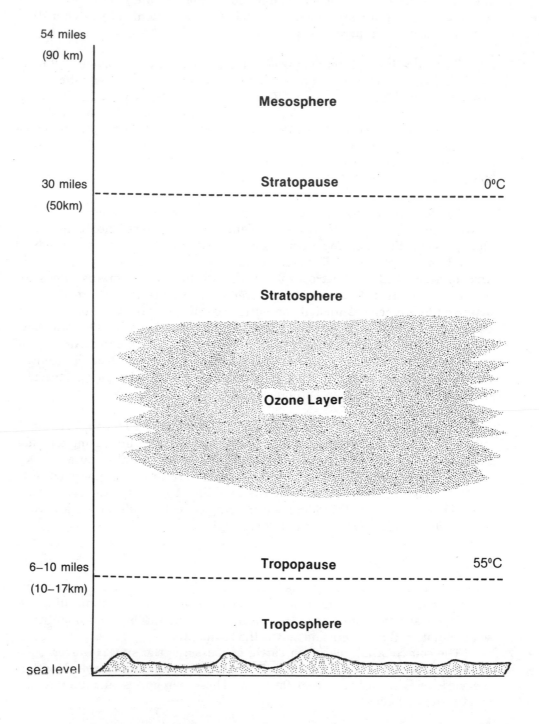

Type of Radiation	% of Total Energy	Wavelength (in micrometers)
Ultraviolet rays	9	0.1–0.4
Visible light rays	41	0.4–0.7
Infrared rays (heat)	50	0.7–3000

These forms of electromagnetic radiation travel outward from the sun at a rate of 186,000 miles (300,000 km) per second, taking slightly over nine minutes to reach the earth. Although none of the sun's energy is lost as it travels through space, once it begins to penetrate earth's atmosphere both a depletion and diversion of solar radiation begin to occur.

Most of the ultraviolet radiation present in sunlight is absorbed by the ozone layer as it passes through the stratosphere, though some of the UV wavelengths longer than 0.3 micrometers (the so-called UV-B region) manage to penetrate to the earth's surface where they can produce sunburn and skin cancers. The ozone layer itself is actually created by ultraviolet light, since UV radiant energy causes ordinary oxygen molecules to break apart, releasing single atoms of oxygen which then react with intact oxygen molecules to form ozone. Since, as was explained in chapter 10, ultraviolet radiation can have serious adverse effects on living organisms, the existence of the ozone layer is of great biological significance (Panofsky, 1978).

Visible light rays and infrared radiation penetrate through the upper stratosphere unaffected by the ozone layer. However, as the atmospheric gas molecules increase in density closer to the earth, these molecules cause a random scattering of the incoming visible light waves (infrared waves are not so affected and for the most part continue to stream directly toward the earth). Entering the troposphere, additional scattering and diffuse reflection of visible light waves occur due to contact with dust particles and clouds (a clear sky appears blue because the shorter blue wavelengths are scattered to a greater extent than are the longer red wavelengths and thus reach our eyes from all parts of the sky). Additional amounts of incoming solar radiation are lost by reflection from the upper surfaces of clouds, oceans, or from the land (particularly when covered with snow or ice). Energy losses also occur when carbon dioxide and water vapor absorb infrared radiation (heat waves) as sunlight enters the lower atmosphere. This heat absorption results in an increase in air temperature. Although the carbon dioxide content of the air is constant everywhere, the amount of water vapor varies considerably and is the main factor accounting for differences in the amount of infrared absorption in various climatic regions (e.g. arid regions experience greater temperature extremes during a 24-hour period than do more humid areas at the same latitude because the low water vapor content of desert air minimizes the absorption of the infrared waves). Altogether, scattering, reflection, and absorption of sunlight can result in the loss of as little as 20% of incoming solar radiation when skies are clear to nearly 100% under conditions of heavy cloud cover. On a global yearly average it is estimated that the earth-atmosphere system absorbs about 68% of the total incoming solar radiation, 32% being lost due to the factors just mentioned.

Figure 11-2   Reflection and Absorption of Solar Radiation

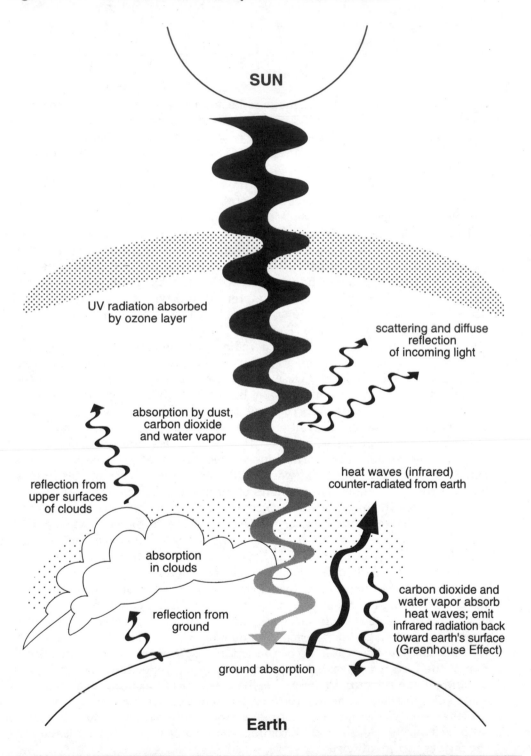

SUN

UV radiation absorbed
by ozone layer

scattering and diffuse
reflection
of incoming light

absorption by dust,
carbon dioxide
and water vapor

heat waves (infrared)
counter-radiated from earth

reflection from
upper surfaces
of clouds

absorption
in clouds

carbon dioxide and
water vapor absorb
heat waves; emit
infrared radiation back
toward earth's surface
(Greenhouse Effect)

reflection from
ground

ground absorption

Earth

In order to maintain a global radiation balance, energy absorbed by the earth from incoming sunlight must be equalled by outward radiation of energy from the earth's surface. This so-called "ground radiation" occurs in the form of infrared waves longer than 3 or 4 micrometers (referred to as "long wave radiation"), which are continually being radiated back into the atmosphere, even at night when no solar radiation is being received. Some of the infrared waves leaving the earth (those in the 5–8 and 12–20 micrometer range) are absorbed by water vapor and carbon dioxide in the atmosphere, a portion of which are reradiated back to the earth's surface, thereby keeping the earth's climate warmer than it would otherwise be. This phenomenon, known as the greenhouse effect, has extremely important climatic implications that will be discussed in more detail later in this chapter.

While incoming and outgoing units of radiation are often not in balance at any one particular time and place (indeed, such imbalances provide the forces behind our constantly changing weather patterns), an equilibrium of such units for the world as a whole during any given year exists, resulting in the maintenance of annual average global temperatures which fluctuate very little from year to year (Strahler and Strahler, 1973). One of the most pressing concerns among atmospheric scientists today is that human activities may be altering the global radiation balance in ways which may have far-reaching climatic consequences.

Human Impact on the Earth-Atmosphere System

Geologic records give ample indication of drastic climatic changes at various times in Earth's long history, the most recent being four successive periods of widespread glaciation (the "Ice Ages"), the last of which ended only 10,000 years ago. Obviously humans had nothing to do with past fluctuations in the global heat balance, but our impact today may no longer be so negligible. Temperature measurements compiled over many decades clearly indicate that possibly significant changes in climate are already underway; the extent to which human activities are provoking or enhancing such trends is presently the topic of heated academic debate.

The major causes of human-induced atmospheric change are:

1. introduction into the atmosphere of pollutant gases and particles not usually found there in significant amounts, and

2. changes in the concentrations of natural atmospheric components.

The following sections illustrate two of the most difficult issues we must confront as the impact of human activities on the earth-atmosphere system inexorably intensifies—depletion of the ozone layer and rising levels of atmospheric CO_2 (global warming).

Depletion of the Ozone Layer

Although ozone is one of the rarest of atmospheric gases, its presence in the stratosphere is of vital importance in protecting life on earth from the

Figure 11-3   Formation of Ozone in the Stratosphere

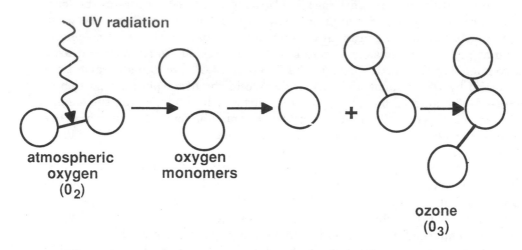

UV radiation

atmospheric
oxygen
(O_2)

oxygen
monomers

+

ozone
(O_3)

damaging effects of solar ultraviolet radiation. As mentioned earlier, the ozone layer is created when UV energy splits the oxygen molecule and the freed atoms rejoin other oxygen molecules to form ozone (O_3). At the same time, the highly reactive ozone is being broken down again to normal oxygen (O_2); thus the ozone layer is maintained in a state of dynamic equilibrium, daytime increases being balanced by nighttime decreases.

In 1974 atmospheric chemists advanced a hypothesis that certain pollutant emissions into the atmosphere had the potential to disrupt this equilibrium, threatening the long-term integrity of the ozone layer. Initially attention focused on the damage potential of nitrous oxides emitted with jet airplane exhausts (particularly from supersonic transports such as the Anglo-French Concorde) and the use of nitrogen fertilizers. It gradually became apparent, however, that a far more serious threat to the ozone layer is posed by the widespread use of a group of synthetic chemicals called chlorofluorocarbons (CFCs), one of the best known of which is the refrigerant Freon. Used in a number of industrial processes, as solvents and refrigerants, in making plastic foams, and as spray can aerosol propellants until their use for this purpose was banned in 1978, CFCs are particularly troublesome because they are such stable chemicals; when released into the environment through vaporization or leakage from enclosed systems or by direct spraying into the air, as in the case of aerosol containers, CFCs do not break down but instead drift upward through the troposphere into the stratosphere where the molecules are finally broken down by solar radiation, releasing atoms of chlorine that react with and destroy ozone. The chlorine-ozone reaction is a catalytic one, meaning that the same chlorine atom can repeat the reaction with tens of thousands of ozone molecules. This, plus the fact that the chlorine atoms will remain in the atmosphere for 100 years or more, explains why CFCs' destructive impact on the ozone layer will be much greater than emission levels might suggest.

Depletion of the ozone layer is worrisome from a human health perspective because of stratospheric ozone's role in absorbing biologically damaging ultraviolet radiation. It is now well-established that for each 1% decrease in atmospheric ozone, penetration of UV radiation to the earth's surface will increase by 2%. Since more than 90% of nonmelanoma skin cancers are associated with exposure to UV radiation in sunlight, any increase in ultraviolet exposure is expected to result in a rising incidence of skin malignancies. A National Academy of Sciences report in 1982 estimated that for every 1% decrease in the concentration of atmospheric ozone, there will be a 2–5% increase in cases of basal cell carcinomas and a 4–10% increase in squamous cell carcinomas. The impact of rising UV exposure on the incidence of more dangerous malignant melanomas is unclear (Maugh, 1982). An EPA analysis concluded that between now and 2075, increasing levels of UV exposure due to ozone layer depletion could result in as many as 200 million additional cases of skin cancer among Americans, as well as damage to the body's immune system. In 1992, estimates released by the United Nations Environment Program forecast a 26% worldwide increase in nonmelanoma skin cancers if stratospheric ozone levels fall by 10%.

The "Hole in the Sky"

During the early 1980s, both government and many scientists downplayed the ozone depletion threat, asserting that earlier forecasts of ozone loss had been exaggerated and assuring skeptics that CFC production had leveled off and thus presented little cause for concern. This sense of complacency was suddenly shattered in 1985 when members of the British Antarctic Survey announced the existence of a large hole in the ozone layer over the South Pole. Although the gap was temporary, opening in early September (Antarctic spring) and closing by mid-October as the southern atmosphere grew warmer, it had been increasing in size each year since the British researchers first noticed it in 1981; by the time of their startling revelation, the "hole" represented a 40% decline in ozone concentrations. Subsequent confirmation by NASA that the ozone hole was real led to intensified research efforts to learn what was going wrong in the polar skies. United States scientists sent to McMurdo Bay in the years following discovery of the "hole in the sky" revealed that the springtime depletion of ozone was steadily getting larger, appearing earlier, and lasting longer. In 1987, ozone losses totalled 50%; by 1991 they reached 70% over an area four times the size of the United States and measurements of UV radiation reaching the ground were the highest ever recorded in Antarctica up to that time. During the 1990s the Antarctic "ozone hole" grew ever larger. In 1998 it broke all previous records, encompassing 26 million square kilometers—an area larger than North America. The vertical zone of total ozone destruction extended from a region 15 km above the earth's surface to an altitude of 21 km, the highest yet recorded (Kerr, 1998). The 1998 ozone hole also remained in place longer than usual, not breaking up until early December.

During the late 1980s and early 1990s conflicting theories regarding the cause of this depletion were vigorously debated by researchers. Chemical pollution, cyclical solar flares, and natural atmospheric variation were the main contenders for chief villain. Within a few years the weight of evidence tilted toward the chemical pollution theory with the discovery that concentrations of ozone-destroying chlorine molecules were 400–500 times higher within the ozone hole than outside. The presence of chlorine was widely regarded as a "smoking gun"—evidence establishing a direct cause-and-effect link between CFC emissions and ozone layer destruction.

Since the late 1980s, evidence has continued to mount that the pace of ozone loss is accelerating, not only over the South Pole but also above the more populous regions of the Northern Hemisphere. Since 1979 the U.S. government has been collecting data on atmospheric ozone from ground-based survey stations and the Nimbus-7 satellite. By 1993 NASA scientists were reporting record low concentrations of stratospheric ozone above the middle latitudes of North America and Eurasia—down by as much as 20% from their normal levels. While this dramatic drop in ozone may be blamed, at least in part, on debris hurled into the upper atmosphere by the massive 1991 eruption of the Philippine volcano, Mt. Pinatubo, researchers point out that even prior to this event about 3% of the ozone layer above the United States, Europe, Russia, Japan, and China had been lost. Moreover, when the ozone dipped by 3% over the United States, it dropped by 4% over Australia and New Zealand, and 6% in Scandinavia. More ominously, this loss was occurring in the spring and summer when human exposure to sunlight is at peak levels ("Ozone Takes"... 1993; World Resources Institute, 1992). While winter ozone losses over the Arctic haven't occurred as predictably year after year as they have over the South Pole, the winter of 1997 saw the highest Arctic ozone depletion yet recorded, a reminder that the problem is still very much with us.

Until recently, a major weakness in the claim that observed declines in stratospheric ozone levels represent a serious environmental health threat was the scarcity of data documenting an actual increase in ultraviolet light penetration anywhere except in Antarctica—where the number of exposed humans is negligible. That data gap was essentially closed in November 1993, with the publication of a five-year study conducted in Toronto by two scientists working with Environment Canada (Canadian equivalent of EPA). From 1989 to 1993, the researchers took ground-level measurements of UV radiation every hour from sunrise to sunset during winter and summer (seasons when UV levels are at their highest and lowest, respectively). They found that at wavelengths around 300 nanometers (the portion of the UV spectrum most strongly absorbed by stratospheric ozone), ultraviolet radiation increased by 35% per year in winter, 6–7% per year in summer. Since measurements of stratospheric ozone concentrations above Toronto had documented a 4% annual decrease in winter and a 2% summer decline each year during the study period, skeptics' arguments that air pollution or cloud cover will counteract the effect of ozone loss have been proven wrong (Kerr and McElroy, 1993).

Policy Response—The Montreal Protocol

After years of controversy among scientists, the chemical industry, and government policymakers as to the extent of ozone depletion, the identity of the main culprits, and the most effective approach for halting—or at least slowing down—the process, consensus has emerged that ozone depletion is real, that it presents a major threat to life on this planet, and that global cooperation is required to combat a phenomenon that threatens us all. A major step forward to meet this challenge was taken in September 1987, when diplomats from 29 nations, meeting in Montreal, Canada, signed an international accord aimed at controlling the chemicals most responsible for ozone layer depletion. As originally ratified, the Montreal Protocol called for the freezing of CFC consumption at 1986 levels by 1990, to be followed by a 50% reduction in the production of these chemicals by the end of the century. The treaty went into effect in January 1989, after ratification by nations representing more than two-thirds of the world's CFC production (eventually over 140 nations signed the Montreal Protocol). By the early 1990s, scientific evidence that ozone depletion was occurring much more rapidly than anticipated prompted several strengthening amendments to the international treaty. The list of chemicals targeted for controls was expanded to include halons, carbon tetrachloride, methyl chloroform, hydrochlorofluorocarbons (HCFCs), and methyl bromide; in addition, the timetable for phasing out production and use of ozone-depleting substances was advanced. For industrialized nations, the CFC ban took effect on January 1, 1996; developing countries, whose production and use of these chemicals has risen rapidly during the 1990s, were required under the Montreal Protocol to freeze production at their 1995–1997 levels by 1999 and to halt production completely by 2010. Industrialized countries ceased manufacturing halons in 1994, an action developing nations are not required to take until 2010. Phaseout of other ozone-depleters will follow in the early decades of the 21st century.

Unfortunately, even full implementation of the treaty's requirements will not prevent further losses of ozone. Millions of pounds of CFCs already released are gradually drifting up toward the ozone layer and will remain in the atmosphere for many decades. Nevertheless, the cutbacks in CFC production called for in the Montreal Protocol are already having an impact. In August 1993, atmospheric physicists working for the National Oceanic and Atmospheric Administration (NOAA) announced that the unexpectedly rapid drop in industrial production of CFCs even prior to the implementation deadlines set by the treaty had resulted in a substantial slowdown in the rate at which ozone-depleting chemicals were accumulating in the atmosphere. Most developed nations met the 1996 deadline to halt CFC production, and atmospheric levels of these chemicals are beginning to stabilize. Scientists were hopeful that if efforts to phase out the other ozone depleters were equally successful, the ozone layer would begin a gradual regeneration, starting soon after the turn of the century and would return to its former level within 50–100 years. In 1999, Australian scientists at the Commonwealth Scientific and Industrial Research Organisation (CSIRO) Atmospheric Research Center reported that emissions of halons, assumed to have peaked in the late 1980s, instead have risen by about 25% and are now responsible for 20% of ozone layer destruction. Used primarily as fire retardants, halons were scheduled for a production ban in 1994, two years earlier than CFCs, because they are 3–10 times more destructive than are the chlorofluorocarbons. However, as previously mentioned, developing nations can legally produce and use halons until 2010, and China, India, Korea, and Russia continue to do so. China is currently the world's largest halon producer (about 90% of total world produc-

BOX 11-1
Thwarting Ozone Recovery Efforts: CFC Smuggling

Optimistic assurances that the 1996 ban on CFCs will result in a return to normal conditions in the stratosphere sometime around the middle of the 21st century are regularly qualified by the phrase, "If the plan to eliminate all ozone-depleting substances proceeds as set forth in the Montreal Protocol." The United States and other western industrialized nations have, indeed, been making the transition from CFCs to more ozone-friendly chemicals more rapidly than many skeptics thought possible in 1987 when the Protocol was signed. Although the changeover has cost industry billions of dollars to retool manufacturing processes and products, cooperation by CFC producers, industry, and government has enabled most developed countries to meet the 1996 deadline. With a 70% drop in global consumption levels of ozone-depleting chemicals since 1987, researchers have already detected a leveling-off of atmospheric CFC concentrations. Unfortunately, several unexpected developments, made possible by loopholes in the Montreal Protocol, are undermining the spirit of the treaty.

One of these problems is the sharp *increase* in CFC production and use in several developing nations, notably China, India, Mexico, and Brazil. Under the Montreal Protocol, such increases in developing nations were legal until 1999, at which time production levels were to be frozen at their 1995–1997 levels; after 1999, developing countries are supposed to cut production gradually, with complete termination by 2010. However, framers of the Protocol didn't anticipate the sharp surge in production that, in fact, occurred. Between 1986–1995, developing world production of CFCs more than doubled,

while consumption rose by 40%. This means that the baseline level (1995–97 figures) at which production must stabilize is considerably higher than that originally envisioned.

Equally unexpected has been the sudden explosion in CFC black marketeering—a situation so out-of-control that among illegal imports to the U.S., only cocaine is entering in larger quantities. On a worldwide basis, it's estimated that 20,000–30,000 tons of CFCs, with a street value in the billions of dollars, are traded on the black market each year. From its inception, CFC smuggling focused primarily on the United States where, since 1990, progressively higher excise taxes have been imposed on these chemicals to encourage recycling of those still in use and to provide a cost incentive for converting equipment to use CFC substitutes. These excise taxes substantially increased the cost of U.S.-produced CFCs even before the 1996 ban took effect. After 1996, not only could CFCs not be manufactured in the U.S., it was also illegal to import and use foreign-made CFCs (with a few minor exceptions, such as propellants for anti-asthma inhalers).

For the most part, such restrictions posed no major problems; planning ahead, companies once dependent on CFCs had replaced them with safer substances well before the ban took effect. New refrigerators and air conditioning units were being manufactured with non-freon refrigerants by the early to mid-1990s and older models were easily retrofitted to use the CFC substitutes. Automobiles rolling off the assembly lines after 1993 were equipped with air conditioners using HCFCs rather than freon. The major problem, however, and the one that continues to support a booming CFC black market, is the millions of older vehicles equipped with air conditioners that require replacement coolant every 2–3 years. Owners of these cars can legally purchase domestically produced freon from a dwindling amount stockpiled before the 1996 production halt; however, due to growing scarcity and stiff taxes, such refills can cost several hundred dollars. Alternatively, an older car can be refitted with a new air conditioner, but this is even more expensive. The visionaries who hammered out the terms of the Montreal Protocol idealistically assumed that as the cost of legal freon replacements steadily increased, vehicle owners would have a cost incentive to retrofit their cars with newer, CFC-free air conditioners. Unfortunately, they overlooked the Protocol's built-in incentives for smuggling.

Primary sources of contraband freon are the developing nations, where ironically, the main producers of the chemicals involved in black market dealings sometimes are American-owned firms (Allied Signal's *Quimobasicos* plant in Monterrey, Mexico, is but one example). Currently the largest quantities of illicit CFCs in both the U.S. and Europe originate in China, where production is still legal, and in Russia, where it isn't (the Russian Mafia is now deeply involved in freon trafficking). Other consignments are crossing the border from Mexico, India, and various other nations. Once inside the country, smugglers sell their black market goods to auto-parts stores or go-betweens who then resell them to air conditioning repair shops and service stations. Hefty profits are made with each transaction of the bootleg merchandise; a service station manager might pay $400 for a 30–pound canister of freon and then re-sell it to his customers for $80 per pound—still cheaper to the customer, however, than the price of legal product.

While many smugglers are small-time crooks who view peddling CFCs as a harmless, easy way to make a lot of money, law enforcement officials are responding to this situation with the seriousness it deserves. The federal government has launched an on-going effort dubbed "Operation Cool Breeze" to interdict illegal CFC shipments and to prosecute those responsible. Mustering the combined forces of EPA, the FBI, Customs Service, the CIA, and Interpol, federal officials have confiscated thousands of cylinders of CFCs, targeted dozens of companies for investigation, raided suspected smuggling centers, and made numerous arrests. Law enforcement activity is also gathering steam in Europe, where contraband has been seized and arrests made in both the Netherlands and the United Kingdom. Officials admit that until better CFC tracking mechanisms are in place, substantially curtailing black market activities will be difficult. To this end, the Montreal Protocol was recently amended to set up a licensing system for CFC exports and imports. For the system to work effectively, however, much more needs to be done to train customs officials, to improve cooperation among agencies—both within the U.S. and internationally—and to impose stricter penalties on individuals convicted of CFC smuggling. To do less would be to sacrifice the hard-won gains achieved over the past decade and to prolong the environmental risks posed by the continued loss of stratospheric ozone.

References

Sheff, David. 1997. "The Chilling Effect." *Outside* (Aug).

World Resource Institute. 1998. *World Resources 1998–99*. Oxford University Press.

tion) and the Australian researchers assume halon use in China is primarily responsible for the observed increase in emissions. This development is profoundly disappointing because it means that ozone layer recovery will now take many more years than had been anticipated. Although the conversion from CFCs and other ozone-destroying chemicals to more environmentally benign substitutes is still incomplete, scientists and policymakers are pleased with progress to date. The international efforts to protect the ozone layer exemplified by the Montreal Protocol are extremely significant in that they represent the first time in history that the nations of the world have agreed to work together to prevent a disaster of global proportions before it's too late. Initial indications of the success of this approach offer hope for similar cooperation in tackling even more difficult environmental challenges—such as global climate change.

Rising Levels of Atmospheric CO_2—Moving Toward a Warmer World?

> The inhabitants of Planet Earth are quietly conducting a gigantic environmental experiment. So vast and so sweeping will be the impacts of this experiment that, were it brought before any responsible council for approval, it would be firmly rejected as having potentially dangerous consequences. Yet, the experiment goes on with no significant interference from any jurisdiction or nation. The experiment in question is the release of carbon dioxide and other so-called greenhouse gases to the atmosphere.
>
> —Wallace S. Broecker, geochemist, Columbia University
> (Mintzer, 1987)

As mentioned earlier in this chapter, the relative concentrations of the four major atmospheric gases—nitrogen, oxygen, argon, and carbon dioxide—have remained constant for at least several hundred million years. Within recent decades, however, scientists have been expressing concern that a decrease in oxygen levels and an increase in the amount of atmospheric carbon dioxide might be occurring due to the sharp rise in fossil fuel combustion (a process that consumes O_2 and releases CO_2), the worldwide destruction of forest cover, and the poisoning of oceanic photoplankton by pollution of the seas. (Plants are the source of atmospheric oxygen and also capture and store huge amounts of CO_2, thereby removing it from the atmosphere.) Fortunately, recent studies of the oxygen balance have shown that no oxygen depletion has yet occurred and forces operating at the present time are deemed far too insignificant to constitute a real threat so far as oxygen supply is concerned (Broecker, 1970).

The fears regarding carbon dioxide increase, on the other hand, have proven to be well founded and the prospect of a long-term global warming due to CO_2-induced enhancement of the greenhouse effect has become one of the most pressing and politically charged global environmental issues. Levels of atmospheric CO_2 have been gradually rising ever since the dawn of the Industrial Revolution as a result of the ever-increasing use of coal, oil, and gas to

Table 11-1   Countries With the Highest Industrial Emissions of CO_2

Country	Total CO_2 Emissions (000 metric tons)
United States	5,468,564
China	3,192,484
Russian Federation	1,818,011
Japan	1,126,753
India	908,734
Germany	835,099
United Kingdom	542,140
Ukraine	438,211
Canada	435,749
Italy	409,900
Korea, Rep	373,592
Mexico	357,834
France	340,085
Poland, Rep	338,044
South Africa	305,805

Source: World Resources Institute, World Resources 1998–99.

power the world's factories and vehicles. When fossil fuels are burned, one of the primary combustion products is carbon dioxide; the combustion of one ton of coal, for example, releases three tons of CO_2. In past ages, excess carbon dioxide released through volcanic outgassing was gradually absorbed into the oceans and eventually incorporated into carbonate rock or was photosynthetically "fixed" by green plants. These natural processes, however, are now being overwhelmed by the sheer volume of excess carbon dioxide being released. Since 1950, annual carbon emissions worldwide have risen four-fold, reaching a record-high 6.3 billion tons in 1997 (Brown et al., 1998).

While fossil fuel combustion has received most of the attention—and blame—in relation to rising CO_2 concentrations, the widescale destruction of natural vegetation, particularly deforestation in the tropics, contributes nearly one-fourth (23%) of all global CO_2 emissions. Both forests and the organic matter in soil humus hold immense quantities of carbon that are oxidized and released as carbon dioxide when vegetation is destroyed. Space satellite monitors have revealed that the impact of forest destruction on CO_2 release may be even greater than previously realized. Data collected over the Amazon basin indicate that the thousands of fires deliberately set every year by settlers and ranchers clearing the Brazilian rain forest are generating such enormous quantities of gases and particles that they alone may account for at least one-tenth of the carbon dioxide released by human activities each year (Watson et al., 1990). The equilibrium that has prevailed for millennia has been disrupted, with the result that atmospheric CO_2 levels are now sharply increasing.

Figure 11-4   Per Capita CO$_2$ Emissions for the Countries with the Highest Total Industrial Emissions, 1995

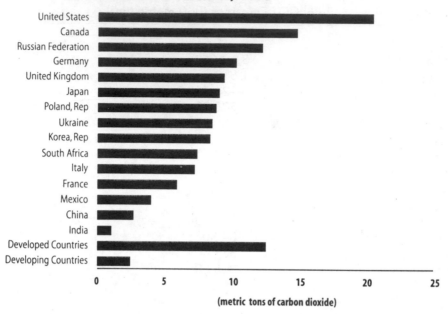

(metric tons of carbon dioxide)

Source: World Resources Institute, *World Resources 1998–99.*

In 1999, a team of Russian, French, and U.S. scientists working at Russia's Vostok research station in Antarctica published data showing that current greenhouse gas levels are higher than any in the past 420,000 years. By chemically analyzing air bubbles trapped in ice cores drilled two miles into the Antarctic ice sheet, the researchers were able to construct a record of past climatic conditions, demonstrating increases and decreases of carbon dioxide and methane as warm interglacial periods alternated with colder glacial epochs. They found that even the highest concentrations of greenhouse gases in past millennia, present during the warm interglacial years, were well below present-day levels, strongly suggesting that humans are strongly influencing today's climatic patterns (Petit et al., 1999). Since the beginning of the Industrial Revolution two centuries ago, concentrations of atmospheric CO$_2$ have risen by nearly 30%, from 280 ppm to 366 ppm in 1999; throughout the preindustrial portion of the past millennium, atmospheric CO$_2$ concentrations never varied by more than 5 ppm (Indermühle et al., 1999). At present, CO$_2$ levels in the atmosphere continue to rise at a rate of 0.4% (1.5 ppm) per year. If current rates of emission persist, atmospheric CO$_2$ concentrations will more than double by 2100 (IPCC, 1994).

The sense of alarm felt by those monitoring this situation relates not to any adverse effect that CO$_2$ might exert on human health—the gas is not a toxic pollutant but a natural and necessary constituent of the biosphere—but rather is due to the impact increasing levels of carbon dioxide will have on global climate. As mentioned earlier in this chapter, atmospheric CO$_2$ plays a vital role in moderating the earth's temperature, a phenomenon known as the **greenhouse effect.** Just as the glass in a greenhouse permits light to enter but prevents the escape of heat, thereby warming the air within, so the absorption of infrared ground radiation by carbon dioxide and its subsequent re-radiation back toward the earth helps to maintain an average global temperature of 59 °F (15 °C). Without CO_2 in the atmosphere, the earth's average surface temperature would fall to about O °F, making the existence of life as we know it impossible. By way of comparison, the planet Venus, with a dense, CO_2-rich atmosphere, has a surface temperature of 890 °F—hot enough to melt lead—while Mars, whose atmosphere consists primarily of CO_2 but is very diffuse and contains but a trace of water vapor, is colder than Antarctica, with an average temperature of -53 °F (Revkin, 1992; Houghton, Jenkins, and Ephraums, 1990). However, as carbon dioxide levels increase, more infrared radiation will be absorbed and over time average global temperatures will correspondingly rise.

Comprehensive scientific efforts to determine whether global warming is actually occurring as a result of human activities have been underway since the late 1970s, drawing on evidence derived from such diverse sources as ice core analyses, orbiting satellites, ocean current studies, and computer modeling. The result of these wide-ranging investigations has been an evolving scientific consensus that rising greenhouse gas concentrations are, indeed, likely to alter the global energy balance enough to cause a 2 °C increase in average world temperature, relative to its 1990 value, before the end of the 21st century. This would be in addition to the 0.5 °C (1 °F) increase already documented since the late 1800s. Uncertainties associated with making emissions projections far into the future mean that actual temperature increases could be slightly higher or lower than the 2 °C "best guess." However, any of the temperatures within the estimated range of 1 to 3.5 °C (1.4 to 6.3 °F) represent a global climate warmer than anything experienced during the last 10,000 years. Until a few years ago, the international scientific community was hesitant to attribute incipient signs of climate change to human causes, pointing out that natural fluctuations in the past had resulted in alternating cycles of warming and cooling and could be doing so again. Such reticence ended in 1995 when an exhaustive report by the Intergovernmental Panel on Climate Change (IPCC) concluded that "human activities are changing the atmospheric concentrations and distribution of greenhouse gases and aerosols." This statement carries considerable weight since the IPCC was jointly established by the United Nations Environment Programme and the World Meteorological Organization to assess information related to climate change. Comprising 2,500 scientists representing some 60 countries, the IPCC is regarded as the official advisory body on issues pertaining to global warming by governments around the world. Although a small minority of dissident scientists still argue to the contrary, the IPCC statement, published as part of the group's Second Assessment Report, represents an important affirmation of the breadth and depth of agreement within the scientific community about the reality of global climate change. (Note: IPCC's First Assessment Report, issued in 1990, concluded that global warming is occurring but didn't establish whether human or natural forces were to blame; IPCC's Third Assessment Report, reflecting the most recent experimental evidence, is due in 2000.)

Turning up the Heat: Other Greenhouse Gases

As if humanity doesn't have enough to worry about with the seemingly inexorable rise in carbon dioxide levels, climatologists now warn that increasing atmospheric concentrations of several other gases—specifically, methane, nitrous oxide, and chlorofluorocarbons (CFCs)—are further enhancing the greenhouse effect by capturing wavelengths of infrared radiation not readily absorbed by CO_2. Although present in concentrations far below that of carbon dioxide, these trace gases are much more efficient than CO_2 in absorbing outgoing heat waves. A molecule of methane, for example, can trap 20–30 times more infrared radiation than does a molecule of CO_2. Equally worrisome is the fact that emissions of trace gases are increasing at a substantially faster rate than CO_2 and originate from sources that may be even more difficult to control. A brief look at the situation regarding the other "greenhouse gases" reveals the following picture.

Methane (CH_4). Although current atmospheric concentrations of this gas are less than 2 ppm, as opposed to CO_2 levels of 366 ppm, methane is far more potent as a greenhouse gas and is increasing at a 0.6% annual rate. Curtailing methane emissions will not be easy, since over half originate from rice cultivation (due to the respiration of anaerobic bacteria in waterlogged paddy fields) and from microbial activity in the intestines of cattle and termites (it is estimated that a cow belches methane approximately twice a minute!). Other significant sources more amenable to controls include emissions from gas and coal production, flares on oil rigs, landfills, and tropical deforestation (when vegetation is burned during clearing activities).

Nitrous Oxide (N_2O). Up by 8% since the beginning of the 20th century and increasing at a rate of 0.25% annually, the so-called "laughing gas" once used as a painkiller by dentists is a more efficient greenhouse gas than CO_2 but because its total atmospheric concentrations are in the parts per billion range, its overall contribution to global warming is still fairly limited. Nitrous oxide is a natural by-product of the metabolism of certain soil microbes, but the generation of this gas has been boosted significantly by the increased worldwide use of nitrogen fertilizers. Combustion of fossil fuels, increased land cultivation, burning of biomass, and the decomposition of agricultural wastes and sewage are presumed to be additional sources of N_2O.

Chlorofluorocarbons (CFCs). The prime villains in ozone layer destruction, CFCs are also potent greenhouse gases, each molecule of which has a direct warming effect 12,000–20,000 times greater than that of a CO_2 molecule. While atmospheric concentrations of CFCs are considerably lower than those of other greenhouse gases, they have been rising at a rapid rate. It is assumed that the 1996 halt in CFC production in the developed countries will, over time, reduce the contribution of these chemicals to global warming.

Several other substances targeted for emissions reductions due to their role as powerful greenhouse gases include **sulfur hexafluoride (SF_6)**, used primarily in electrical transmission and distribution systems, and **perfluoro-**

carbons (**PFCs**) and **hydrofluorocarbons (HFCs)**—both on the rise due to their increasing commercial and industrial use as substitutes for CFCs and other now-banned, ozone-depleting chemicals.

It should be noted that water vapor is another important greenhouse gas, but because human activities have negligible impact on its atmospheric concentrations and because the amount of water in the air varies widely from place to place and day to day, levels of this atmospheric constituent are not taken into consideration when discussing global warming scenarios.

While the lion's share of public attention regarding climate change has thus far focused on carbon dioxide emissions, it is now agreed that the cumulative effect of the other greenhouse gases will be nearly equivalent to that of CO_2. Ironically, air pollution may help to counteract the heat-capturing potential of greenhouse gases to some extent. Airborne soot and sulfate particles released when fossil fuels and other organic materials are burned directly absorb and reflect solar radiation, thereby exerting a cooling effect on climate. Based on what is now known about the impact of these particles on the global radiation balance, researchers have scaled back earlier warming rate projections that failed to take into account the cooling effect of sulfate aerosols. Nevertheless, because these pollutants are unevenly distributed in the atmosphere and settle out relatively quickly, their overall impact on climate is difficult to assess (Houghton et al., 1996).

Impacts of Global Warming

To many people, the prospect of temperatures a few degrees higher than they are at present seems little cause for dismay—particularly when they happen to be contemplating such a scenario during a January blizzard. The major impact of a global warming trend, however, would not be felt in terms of human physical discomfort but rather in a possibly drastic alteration of worldwide rainfall and temperature patterns.

While climatologists are unable to make accurate detailed predictions regarding CO_2-induced climatic changes in specific areas of the globe, their computer modeling studies support widespread agreement that while temperatures everywhere are rising to some extent, the global warming trend is not evenly distributed. The high latitude regions of the Northern Hemisphere are expected to experience the greatest temperature increases (perhaps twice as high as the world average), particularly during the winter months. In mid-latitude regions also (including the continental United States) greenhouse warming will exceed the global average, with winter temperatures increasing more than summer temperatures. Regional changes in rainfall patterns are even more difficult to predict, but computer models suggest that our grandchildren's generation may witness heavier precipitation in the already-wet equatorial regions, more winter precipitation in the polar regions, much drier summers in the midwestern United States, and drier winters in California. Along with such widespread regional climatic alteration, more localized weather changes such as the frequency and intensity of storms and hurricanes will also be pronounced. More frequent "January thaws" during winter and more unusually hot days during the summer may become commonplace. Whereas Washington, D.C. now averages only one day each year when the mercury tops 100 °F, a doubling of CO_2

BOX 11-2

Has Global Warming Begun?

The reality of global climate change has been vigorously debated for years. Although the experts continue to wrangle over the question, a majority of Americans, according to opinion surveys, are convinced that climate has changed already. Such convictions are based on personal observation of less predictable weather patterns and milder winters today than in years gone by. These attitudes are further reinforced by widespread media reference to record-breaking temperatures during the 1990s. Scientists and policymakers, however, demand more than anecdotal evidence and one of the serious hindrances in formulating a comprehensive government response to the threat of greenhouse warming has been the lack of conclusive proof that global warming has begun. Nevertheless, an ever-increasing flood of research data from a wide variety of sources around the world is providing ample grounds for concern and suggests the public's "gut reaction" may be correct. A sampling of recent findings includes the following:

1. Spring in the far North is now arriving a week earlier than it did in the 1970s and autumn lasts 2–4 days longer, according to researchers at the Scripps Institution of Oceanography in San Diego. As a result, plant growth has been stimulated over wide areas of Alaska, northern Canada, Siberia, and northern Europe. The increase in plant growth—as great as 10% in some regions—is pointed to as one of the best indicators yet of ecosystem response to a warming climate.

2. Mountain glaciers are melting. Switzerland's Aletsch glacier, the largest in mainland Europe, has retreated more than a mile since the mid-1800s and has shrunk by more than 300 feet in thickness. Alpine glaciers as a group have lost one-third to one-half their ice volume during the past century. Half a world away in the mountains of New Guinea, glaciers have also been steadily dwindling in size, despite receiving heavy snow cover. Researchers conclude the shrinking can only be explained by a general increase in temperature.

3. Ocean water temperature is rising. Deep-water temperature increases of about 0.5 °C (0.9 °F) have been recorded in the southwestern Pacific, the Indian Ocean, and in the North Atlantic. More dramatic increases have occurred in the Arctic Ocean, where a rise of 1°C (1.8 °F) since the mid-1980s has been documented. This increase may already be having a detrimental impact on salmon in the North Pacific, where populations of several species of this commercially valuable fish crashed during the exceptionally warm years of 1997 and 1998. When water temperatures rise, salmon need more food just to survive and above a certain threshold they starve. Another valuable marine resource, coral reefs, are similarly devastated when water temperatures increase. The epidemic of coral "bleaching" currently being witnessed in tropical waters around the globe is another suggestive indicator that global warming may already have begun.

4. Air temperatures in the far North are noticeably rising. Fairbanks, Alaska, now experiences half as many days with −40 °F temperature readings as it did in the 1950s. As a result, permafrost is beginning to thaw, releasing more CO_2 from decaying plant material into the atmo-

sphere, thereby constituting a "positive feedback mechanism" that stimulates even more climatic warming.

5. Sea ice is melting, thanks to the rise in both air and water temperatures in polar regions. In the Bering Sea, north of Alaska, sea ice has been reduced approximately 5% in the past 40 years, retreating many miles north of its historical southward extent. Dwindling sea ice has had a devastating impact for such Arctic species as walruses, polar bears, and certain sea birds that rely on ice floes for hunting grounds and breeding sites. Worrisome population declines of several Arctic species have been documented in recent years as ice cover has dwindled. Similar trends in western Antarctica, where midwinter temperatures have risen by 4–5 °C over the past half century, have led to a 40% drop in Adelie penguin numbers. Biologists attribute the problem to a decline in the penguins' main food, krill, which normally thrives in plankton-rich areas near sea ice. Melting of the ice has resulted in a crash in krill populations, depriving the Adelies of a food staple. Compounding the penguins' problems, warmer temperatures have increased spring snowfall, and scientists studying the birds worry about reproductive failure as penguin eggs are buried under unaccustomed piles of snow.

6. Distribution patterns of plants and animals are shifting. Scientists have long predicted that if climate changes, the established range of various wildlife species will shift in response. Ecologists are now witnessing the accuracy of that prediction. A researcher at the University of California has documented a 160–kilometer northward shift in the population of the Edith's checkerspot butterfly, with the insect vanishing from the southern extreme of its traditional range and expanding from its northern boundary. She has also found the same phenomenon occurring in Europe, where 22 species of butterflies have either died out at the southern edge of their range, expanded beyond the northern edge, or both. One species, the sooty copper butterfly, has now disappeared from Spain but has shown up in Estonia. Plants, too, are on the move. In eastern Switzerland and western Austria, nine species of alpine plants have been moving up mountainsides at a rate of about 12 feet (4 meters) per decade since the early years of the 20th century. More troubling than the migration of butterflies or wildflowers has been the spread of disease-carrying mosquitoes, both northward and to higher altitudes, where temperatures previously were too cool for them to survive. Already yellow fever mosquitoes are appearing in certain mountainous regions of South America where they were never encountered in the past.

All these converging lines of evidence should provide food for thought to those still inclined to debunk the urgency of global climate change in the absence of overwhelming catastrophe.

levels could result in two sweltering weeks of triple-digit temperatures in our nation's capital; residents of Dallas, who currently suffer through 100 °F heat approximately 19 days each year, can look forward to 78 such days in the warmer world projected by climatologists.

Scientists and policymakers alike are now striving to determine what changes are likely to occur as temperatures climb and to formulate strategies to ameliorate detrimental effects as much as possible. The more significant potential impacts of global warming are discussed in the following sections.

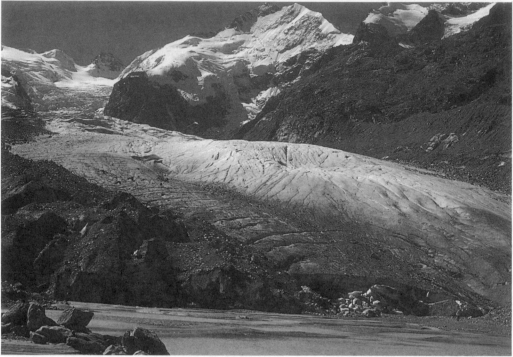

The retreating Monteratsch glacier in the Swiss Alps is one of many Alpine glaciers that has shrunk during the past century. *[Author's photo]*

Diminishing Crop Yields

The hotter, drier weather forecast for some of the world's most productive agricultural lands is bad news at a time when global food demand is steadily increasing. For farmers, major climatic change could bring benefits to some regions, severe hardship to others. Climate models predict that greenhouse warming would result in shifting rainfall patterns that could bring substantially heavier monsoon rains to India but 30–60% less summer precipitation to the American Midwest. Higher temperatures could force a northward shift of agricultural zones, perhaps boosting crop yields in Canada and Russia while turning the American "Breadbasket" into a dustbowl. Although some observers have suggested that rising concentrations of CO_2 might actually enhance food production by increasing photosynthetic rates, the combined impact of excessive heat and drought could counteract this effect. Similarly, soils in the northern latitudes that may benefit from increasing temperatures are generally too acidic and not fertile enough to support intensive grain production.

Global warming could have other less obvious impacts on agricultural productivity. Livestock production will suffer due to heat-induced declines in animal fertility; pastures and rangelands can be expected to sustain heat damage. As temperatures rise, the range of plant pathogens and crop destroying insects expand considerably; pests currently confined to southern latitudes may spread northward, causing serious agricultural losses. A shift in the balance between pest and predator species, prompted by changing environmental conditions, could also have adverse repercussions for farming by favoring the survival of more resilient pest species over that of their natural enemies. These increased pest infestations may prompt farmers to increase applications of chemical pesticides, raising the probability of more surface and groundwater pollution problems. Crop losses are likely to be further compounded by increasing levels of tropospheric ozone, a pollutant gas that forms most readily on hot, sunny days. Conflicts over access to irrigation water is bound to increase, pitting farmers against city dwellers within nations and heightening international tensions where disputed water supplies cross national borders. In the U.S. this problem may become particularly contentious in California, where EPA predicts that climate change produced by a doubling of CO_2 will result in a 7–16% reduction in annual water supplies to the now highly-productive Central Valley—a region already beset by burgeoning water demand.

The extent to which greenhouse warming will affect agricultural production will depend in large measure on the rate at which these climatic changes occur. Most of the world's major food crops are already adapted to a wide range of environmental conditions and if climatic change is gradual, agricultural scientists will have time to develop new, even more tolerant varieties. IPCC scientists are optimistic that on a worldwide basis, harvests can be maintained relative to baseline production levels despite global warming, but warn that regional food production—particularly in the tropics and subtropics—may suffer. A study commissioned by EPA concluded that by 2060, grain production in the developing countries may fall by 9–11% as a result of global climate change. Like so many other environmental problems, global warming is likely to have its greatest impact on those already living a marginal existence.

Loss of Biodiversity

Climate change will impose even greater stresses on natural ecosystems than on domesticated plants and animals, since many nonagricultural species have gradually become adapted to life in a specific habitat and have a rather narrow range of tolerance to changing environmental conditions. Plants and animals, particularly those living in temperate regions, will be forced to move hundreds of miles toward the poles (or thousands of feet up mountainsides) in order to maintain the temperature conditions to which they have become adapted. For many species such migration will be virtually impossible. Plants, for example, can shift location only as far as their seeds are dispersed. A gradual poleward migration might be conceivable if the rate of climate change is very slow, but if warming is so rapid that the present habitat becomes unsuitable before a new area can be colonized, then the species will die out.

One might assume that animals, capable of moving under their own power, would find migration to more congenial climes relatively easy. In today's world, however, barriers to migration in the form of cities, highways, dams, and so on make large-scale movements of many species highly problematic (visualize the challenges faced by a group of alligators heading north out of Okefenokee Swamp as they attempt to traverse Atlanta!). While some animal species migrate easily, others are genetically programmed to be highly territorial and wouldn't even try to move as their environment became uninhabitable; others might be capable of migrating, but if the plant species on which they feed don't move also, they would perish of starvation. Biodiversity, already suffering severely from pressures imposed by overhunting, pollution, and habitat destruction, may find greenhouse warming the most devastating blow of all.

Rising Sea Levels

The most dramatic consequence of global warming will be a worldwide rise in sea level due to both the thermal expansion of water as temperatures in the ocean rise and to the melting of the Greenland and Antarctic ice sheets. Although this development could be a boon to navigation in the Arctic (the fabled "Northwest Passage" might become a practical alternative to the Panama Canal!), its impact on densely populated coastal regions worldwide will be devastating. In its 1995 Second Assessment Report, the IPCC estimates a global average rise in sea level of about 1½ feet (50 cm) by 2100, with an upper range of nearly 3 feet (95 cm) considered an outside possibility. At particular risk are the inhabitants of low-lying coral atolls. Residents of small island nations such as the Bahamas, Maldives, and Marshall Islands have been the most vociferous proponents of measures to curb greenhouse gas emissions as they confront the prospect of their homelands disappearing beneath the waves. Along the edges of continents, towns and cities built on barrier islands, river deltas, or low-lying shorelines can anticipate a similar scenario unless they soon embark on multi-billion dollar coastal defense construction projects. In many desperately poor, densely populated regions of the world, such expenditures are obviously impossible. It is anticipated that Egypt may lose 15% of its arable land to encroaching seas by the mid-21st century; in Bangladesh even a three-foot rise in sea level would inundate one-sixth of the country's land area. When one pauses to consider the number of major world cities now located at or near sea level, the impact of such a rise on human settlement patterns becomes clear. Although sea level will advance gradually (no one foresees the likelihood of Boston or Galveston or Miami being submerged overnight!), even a slight increase can have significant consequences. Some experts feel that a six-inch rise during the 20th century has been responsible for much of the coastal erosion that has occurred, and experts contend that a continuation of present trends will obliterate most beaches along the eastern coast of the U.S. by 2020. Greenhouse warming of ocean waters will also exacerbate coastal problems by provoking more severe hurricanes and storm surges—a serious concern, considering that by 2010 three-fourths of the world's people will be living within 36 miles (60 km) of a coastline.

Human Illness

Although global warming is primarily an environmental problem rather than a human health issue, the increasing frequency of heat waves will have an impact on morbidity and mortality rates. Extreme heat will result in some excess deaths, mainly due to heart attacks and strokes. However, the most significant public health problem associated with global warming is the likely spread of certain vectorborne tropical diseases such as malaria and dengue fever into regions where they are currently unknown. As a possible portent of things to come, unusually hot, humid weather during the mid-1990s sparked a dengue epidemic in Mexico and Central America when virus-carrying mosquitoes moved from endemic coastal areas into the usually cool highlands. An Asian Development Bank survey predicts a similar scenario in Indonesia, projecting a quadrupling of dengue cases in the years ahead as a warming climate facilitates the spread of mosquitoes from the lowlands into Indonesia's mountain regions (O'Meara, 1997).

Rate of Global Warming

As mentioned earlier, the rate at which global temperatures rise will be extremely important in determining how serious the impacts of climate change will be. Humanity may be able to adjust reasonably well to a very gradual warming trend, whereas a more rapid change could be catastrophic. Which of these two scenarios is more likely? Several years ago Columbia University geochemist Wallace Broecker, in testimony submitted to a congressional hearing, remarked that:

> Earth's climate does not respond in a smooth and gradual way; rather it responds in sharp jumps. If this reading of the natural record is correct, then we must consider the possibility that the major responses of the system to our greenhouse provocation will come in jumps whose timing and magnitude are unpredictable. Coping with this type of change is clearly a far more serious matter than coping with a gradual warming.

In this context, reports from scientists working in Greenland provide considerable cause for alarm. Analysis of air bubbles in layers of ice from cores drilled deep into the island's massive ice cap provides evidence for the rate of climate change in the distant past. University of Rhode Island researchers have found that the end of the last ice age, slightly over 11,000 years ago, occurred much more rapidly than previously thought possible. In just a few decades or less, average temperatures in Greenland suddenly rose 9–18 °F. A similarly abrupt, though less extreme, warming trend occurred over much of the Northern Hemisphere at this time (Severinghaus et al., 1998). Another research team working with ice core evidence found that the transition from the last period of glaciation to the warmer modern era came in two sudden temperature increases, each of about 10 degrees Fahrenheit and each occurring within less than 10 years. Yet a third study conducted by researchers from Columbia University's Lamont Doherty Earth Observatory focused on Atlantic Ocean sediments for clues to how quickly climate change might occur. Working off the northwestern coast of Africa, researchers discovered that since the end of the last ice age, ocean temperatures there have experienced wide, abrupt fluctuations roughly every 1,500 years. These changes, and their consequent impact on regional climate, occurred within a period of about 50 years—a finding that lends additional support to the hypothesis of climatic thresholds that can suddenly be tripped. Converging lines of evidence from these and similar investigations suggest that the relatively stable climate of the past 10,000 years, the period during which human civilizations developed

Figure 11-5   Average Global Temperature for the Last Century

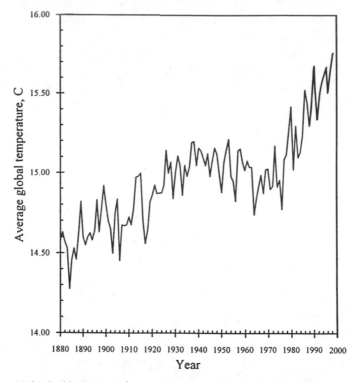

Source: Adapted from NASA Goddard Institute for Space Studies and National Climatic Data Center.

and flourished, is an anomaly—an exception to the rule of frequent and sudden change throughout much of geologic time. Again quoting Dr. Broecker: "The climate system is an angry beast and we are poking it with sticks. We don't know whether it's going to pay attention to the pokes. But if it does, it might rise up and do something we don't like."

The Greenhouse Policy Debate

Since the early 1970s, climatologists have been raising increasingly strident warnings about the impending greenhouse warming, urging policymakers to take action to forestall this so-called "Doomsday Issue." While the general public until recently tended either to ignore such predictions or to regard them as plot material for a science fiction novel, there has been a steadily growing chorus of experts who claim that global climate change has already begun. Testifying before a Senate subcommittee during the torrid summer of 1988, James Hansen of the NASA Goddard Institute for Space Studies told the assembled lawmakers that "the greenhouse effect has been detected and is changing our climate now." Hansen cited the fact that the four hottest years then on record had all occurred in the 1980s. In retrospect, the weather of the 1980s looks mild when compared with the 1990s, which witnessed the six hottest years since record-keeping began in 1860. Average sur-

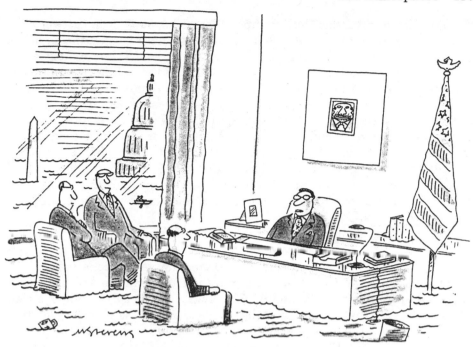

"Gentlemen, it's time we gave some serious thought
to the effects of global warming."

face air temperatures in 1998 were the warmest ever, each month breaking every previous record for that date. Average sea surface temperatures also hit new highs during the 1990s. Such developments add a sense of urgency to demands that governments shake off their inertia and launch efforts to reduce the continued emission of greenhouse gases. As Howard Ferguson, a meteorologist with the Canadian Atmospheric Environmental Service, remarked: "All the greenhouse scenarios are consistent. These numbers are real. We have to start behaving as if this is going to happen. Those who advocate a program consisting only of additional research are missing the boat."

Calling for action is easier than implementing such changes, however. Delegates to the United Nations' Earth Summit, held in Rio de Janeiro in 1992, took the first substantive steps toward tackling the global warming issue when they endorsed the **United Nations Framework Convention on Climate Control (UNFCCC)**. This treaty, which by 1999 had been ratified by 175 countries, calls for a voluntary reduction in greenhouse gas emissions to 1990 levels by 2000. It also calls for the rich nations whose greenhouse gas emissions are largely responsible for the present state of affairs to take the lead in emissions reductions. Progress toward attaining UNFCCC's voluntary goals has been dismal, however. Although the European Union has been able to reduce carbon emissions to a level just 1% above the 1990 benchmark, the U.S. witnessed an 8.8% increase in CO_2 emissions between 1990 and 1996, due to a booming economy, low fuel prices, and lack of progress in improving energy efficiency standards. (The United States has long been the world's top carbon emitter, contributing 23% of the world's total.) During the same time period, Japanese carbon emissions rose by 12.5% and those of Australia by 9.6% (Brown et al., 1998). The obvious failure of the voluntary approach to curbing CO_2 emissions led to another set of international negotiations, held in Kyoto, Japan, in December 1997. Attended by representatives from 171 nations, the conference concluded with the signing of the **Kyoto Protocol**, which sets *mandatory* emissions reductions for 38 industrial nations. Aimed at reducing emissions of six greenhouse gases (CO_2, CH_4, N_2O, HFCs, PFCs, and SF_6) by industrialized countries as a group to 5.2% below 1990 levels, the Protocol assigns each individual country its own goal: United States, 7%; Japan, 6%; European Union, 8%; Russia, 0%. Such cuts are to be made gradually, between 2008–2012.

Whether achieving these goals is even attempted remains in doubt, however. Terms of the Kyoto Protocol become legally binding only after 55 countries representing 55% of the world's 1990 greenhouse gas emissions ratify it. In the United States, strong opposition in the U.S. Senate makes ratification any time in the near future highly unlikely (see Box 11-3). A major sticking point is the fact that the Protocol does not *require* developing nations to cut their emissions but merely "encourages" them to do so. Although the industrialized nations currently are responsible for over half (i.e. 55%) of all carbon emissions since 1950 and still contribute 45% of the annual total, developing nations are rapidly becoming major players in the global warming drama. As efforts to modernize their economies and raise living standards gain momentum, countries such as China, India, and Mexico are witnessing a sharp rise in greenhouse gas emissions. Already the People's Republic of China is the world's second-highest CO_2 emitter (14% of total), with a rate of increase faster than anywhere else in the world (Brown et al., 1998). As China strives to promote rapid industrialization and electrification for its still-growing population, the need to exploit its vast coal reserves to fuel development goals will doubtless take precedence over international commitments to cap greenhouse gas emissions. And if the populations of demographic giants such as China and India achieve levels of affluence even remotely resembling those of more industrialized countries, the impact of emissions from millions of additional cars, refrigerators, and so on would be far higher than those currently generated in the West. While China argues that it would be unfair for the Kyoto Protocol to impose equal restrictions on its "survival emissions" (as opposed to the United States' "luxury emissions"), members of the U.S. Senate are adamant that without mandatory developing country participation, CO_2 reductions achieved by industrialized nations will be to no avail. At a follow-up meeting in Buenos Aires, Argentina, in November 1998, negotiators from 160 countries attempted to reach agreement on implementation of the Kyoto Protocol but made little progress beyond agreeing to set rules for compliance and enforcement of the treaty by the end of 2000. Without U.S. participation, it is doubtful how effective international efforts to control greenhouse gases can be, and the longer meaningful action is delayed, the more difficult it will be to achieve emission goals. The U.S. Department of Energy estimates that, in the absence of any significant change in consumer behavior and national energy policy, U.S. carbon emissions in 2010 will be 34% higher than they were in

BOX 11-3

The Politics of Global Warming

The Kyoto agreement...is deader than a Costa Rican golden toad.

—David Ignatius
("As Temperatures Rise,"
Washington Post, May 30, 1999)

Castigating congressional refusal even to consider meaningful policy initiatives to combat global climate change, columnist David Ignatius echoes the dismay of scientists and environmentalists, incredulous that the U.S. government has sidestepped meaningful action on what some observers have called "the greatest challenge of human history."

A coherent international response to global warming, unfortunately, involves far more than collecting scientific data and crafting a "technological fix." The current policy debate, initially prompted by warnings from scientists and pushed into the media's glare by a series of extreme weather events, is now mired in controversy both at the national and international levels. Although remaining scientific uncertainties regarding evidence for global warming are important to resolve, doing so will not erase opposition to action. Of equal, if not greater, importance than scientific facts are economic and political realities which may be even more difficult to reconcile.

Because any effective strategy to reduce greenhouse gas emissions must, by necessity, focus on reducing fossil fuel combustion, it shouldn't be surprising that the loudest voices against concerted action on global warming are those of the major producers of oil, gas, and coal. Internationally, countries such as Saudi Arabia and other petroleum-rich nations regularly try to block action by world bodies; within the U.S., lobbyists for the fossil fuel industry and their congressional allies from resource-rich states are outspoken foes of the issue. Big Coal and Big Oil are formidable opponents for the cash-strapped environmental organizations trying to raise public awareness and legislative support for policies to reduce CO_2 emissions. Using the misleading name "Global Climate Coalition," an industrial lobbying group for fossil fuel interests has been pouring millions of dollars into an effective public relations effort to persuade Americans that global warming is a nonissue. The group also has funneled prodigious sums of money to a handful of university scientists who regularly testify before Congress and appear as "experts" on media newscasts and talk shows, questioning the validity of research results that support the global warming thesis. While there is virtually no argument today among recognized authorities in the field that climate change is real, these hired-gun "greenhouse skeptics" have misled both the public and the media into believing that there is still serious disagreement among the scientific experts—and hence no need to take action. Since most citizens (and most legislators) are not sufficiently knowledgeable about the complexities of greenhouse warming to evaluate the claims and counter-claims critically, public confusion about what, if anything, should be done is understandable.

The economic implications of policy initiatives to prevent global climate change worry more than just coal and oil interests, however. Utility executives and auto manufacturers foresee problems for their industries if CO_2 emission reductions are mandated. Labor unions, too, have expressed strong reservations to U.S. ratification of the Kyoto Protocol, anticipating major job losses among coal miners. Moreover, without conclusive proof of immediate danger, most policymakers are reluctant to advocate measures that might negatively affect current U.S. economic prosperity. The public bears a substantial share of the blame for this, since its concern about global warming has not translated into voter support for the single most effective policy approach to reducing CO_2 emissions—a hefty tax hike on gasoline and other fossil fuels. Public antipathy to *any* tax increase, however worthy the cause, would render such action political suicide—and few lawmakers exhibit suicidal tendencies.

Political ideology is also limiting the ability of the U.S. government to act decisively on climate change issues. By the late 1990s, the global warming debate had become sharply partisan, with most congressional Republicans viewing it as a Democratic issue. Because Vice President Gore was the nation's leading advocate for action on climate change—and also harbored presidential ambitions—Republicans vowed to oppose any pro-environment greenhouse policy initiatives, emphasizing economic and social costs while downplaying scientific evidence supporting action. A growing antagonism within Congress toward the United Nations and other international bodies also fueled legislators' refusal to consider ratification of Kyoto Protocol mandates. Many lawmakers are unwilling to support any efforts that are not U.S.-led and dominated. Refusal of delegates at the Kyoto meetings to require that developing countries comply with binding emissions reductions similar to those imposed on industrialized countries further alienated members of the U.S. Senate. Citing the adverse effects this unequal arrangement will have on U.S. employment, growth in certain industries, and international competitiveness, senators passed a resolution, on a 95–0 vote, asking President Clinton not to submit the Kyoto Protocol for ratification unless and until developing nations agreed to mandatory emissions limitations. For politicians concerned about the next election, strong support for policies to deter global warming lacks practical appeal. While the cost of acting now will be incurred by today's constituents who might take revenge at the polls, benefits in the sense of disaster avoided will only be evident to future generations. The inability of most elected officials to deal meaningfully with issues whose ultimate payback lies far beyond the standard election-year cycle is a major roadblock to action.

It is anticipated that within the first decade or two of the 21st century, most of the remaining scientific uncertainties about global climate change will be resolved. Scientific facts, however, almost never determine public policy: they can push an issue onto lawmakers' agenda and stimulate the debate, but they take a back seat to economic considerations, influential constituents, and political ideology and ambitions. Given the current unwillingness of Congress to deal seriously with the global warming issue, environmentalists can only hope for a succession of long hot summers (and a total collapse of air conditioning systems!) to convince voters that the time to respond is now.

References
Gelbspan, Ross. 1997. *The Heat is On: The High-Stakes Battle Over Earth's Threatened Climate*. Addison Wesley.

Skolnikoff, Eugene B. 1999. "The Role of Science in Policy." *Environment* 41, no. 5 (June):16–20, 42–45.

1990 (WRI, 1998). Achieving the 7% *reduction* called for under the Kyoto Protocol thus appears highly unlikely.

Unfortunately, even if all nations were to move immediately and wholeheartedly to fulfill treaty commitments, capping emissions at or near their present levels will not be sufficient to forestall global warming. This is because current rates of CO_2 emissions, stable or not, are so much higher than those of the pre-industrial period that natural processes of absorption or destruction—which formerly maintained a rough equilibrium—cannot keep pace and the atmospheric reservoir of CO_2 continues to increase. Merely stabilizing atmospheric CO_2 concentrations at double their pre-industrial level (*i.e.* at 560 ppm) would require a worldwide slashing of emissions by more than 60%—a drastic step no government is currently contemplating. Even then, there is no assurance that this would be a safe level; what *is* certain is that the longer we postpone sharp emission reductions, the deeper future cuts will have to be in order to achieve the same ultimate effect (WRI, 1998).

Policy Options

A number of approaches for reducing greenhouse gas emissions have been proposed and need to be pursued simultaneously if the world is to have any hope of achieving climate stability. Several of the most important initiatives are outlined in the following sections.

Improving Energy Efficiency. Contrary to the belief of most Americans that the best way to prevent global warming is to reduce pollution (Kempton, 1997), experts unanimously agree that one of the two most effective approaches to the problem is to improve the efficiency of energy use. End-of-pipe pollution control technologies, in fact, do nothing to reduce emissions of CO_2, a non-pollutant gas that is the natural by-product of burning any carbon-containing material. Improvements in energy efficiency, along with related energy conservation measures, result in less fuel combustion and hence fewer CO_2 emissions. Since fully 5% of all the carbon dioxide released worldwide each year comes from U.S. motor vehicles (TRB, 1997), simply improving gas mileage on automobiles could have an enormous impact on atmospheric carbon levels. It has been calculated that raising the fuel efficiency of the average American car to just 45 mpg would result in a 40% drop in vehicle CO_2 emissions. Similarly, mandated efficiency standards for electrical appliances, power tools, and lighting, or tax credits for manufacturers who invest in new, more efficient plants are examples of ways government could promote CO_2 reductions. While U.S. energy efficiency is higher than that of China, India, or eastern Europe, American efforts lag far behind those of western Europe. A serious national undertaking to boost energy efficiency is essential if we ever hope to attain the CO_2 emission reduction goals required under the Kyoto Protocol.

Replacing Fossil Fuels with "Soft Energy Path" Technologies. Breaking modern society's addiction to fossil fuels is the other most significant action that must be taken if efforts to forestall greenhouse warming are to be successful. Switching to solar, wind, or wave power to heat homes and generate electricity could provide an infinitely renewable source of energy with zero

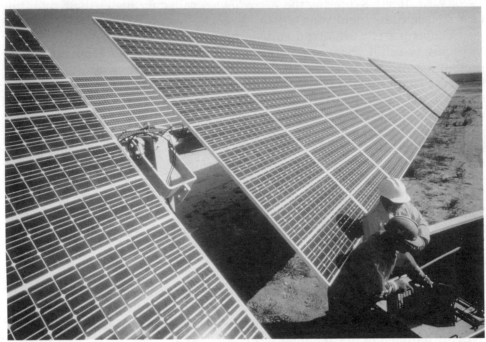

Solar energy panels are one of several alternative energy sources that produce no carbon dioxide emissions. *[Courtesy of Siemens Solar Industries]*

emissions of carbon dioxide. But greatly increased funding for research and development is urgently needed to facilitate rapid development of these promising energy alternatives. Although nuclear power generation also avoids the CO_2 emissions problem, scientists do not generally regard the rapid expansion of nuclear capacity as a viable response to thwart global warming. Aside from the fact that the nuclear power industry still confronts some serious unresolved problems, the economic obstacles to a massive program to build nuclear power plants appear insurmountable at present.

Reversing Forest Loss. Since forests act as carbon "sinks," removing CO_2 from the air during photosynthesis, the worldwide destruction of forests has had a significant contributory impact on rising levels of atmospheric CO_2. Reversing the ongoing loss of tree cover through massive reforestation efforts has been a widely discussed option, though skeptics claim that it would be necessary to replant an area larger than the continent of Australia simply to offset the CO_2 emitted over the next four to five decades, assuming that annual emission rates during those years remain at current levels. Attempting to prove the naysayers wrong, a Connecticut-based utility, Applied Energy Services, has undertaken a "carbon offset" project in Guatemala where, with the help of the Guatemalan forestry department, Peace Corps volunteers, CARE, and the U.S. Agency for International Development, the company donated $2 million for the planting of 52 million trees. Project sponsors are hopeful that the amount of carbon dioxide removed from the atmosphere by this enormous woodlot will exceed that emitted by a new fossil fuel plant the company constructed in Connecticut.

Reducing CFC Emissions and Other Greenhouse Gases. Full implementation of the terms of the Montreal Protocol should result in an eventual decline in atmospheric CFC concentrations, though the longevity of these chemicals guarantees that they will continue to exert an influence for nearly a century after emissions cease. Strategies for reducing emissions of methane and nitrous oxide, two other potent heat-trapping gases, are less well-defined. Developing rice varieties that don't require flooding could help to eliminate the methane-generating anaerobic microbes that currently make rice cultivation the single largest source of this greenhouse gas. Certain additives to livestock fodder could reduce belching of methane by modifying fermentation in the rumen of cattle. Capping manure piles to capture methane (which can then be converted to fuel in biogas plants) and repairing leaks in natural gas pipelines could further reduce emissions of methane to the atmosphere. Lowering nitrous oxide emissions would require cutting back on the use of nitrogen fertilizers. Curbing emissions of perfluorocarbons and hydrofluorocarbons depends on finding benign substitutes for these synthetic chemicals that have partially filled the gap left by now-banished CFCs. Similarly, reductions of sulfur hexafluoride emissions can be achieved by replacing SF_6 with alternative chemicals in the electrical transmission and distribution systems where they are now used.

Taxing the Use of Fossil Fuels. In his best-selling book, *Earth in the Balance,* then-Senator Al Gore advocated imposition of a so-called "carbon tax," in which production of gasoline, heating oil, coal, natural gas, and electricity generated from fossil fuels would be taxed incrementally according to their carbon content. Such a tax scheme recognizes that not all fossil fuels pollute equally: coal burning emits twice as much CO_2 as does natural gas, 1.5 times more than oil. A differential tax would provide financial motivation for energy purchasers to choose less-polluting fuels and would incorporate the environmental costs of energy use into energy prices. Alternatively, increasing the tax on gasoline alone would have a positive impact in reducing carbon emissions from motor vehicles. The exceptionally low gasoline prices enjoyed by American motorists take away any incentive to drive less or to purchase fuel-efficient automobiles. In Germany, where taxes in 1995 comprised 78% of the cost of gasoline, energy consumption dropped by 1.5% a year during the early 1990s, while the economy grew by 1.1% (WRI, 1998). Nevertheless, although taxing fossil fuels would undoubtedly curtail their use, doing so is politically unpopular and policymakers tend to shun this approach.

Obstacles to Success

Action to implement these long-term strategies must begin immediately on a global scale if the changes already underway are to be minimized. The obstacles to success are great, since the basic problem stems from the energy use decisions of billions of individuals in every nation of the world. Some observers conclude that it is already too late; the degree of worldwide cooperation and coordination necessary to achieve any meaningful reduction in CO_2 releases would, in their view, be impossible to attain in a world "hooked" on fossil fuels. Instead of a crash fuel-switching effort, such voices call for accelerating research on CO_2 and its effects and for a policy to improve society's ability to adapt to changing circumstances, preparing the economy for the consequences of global warming. Perhaps the best summation of the differing assessments of what society's response to greenhouse warming ought to be is that given more than a decade ago by Harvard planetary scientist Michael McElroy:

> If we choose to take on this challenge, it appears we can slow the rate of change substantially, giving us time to develop mechanisms so that the cost to society and the damage to ecosystems can be minimized. We could alternatively close our eyes, hope for the best, and pay the cost when the bill comes due (Lyman et al., 1990; Revkin, 1992; EPA, 1992).

References

Broecker, Wallace S. 1970. "Man's Oxygen Reserves." *Science* 168 (June 26).

Brown, Lester R., Michael Renner, and Christopher Flavin. 1998. *Vital Signs 1998*. Worldwatch Institute, W.W. Norton.

Budyko, M. I. 1986. *The Evolution of the Biosphere*. D. Reidel Publishing.

Environmental Protection Agency. 1992. *Climate Change Discussion Series: Agriculture*. Office of Policy Planning and Evaluation, May.

————. 1990. *Policy Options for Stabilizing Global Climate: Report to Congress*. Washington, D.C.

Gribbin, John. 1982. "Carbon Dioxide, Ammonia—and Life." *New Scientist* 94(May 13):413–16.

Houghton, J.T., L.G. Meira Filho, B.A. Callander, N. Harris, A. Kattenberg, and K. Maskell, eds. 1996. *Climate Change 1995: The Science of Climate Change*. Cambridge University Press.

Houghton, J.T., G.J. Jenkins, and J.J. Ephraums, eds. 1990. *Climate Change: The IPCC Scientific Assessment*. Cambridge University Press.

Indermühle, A., T.F. Stocker, F. Joos, H. Fischer, H.J. Smith, M. Wahlen, B. Deck, D. Mastroianni, J. Tschumi, T. Blunier, R. Meyer, and B. Stouffer. 1999. "Holocene Carboncycle Dynamics Based on CO_2 Trapped in Ice at Taylor Dome, Antarctica." *Nature* 398 (March 11):121–126.

Intergovernmental Panel on Climate Change (IPCC). 1994. *Radiative Forcing of Climate Change: The 1994 Report of the Scientific Assessment Working Group of IPCC*. World Meteorological Organization/United Nations Environment Programme.

Kempton, Willett. 1997. "How the Public Views Climate Change." *Environment* 39, no. 9 (Nov):12–21.

Kerr, J. B., and C. T. McElroy. 1993. "Evidence for Large Upward Trends of Ultraviolet-B Radiation Linked to Ozone Depletion." *Science* 262 (Nov).

Kerr, Richard A. 1998. "Deep Chill Triggers Record Ozone Hole." *Science* 282 (Oct. 16):391.

Maugh, Thomas H. 1982. "New Link Between Ozone and Cancer." *Science* 216 (April 23).

Mintzer, Irving M. 1987. "A Matter of Degrees: The Potential for Controlling the Greenhouse Effect." World Resources Institute, Research Report 5, April.

O'Meara, Molly. 1997. "The Risks of Disrupting Climate." *World Watch* 10, no. 6 (Nov/Dec):10–24.

"Ozone Takes a Nose Dive After the Eruption of Mt. Pinatubo." *Science* 260 (April 23, 1993).

Panofsky, Hans A. 1978. "Earth's Endangered Ozone." *Environment* 20, no. 3 (April).

Petit, J.R, J. Jouzel, D. Raynaud, N.I. Barkov, J.M. Barnola, I. Basile, M. Bender, J. Chappellaz, M. Davis, G. Delaygue, M. Delmotte, V.M. Kotlyakov, M. Legrand, V.Y. Lipenkov, C. Lorius, L. Pépin, C. Ritz, E. Saltzman, and M. Stievenard. 1999. "Climate and Atmospheric History of the past 420,000 Years from the Vostok Ice Core, Antarctica." *Nature* 399 (June 3):429–436.

Revkin, Andrew. 1992. *Global Warming: Understanding the Forecast*. Abbeville Press.

Severinghaus, J.P., T. Sowers, E.J. Brooke, R.B. Alley, and M.L. Bender. 1998. "Timing of Abrupt Climate Change at the End of the Younger Dryas Interval from Thermally Fractionated Gases in Polar Ice." *Nature* 391 (Jan. 8):141–146.

Stern, Paul C., Oran R. Young, and Daniel Druckman, eds. 1992. *Global Environmental Change: Understanding the Human Dimensions*. National Academy Press.

Strahler, Arthur N., and Alan H. Strahler. 1973. *Environmental Geoscience*. Hamilton Publishing Company.

Transportation Research Board (TRB) and National Research Council (NRC). 1997. *Toward a Sustainable Future: Addressing the Long-Term Effects of Motor Vehicle Transportation on Climate and Ecology*. National Academy Press.

Watson, R. T., H. Rohde, H. Oeschger, and U. Siegenthaler. 1990. "Greenhouse Gases and Aerosols." In *Climate Change: The IPCC Scientific Assessment*, edited by J. T. Houghton, G. J. Jenkins, and J. J. Ephraums. Cambridge University Press.

World Resources Institute (WRI). 1998. *World Resources 1998–99: Environmental Change and Human Health*. Oxford University Press.

———. 1992. *World Resources 1992–93*. Oxford University Press.

———. 1990. *World Resources 1990–91*. Oxford University Press.

CHAPTER 12

Air Pollution

...why, it appears no other thing to me
but a foul and pestilent congregation of vapors.
—William Shakespeare (*Hamlet*)

Humans have undoubtedly been coping with a certain amount of polluted air ever since primitive *Homo sapiens* sat crouched by the warmth of a smoky fire in their Paleolithic caves. An inevitable consequence of fuel combustion, air pollution mounted as a source of human discomfort as soon as people began to live in towns and cities. More recently it has become an extremely serious problem on a worldwide basis for two primary reasons: 1) there has been an enormous increase in world population, particularly in urban areas, and 2) since the early 1800s the rapid growth of energy-intensive industries and rising levels of affluence in the developed countries have led to record levels of fossil fuel combustion.

Prior to the 20th century problems related to air pollution were primarily associated, in the public mind at least, with the city of London. As early as the 13th century small amounts of coal from Newcastle were being shipped into London for fuel. As the population and manufacturing enterprises grew, wood supplies diminished and coal burning increased, in spite of the protestations of a long series of both monarchs and private citizens who objected to the odor of coal smoke. One petitioner to King Charles II in 1661 complained that due to the greed of manufacturers, inhabitants of London were forced to "breathe nothing but an impure and thick Mist, accompanied by a fuliginous (sooty) and filthy vapour, which renders them obnoxious to a thousand inconveniences, the Lungs, and disordering the entire habit of their Bodies. . . ." (Evelyn, 1661).

In spite of such railings, English coal consumption increased even faster than the rate of population growth and by the 19th century London's thick, "pea-soup" fogs had become a notorious trademark of the city. Numerous well-meaning attempts at smoke abatement were largely ignored during the hey-

447

day of laissez-faire capitalism, epitomized by the industrialists' slogan, "Where there's muck, there's money."

The same conditions that had made London the air pollution capital of the world began to prevail in the United States as well during the 19th and early 20th centuries. St. Louis, plagued by smoky conditions, passed an ordinance as early as 1867 mandating that smokestacks be at least 20 feet higher than adjacent buildings. The Chicago City Council in 1881 passed the nation's first smoke abatement ordinance. Pittsburgh, once one of the smokiest cities in the United States, was the site of pioneer work at the Mellon Institute on the harmful impact of smoke both on property and human health. In spite of gradually increasing public awareness of the problem, levels of air pollution and the geographical extent of the areas affected continued to increase. Although by the late 1950s and 1960s large-scale fuel-switching from coal to natural gas and oil had significantly reduced smoky conditions in many American cities, other newer pollutants—products of the now-ubiquitous automobile—had assumed worrisome levels. Today foul air has become a problem of global proportions; no longer does one have to travel to London or Pittsburgh or Los Angeles to experience the respiratory irritation or the aesthetic distress which a hazy, contaminated atmosphere can provoke. As the 21st century dawns, from Beijing to Bangkok, New Delhi, Athens, Moscow, Mexico City— virtually every metropolitan area in the world is grappling with the problem of how to halt further deterioration of air quality without impeding industrial productivity and industrial development.

Sources of Air Pollution

Where is all this dirty air coming from? Not surprisingly, the sources of air pollution are quite diverse and vary in importance from one region to another. Some air contaminants are of natural origin; volcanic eruptions, forest fires, and dust storms periodically contribute large quantities of pollutant gases and particles to the atmosphere. In June 1991, immense quantities of volcanic ash and an estimated 18 million metric tons of sulfur dioxide (roughly equivalent to U.S. emissions of this pollutant gas during an entire year) were spewed into the atmosphere during a single massive eruption of Mt. Pinatubo in the Philippines. For several months during the fall of 1997, fires deliberately set by farmers and loggers to clear land on the Indonesian island of Sumatra burned out of control, creating a pall of pollution over much of Southeast Asia. Covering an area inhabited by 200 million people, the smoke provoked acute respiratory problems throughout the region, caused transportation accidents that killed hundreds, devastated the tourist trade, and severely damaged the economies of the nations affected. British experts estimate that the burning forests released more greenhouse gases than were emitted in an entire year by all the cars in Europe. Less dramatic but worthy of note, considerable amounts of methane gas are released into the air when organic matter decays in the absence of oxygen, and some plant species produce volatile hydrocarbons that are thought to be responsible for the blue haze observed in the Smoky Mountains and other forest regions. However, most of the pollutants befouling our air today come from emission sources that have proliferated with the development of industries and transportation networks.

At present in the industrialized world the largest sources of air pollution, in order of importance, are 1) transportation, primarily automobiles and trucks; 2) electric power plants that burn coal or oil; and 3) industry, the major offenders being steel mills, metal smelters, oil refineries, and pulp and paper mills. Of less importance now than in past decades is the contribution made from heating homes and buildings and burning refuse. The general trend toward heating with oil, gas, or electricity instead of with coal greatly reduced pollution from space heating. At the same time, increasingly common municipal bans on home refuse burning, along with the utilization of sanitary landfills or incinerators equipped with pollution control devices for community solid waste disposal, have accounted for a marked decline in emissions from trash combustion. Within any one region or community, of course, the relative importance of various emission sources may differ from the overall national rankings noted here. In most metropolitan areas, automobiles contribute by far the largest amount of air pollutants, in small towns, by contrast, significant levels of contamination may be caused by just one polluting factory.

Criteria Air Pollutants

Air pollution, of course, is no single entity; thousands of gaseous, liquid, and solid compounds contribute to the atmospheric mess. The nature of some of these substances is well known while others are only now being studied and their threat to human health assessed. The most common and widespread air pollutants include six that the federal government has designated **criteria pollutants,** requiring the Environmental Protection Agency to gather scientific and medical information on their environmental and human health effects. These are the pollutants for which **National Ambient Air Quality Standards (NAAQS**—familiarly referred to as "nax") have been set, specifying the maximum levels of concentration of these pollutants allowable in the outdoor air. The six criteria air pollutants are discussed in the following sections (it should be noted that most industrialized countries, and some developing nations as well, now have regulations controlling these same air contaminants).

Particulate Matter (PM$_{10}$ and PM$_{2.5}$). All airborne pollutants that occur in either liquid or solid form, including pollen, dust, soot, smoke, acid condensates, and sulfate and nitrate particles are referred to as particulate matter. Particulates range in size from pieces of fly ash as large as a thumbnail to tiny aerosols less than 1 micrometer in diameter—so small that they remain suspended in the air and are transported on wind currents as easily as are gases. To many people, particulate matter and "air pollution" are synonymous, since easily visible dark plumes of smoke and soot or clouds of dust are the only forms of air pollution of which they are aware. Marked reductions in particulate levels in a number of urban areas in recent years have led many citizens to conclude erroneously that air quality is no longer a problem, since most other air pollutants are invisible.

Particulate matter is generated by a wide variety of activities—fuel combustion, road traffic, agricultural activities, certain industrial processes, and natural abrasion. The most visible damage caused by particulate matter is the layer of grime deposited on buildings, streets, clothing, and so on. Prior to pollution-control efforts launched during the 1970s, it was estimated that in the most polluted areas of big cities as much as 50–100 tons of particulate matter per square mile fell each month (Air Pollution Primer, 1969). Particulate matter can obscure visibility and corrode metals; more important is the fact that when inhaled, particulates irritate the respiratory tract. Most dangerous in this regard are the tiny aerosols that, because of their very small size, can evade the body's natural defense mechanisms and penetrate deeply into the lungs (in most cities, these very small particles comprise 50–60% of suspended particulates). In recognition of this fact, the EPA in 1987 replaced the original standard for total particulates with a revised standard that applies to those particles with a diameter of 10 micrometers or less (PM_{10}) that are small enough to penetrate to the highly sensitive alveolar region of the lungs. In 1997, EPA again revised the standards for particulate matter, adding new requirements for particles smaller than 2.5 micrometers in diameter. This action was taken in response to recent studies indicating that the characteristics, sources, and health effects of these smaller particles are substantially different from those in the PM_{10} category.

Sulfur Dioxide (SO_2). The major source of this colorless pollutant gas is fuel combustion, inasmuch as sulfur is present to a greater or lesser degree as an impurity in coal and fuel oil. When these sulfur-containing fuels are burned, the sulfur is oxidized to form SO_2. By itself sulfur dioxide is not particularly harmful, but it readily reacts with water vapor in the atmosphere to form other sulfur compounds such as sulfuric acid, sulfates, and sulfites which irritate the respiratory system, corrode metals and statuary, harm textiles, impair visibility, and kill or stunt the growth of plants. Sulfur dioxide is also one of the main precursors of acid precipitation, recognized now as an environmental threat of major proportions and a subject which will be dealt with in greater detail later in this chapter.

Carbon Monoxide (CO). No other pollutant gas is found at such high concentrations in the urban atmosphere as is the extremely toxic, odorless, and colorless carbon monoxide. Any type of incomplete combustion produces CO, but the most significant source in terms of urban air pollution is automobile emissions; according to EPA, in the mid-1990s motor vehicles accounted for fully 81% of all CO emissions to the ambient air (in indoor situations, cigarette smoking is a major source of carbon monoxide). When inhaled, CO binds to hemoglobin in the blood, displacing oxygen and thereby reducing the amount of oxygen carried in the bloodstream to the various body tissues. For this reason, carbon monoxide is the air pollutant that provokes the most severe reactions among heart patients. Studies have shown that more deaths among heart attack victims occur during periods of high CO concentrations than at other times. Patients suffering from angina pectoris, a coronary disease in which there is an insufficient supply of oxygen to the heart during exercise, experience a much more rapid onset of pain during periods of increased carbon monoxide pollution. Depending on the concentration of CO in the air and the length of exposure, inhalation of carbon monoxide can result in adverse health effects ranging from mild headaches or dizziness at rela-

Table 12-1   Criteria Pollutants

Pollutant	Form	Major Source	Effects
PM_{10}, $PM_{2.5}$ (or simply Particulate Matter)	solid or liquid	Combustion, industrial processes, vehicle exhaust	1. grime deposits 2. obscures visibility 3. corrodes metals 4. respiratory disease
SULFUR DIOXIDE (SO_2)	gas	Coal-burning power plants, metal smelters, industrial boilers, oil refineries	1. respiratory irritant 2. corrodes metal & stone 3. damages textiles 4. toxic to plants 5. precursor of acid rain
CARBON MONOXIDE (CO)	gas	Motor vehicles	1. aggravates cardiovascular disease 2. impairs perception and mental processes 3. fatal at high concentrations
NITROGEN DIOXIDE (NO_2)	gas	Motor vehicles, power plants	1. respiratory irritant 2. toxic to plants 3. reduces visibility 4. precursor of ozone 5. precursor of acid rain
OZONE (O_3)	gas	Motor vehicles, (indirectly)	1. respiratory irritant 2. toxic to plants 3. corrodes rubber, paint
LEAD (Pb)	metal aerosol	Motor vehicles	1. damage to nervous system, blood, kidneys

tively low levels of exposure to death at high levels. Fortunately, the health effects of short-term carbon monoxide exposure are reversible, but people who work for many hours in areas of heavy traffic (e.g. police officers, toll collectors, parking garage attendants) are obviously receiving substantial doses. Some evidence indicates that blood absorption of CO slows down mental processes and reaction time, raising the suspicion that many rush-hour traffic accidents can be at least partially attributed to low-level carbon monoxide poisoning.

Nitrogen Oxides (NO_x). Consisting primarily of nitric oxide (NO) and nitrogen dioxide (NO_2), oxides of nitrogen are formed when combustion occurs at very high temperatures. Nitrogen oxides enter the atmosphere in approximately equal amounts from auto emissions and power plants (in urban areas, cars are generally the predominant source of NO_x emissions). Nitrogen dioxide is the only criteria pollutant gas that is colored. The yellow brown "smoggy" appearance typical of southern California on bad days is due to the high concentrations of NO_2 in the air. At high levels of pollution, nitrogen dioxide has a pungent, sweetish odor. At commonly encountered ambient levels, NO_2 causes lung irritation and can increase susceptibility to acute respiratory ailments such as pneumonia and influenza. Nitrogen dioxide stunts plant growth and visibly damages leaves. It reduces visibility and, like sulfur dioxide, contributes to the formation of acid rain.

Ozone (O_3). The main constituent of a group of chemical compounds known as **photochemical oxidants,** ozone and such fellow travelers as peroxyacetylnitrate (PAN) and various aldehydes are considered to be auto-associated pollutants even though they are not emitted directly from the tailpipe into the atmosphere. Instead, these substances form in a complex series of chemical reactions when nitrogen dioxide and **volatile organic compounds (VOCs),** especially certain hydrocarbons from both auto exhausts and a variety of stationary sources, react with oxygen and sunlight to produce a witch's brew of chemicals dubbed **photochemical smog.** First observed in the Los Angeles area in the 1940s (the bright sunlight, warm temperatures, frequent atmospheric inversions, and heavy traffic make southern California particularly well-suited for photochemical smog formation), photochemical smog is now often observed in other cities as well, especially on bright summer days ("ozone season" is considered to extend from May 1 through September 30). Ozone, an early and continuing product of the photochemical smog reaction, is the chemical whose presence is used to measure the oxidant level of the atmosphere at any given time. This pungent, colorless gas irritates the mucous membranes of the respiratory system, causing coughing, choking, and reduced lung capacity. Heart patients, asthmatics, and those suffering from bronchitis or emphysema are at special risk during periods of high O_3 levels. Ozone also cracks rubber, deteriorates fabrics, and causes paint to fade. The eye irritation and watery eyes frequently experienced during smog episodes is caused both by ozone and by PAN. Photochemical smog has caused extensive plant damage, killing or injuring plants directly or increasing their vulnerability to attack by insects. A classic example of photochemical oxidant damage to plants can be seen in the ailing ponderosa pine forests of the San Bernardino Mountains, about 70 miles downwind from Los Angeles. The profound impact of photochemical oxidants on agricultural yields was highlighted in a report issued by the World Resources Institute which documented crop damage due to air pollution, primarily ozone, as costing U.S. farmers up to $5 billion a year. Crops most seriously affected included soybeans, cotton, winter wheat, kidney beans, and peanuts.

Lead (Pb). The adverse impact of this toxic metal on the intellectual development of children (see chapter 7) caused it to be added to the list of criteria pollutants when the Clean Air Act was reauthorized in 1977. Since most airborne lead can be traced to automobile emissions, the major control strategy for this pollutant was to phase out the use of leaded gasoline, a process completed in the United States by the end of 1995. Thirteen other countries, including Canada, Japan, Sweden, and several South American nations, have

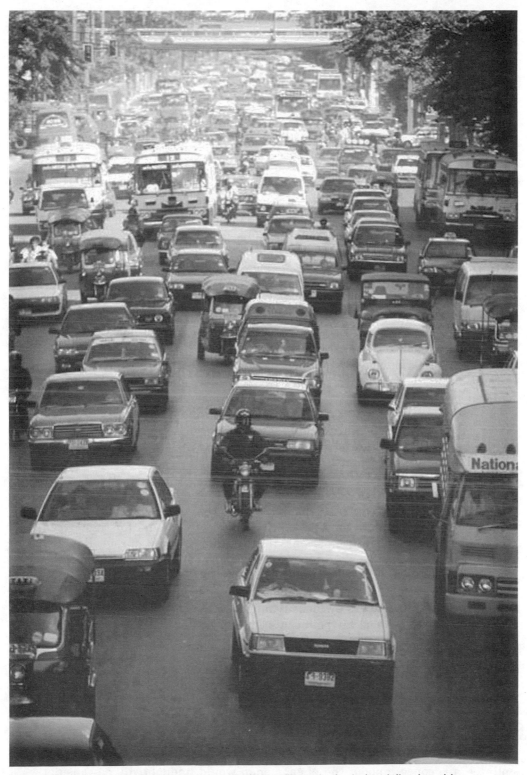

Motor vehicles constitute the largest source of air pollution in the industrialized world.

now joined the U.S. in completely ending the use of leaded gasoline (China has declared its intention to follow suit by mid-2000), but in approximately 100 nations people are still exposed to airborne lead from this source.

Hazardous Air Pollutants (HAPs)

In addition to the criteria air pollutants, a large number of less common, but much more hazardous, chemicals are released into the atmosphere from a wide range of industries and manufacturing processes, as well as from motor vehicles. Although the sources of these emissions are more localized than are those of the criteria pollutants, the fact that many of them are either toxic or carcinogenic suggests that they deserve special attention. In 1970 Congress directed the EPA to develop a list of industrial air pollutants that can cause serious health damage even at relatively low concentrations and to establish protective emission standards for those so listed. No deadline date for listing substances as hazardous was mandated, however, and implementation of the congressional directive was exceedingly slow.

By 1990, twenty years after the original congressional mandate, only eight toxic air pollutants had been listed—**asbestos, mercury, beryllium, benzene, vinyl chloride, arsenic, radionuclides, and coke oven emissions**—and standards had been set only for the first seven (a standard for coke oven emissions was finally promulgated in 1993). Frustrated with this snail's pace, environmentalists for years had prodded EPA to speed up the evaluation process, urging the agency to list and set standards for additional toxic air pollutants which pose a special hazard to public health. In 1986, congressional passage of the Emergency Planning and Community Right-to-Know Act (Superfund Amendments and Reauthorization Act, commonly referred to as SARA Title III), prompted by a tragic chemical accident in Bhopal, India two years earlier, led to heightened public awareness of the toxic threats lurking in hundreds of communities across the nation. By requiring that manufacturers disclose information on the kinds and amounts of toxic pollutants they discharge into the local environment each year, this law prompted demands from community activists and the media for tighter controls on health-threatening emissions. In turn, the necessity of revealing data that might alarm previously complacent local residents prompted voluntary emissions reductions by a number of firms eager to maintain a positive corporate image. In 1990 Congress responded to the mounting pressure to "do something" about air toxics by identifying 189 chemicals that it ordered EPA to regulate as hazardous air pollutants and by establishing comprehensive, technology-based controls for dealing with this largely ignored public health threat (one of these air toxics, caprolactam, was removed from the list in 1996, leaving 188 regulated HAPs). The new regulatory approach to controlling air toxics will be discussed in greater detail later in this chapter.

Impact of Air Pollution on Human Health

If dirty skyscrapers or sick ponderosa pines were the only consequence of polluted air, concern about the phenomenon would undoubtedly be considerably less than it is today. The unfortunate fact is, however, that over the years there has been a steadily growing mass of evidence indicating that the quality of the air we breathe has a measurable impact on human health.

Some of the ill effects of air pollution have, of course, been known for a long time: Los Angelenos knowingly curse the smog as they wipe tears from their burning eyes; motorists hopefully roll up their car windows in heavy traffic, trying to avert a carbon monoxide-induced headache; and asthmatics resignedly brace for an attack when the weather forecaster proclaims an ozone alert. For many years discomforts such as these were shrugged off as necessary consequences of economic growth. Only after several air pollution "disasters" made world headlines did the general public begin to realize the extent of the threat posed by dirty air. The great London smog of 1952 (see Box 12-1) involved the largest number of casualties, but it wasn't the first such episode. Eighteen years earlier a very similar scenario unfolded in the heavily industrialized Meuse River Valley of Belgium. During a three-day inversion, 60 people died of the foul air, while thousands of others became seriously ill, coughing and gasping for breath. In the fall of 1948, the small (pop. 14,000) Pennsylvania town of Donora, near Pittsburgh, fell victim to a five-day inversion. Situated in a heavily industrialized valley, Donora was enveloped in a cold, damp blanket of smoggy air, permeated with the smell of sulfur. During this time, fully 42% of the town's population suffered eye, nose, and throat irritation; chest pains; coughing; difficulty in breathing; headaches; nausea; and vomiting. When the inversion finally lifted, it was found that 20 people had died during the period (Waldbott, 1978).

The dramatic examples of pollution-induced death and disease described above were all associated with levels of air contamination considerably worse than those experienced by most urban residents today, even those living in visibly smoggy cities. For many years researchers have been trying to determine whether air pollution at levels typically encountered in metropolitan areas can, by itself, increase mortality and morbidity rates and, if so, which specific pollutants pose the greatest hazard. Results obtained from a number of studies now confirm fears long suspected—air pollution kills, and at levels of pollutant concentration well within the legally allowable limits established by the NAAQS.

The Air Pollution-Health Connection

Investigations aimed at determining precise cause-and-effect relationships linking given levels of pollution with specific health responses have encountered numerous difficulties. One such problem relates to scientific ethics: it simply isn't acceptable to expose the most vulnerable members of society—children, the elderly, asthmatics, etc.—to high levels of air pollution and then watch to see what happens to them. In addition, because urban air contains so many different pollutants, determining with certainty *which* pollutant at *what level* is causing an observed health effect has been problematic. The likelihood that synergistic effects play a role in determining the response to polluted air is a further complicating factor, as is the possibility of contributory occupational exposure. Particularly troublesome to researchers has been the overwhelming influence of cigarette smoking—i.e. how much is due to the pollutants in city air and how much is due to self-inflicted tobacco pollutants?

BOX 12-1

Atmospheric Inversions

Shortly before Christmas of 1952, the city of London experienced a killer smog that even in that notoriously polluted metropolis was exceptionally severe. For a period of five days the cold, moist air hung over the city like a heavy wet blanket, with scarcely a trace of breeze to carry away the thickening cloud of smoke and fumes from millions of coal-burning fireplaces, factories, and motor vehicles. Even in the middle of the day, the pervading gloom was so thick that car-train collisions were common and a steam ferry ran into an anchored ship along the Thames River. When the fog finally lifted, health officials revealed the grim human toll of this episode—nearly 3,000 excess deaths, most of them due to respiratory or heart disease, had occurred during the week of foul air. The London situation was not solely a result of pollutants being dumped into an overburdened atmosphere. The volume of emissions during the time period in question was not substantially different than at many other times during the year. The chief villain in this situation, and in virtually every other air pollution "disaster" on record, was an atmospheric anomaly known as an **inversion**.

Under normal conditions air is in a constant state of flux. As the air near the earth's surface is warmed it expands and rises, carrying with it pollutant particles and gases. Cooler, cleaner air moves in to replace it, setting up convection currents. These forces, combined with the earth's rotation, generate winds that further aid in dispersing pollutants.

The vertical extent to which warm air rises until it cools to the same temperature as the air above is referred to as the **mixing depth**—an expanse that corresponds with the upper boundary for pollution dispersal. The amount of mixing depth varies depending on the time of day and the season of the year, being greater during daytime and in summer than it is at night and during winter.

A reversal of this normal pattern can occur when the air closest to the surface of the ground is cooler than the layer above it. In such a situation the cool air, being heavier than warm air, is unable to rise and mix and remains atypically stable. This state of affairs is known as an **atmospheric inversion**—a condition where a layer of cool surface air is trapped by an overlying layer of warmer air. In such a case, the mixing depth will be minimal and pollutant emissions, if any, within the affected area can accumulate to levels that may threaten human health.

The two most important types of inversions are:

1. **Radiation inversion.** This normal nocturnal situation often occurs on clear nights when absorbed daytime heat is radiated quickly out into space and the temperature of surface air drops below that of the air above it. Generally a radiation inversion presents little health threat because it breaks up as soon as the morning sun warms the earth, reestablishing normal convection currents. In most cases a radiation inversion simply doesn't persist long enough to permit build-up of dangerously high concentrations of pollutants.

2. **Subsidence inversion.** More troublesome than radiation inversions are subsidence inversions, caused when a layer of air within a high-pressure mass settles down over a region, being compressed and thereby heated by the high pressure area above. At ground level the air temperature remains unchanged and

hence is relatively cooler than the air layer directly above. Subsidence inversions are particularly worrisome because they may remain in place for days, the surface air becoming increasingly foul as time passes. While inversions can occur at any time (southern California experiences inversions as often as 340 days of the year), they are more frequent and last longer during the fall and winter months. They are particularly common in valleys, since at night cool air flows down the hillsides and is trapped at the bottom. Not until the sun is directly overhead will the

surface air be sufficiently warmed to break up the inversion layer, and in winter such an inversion may persist all day.

It should be pointed out that an atmospheric inversion per se is a perfectly natural occurrence and presents no threat to human health if there are few sources of pollutants within the affected region. Inversions become major problems only when they occur in industrialized or densely settled areas where noxious pollutants can steadily accumulate to dangerous concentrations.

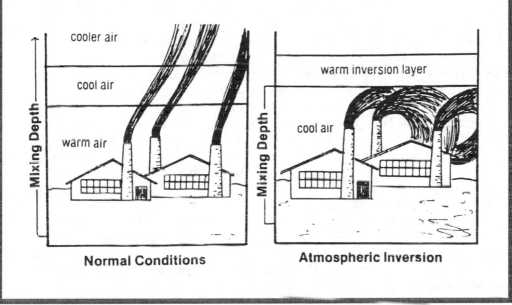

Normal Conditions   **Atmospheric Inversion**

In spite of these challenges, a substantial body of evidence documenting the health effects of air pollutants has been compiled by researchers in many parts of the world. Epidemiological data collected in the United States since the 1970s supports environmentalists' contention that air pollution can be deadly. An estimated 2–3% of all deaths in the U.S. each year are attributed to air pollution-induced respiratory or cardiovascular disease. Similar levels of mortality due to dirty air have been reported in Poland and the Czech Republic (WRI, 1996). In urban areas of the developing world, where levels of ambient air pollution are much higher than those encountered in cities of the industrialized nations, the World Bank estimates that 2–5% of all deaths are due to particulate pollution alone. This well-documented toll of death and disease provides ample justification for government regulation of air pollution in order to protect human health.

Major Health Effects

Not surprisingly, air pollution's major impact on health is the result of irritants acting on the respiratory tract. Not all air pollutants are equally harmful, however. Research indicates that the most serious health effects associated with polluted air can be attributed to elevated levels of very fine particulates—those with an aerodynamic diameter of 2.5 micrometers or less—and to sulfate particles. These pollutants have been more directly associated with heightened risk of death and disease than have any other contaminants in the ambient air; the fatalities that occurred during the air pollution disasters previously described have all been attributed to this group of pollutants. These tiny aerosols, generated primarily by the combustion of fossil fuels, present a particularly serious threat to human health because they tend to be more toxic than larger particles and can be inhaled deeply into the lungs where they lodge in sensitive pulmonary tissue and constitute a chronic source of irritation. Epidemiologic studies conducted from 1975–1988 in six U.S. cities have convincingly demonstrated the link between high levels of particulate air pollution and death due to lung cancer, respiratory disease, and heart ailments—even after controlling for individual risk factors such as smoking, occupational exposure, excessive weight gain, and so on. The correlation was most dramatically evident in Steubenville, Ohio, the most polluted city in the survey group, where adjusted mortality rates were 26% higher than in Portage, Wisconsin, the least polluted of the six communities studied. Interestingly, the link between pollution levels and increased risk of premature death was statistically significant only in relation to concentrations of fine, inhalable particles; varying levels of total suspended particulates, NO_x, SO_2, or ozone appeared to have no measurable impact on death rates—an indication that fine particulates constitute the most dangerous form of air pollution in terms of human health impact (Dockery, 1993).

When polluted air is inhaled, both the structure and the functioning of the respiratory tract can be altered. Although much remains to be learned about the precise physiologic mechanisms by which exposure to air pollution can kill, some of the ways in which air pollutants can induce illness include the following.

Inhibit or Inactivate Natural Body Defenses. The human respiratory system is well constructed to restrict entry of foreign particles and to rid the body of such intruders if they succeed in penetrating the first lines of defense. As a result, the approximately 10,000–20,000 liters of germ- and particle-laden air inhaled by a person each day are effectively cleansed by the time they reach the lungs. Particles are removed both by deposition and by clearance, the precise site at which this occurs depending on particle size. Large particles may be trapped by nasal hairs or are deposited on the walls of the nose or throat, while smaller particulates generally escape these defenses and travel deeper into the respiratory tract where the slower air movement causes all but the smallest to settle out on the surface of the trachea or bronchi (the conducting airways). Upon settling, the invading particles are trapped by mucus produced by cells lining the airways. They are then swept upward by the constant beating movement of millions of tiny **cilia,** hair-like projections of epithelial

Figure 12-1 Human Respiratory System

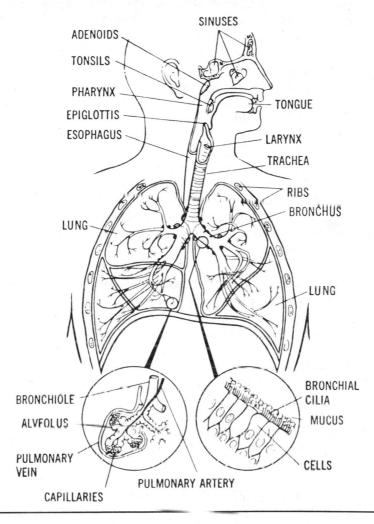

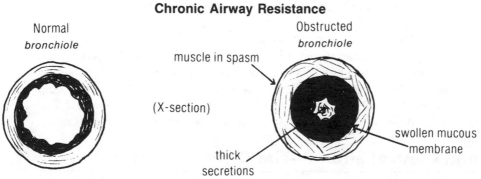

Chronic Airway Resistance

Normal
bronchiole

Obstructed
bronchiole

muscle in spasm

(X-section)

thick
secretions

swollen mucous
membrane

Source: American Lung Association.

cells lining the respiratory tract. This mucociliary action transports dirt and pathogens to the upper respiratory passages from whence they are expelled by nose-blowing, coughing, sneezing, or swallowing. The tiniest aerosol particulates that evade removal in this manner and are deposited on the lining of the **alveoli** (terminal air sacs) may be attacked and devoured by specialized scavenger cells called **macrophages,** thus removing them from the lungs. Although not always successful, these defense mechanisms are extremely important in shielding the respiratory system from assault. Research has shown that exposure to certain air pollutants can induce health problems due to the effect of these contaminants on the body's natural defenses. When pollutant gases, especially ozone, NO_2, or SO_2 are inhaled, the action of the cilia lining the airways may be slowed down or halted altogether. At high pollutant concentrations, patches of ciliated cells may be killed and slough off; function of the macrophage cells in the alveoli also may be inhibited. Any of these effects greatly reduces the body's ability to withstand invasion from pathogenic organisms such as bacteria or viruses. Thus a common health consequence of breathing polluted air is increased susceptibility to infectious airborne diseases such as pneumonia or acute bronchitis.

Cause Constriction of the Airways ("chronic airway resistance"). Exposure to gases such as O_3 or SO_2 may result in a swelling of the membrane lining the airways, thereby reducing the diameter of the opening and resulting in more labored breathing.

Induce Fibrosis and Thickening of Alveolar Walls. Ozone is particularly effective in altering the wall structure of the delicate terminal air sacs. When ozone comes into contact with sensitive alveolar cells, tiny lesions are formed. The breaks subsequently heal, but in the process scar tissue is formed. Lung tissue becomes thicker and stiffer, making it more difficult for air to penetrate and thereby reducing functional lung capacity ("Health Effects," 1978).

Fortunately, in most of the industrial democracies, the public has recognized the serious health hazards posed by air pollution and has demanded air quality controls that have significantly reduced levels of contamination. Although air quality continues to worsen in many developing nations, today in most parts of the United States, Japan, and western Europe it is very unlikely that another air pollution disaster such as that of Donora in 1948 or London in 1952 could occur again. For this we can thank the persistent efforts of a dedicated coalition of citizens and scientists who wouldn't allow the public to ignore the air pollution-health connection and the legislators, both state and federal, who had the political courage to impose mandatory controls on polluters.

Pollution Control Efforts—The Clean Air Act

As air quality in the United States steadily deteriorated during the 1950s and 1960s, it became increasingly evident that a broad-based, concerted effort was needed to deal with what was increasingly perceived as a problem

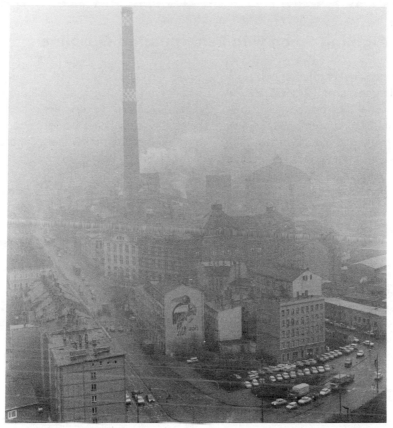

Heavy smog settles on downtown Leipzig, Germany. Decades of author-
itarian government and central planning have resulted in severe pollution
problems throughout the former Soviet Union and the former communist
states of eastern and central Europe. *[Reuters/Bettman]*

of national scope. Until 1955 any attempts to regulate pollutant emissions
were based solely at the local or state level; in that year the first federal law
dealing exclusively with air pollution offered research and technical support
to states and municipalities, thereby initiating a policy of federal-state-local
partnership in the pollution control effort. By 1963, worsening levels of air
pollution generated pressure for more effective action and led to passage of the
first Clean Air Act, which gave the federal government a modest degree of
authority to attack interstate air pollution problems and which further
increased the flow of federal dollars to state and local pollution control agencies. By 1965 recognition of the automobile's contribution to air quality problems precipitated the first emission standards for automobiles (these
standards, set for carbon monoxide and hydrocarbon emissions, took effect
with 1968 model year cars). In 1967 the comprehensive Air Quality Act established a regional approach for establishing and enforcing air quality standards, though the main responsibility for control of emission sources (except
for automobiles) remained at the state and local levels of government. This

BOX 12-2
Fighting Smog with Reformulated Gasoline

All gasoline is not created equal. Hundreds of different formulations are used to make the fuel that powers the spark-ignited engines found in the vast majority of automobiles and small trucks. The composition of these various blends is periodically altered to conform with the power and performance requirements of the vehicles in which the gasoline is burned. However, prior to passage of the 1990 Clean Air Act Amendments, the emissions performance of a particular gasoline formulation was not an issue.

During the congressional debate that preceded enactment of the new law, the petroleum industry advanced the idea that **reformulated gasoline (RFG)** could be a valuable weapon in the war against air pollution. In comparison with conventional gasoline, RFG has lower levels of certain compounds that contribute to air pollution and doesn't evaporate as easily; thus, industry argued, reformulated fuels can have a major impact on the amount of pollutant emissions released by fuel combustion. In pushing RFG, oil industry lobbyists were protecting their own interests, since federal legislators were on the verge of requiring the use of alternative, nonpetroleum fuels as a means of improving air quality, something the petroleum industry was not eager to see happen. By the late 1980s, oil companies were already marketing a type of RFG in California that reduced emissions from older vehicles no longer able to use leaded gasoline, and they managed to persuade lawmakers that RFG was a more practical alternative than nongasoline fuels. Industrial spokespersons argued that RFG could immediately be used in the nation's existing car fleet, while alternative fuels, by contrast,

could only be phased in as new cars engineered to use them rolled off the assembly lines. In the end, they succeeded in convincing Congress to scuttle most of the alternative fuel proposals in favor of RFG.

The reformulated gasoline program mandated in 1990 targeted urban areas that were consistently in violation of the national ambient air quality standards for ozone (i.e. smog) and carbon monoxide, developing specific RFG requirements to deal with each of these problems. In the nation's smoggiest cities, the government ruled that RFG must contain a minimum oxygen content of 2% by weight, no more than 1% benzene, and must be free of lead, manganese, and other heavy metals. Although several compounds potentially could be used to meet the oxygen requirement, in most formulations developed for ozone-plagued regions the oxygenate of choice has been **methyl tertiary butyl ether (MTBE)**, an additive first introduced in the 1970s as an octane enhancer to replace lead. Currently ten major metropolitan areas are required by federal law to use RFG as a means of reducing ozone pollution: Los Angeles, San Diego, Sacramento, Houston, Milwaukee, Chicago, Baltimore, Philadelphia, New York, and Hartford. In addition, numerous other cities experiencing smog problems have voluntarily opted to use RFG. As a result, reformulated gasoline is now being sold in 17 states and the District of Columbia.

In regions of the country where attainment of the NAAQS for carbon monoxide has been problematic, the Clean Air Act Amendments require the *wintertime* use of RFG containing higher oxygenate levels than those required for ozone nonattainment areas—in this case a minimum of 2.7% by weight. **Ethanol** is the oxygen additive most commonly used in the wintertime program, though a few of the affected cities have chosen MTBE instead. Added to RFG, both ethanol and MTBE have the effect of "leaning-out" the air-to-fuel ratio, promoting more complete combustion during cold temperature months when cars need additional fuel to start and when catalytic converters operate less efficiently. Some of the cities participating in the Wintertime Oxygenated Fuels Program, launched in 1992, are: Denver, Las Vegas, Phoenix, Los Angeles, San Diego, Seattle, Portland, Salt Lake City, Minneapolis-St. Paul, Raleigh-Durham, New York, Philadelphia, and Washington, DC.

By the late 1990s, several controversies over oxygenates used in RFG raised questions about their safety and effectiveness. In 1999, the California Energy Commission voted unanimously to end the use of MTBE in that state by Dec. 31, 2002 (this deadline was later dropped). Sold in California since the 1970s, MTBE was targeted for phaseout because an estimated 10,000 wells in that state show evidence of MTBE contamination, a result of leaks from underground storage tanks and accidental spills. Maine pulled out of the program as well, citing similar concerns. Several months later MTBE producers got more bad news when an EPA advisory panel recommended that the agency promptly begin reducing MTBE use across the country because of the contamination threat to groundwater supplies. While not calling for an immediate ban, panel members urged that alternatives to MTBE be brought onto the market as soon as possible. Congressional action is necessary for altering the government's RFG requirements and MTBE manufacturers are hotly contest-

ing the panel's recommendation, but most observers anticipate that MTBE's share of the reformulated gasoline market will decline significantly in the years ahead.

Manufacturers of ethanol, MTBE's main commercial rival, would appear to be major beneficiaries of California's action, but the ethanol industry itself is facing a potential problem as the EPA steps up its war on ozone pollution. Although ethanol additives help gasoline burn cleaner during the winter, it also increases vapor pressure during the warmer months of the year—an ozone-enhancing feature that MTBE doesn't share. As perennial competitors for the oxygen additive market, producers of ethanol and MTBE have a considerable financial stake in EPA's ultimate decision regarding legally allowable limits for vapor pressure. In the meantime, neither industry was happy with a report issued by the National Research Council (NRC) in the spring of 1999, which concluded that *neither* ethanol nor MTBE had much impact on reducing emissions that contribute to ozone formation. The real heroes in accounting for the demonstrated improvement in urban air quality, according to the NRC report are (1) better emissions control equipment on motor vehicles, (2) other non-oxygenate additives to RFG, (3) improved auto engine design, and (4) increasingly stringent air quality regulations. The NRC predicted further improvements in urban air quality in the years ahead, not due to ethanol or MTBE use, but as a result of new technology. Not surprisingly, the Oxygenated Fuels Association takes strong exception to NRC's conclusions, pointing out that the report failed to acknowledge the role oxygenates play in reducing wintertime carbon monoxide levels. EPA also defended the use of oxygenates in reformulated gasoline, stating that they significantly reduce air toxics such as benzene and dilute or displace other fuel components such as sulfur, which then reduces emissions of VOC and NO_X, major precursors of smog formation.

For motorists, the pros and cons associated with various gasoline additives for enhancing air quality are probably of less immediate interest than the effect of reformulated gasoline on car performance and fuel efficiency. Fortunately, on this score the news is mostly good. Requirements for fuel formulations that burn cleaner have simply been added to long-standing considerations regarding vehicle performance. As a result, RFG has no adverse impact on a car's performance or on the durability of the engine and fuel system components. In terms of fuel efficiency, however, RFG may lower gas mileage in some cars by 1–2% compared to oxygenate-free gasoline, and RFG costs a few cents more per gallon than conventional blends. Residents of RFG marketing areas who travel to parts of the country where the reformulated product is not sold need have no concerns about filling up with conventional gasoline—mixing the two won't have any effect on a car's performance.

Overall, environmental officials regard the reformulated fuels program as a big step forward in clearing the nation's urban air. EPA credits reformulated gasoline with eliminating almost 300 million tons of pollutants from being emitted to the atmosphere since 1995. For drivers it's a win-win situation: improved, cleaner-burning gasoline, no change in vehicle performance, and more healthful air for everyone to breathe.

Reference

U.S. Environmental Protection Agency, Office of Mobile Sources. 1999.

gradual transition from total reliance on state and local authorities to an increasing federal involvement grew out of general recognition that the problems of air pollution were so immense, diverse, and complex that environmental improvement could be achieved only through intergovernmental cooperation at all levels.

Although such laws were well intentioned, they relied on voluntary compliance by states, many of which were reluctant to adopt strict controls for fear of driving away industry, thereby forfeiting jobs and tax revenues. As a result, pollutant levels continued to rise and public outcry mounted. By 1970, spurred by a grassroots demand that something be done about the environmental crisis facing the nation (a public outcry that culminated in the first national observance of "Earth Day" on April 22, 1970), an historic turning point was reached with congressional passage of the **Clean Air Act Amendments of 1970** (henceforth referred to here simply as the Clean Air Act). This landmark piece of environmental legislation provided the first comprehensive program for attacking air pollution on an effective nationwide basis.

The 1970 Clean Air Act established a number of legal precedents that form the basis of U.S. air quality control regulations in effect today—and, coincidentally, served as a model subsequently adopted by many other nations. Some minor modifications to the law, primarily in the form of deadline extensions for meeting stringent new auto emission requirements, were made in 1977. However, by the early 1980s, continuing problems with high levels of certain auto-related pollutants, complaints that portions of the act had not been implemented with sufficient vigor, and the emergence of acid rain as a troublesome new issue not even addressed by the 1970 mandate, gave rise to vociferous demands from the environmental community for changes that would make the Clean Air Act both stronger and more comprehensive. At the same time, the new Reagan Administration viewed its mission as one of dismantling many of the environmental programs enacted during the 1970s. Although Congress refused to approve most of the changes proposed, decisions by the Reagan EPA to waive implementation of certain regulations deemed burdensome to industry resulted in a gradual reversal of air quality improvements that had been on the upswing during the decade of the 1970s. On the most contentious issue of all—what to do about acid rain—the Reagan White House adamantly opposed any new initiatives other than further study, remaining steadfastly unconvinced that the phenomenon posed any real problems.

As a result of this impasse, efforts to reauthorize the Clean Air Act as required by law languished throughout the 1980s, in spite of continued public support for improving air quality. The legislative logjam remained unbroken until 1988 when newly elected President George Bush, citing his desire to be remembered as the "Environmental President," threw his active support behind efforts to resolve the clean air controversy. Within Congress the clash among regional interests and competing ideologies frequently threatened to derail negotiations, but eventually, after months of heated debate, the differences were resolved. Passage of the Clean Air Act Amendments of 1990, signed into law by President Bush in November of that year, marked a significant strengthening of U.S. air quality legislation. The amendments expanded the scope of regulatory requirements, addressed new issues ignored by the 1970 act, and made the law more consistent with other environmental mandates. Although these amendments won't be fully implemented until 2010, they should result in major measurable improvements in U.S. air quality. Some of the most significant provisions of the Clean Air Act are discussed in the following paragraphs.

National Ambient Air Quality Standards (NAAQS)

In setting national ambient air quality standards for the six criteria air pollutants, the EPA reviews the existing medical and scientific literature to establish **primary standards** at levels intended to safeguard human health, allowing a margin of safety to protect more vulnerable segments of the population such as young children, asthmatics, and the elderly. These standards are subject to periodic revision as new data become available. In 1997, studies demonstrating elevated mortality rates in cities where PM_{10} levels were well below the legal limit prompted EPA to promulgate a new $PM_{2.5}$ standard for the tiniest—and most harmful—particulates. At the same time, the agency also issued a more stringent standard for ozone, citing scientific evidence that long-term exposure to O_3 at levels below the existing standard could provoke asthma attacks, loss of lung function, and respiratory problems. The Clean Air Act differs from other major environmental laws in requiring that primary standards be set solely on the basis of protecting health, without regard for the costs of pollution control.

The primary standards were originally mandated to be attained by 1975, with penalties (e.g. bans on the construction of new sources of pollution, cutoff of federal highway construction funds, etc.) to be imposed on those **nonattainment areas** which failed to bring their pollution levels into conformance with the NAAQS. Twenty years after passage of the original legislation, numerous urban areas were still in violation of the primary standard for ozone, historically the most difficult-to-control pollutant, and many cities also exceeded the standard for carbon monoxide as well. Therefore, with the enactment of the 1990 amendments, Congress revised its approach for dealing with nonattainment areas. Under the current program, regions still in violation of any of the air quality standards are classified according to the seriousness of their pollution problems (categories range from "marginal" to "extreme"), and are given varying amounts of time—anywhere from 3–20 years, depending on the severity of nonattainment—to come into compliance with the standards. The higher the pollution levels, the more regulatory steps states must take in dealing with the problem. Lest affected areas postpone action until deadlines are imminent, the 1990 amendments require specified annual emission reduction goals to ensure steady progress toward the ultimate objective of full compliance with NAAQS primary standards.

Table 12-2 National Ambient Air Quality Primary Standards

Pollutant	Averaging Time	Maximum Concentration (approximate equivalent)
Particulate matter (PM_{10})	Annual arithmetic mean 24-hour	$50\ \mu g/m^3$ $150\ \mu g/m^3$
Particulate matter ($PM_{2.5}$)*	Annual arithmetic mean 24-hour	$15\ \mu g/m^3$ $65\ \mu g/m^3$
Sulfur dioxide (SO_2)	Annual arithmetic mean 24-hour	$80\ \mu g/m^3$ (0.03 ppm) $365\ \mu g/m^3$ (0.14 ppm)
Carbon monoxide (CO)	8-hour 1-hour	$10\ mg/m^3$ (9 ppm) $40\ mg/m^3$ (35 ppm)
Nitrogen dioxide (NO_2)	Annual arithmetic mean	$100\ \mu g/m^3$ (0.053 ppm)
Ozone (O_3)*	Maximum daily 8-hour average	$157\ \mu g/m^3$ (0.08 ppm)
Lead (Pb)	Maximum quarterly average	$1.5\ \mu g/m^3$

*Note: These standards have been called into question by a controversial 1999 Federal appeals panel decision which sent them back to EPA for review and revision. EPA is appealing the ruling, but at the time this book went to press, the matter had not yet been resolved.

Table 12-3 Selected Ozone Nonattainment Areas

Classification	Metro Area	Attainment Date
Extreme	Los Angeles, CA	2010
Severe 2	Chicago-Gary, IL-IN	2007
Severe 2	Houston-Galveston	2007
Severe 2	Milwaukee-Racine, WI	2007
Severe 2	New York-Newark, NJ	2007
Severe 1	Baltimore, MD	2005
Severe 1	Philadelphia, PA	2005
Severe 1	Sacramento, CA	2005
Severe 1	Ventura County, CA	2005
Serious	Atlanta, GA	1999
Serious	Boston, MA	1999
Serious	Greater Connecticut	1999
Serious	Providence, RI	1999
Serious	San Diego, CA	1999
Serious	Washington, DC	1999
Moderate	Cincinnati, OH	1996
Moderate	Dallas-Fort Worth, TX	1996
Moderate	Phoenix, AZ	1996
Moderate	St. Lous, MO	1996
Marginal	Birmingham, AL	1993
Marginal	Buffalo-Niagara Falls, NY	1993
Marginal	Reno, NV	1993
Marginal	Scranton, PA	1993

In addition to the primary standards, EPA was told to set more stringent **secondary standards** that would promote human welfare by protecting agricultural crops, livestock, property, and the environment in general. No timetable for compliance with secondary standards has been set. However, since the secondary standards set by the EPA are, in most cases, identical to the primary standards, the lack of a deadline date is largely irrelevant.

It is difficult to over-emphasize the importance of national (as opposed to state or local) air quality standards. As experience prior to 1970 amply demonstrated, drifting air pollutants pay little heed to political boundaries, a fact that largely nullified feeble state attempts at improving air quality within their own borders. States or cities that tried to impose emission controls on polluters within their jurisdictions found that air quality gains were minimal due to airborne pollutants arriving from less concerned—or less courageous— states upwind. Threats by polluting industries to leave a particular state and relocate in a more lenient regulatory environment made many state legislatures extremely reluctant to get tough with polluters. Thus, establishing uniform nationwide standards has been a key element in improving air quality since 1970.

Emission Limitations for New Stationary Sources of Pollution

The intent in establishing **new source performance standards (NSPS)** for factories and power plants is to reduce pollutants at their point of origin by ensuring that pollution controls are built in when factories and plants are newly constructed or substantially modified. Note that this requirement is not retroactive; that is, polluting power plants or factories already in operation at the time the Clean Air Act was passed are not affected by the NSPS guidelines. The new source performance standards are set on an industry-by-industry basis, taking into account such factors as economic costs, energy requirements, and total environmental impacts such as waste generation and water quality considerations. The 1990 amendments strengthened this provision by adding a requirement for all stationary sources to obtain operating permits from the state regulatory agency, specifying allowable levels of pollutant emissions, as well as required control measures.

Strict Emission Standards for Automobiles

Emission standards for automobiles and other mobile sources form an integral part of Clean Air Act requirements, inasmuch as motor vehicles spew more pollutant emissions into the outdoor air than any other single source. In traffic-congested metropolitan areas, 90–95% of CO concentrations, 80–90% of NO_x and hydrocarbons, and a significant percentage of airborne particulates originate from an ever-expanding fleet of cars, trucks, and buses (WRI, 1996). Detroit eventually settled upon modified engine design plus installation of catalytic converters as the chief means by which American car manufacturers would reduce emissions. Claiming financial difficulties and the impossibility of meeting the deadline imposed by Congress, the auto industry won several deadline extensions and a relaxed standard for NO_x emissions. In spite of much foot-dragging on the part of industry, new model automobiles can now meet federal standards and average emission levels are steadily dropping. According to the EPA, automobiles coming off the assembly lines today emit 90% less carbon monoxide, 80–90% fewer hydrocarbons, and 70% less nitrogen oxides than did cars manufactured prior to passage of the Clean Air Act.

Improvements in urban air quality resulting from reduced auto emissions since the mid-1970s have been dramatic, but a shift in vehicle preference among American motorists in recent years threatens to reverse these gains. Sports utility vehicles (SUVs), minivans, and light-duty trucks now comprise almost half of all new vehicle purchases and account for a steadily increasing proportion of vehicle miles traveled. This fact poses serious air quality concerns because a loophole in the 1970 Clean Air Act, enacted when these types of vehicles comprised a small percentage of the nation's fleet, permitted such vehicles to emit 2–3 times as much pollution as ordinary passenger cars. In an effort to rectify this omission and to protect clean air progress,

Figure 12-2 Per Vehicle Emissions vs. Vehicle Miles Traveled

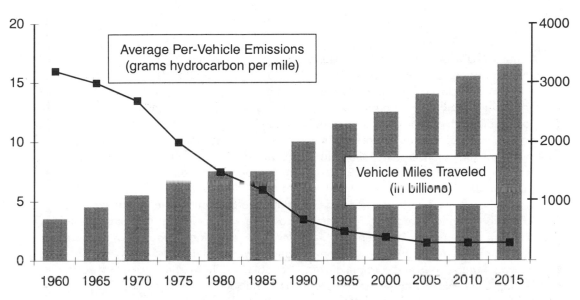

Source: U.S. Environmental Protection Agency.

the EPA in 1999 issued a proposal to require that SUVs and pickup trucks meet the same tailpipe emissions standards as cars (an action taken by California's Air Resources Board in 1998). EPA's proposal also called for both passenger cars and SUVs to meet significant new reductions on tailpipe emissions of NO_x as a means of reducing urban smog levels. Auto manufacturers must begin improvements to meet the tougher emission requirements for passenger cars by 2004. All cars, as well as smaller-model SUVs and minivans, must be in full compliance by 2007, while large SUVs and pickup trucks have until 2009 to achieve the mandated emissions reductions. Although some auto manufacturers complain that they need more time to engineer the mandated improvements, Ford Motor Company—the world's second-largest auto company—decided not to wait for the federal deadline. In 1998, Ford executives announced that all of the company's 1999 model-year SUVs, as well as its Windstar minivan, would meet the same emission standards required for passenger cars; Ford's 2000 model-year pickup trucks similarly comply with passenger car standards. Several other automakers are now striving to follow Ford's example and hope to meet the required emissions reductions on at least some of their models ahead of schedule.

While reducing tailpipe emissions has been a key component of efforts to curb mobile source pollution, other approaches are being pursued as well. Altering the relative proportions of the ingredients used in making gasoline can have a major impact in reducing emissions of ozone-forming chemicals and toxic air pollutants such as benzene. Recognizing the pollution-reducing potential of such reconfigured fuels, the 1990 amendments to the Clean Air Act mandated the use of so-called **reformulated gasoline** (see Box 12-2) in

BOX 12-3

Fighting Smog: The I/M Approach

Much of the documented improvement in urban air quality since passage of the 1970 Clean Air Act has been achieved through strict pollution controls on motor vehicles—a prime source of carbon monoxide, nitrogen oxides, ozone, volatile hydrocarbons, and lead. The device chosen by auto manufacturers to limit such emissions was the catalytic converter, installed in all nondiesel American cars since 1975. Within the catalytic converter carbon monoxide, hydrocarbons, and nitrogen oxides are burned at temperatures between 2000–3000 °F and thereby converted to nonpolluting water vapor and carbon dioxide. Improvements in catalytic converters over the years since they were first introduced have made these devices highly efficient, reducing pollutant emissions of carbon monoxide and hydrocarbons approximately 90% below those of vehicles without emissions controls. Emissions of nitrogen oxides have also been sharply curtailed.

Unfortunately, the theoretical air quality gains achievable if all vehicles were equipped with properly functioning catalytic converters have not been fully realized. Poor auto maintenance and illegal tampering with pollution control devices (due to the mistaken belief that catalytic converters reduce gasoline mileage and engine efficiency) has impaired the effectiveness of catalytic converters to the extent that air quality gains in many metropolitan regions are being seriously jeopardized.

Because of excessive auto emission levels, a number of metropolitan areas consistently violate the NAAQS for ozone and carbon monoxide, resulting in the threat of federal sanctions. Recognizing

that just 15% of cars in the United States are responsible for 75% of troublesome emissions and that further reductions in auto-related pollutants in congested urban areas are unlikely to be achieved without strict transportation controls, Washington has pushed states to implement auto **inspection and maintenance (I/M)** programs within nonattainment areas. Such programs require motorists to bring their cars to an approved testing station to determine whether the catalytic converter is achieving the appropriate level of emissions reduction. Because only newer-model catalytic converters are capable of achieving the pollution reduction efficiency mandated by EPA, the exact level of emissions that determine whether a car passes or fails the test differs, depending on its make and model-year. Older vehicles have less stringent requirements than newer models and pre-1968 autos are exempt from testing altogether. Many I/M programs also include a tamper inspection and require that any missing or tampered pollution control devices be replaced before a car is certified as passing the test.

Beginning in 1974 when New Jersey became the first state to institute an I/M program, the concept has spread nationwide. The 1990 Clean Air Act Amendments made what had been a strongly recommended effort mandatory by requiring all of the approximately 154 nonattainment areas in the country to begin emissions inspection programs. Over 30 states now have I/M programs, with approximately one-third of all cars in the United States subject to periodic testing.

Depending on the extent of air quality problems within designated nonattainment areas, EPA requires either a "basic" or "enhanced" testing protocol. Basic I/M, sufficient for regions in "moderate" or "marginal" nonattainment, involves the insertion of a computer-linked probe into the exhaust pipe to measure emissions of CO and hydrocarbons while the engine is idling. Enhanced testing, required in areas where pollution levels are categorized as "extreme," "severe," or "serious," provides a more accurate assessment of pollutant emissions under realistic city driving conditions. Unlike basic testing, where the driver remains in the car, enhanced testing requires a certified inspector to drive the vehicle onto a treadmill-type device called a dynamometer. This device accelerates and decelerates, capturing the pollutant emissions produced by various driving modes—important because malfunctioning vehicles can emit large amounts of pollutants when changing speed. Whereas the basic test only measures CO and hydrocarbon emissions, enhanced testing also measures NO_x, a prime contributor to smog formation. In addition, enhanced testing measures the total mass of pollutants emitted (results from the basic test are expressed simply as the concentration of pollutants as a percentage of exhaust gases), thus providing a clearer picture of that car's overall contribution to air pollution. The dynamometer is also capable of measuring a vehicle's fuel economy. Additional procedures carried out during enhanced testing that are not possible under the basic program include purge and pressure tests that monitor the proper functioning of the car's evaporative emission system. This is important because during hot weather, fuel vapors escaping into the air can be a greater source of hydrocarbon pollution than exhaust emissions. Enhanced I/M programs also include a requirement for on-road remote sensing devices (RSDs) to

identify passing vehicles whose emission control systems malfunction during the period between scheduled tests. Such RSD systems, which can easily be moved from one location to another, have proven more useful than random roadside pull-overs for detecting vehicles whose catalytic converters have been tampered with between tests. They also aid officials in identifying drivers who cheat on registration or register outside the affected area in order to avoid participation in the I/M program. RSDs employ laser beams or beams of UV light projected across the roadway to detect violators; a freeze-frame video camera and digitizer is part of the RSD system, making it possible to capture the license plate number of the offending car and to store emissions information. Authorities can then contact the vehicle owner and order the car to be taken immediately to a testing station for an out-of-schedule I/M emissions check. Repairs are then required for cars failing to pass this test.

Vehicle inspection/maintenance programs represent one of the most effective and least costly means of combating urban smog, short of prohibiting driving altogether. EPA estimates that a well-run I/M program can reduce levels of air pollution in a traffic-congested city by as much as 30%. The cost of such air quality improvement will be borne largely by motorists whose cars fail to pass inspection; the government estimates out-of-pocket expenses to drivers for repairing a vehicle with excessive emissions could be as low as $25 (sometimes a simple engine tuneup is all that's needed) or as high as $450. If a vehicle still fails to pass inspection after the owner has spent $450 or more on repair costs, emission requirements will automatically be waived.

A concept pioneered in the U.S., the

I/M approach to reducing pollution from motor vehicles is now being adopted to a limited extent in Mexico, Chile, India, and in several Southeast Asian nations. Inspection/maintenance programs are particularly needed in developing countries because such a large proportion of their total car fleet is made up of older, more polluting vehicles (poorly maintained older cars emit up to 100 times more pollutants than well-tuned, newer models).

Although I/M programs impose a modicum of inconvenience and expense on motorists within affected areas, public response has generally been one of acceptance. As an official with the Automobile Club of New York remarked, "Everybody is for cleaner air; this is a way for motorists to do their bit."

References

U.S. Environmental Protection Agency. 1994. "High-Tech Inspection and Maintenance Tests (Procedures and Equipment)." EPA 400-F-93-005 (July), Fact Sheet OMS-16.

U.S. Environmental Protection Agency. 1993. "Clean Cars for Clean Air: Inspection and Maintenance Programs." EPA 400-F-92-016 (January), Fact Sheet CMS-14.

the major metropolitan areas experiencing the most severe ozone problems. In addition, service stations in such areas were told to install vapor recovery systems on gasoline pumps to capture hydrocarbons that would otherwise be released during refueling. Cities in violation of carbon monoxide standards were required to use reformulated gasoline containing oxygen additives ("oxygenates") during winter months to increase the combustion efficiency of gasoline, thereby reducing tailpipe emissions of CO.

Looking to the future and the ultimate solution of a zero-emissions vehicle, the law also established a pilot program in California requiring car manufacturers to produce and market clean fuel cars. Under rules promulgated by the California Air Resources Board, by the year 2003, 10% of all new cars sold or leased in that state by the seven largest auto companies must be zero-emissions vehicles (New York State subsequently adopted a similar rule). Many observers think this goal will be impossible to attain and predict a relaxation of the California requirement; nevertheless, several major automakers have announced their intention to have nonpolluting fuel-cell vehicles in production by 2004. Development of electric cars, by contrast, has stalled due to manufacturers' concerns that the high sticker price and need for frequent recharging of these cars will translate into minimal market demand.

The success or failure of these initiatives holds important implications for the future because there is little hope of solving auto-related air quality problems solely through reliance on catalytic converters. Even with extremely strict standards for tailpipe emissions, the sheer increase in numbers of cars on the road (some experts predict this figure will exceed 600 million worldwide by the year 2000 and reach one billion by 2030) guarantees a reversal of air quality gains in the years ahead unless a radically different approach to curbing emissions is adopted.

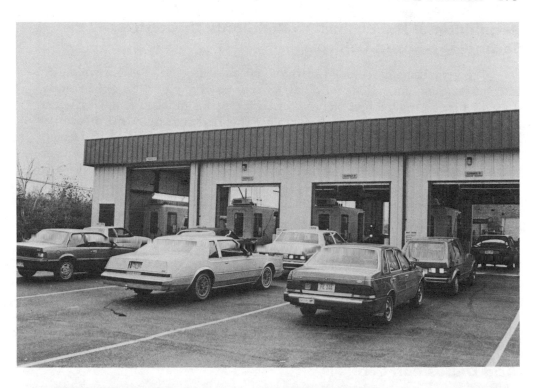

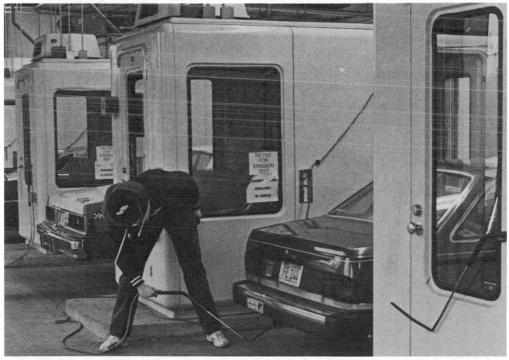

Inspection/Maintenance program: (top) vehicles await their turn for emissions testing in Chicago; (bottom) a monitor inserted into the tailpipe of an automobile measures emissions of carbon monoxide and hydrocarbons. *[Illinois Environmental Protection Agency]*

Regulation of Hazardous Air Pollutants Through Technology-Based Controls

The requirement included in the 1990 amendments that EPA identify and set emission limitations for all major sources of any of the 189 (currently 188) air toxics targeted by Congress for such controls marked a major change in the existing Clean Air Act legislation. The **Hazardous Air Pollutants (HAPs)** mandate impacts thousands of manufacturing facilities and small businesses never previously affected by requirements for operating permits or emission controls. After issuing standards for HAP source categories, EPA is required to promulgate health-based standards for those chemicals believed to present a cancer risk of 1:1,000,000 exposed persons or greater. Emission reductions began in 1995 and by 2005 the level of airborne toxics should be down by as much as 75% from pre-control levels. A requirement that EPA subsequently reevaluate health threats that may persist (i.e. "residual risk") after controls have been established means that publication of final emission standards may not be truly final—a further tightening of restrictions on HAP emissions may be ordered if conditions call for such action. Finally, the 1990 air toxics regulations also created an independent Chemical Safety Board, charged with investigating the cause of chemical accidents.

Acid Deposition Controls

Perhaps the most bitterly debated issue during the Clean Air Act reauthorization process was acid rain controls. Such controls became a part of federal clean air legislation only after passage of the 1990 amendments. The main focus of the new program was a mandate to cut sulfur dioxide emissions in half—a 10 million ton annual reduction from 1980 levels by the year 2000, with an interim SO_2 reduction target of 5 million tons by January 1, 1995. Nitrogen oxides, another major contributor to acid rain formation, are targeted for emission reductions of 2 million tons annually, based on 1980 emission levels. A novel feature of the acid deposition regulations that is attracting widespread interest and attention is a market-oriented system of emissions allowances that utilities can buy, sell, or trade to help finance the costs of pollution controls (see Box 12-4).

The provisions described here represent only the highlights of this extremely complex piece of legislation. Responsibility for implementing and enforcing the federal mandate falls primarily on the environmental agencies of state government, which must develop **State Implementation Plans (SIPs)**, detailing strategies for compliance with Clean Air Act requirements. SIPs must list all the pollution sources within the state, estimating the quantities of each pollutant emitted annually, including both mobile and stationary sources. They must issue operating permits for stationary sources, as well as timetables for compliance, and must include some kind of transportation control strategy for dealing with auto-related pollutants in areas of heavy traffic. States must have their SIPs approved by the federal EPA or be working with the agency to improve a conditionally approved plan before they can issue a construction permit for any new polluting facility.

Enforcement provisions under the Clean Air Act, and the civil and criminal penalties for violation of the law, were significantly strengthened under the 1990 amendments. EPA can levy large financial penalties against facilities in violation of air quality requirements—penalties sufficiently stiff to cancel any economic benefits a firm might derive from delaying compliance. Criminal liability, which may be imposed on persons *knowingly* violating the law, can result in fines, imprisonment, or both. The Clean Air Act gives citizens the right to file suit against polluters if the EPA fails to take action. To encourage "whistle-blowing" by persons aware of Clean Air Act violations, Congress has authorized EPA to pay informants up to $10,000 for information leading to a civil penalty or criminal conviction (Bryner, 1993; "Easy Guide," 1993; *Environmental Law Handbook,* 1993).

Global Air Quality Trends

Deadline dates have come and gone, hot summers are punctuated with ozone alerts, and a haze of smog still hovers over many of our cities. Nevertheless, 30 years after the Clean Air Act ushered in a "get tough" approach regarding air pollution control, overall trends in American skies are favorable. Elsewhere in the world, progress in cleaning up dirty air varies considerably from one country to another.

A comprehensive assessment of international air quality trends is complicated by the fact that scarcely any routine monitoring has been conducted in the developing nations that comprise the bulk of world population. Anecdotal information suggests that pollution levels in Third World cities are far higher than in most industrialized countries—and getting steadily worse. Problems appear especially serious in terms of particulate pollution, known to have the most serious adverse health impact of all air contaminants. According to the World Resources Institute, the 15 most polluted cities in the world in terms of airborne particulates are all in Asia. In Lanzhou, China, a city of 2 million people, the air is so foul that simply breathing is the equivalent of smoking a pack of cigarettes daily. A report issued by the World Health Organization (WHO) estimates that 70% of the entire world population, primarily residents of developing nations, breathe air that contains health-threatening levels of particulates. Concentrations of sulfur dioxide, another pollutant known as a respiratory irritant and a precursor of acid rain, are increasing dramatically in a number of developing nations, as well as in Russia and eastern Europe, as plentiful supplies of sulfur-laden coal are burned without pollution controls. A 1995 survey revealed that of 88 cities monitored for SO_2 levels, over half were above WHO guidelines (of 87 cities monitored for particulate matter, 85 exceeded WHO limits). In Lanzhou, SO_2 concentrations were almost 10 times above the level WHO considers acceptable. Residents of Tehran, Istanbul, Rio de Janeiro, and Moscow similarly suffer levels of sulfur dioxide exposure more than double WHO guidelines.

Auto-related pollutants are also mounting rapidly in Third World cities as car ownership becomes synonymous with "the good life." Few developing nations require that vehicles be equipped with emission controls and most continue to sell leaded gasoline (two notable exceptions are Thailand, which banned its sale in 1996, and China, where the phaseout of leaded gasoline

Figure 12-3   Percent Decrease in Ambient Air Concentrations of Criteria Pollutants (1986–1995)

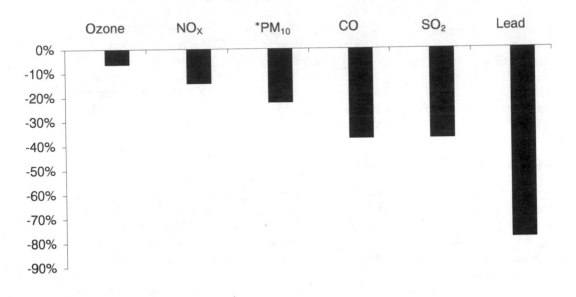

*Measurements began in 1988.

Source: EPA Office of Air and Radiation. 1995. *National Air Quality Status and Trends.*

should be complete by July 2000). In most developing countries, and particularly in Asia, the number of cars on the road is increasing exponentially and the fact that many are old and poorly maintained—and frequently fueled with adulterated gasoline—ensures choking levels of pollutant emissions that can scarcely be imagined by motorists in Los Angeles or London.

In contrast with the downward trends in air quality evident in many developing countries, in parts of the industrialized world emission levels from both stationary sources and motor vehicles have been drastically cut in recent years. While the United States was the pace-setter in air pollution control initiatives until the early 1980s, since then several European nations and Japan have equalled or surpassed the American record. Prompted by international treaty obligations, the European nations reduced sulfur dioxide emissions by 32% between 1980–1990 (McDonald, 1999). Japan requires state-of-the-art controls on automobiles, incinerators, power plants, and steel mills and is the only country in the world that compensates victims of air pollution—deriving monies for those so injured from a tax on SO_2 emissions. The Canadian province of Ontario has an ambient air standard for SO_2 considerably more stringent than that of the United States. Germany, jolted out of complacency in the early 1980s by reports of widespread forest damage due to acid rain, since 1983 has implemented one of the world's most vigorous air quality control programs. Unlike the situation in the United States, where power plants in operation prior to promulgation of New Source Performance Standards were exempted from the requirement for the best available technological controls, Germany has mandated the retro-fitting of all its medium and large-size power plants, regardless of age, with state-of-the-art pollution control devices. The Swiss and Austrians, similarly concerned about dying forests, have adopted what may be the most stringent air quality regulations in the world, setting emission standards even for motorcycles!

The trend toward tighter controls on mobile sources has been relatively recent outside the United States. In 1980 Japan was the only other country with strict requirements for automobiles. Within a decade, however, all major industrialized nations, with the exception of Russia and the eastern European countries, were regulating tailpipe emissions, many of them with standards equivalent to those in America. Several developing nations—Mexico, Brazil, Taiwan, and South Korea—also have adopted U.S. emission standards (World Resources Institute, 1990).

In the United States, air quality in most parts of the country has improved significantly since passage of the Clean Air Act. In spite of population growth, increased traffic volume, and continued industrial development, emissions of most pollutants have declined and the number of days rated as "unhealthy" has dropped dramatically since the 1970s. Progress in cleaning up the nation's air has not been uniform—concentrations of some pollutants have declined more than others and some regions of the country have experienced air quality trends better or worse than national averages would indicate. Of the criteria air pollutants, since 1970 ambient levels of lead have dropped by a precipitous 97%, but nitrogen oxides have actually risen slightly due to increased fossil fuel combustion. Emissions of particulates, SO_2, CO, and the volatile organic compounds that contribute to ozone formation have all declined measurably since passage of the Clean Air Act. An indirect indication of progress in reducing CO emissions, due primarily to improvements in automobile control systems, is the sharp drop in accidental carbon monoxide fatalities, over 80% of which are caused by inhalation of car exhausts. Since the number of people, the number of cars, and the amount of fuel consumed are all increasing, it would be logical to expect the number of auto-associated CO poisonings to increase as well. However, the reverse has been the case. In 1979, accidental CO-related fatalities in the United States totalled 1,513—a number that dropped steadily to 878 in 1988. Researchers attribute this welcome news to the fact that catalytic converters have achieved CO emission reductions of more than 90% over levels prevailing prior to imposition of pollution controls (CO in the ambient air fell by 28% during this period, in spite of a 39% increase in vehicle miles traveled). As a consequence, it now takes much longer for CO emissions from a car left idling in an enclosed space to reach life-threatening concentrations (Cobb and Etzel, 1991).

However, levels of the criteria pollutants in a number of urban areas still remain high enough to endanger the health of their residents. EPA, which gathers information on air concentrations of the various criteria pollutants from over 4,000 monitoring stations across the United States, reports that in 1995 nearly 80 million people lived in areas that still exceeded the NAAQS for at least one pollutant. In that year almost 71 million resided in areas where ozone levels violated federal standards. It should be noted, however, that smog levels within a region vary considerably from year to year, depending on weather conditions; increases in 1995 ozone concentrations were due in part to very hot temperatures during the summer of that year. Ozone remains by far our most troublesome pollutant in terms of numbers of people affected. It is likely that in the years immediately ahead there will be much more aggressive efforts to tighten controls for nitrogen oxides, whose emissions appear to be more important contributors to ozone formation than previously realized. Controls are likely to expand over a wide range of formerly unregulated sources of VOCs such as dry cleaning establishments, furniture refinishers, auto body shops—and possibly even consumer items such as charcoal lighter fuel, spray starch, and power lawn mowers! Of all regions of the United States, the Los Angeles area will be most heavily impacted by stricter air quality regulations. A nonattainment area for four of the six criteria pollutants, southern California is in violation of the NAAQS more frequently than New York, Houston, Chicago, Denver, and Pittsburgh (other nonattainment areas) combined. Although present ozone levels in Los Angeles are only one-quarter of the choking, eye-watering levels prevailing in the mid-1950s, they still must be cut by half to comply with existing standards. As a result, California has adopted the toughest, most aggressive air quality regulations in the nation—some of which are now being copied by several northeastern states grappling with smog problems of their own.

In spite of these remaining challenges, air quality trends in the United States overall are very encouraging. While declining levels of pollutant emissions are due in some measure to energy conservation, fuel-switching, and the demise of many smokestack industries, a large share of the credit must be given to the regulatory programs that have mandated significant investment in pollution control technologies. Although the battle to control air pollution is by no means over, progress to date proves that the Clean Air Act is working.

Acid Deposition

An air quality problem virtually unrecognized and unmentioned at the time the 1970 Clean Air Act was passed, the issue of acid deposition (commonly referred to in popular jargon as "acid rain," though the phenomenon includes not only rain but also snow, fog, dry SO_2 and NO_2 gas, and sulfate and nitrate aerosols) became political dynamite during the 1980s, pitting region against region, nation against nation. Although the domestic policy battles generated by the debate over acid rain controls were largely resolved by key provisions of the 1990 Clean Air Act Amendments and by the Canada-United States Air Quality Agreement of 1991, the problem itself persists and the damage toll continues to climb. Nor are all the facts concerning acid deposition completely understood even today. To comprehend what the fuss is all about requires a brief look at the nature of acid deposition, how it is formed, and the types of damage it causes.

What Is Acid Deposition?

On a pH scale, distilled water has a pH of 7.0, considered "neutral" because the number of hydrogen (H^+) and hydroxyl (OH^-) ions is equal, making the solution neither acidic nor basic. However, since atmospheric CO_2 tends to dissolve in water, forming a weak solution of carbonic acid, rainfall is slightly acidic by nature. Measurements of the pH of precipitation in many parts of the world have led researchers to conclude that natural, unpolluted rain has a pH around 5.0. Thus, by definition, any precipitation measuring **less than 5.0** on the pH scale is considered acid deposition. Since the pH scale is logarithmic, rainfall with a pH of 4.0 is ten times more acid than precipitation with a pH of 5.0 and 100 times more acid than that of pH 6. A reading below 2.0, such as that recorded during a three-day drizzle in the fall of 1978 at Wheeling, West Virginia, represented a level 10,000 times more acid than unpolluted rainfall.

Extent of the Problem

Acid precipitation has been observed as a local phenomenon in the vicinity of coal-burning facilities for more than a century. In fact, the term "acid rain" was first coined by an English chemist, Robert Angus Smith, to describe the corrosive brew falling on industrial Manchester more than 100 years ago. In the early 1960s Canadian ecologist Eville Graham, a pioneer of acid rain research in North America, described the acidification of lakes in northern Ontario in the vicinity of the huge Sudbury smelting complex, then the world's largest single source of sulfur emissions (Munton, 1998). Not until the 1970s, however, did acid rain emerge as a regional problem, affecting areas far from the source of pollutant emissions. The alarm was first raised in 1972 by Swedish delegates attending the U.N. Conference on the Human Environment in Stockholm. After initial disbelief by many national governments, Swedish views about the extent and seriousness of this newly recognized environmental threat have become widely accepted. On the basis of measurements taken during the past few decades, scientists have shown that until the late 1990s, when government-mandated controls began to take effect, the pH of rainfall steadily dropped throughout large areas of North America and Europe. Not only did rainfall become more acid in the affected areas, but the geographical extent of the problem has widened also. Early measurements of rainfall pH indicated that in the years 1955–1956 only 12 northeastern states were experiencing acid precipitation. By 1972–1973 the number of states experiencing excessive rainfall acidity extended over the entire eastern portion of North America, except for the southern tip of Florida and the far northern regions of Canada. In addition, acid rain was detected in several of the major urban areas of California and in the Rocky Mountain region of Colorado.

Today the pH of rainfall averages 4.4 throughout the United States east of the Mississippi River, with substantially lower readings being obtained during some individual storm episodes. However, encouraging news has been reported by scientists working for the U.S. Geological Survey who documented a steady drop in the concentrations of acid-forming sulfates in precipitation from 1980 to 1991—a decline that has accelerated since the 1990 Clean Air Act imposed strict SO_2 reduction requirements on coal-burning power plants. As a result, in many of the affected regions, the average pH of rainfall has gradually been rising. Such field data are hailed as evidence that pollution control technologies aimed at curbing SO_2 emissions are having the intended impact. Unfortunately, USGS monitoring stations have not seen an equivalent decline in rainfall nitrate concentrations, nor has a nearly 35-year trend toward increasing acidification of waterways been reversed. Indeed, in the streams being monitored, pH levels have continued to fall year after year (Hilchey, 1993).

Beyond North America, acid deposition today also affects most countries of Europe, although on that continent, as in North America, increasingly stringent controls on sulfur dioxide emissions reduced the seriousness of the problem during the decade of the 1990s. By contrast, acid rain has emerged as a growing environmental threat in Asia, particularly in the rapidly industrializing provinces of southeastern China. Japan is reporting acidification problems, and high levels of acid precipitation are now being experienced in northeastern India, northern and central Thailand, and throughout the Korean peninsula (WRI, 1998).

Mystery of the Dying Lakes

During the 1960s and 1970s anglers, campers, and resort owners raised the first alarms concerning what was to become a major environmental tragedy. From the sparkling lakes of the remote Adirondacks, to the popular vacationlands of Ontario and Quebec, to the waterways of Scandinavia, reports of the mysterious disappearance of once-abundant fish, amphibians, and aquatic insects began to generate public concern. The fact that such lakes and streams were far from any of the usual sources of water pollution which have traditionally been associated with fish kills only increased the bewilderment. To a casual observer the water remained blue and clear, uncontaminated by chemical spills or sewage overflows; beneath the surface, however, the affected lakes had become watery deserts, devoid of life. By 1999, EPA data reported that 26% of Adirondacks lakes are acidified, as are 580 streams on the mid-Atlantic coastal plain and 1,350 streams in the mid-Appalachian highlands. In New Jersey's Pine Barrens, fully 90% of all streams are acidic—the highest percentage in the nation. In eastern Canada the toll is even higher—acidified lakes total 14,000, with approximately 150 now fishless. Such lakes are acid dead, poisoned by pollutants falling from the sky in the form of sulfuric and nitric acid.

Formation of Acid Rain

Acid precipitation forms when its major precursors, sulfur dioxide and nitrogen dioxide, are chemically converted through a complex series of reactions involving certain reactive hydrocarbons and oxidizing agents such as ozone to become sulfuric or nitric acid. The reactions involved can take place either within clouds or rain droplets, in the gas phase, on the surface of fine particulates in the air, or on soil or water surfaces after deposition (Rhodes and Middleton, 1983).

Sulfur dioxide, one of the two pollutants primarily responsible for acid rain formation, is discharged into the atmosphere in amounts averaging 15 million tons annually in the United States. Of this amount, approximately two-thirds originates from coal- and oil-burning power plants; the remainder is primarily from smelters and industrial boilers. A certain amount of SO_2 enters the atmosphere from natural sources such as volcanoes or mud flats, but such emissions contribute relatively little to the problem of acid rain; it is estimated that in the northeastern U.S., 90% of the sulfur in the air comes from human sources of pollution.

Nitrogen oxides, of which about 20 million tons per year are currently emitted in the United States, come predominantly from auto emissions, power plants, and industry. NO_x emissions have declined by only about 3% since 1986, considerably less than reductions achieved for SO_2. Some observers worry that, unless additional controls are imposed, NO_x levels will once again begin to climb as the automobile fleet continues to grow and as new factories and power plants come on line. Until recently, SO_2 emissions have widely been perceived as posing a more serious problem than NO_x in terms of acid rain formation; however, as technological controls are increasingly successful at reducing levels of airborne sulfur compounds, the role of nitrogen oxides as acid rain precursors will grow in importance. The most recent assessment of national acid precipitation trends reports that sharp reductions in rainfall sulfate concentrations since the early 1990s have not been matched by any statistically significant decline in nitrate concentrations (NSTC, 1998).

Long-Distance Transport

The aspect of acid rainfall that makes it such a politically charged issue is the fact that the pollutant emissions that are the precursors of acid rain formation may be produced hundreds of miles from the regions suffering the effects of acid deposition. Because some pollutants can remain in the air for a relatively long period of time, they can be carried on the prevailing winds across geographical and political boundaries far from their place of origin—a phenomenon known as **long-distance transport**. There are documented examples of acid rain-forming pollutants being carried more than 600 miles before being deposited on the earth's surface.

Ironically, pollution control technologies adopted early in the 1970s to reduce *local* levels of ambient air pollution had the unintended effect of increasing the long-distance transport problem. The approach adopted most often by utilities striving to lower SO_2 concentrations in the vicinity of their plants was to pursue a **tall stack strategy**; that is, to build extremely tall "superstacks" that discharged pollutant gases into the persistent air currents more than 500 feet above the ground. This approach was indeed effective in reducing local pollution levels, but it promoted long-distance transport and thereby increased the range and severity of acid deposition in regions downwind. Until the 1990 Clean Air Act Amendments committed the United States to aggressive acid rain control efforts, relations between Canada and the United States were seriously strained because half of the corrosive rain falling over southeastern Canada originates in the heavily industrialized Ohio River Valley and upper Midwest. New York and the New England states harbored a similar grudge against Illinois, Indiana, and Ohio—the source of fully one-fourth of all U.S. sulfur emissions. In the same way, much of the acid rain now damaging vegetation and aquatic environments in Japan originated in China, whose sulfur emissions in 1990 were 40–45 times higher than those during Japan's worst air pollution years in the mid-1970s. Japanese authorities estimate that at least 37% of the sulfur deposition over their country is "made in China" and have offered the Chinese low-interest loans to purchase pollution control equipment for reducing SO_2 emissions (Brown et al., 1998). Prior to the 1980s, acid rain provoked harsh words among neighboring European countries as well, since the corrosive precipitation wreaking havoc on lakes and forests in Norway and Sweden was produced primarily in central Europe and Great Britain. Such circumstances make the formulation of acid rain control policies politically difficult because those bearing the cost of pollution abatement strategies and those reaping the benefits are not one and the same. Effective action toward resolving this dilemma was taken first in Europe where 35 countries in 1979 signed the **Convention on Long-Range Transboundary Air Pollution,** an agreement requiring the signatory nations to achieve a 30% reduction in SO_2 emissions from 1980 levels by 1993. Targets have subsequently been set for reducing NO_x and VOC emissions as well. In the United States, the acid rain debate raged in Congress for years. Legislators from the Midwest were nearly unanimous in their opposition to proposed federal rules that would impose more stringent sulfur emission controls on coal-burning power plants in their region. Citing the financial burden that would be passed along to electric consumers and the inherent threat controls would pose to coal-mining interests in states like Illinois and West Virginia, Midwestern representatives were acutely aware that the environmental gains achieved by tougher regulations would be enjoyed by citizens outside their own constituencies. Conversely, legislators from such states as New Hampshire and Maine, areas that had few large sources of emissions yet were suffering severe economic and ecological damage due to acid rain, were among the most vocal in demanding regulatory action.

Regional Vulnerability to Acid Rain

Although the entire eastern United States is now experiencing acid rainfall, not all areas are suffering adverse ecological effects. An ecosystem's sensitivity to acid precipitation is determined primarily by the chemical composition of the soil and bedrock—an attribute referred to as the **buffering capacity** of that environment.

Buffering capacity refers to an ability to neutralize acids, the buffer acting to maintain the natural pH of an environment by tying up the excess hydrogen ions introduced by acid rain. Regions such as New England, the Mid-Atlantic states, the Southeast, northern Minnesota and Wisconsin, the Rocky Mountain states, and parts of the Pacific Northwest are characterized by soils that are naturally already acidic or underlain by granitic bedrock; these areas are said to have a low buffering capacity and hence are very sensitive to acid rain. By contrast, most parts of the Midwest, the Great Plains, and portions of the Southwest have predominantly alkaline soils and bedrock of limestone, giving them a high buffering capacity. This fact explains why a state such as Illinois, which is currently experiencing rainfall almost as acid as that falling in New York or New England, is not suffering comparable ecological damage. Nevertheless, such apparent invulnerability is not guaranteed to last forever. Over time, a given soil's buffering capacity can be overwhelmed by continual acid inputs, a phenomenon that seems to be occurring already in parts of the upper Midwest. It seems a cruel twist of fate that prevailing wind currents are transporting acid rain-forming pollutants to precisely those regions that are most sensitive to the harmful effects of increased acidification.

Environmental Effects of Acid Rain

Acid precipitation can cause a number of adverse environmental changes, the best-understood of which include the following.

Damage to Aquatic Ecosystems. That acid rain can decimate the biotic communities inhabiting lakes, ponds, and streams in those regions where natural buffering capacity is low has been well documented in numerous studies. Most freshwater organisms do best in waters that are slightly alkaline—about pH 8. As lakes gradually become acidified due to steady inputs of acid rain, one aquatic species after another disappears. The first affected are the tiny invertebrates that constitute a vital link in aquatic food chains; at pH 6.0 the freshwater shrimp are eliminated; at pH 5.5 the bacterial decomposers at the lake bottom begin to die off, as do the phytoplankton, the producer organisms in aquatic ecosystems. Fish populations, the subject of most human attention, are somewhat more tolerant to increasing acidity; little change in their numbers is noticed until the pH drops below 5.5. Under pH 4.5 all fish species disappear, as do most frogs, salamanders, and aquatic insects ("Acid Rain," 1982).

Interestingly, falling pH levels seldom kill adult fish directly. The primary cause of fish de-population is acid-induced reproductive failure; pH values below 5.5 can prevent female fish from laying their eggs, and those eggs which are laid frequently fail to hatch or result in the production of deformed fry. (Just as the early developmental stages of humans are the most vulnerable to the adverse influence of environmental contaminants, the same holds true for the larval stages of lower organisms.) Interference with hatching is accentuated by the fact that the most critical developmental period usually coincides with the time of the annual snow melt when several months' accumulation of acid suddenly inundates the spawning areas in one massive dose, a situation known as **shock loading** or **episodic acidification**. This sort of periodic drop in pH, due either to snow melt or heavy downpours, is much more common than chronic acidification of lakes and streams. Three times as many sensitive Adirondacks lakes are at risk of episodic acidification as are those experiencing on-going acid conditions; in Appalachia, 30% of sensitive streams are likely to suffer temporary acidification during an episodic event— seven times as many as those that are chronically affected. While the abrupt drop in pH levels during such events is generally of short duration, the ecological impact on young fish or fish eggs can be as devastating as chronic exposure. Large-scale reproductive failure leads to a situation in some lakes where the older fish grow larger and larger, thanks to decreased competition for food, and anglers boast of their excellent catches until, with further increases in acidity, all the fish disappear. As a professor at the University of Toronto succinctly states: "There is no muss, there is no fuss, there is no smell. The fish quietly go extinct . . . They simply fail to reproduce and become less and less abundant, and older and older, until they die out" (Weller, 1980).

At one time it was assumed that acid rain's impact on aquatic environments was limited to freshwater ecosystems. It is now recognized, however, that acid precipitation contributes 30–40% of all the nitrates entering Chesapeake Bay. Studies have shown that these airborne nutrients are as important as farmland fertilizer runoff in stimulating the algal blooms that are degrading water quality in that important saltwater estuary.

Mobilization of Toxic Metals. Contact with acidified water can cause tightly bound toxic metals such as aluminum, manganese, lead, zinc, mercury, and cadmium to dissolve out of bottom sediments or soils and leach into the aquatic environment. Such metals, especially aluminum, can kill fish by damaging their gills, thereby causing asphyxiation. Acid-induced release of aluminum, even at concentrations as low as 0.2 mg/L, has resulted in fish kills at water pH levels which wouldn't have been lethal in the absence of the toxic metal. Toxic metals in the water also can bioaccumulate in fish tissues, making them dangerous for humans to eat.

Mobilization of poisonous metals also presents a direct threat to human health if the acidified lakes are a source of drinking water supplies. A resort owner from the Adirondacks testified before a congressional committee that, in response to his children's complaints about the taste of water piped to their lodge, he had the water tested and found it contained 5 times the safe level for lead and 10 times that for copper. In other communities, acidified water that was originally free of toxic metals became contaminated upon passing through lead or copper plumbing systems–the low pH of the water caused corrosion of the pipes, resulting in leaching of toxic metals into the water. Homeowners who obtain their drinking water from roof catchments in areas affected by acid rain are also at special risk (Boyle and Boyle, 1983).

Deterioration of Buildings, Statuary, and Metals. While it is extremely difficult to assign a precise monetary value to the impact of acid rain on materials, it is nevertheless acknowledged that the scope of the damage is large indeed. Most pronounced are the effects of acid deposition on stone and metal buildings and statues, on textiles, leather, and paint, and to some extent on paper and glass. Many monuments of great historic and cultural significance are today slowly disintegrating under the impact of airborne pollutants, of which various sulfur compounds are by far the most important. Corroding surfaces of the Statue of Liberty, the Washington Monument, the Capitol Building in Washington, D.C., Canada's Parliament buildings in Ottawa, and the Field Museum in Chicago all give evidence of the ravages produced by acid rain. In India, the Supreme Court ordered nearly 300 coal-burning facilities near Agra to close by the end of 1997 because their SO_2 emissions were severely corroding the beautiful marble façade of the Taj Mahal (Brown et al., 1997). On a more mundane level, EPA estimates that acid rain increases the cost of each new car by $5.00 due to the necessity of using more expensive acid-resistant paint on vehicles sold in regions where acid rain is a problem.

Reduction of Crop Yields. The extent of acid rain damage to field crops is less clear-cut than with other types of acid-induced environmental damage. Yields of some species appear to be diminished by acid rain, some are stimulated, while others show no change as pH levels of rainfall drop (Cohen, Grothaus, and Perrigan, 1982). In Asia, the increasing acidification of rainfall during the 1990s has been blamed for widespread crop damage. Chinese officials report that approximately 40% of their country's agricultural land is affected by acid precipitation, and the World Bank estimates annual crop and forest losses in China at $5 billion (Brown et al., 1998). In northeastern India, steep reductions in wheat yields in fields downwind of a coal-burning power plant are attributed to acid rain damage (WRI, 1998).

Damage to Forest Productivity. From the wooded slopes of the Adirondacks to the forests of central Europe and Scandinavia, acid-laden rain and fog are contributing to death and reduced growth rates among an ever-increasing number of important tree species. Most affected are conifer forests at high elevations, frequently shrouded in acid fog or mist. At many sites above 850 meters in the White Mountains of New Hampshire or the Green Mountains of Vermont, over half the red spruce have died since the early 1960s. In Germany, the rate at which wide areas of forest have been similarly affected just since the early 1980s has been so dramatic that distraught German scientists have coined a word for the phenomenon—*waldsterben* ("forest death"). By 1989 German scientists were estimating that more than half the trees in the country were suffering some degree of defoliation. Fortunately,

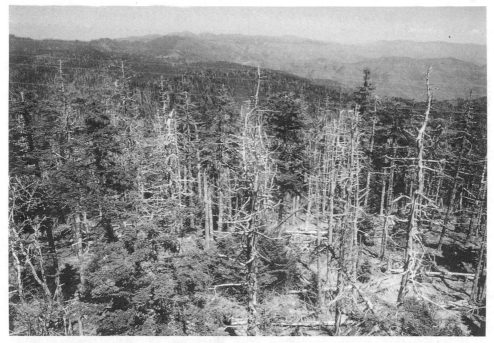

Hundreds of balsam fir trees have been killed or damaged by acid deposition on this mountain ridge in the Great Smoky Mountains National Park. *[Thomas A. Schneider]*

the rate of forest decline in Germany now appears to be slackening, possibly in response to the aggressive pollution control policies enacted specifically for that purpose in 1983. The situation looks less hopeful for Germany's central European neighbors, whose forests are dying at an alarming rate. In the Czech Republic and Poland over a third of all forests are moderately or severely affected (75% of Polish trees show some signs of damage); more than 60% of the conifers in Lithuania are ailing—and the situation is worsening annually. One analysis published in 1990 calculated that three-fourths of European commercial forests were experiencing damage caused by sulfur deposition and 60% were receiving more nitrogen than they could assimilate without harm (World Resources Institute, 1992).

The extent to which acid rain can be blamed for the decline of forests on two continents is currently a subject of intensive investigation by scientists in Europe and North America. In some cases acid rain causes direct damage to leaves, resulting in nutrients being lost from foliage faster than they can be replaced by root absorption. This phenomenon is particularly associated with the acid fog which commonly occurs on ridgetops and it is further enhanced by the presence of ozone. With a pH as low as 2.2, acid fog and clouds with high ozone content are blamed for much of the damage apparent in the red spruce forests at higher elevations. For the most part, however, it appears that acid rain's role in the forest decline drama is less direct. Acid precipitation increases the solubility and migration of soil-bound ions of aluminum, which acts as a poison to the delicate root hairs responsible for nutrient uptake. It also causes the loss of essential plant nutrients—calcium, potassium, magnesium—from forest soils. Calcium depletion in particular is emerging as one of the most significant factors explaining forest decline in eastern North America. An essential element for plant growth, calcium is leached out of forest soils into waterways as precipitation becomes increasingly acidic. Research during the 1990s revealed a marked drop in the calcium content of soils in both the northeastern and southeastern United States since the 1960s—a decline linked to acid rain. This trend is worrisome because calcium loss undermines a tree's ability to resist insect attack, disease, and extreme temperatures. Field investigations have documented a distinct correlation between reduced stress tolerance in ailing red spruce and sugar maple forests to soil calcium deficiencies. Unfortunately, calcium that is leached out of soils by acid precipitation is no longer being replaced at the rate it once was. Studies have shown that rainfall today contains approximately 80% less calcium than it did in the 1950s. As a result, even if the problem of acidification were to vanish overnight, forest recovery would require many decades before the damage is repaired. Researchers working at the Hubbard Brook Experimental Forest in New Hampshire's White Mountains have discovered that the acid-impacted forest essentially stopped growing in 1987, with virtually no new biomass added since that time. Such observations may help to explain why natural ecosystems damaged by past acidification fail to show signs of recovery in spite of recent reductions in acid-rain-forming pollutants. Although by the year 2000 U.S. emissions of SO_2 and NO_x were 50% lower than ten years earlier, researchers warn that both pollutants—and particularly NO_x—must be lowered still further if forests are to recover any time soon (Lawrence and Huntington, 1999; Likens et al., 1996).

Acid Rain Controls

Throughout the 1980s a growing awareness of the extent and severity of the acid rain problem led to increasingly vociferous public demands to "Stop Acid Rain!" through regulatory action, primarily in the form of laws requiring stringent pollution controls on coal-burning power plants. Passage of the 1990 Clean Air Act Amendments, containing the strong acid rain control provisions previously discussed, ended nearly a decade of vituperative debate. The innovative market mechanism devised to make the requirements more financially feasible for the affected utilities permits polluters to choose among numerous options for meeting mandated emission limits (see Box 12-4).

Observers of the acid rain saga are in unanimous agreement that the control program mandated by the 1990 Clean Air Act Amendments has been resoundingly successful in meeting the Phase I goal of a 10-million-ton reduction in SO_2 emissions. All 110 power plants targeted under this phase of the program met the EPA deadline for both sulfur and nitrogen oxide reductions—in fact, by 1995, emissions from these plants were 35% *below* the legally allowable limits. The biggest surprise was the fact that these reductions were achieved at a far lower financial cost than even the most optimistic analysts had predicted—approximately $1 billion per year as opposed to the $3–7 billion cited by industry lobbyists fighting enactment of the legislation. Although market-based allowance trading is frequently credited for this remarkable accomplishment, several other factors were equally, if not more, instrumental in achieving such a favorable outcome. The unusual degree of flexibility built into the program made it possible for power plant managers to take advantage of unexpected opportunities to cut emissions in the most cost-effective manner. EPA's "just do it" directive—setting limits but not specifying the means for achieving them—prompted most of the affected utilities to meet the designated goal by switching to relatively cheap low-sulfur coal rather than by installing expensive flue gas desulfurization systems ("scrubbers"). The small percentage that did opt for scrubbers were pleasantly surprised to discover that, due to new, more efficient technology and manufacturers' need to keep the purchase price competitive, the equipment was both cheaper and more reliable than originally expected. Finally, as described in Box 12-4, the availability of a market-based pollution credit system gave plant operators additional leeway in choosing the most economical way of getting the job done.

Successful as the current approach has been in measurably reducing the acidity of precipitation, however, there is growing doubt that sensitive ecosystems will recover without the imposition of even more stringent controls. Just as particulate pollutants and ozone-laden smog continue to bedevil regulators, so the problem of acid rain promises to remain a challenge for the foreseeable future (Munton, 1998; Kerr, 1998).

Indoor Air Pollution

While the attention of scientists, citizens, and government regulators has until recently been focused almost exclusively on problems of ambient air pollution, recent studies suggest that more serious air quality threats lurk much closer to home. It is now apparent that contaminants within private

BOX 12-4

Marketing Pollution

No longer are the commodities being bought and sold amidst the pandemonium at the Chicago Board of Trade restricted to such mundane items as soybean futures or pork bellies. Thanks to a novel concept known as **allowance trading** created by the 1990 Clean Air Act Amendments, utility companies can now broker government-assigned allowances for SO_2 emissions in an innovative attempt to make acid rain controls more effective and affordable. First proposed by the Environmental Defense Fund, the idea of allowance trading was welcomed by legislators as a means of breaking congressional gridlock over who should pay for rescuing acid-threatened lakes and forests.

Under the strategy devised by Clean Air Act negotiators, EPA has abandoned the traditional regulatory approach that requires polluters to install controls on each piece of equipment. Instead, the agency has set enforceable limits on the amount of sulfur dioxide that power plants can emit each year and has assigned each plant a designated number of emission "allowances." For each allowance granted, the recipient is permitted to discharge one ton of SO_2 annually (the number of allowances assigned to each facility is determined by a complex formula and is specified in the plant's operating permit). The emission limits imposed on individual plants must collectively correspond with the congressionally mandated 10 million ton annual reduction in SO_2 emissions nationwide required by the Clean Air Act to be achieved by the year 2000. Utilities can subsequently adopt any pollution reduction strategy they wish in order to achieve the mandated reductions. A plant's annual emissions cannot exceed the allowances allocated to it for that calendar year—*unless the utility purchases surplus allowances at market rates from another plant whose emissions were below the designated limit.*

The beauty of allowance trading is that it encourages polluting facilities not merely to reduce emissions to the legal limit, but to cut them as low as possible, thereby accumulating unused emissions allowances that can then be sold, at a profit, to another power plant. Thus utilities which choose to install newer, cleaner technologies and make efforts to find the most cost-efficient means of reducing pollutant emissions can help cover the cost of their investment by selling surplus allowances to those facilities—usually older, dirtier plants—for which the cost of installing new equipment substantially exceeds that of purchasing another company's pollution credits. The cost of each credit is, of course, determined by market forces. It was initially expected that the value of an allowance would range between $500–$700, while the EPA-imposed penalty for exceeding allowance allocations is $2000/ton—a fact that makes it much cheaper for utilities with excessive emissions to purchase extra allowances than to pollute the air. This cost differential became even more pronounced when trading officially commenced; in 1993 the price for one allowance averaged just $250 and by the late 1990s had fallen to a bargain-basement price of slightly under $100.

Some critics initially opposed the new program on a philosophical basis, complaining that emissions trading promotes the "right to pollute." Advocates point out, however, that on a nationwide basis the same amount of SO_2 will be removed from the air, thus achieving Clean Air Act goals but at a substantially lower cost than would be possible under the traditional "command-and-control" regimen.

During Phase I of the program, the 110 power plants targeted for emissions reductions had a variety of low-cost options to choose from and didn't employ the allowance system to as great an extent as lawmakers had anticipated, perhaps because of utility executives' unfamiliarity with the concept. Nevertheless, the very existence of an allowance trading mechanism broadened a plant operator's range of choices. For those considering installation of stack gas scrubbers, for example, the availability of emission credits obviated the necessity of purchasing expensive backup equipment. Under the old system, such equipment was mandatory for use during the inevitable "down-time" of the principal scrubber. With the allowance trading option, plant officials know that in an emergency they can simply buy emission credits to cover pollution released when a scrubber has to be shut down for repairs. In such ways, the allowance system is credited with reducing compliance costs by about 30% during the early years of the program. Analysts anticipate more active allowance trading during Phase II of the program, starting in 2000, when more facilities will be required to participate and emission reduction requirements are tightened.

After its successful debut in the United States, allowance trading is generating increased interest abroad. Europeans, whose success at lowering sulfur emissions has come at a much higher price than similar gains in the U.S., are currently exploring the possibility of moving toward American-style allowance trading. Of even greater long-term significance is an initiative by the United States to expand the concept of emissions marketing from SO_2 to carbon dioxide and other greenhouse gases. Government officials are trying to persuade Kyoto Protocol signatories that so-called "flexibility mechanisms" represent the only practical approach to cutting greenhouse gas emissions without devastating national economies. Although developing an international trading system that targets six different gases emitted by millions of sources in over 100 nations will be far more difficult than overseeing a program focused on 100+ power plants in one country, the idea is being aggressively pursued. In the near-term, domestically, it is quite likely that the scope of allowance trading will be broadened to include a market for NO_X emissions, since these have proven much more problematic than SO_2 in recent years.

The success of a more flexible free market approach for meeting acid rain control objectives at surprisingly low cost guarantees that this new problem-solving strategy will be applied to a growing list of environmental challenges in the years ahead.

Reference
Kerr, Richard A. 1998. "Acid Rain Control: Success on the Cheap." *Science* 282 (Nov. 6):1024-1027.

dwellings may pose a greater risk to human health than do outdoor air pollutants. In fact, with the exception of ozone and sulfur dioxide, all the air pollutants regulated under U.S. laws occur at higher concentrations indoors than out, prompting the EPA to rank indoor air pollution among the top five environmental risks to public health. This is particularly worrisome because the majority of people spend more of their time indoors than outside; thus their exposure to indoor air pollutants is nearly continuous. Such pollutants pose a special threat to the very young, the ill, and the elderly—the groups most susceptible to pollution's adverse health effects and also the ones most likely to spend long periods of time inside. Justifiable concerns about energy conservation may have worsened the indoor air pollution problem because thick insulation, triple-glazed windows, and magnetically sealed doors greatly reduce air exchange with the outside, effectively retaining and accumulating contaminants inside the home.

While most people tend to equate the risk of harm they might suffer from toxic pollutants to the total amount and toxicity of such substances, in fact the main determinant of danger is the dose actually received by the individual. Thus in reality large amounts of toxic pollutants such as benzene, formaldehyde, or carbon monoxide, for example, when emitted from a factory smokestack or the tailpipe of a car, pose minimal risk to the average citizen because they break down or are diluted in concentration before he/she is directly exposed to them. By contrast, much smaller amounts of the same chemicals, released in close proximity to individuals inside the confined environs of their homes or offices, have a quick, direct route into the body and hence pose a much greater overall risk of health damage. Studies demonstrate that personal exposures and concentrations of indoor air pollutants exceed those occurring outdoors for all of the 15 most prevalent chemicals studied (Wallace, 1987). In addition, peak pollutant concentrations, as well as overall averages, are generally higher indoors than in the ambient air.

Some of the more common air pollutants known to be present in the home environment include the following.

Radon Gas

When Stanley Watras started radiation-detection alarms ringing at the Limerick nuclear power plant near Philadelphia one December morning in 1984, he didn't realize that he was about to become a national celebrity, alerting Americans to a hitherto unsuspected menace within their own homes. The radioactive contamination that was detected by Watras when he arrived for work that fateful winter morning had obviously come from outside the nuclear facility, so Watras requested Philadelphia Electric, the utility company that owned the plant, to check his home in Colebrookdale Township. To everyone's amazement, tests revealed that the Watras home had levels of radon gas approximately 1,000 times higher than normal. Investigators estimated that Watras, his wife, and two young sons were receiving radiation exposure equivalent to 455,000 chest X-rays a year simply by living in their house. As officials of Pennsylvania's Division of Environmental Radiation hastened to determine the extent of the indoor radon threat, it quickly became apparent that the Watras family was not alone in its predicament. Throughout sections of eastern Pennsylvania, New Jersey, and New York, underlain by a uranium-rich geological formation known as the Reading Prong, thousands of homes exhibit elevated levels of radon. Nor is the problem limited to a few mid-Atlantic states. In the autumn of 1988 the EPA announced that its data indicate radon contamination problems span the country and urged that most homes be tested for the presence of radon. While some scientists feel EPA figures overstate the number of homes affected, there is general agreement that indoor radon exposure represents a serious health hazard.

Radon originates from the natural radioactive decay of uranium. It is present in high concentrations in certain types of soil and rocks (e.g. granite, shale, phosphate, pitchblende), but most soils contain amounts high enough to pose a potential health hazard. Radon dilutes to harmless concentrations in the open air, but when it enters the confined space inside a structure it can accumulate to potentially hazardous levels. Since radon is a gas, it readily moves upward through the soil; small differences in air pressure between indoors and outdoors (very slight negative air pressure inside a heated building results from the "stack effect," created by air's tendency to rise whenever it is warmer than the surrounding atmosphere) cause the gas to seep into homes through dirt floors or crawl spaces, through cracks in cement floors and walls, through floor drains, sump holes, joints, or pores in cinder-block walls. Occasionally, radon gets into wellwater supplies and enters homes when water is used, particularly for showers or baths. Radon is dangerous because it is radioactive, undergoing decay to produce a series of "radon daughters," the most troublesome of which are alpha-emitters polonium-218 and 214. These can be inhaled and deposited in the lungs where they constitute an internal source of alpha radiation exposure, increasing the risk of lung cancer. Radon's contribution to overall human exposure to ionizing radiation is considerable. The National Council on Radiation Protection and Measurement estimates that the average individual receives fully 55% of his or her yearly dose of ionizing radiation from radon inside homes. The health consequences of such exposure, according to EPA estimates, are between 7,000–30,000 lung cancer deaths annually—a number which would make radon the second-leading cause of lung cancer deaths in the United States, behind cigarette smoking. In some parts of the country where radon levels are unusually high, hundreds of thousands of Americans are receiving as much radiation exposure from radon in their homes as that received by the Ukrainian citizens who lived near Chernobyl at the time of the nuclear accident there in 1986. The extent of an individual's chances of developing radon-induced lung cancer depends on radon concentrations inside the home and on the length of time one is exposed. It is thought that long-term exposure to slightly elevated levels of radon poses a greater cancer threat that does short-term exposure to much higher levels. Cigarette smoking has a synergistic effect in enhancing the radon/lung cancer risk by a factor of 10.

Until the 1980s, radon was regarded as a health hazard only to uranium miners, so estimates of risk to residents of radon-contaminated homes have simply been extrapolated from standards set for occupational exposure in the mines. Indoor radon concentrations are measured as the number of picocuries of radiation per liter of air (pCi/L). Outdoors, radon concentrations in the ambient air typically measure about 0.4 pCi/L, while the average indoor level approximates 1.3 pCi/L. Acknowledging that *any* amount of exposure to ionizing radiation entails *some* degree of risk, for practical reasons EPA regards 4 pCi/L as the **action level**—the point at or above which homeowners are advised to take some kind of remedial action (although Congress has established a long-term goal of lowering indoor radon concentrations in every home to a level equivalent to that prevailing outdoors, such a goal is not yet techno-

Figure 12-4

Points Where Radon Can Enter Homes

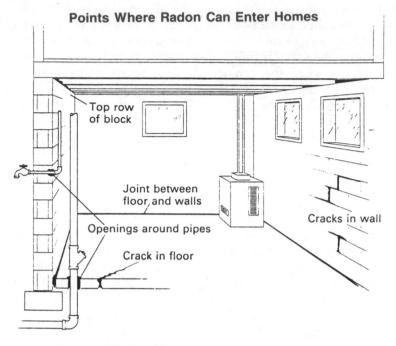

Top row of block

Joint between floor and walls

Openings around pipes

Crack in floor

Cracks in wall

Radon Reduction Methods

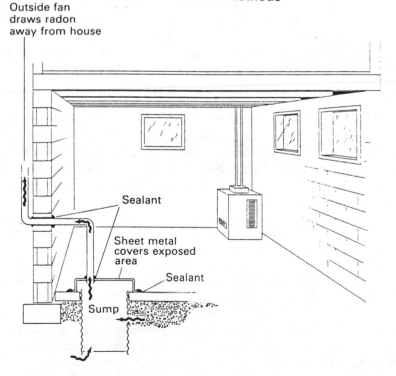

Outside fan draws radon away from house

Sealant

Sheet metal covers exposed area

Sealant

Sump

Source: U.S. Environmental Protection Agency, *Radon Reduction Methods.*

logically achievable; nevertheless, the EPA believes that reducing elevated radon levels to around 2 pCi/L should be possible almost everywhere). Readings above 20 pCi/L are considered cause for serious concern and may require significant abatement measures (as a basis for comparison, radon levels in the Watras home measured 2700 pCi/L).

Results from an EPA-sponsored survey of residential radon levels in nine million homes nationwide revealed that an estimated one out of every 15 homes in the U.S. has average indoor radon levels in excess of 4 pCi/L. Nor is the problem limited to private residences. Another study carried out under the auspices of the 1988 Indoor Radon Abatement Act found that out of 927 public school buildings surveyed throughout the country, 19% had at least one ground floor room where radon concentrations were above EPA's action level. Such findings have prompted a strong EPA recommendation that all homes and schools in the nation should be tested for the presence of radon.

Since it is impossible to predict with certainty which structures are likely to have elevated radon levels (some homes in the Watras neighborhood were essentially radon-free), the need for radon reduction measures can only be determined by actual measurements, which often can be done by the homeowner with relatively inexpensive devices (see Box 12–5). If test results indicate the need for some sort of radon remediation efforts, a variety of options are available. Most require the services of a professional contractor, though some can be as simple as covering sump holes or improving ventilation. More extensive—and expensive—possibilities include installing fans or air-to-air heat exchangers to replace radon-contaminated indoor air with outdoor air; covering any exposed earth inside homes with concrete, gas-proof liner, or sheet metal; sealing all cracks and openings with mortar, polyurethane sealants, or other impermeable materials; installing a drain tile suction system around the outer foundation walls of a house; or by installing a series of exhaust pipes inside hollowblock basement walls or baseboard to draw radon out of the voids within such walls before it can enter the living space. In structures with significantly elevated levels of radon, it may be necessary to utilize several methods to achieve sufficient reductions. For persons planning to build a new home in areas with known radon problems, use of radon-resistant construction techniques is far more cost-effective than installing a radon reduction system after the fact.

Products of Combustion

Carbon monoxide, nitrogen oxides, and particulates can reach very high levels inside homes where gas stoves or other gas appliances are used, where kerosene heaters or wood-burning stoves are operating, where auto emissions from a garage can enter the house, or where there are cigarette smokers. In homes with gas ranges, for example, nitrogen oxide levels are frequently twice as high as those outdoors. Carbon monoxide emissions from wood, coal, or gas stoves often exceed Clean Air Act standards for outside air. The growing popularity of wood-burning stoves is a particular cause for concern, since wood is a much dirtier fuel than either oil or gas. Wood smoke contains approximately 100 different chemicals, at least 14 of which are the same carcinogens found in cigarette smoke.

Cigarette smoking (the by-product of which is now referred to technically as **ETS**—"Environmental Tobacco Smoke") may constitute the most significant source of indoor air pollution in many homes; particulate levels may go as high as 700 micrograms/m^3, far above the primary ambient air quality standard of 50, when there are smokers in a house. A study conducted by researchers at Harvard University found that household tobacco smoke is the main source of exposure to particulate pollutants for most children. It also demonstrated that whereas typical particulate levels in a home without smokers is 10–20 micrograms/m^3, each smoker contributes an additional 25–30 micrograms/m^3, more than doubling the base level amount (Ware et al., 1984). Particulate matter and carbon monoxide are not the only indoor air pollutants generated by smokers—cigarette smoking represents the major source of human exposure to benzene, a known carcinogen and a listed toxic air pollutant. Researchers calculate that fully 45% of Americans' total exposure to benzene comes from inhaling tobacco smoke, while a mere 3% is due to industrial emissions (Ott et al., 1998). Such findings have provided scientific justification for the proliferation of smoking bans in restaurants and other public facilities. Even in the absence of enforceable federal standards, ETS has become a socially unacceptable indoor air pollutant.

Formaldehyde

Known to cause skin and respiratory irritation, formaldehyde is now suspected of being carcinogenic as well. A wide variety of household products contain formaldehyde, most notably particleboard, plywood, and some floor coverings and textiles. Levels of formaldehyde are particularly likely to be high in mobile homes where residents frequently complain of rashes, respiratory irritation, nausea, headaches, dizziness, lethargy, or aggravation of bronchial asthma. Within the same home, formaldehyde levels can fluctuate dramatically, depending on environmental conditions. A 15 °F increase in temperature can result in a doubling of formaldehyde levels, while the lowest formaldehyde concentrations have been recorded on cold winter days; similarly, increases in relative humidity cause a corresponding rise in formaldehyde emissions. In terms of its effect as an irritant, there does not appear to be a threshold level for formaldehyde exposure, though few persons experience symptoms when concentrations are below 0.1 ppm.

The National Academy of Sciences estimates that as many as 10–20% of the population experiences some form of irritation due to formaldehyde exposure even at very low levels of concentration. Since formaldehyde is so ubiquitous in the modern environment, avoiding exposure entirely is almost impossible. Nevertheless, sensitive individuals can reduce exposure and thereby minimize symptoms by substituting metal or lumber products for those containing pressed wood or selectively purchasing low formaldehyde-releasing pressed wood construction materials, cabinets, or furniture. Similarly, those allergic to the chemical should always launder permanent-press fabrics prior to use to remove the formaldehyde finish, since a single wash can reduce textile formaldehyde emissions up to 60% (unfortunately, this approach won't work for draperies, which are also large formaldehyde emitters).

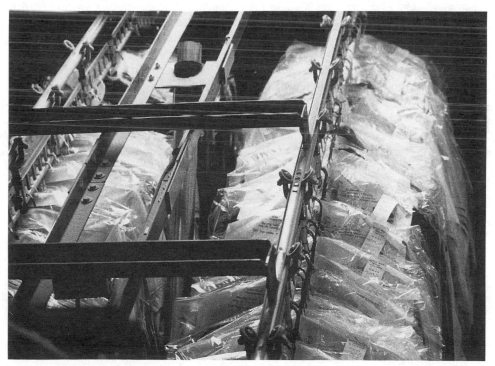

This Is A
"Non-Smoking"
Restaurant.

Thank You. McDonald's

318A

Signs such as this are increasingly being seen in shopping malls, restaurants, and other public places where environmental tobacco smoke has become an unwelcome indoor air pollutant. [Nora Byrne]

Such ordinary items as dry-cleaned clothes can expose household residents to toxic fumes. [Ian Weissman]

BOX 12-5

A Hidden Menace in Your Home?

Radon detection businesses have been proliferating rapidly following EPA's announcement advising that homes nationwide be tested for the presence of this apparently ubiquitous indoor air pollutant. Concerned homeowners, deterred by the hefty fee charged by many entrepreneurs offering radon monitoring services, should be heartened to learn that they can purchase relatively inexpensive devices that will give a reasonably accurate indication of the extent of radon problems in the user's home.

The two most popular do-it-yourself home radon detectors are 1) charcoal canisters—small containers of activated charcoal that should be opened and left in place for three to seven days, then sealed and returned to the manufacturer for analysis and 2) alpha track detectors that are left in place for several weeks to as long as one year. Since radon levels can fluctuate considerably from day to day and season to season, alpha track detectors are good for determining yearly averages; charcoal canisters are useful for short-term screening tests, but since their results are indicative only of radon levels during the few days when the test was performed, they may over- or under-represent the actual extent of hazard. Both devices, however, can be effectively used by nonprofessionals to give a rough approximation of radon pollution. If laboratory analysis reveals that radon levels are high, consultation with a radon abatement specialist would be advisable, but if the screening test indicates negligible amounts of the gas, the homeowner is saved the expense of contracting for a radon survey which might cost several hundred dollars.

Those interested in doing their own radon monitoring can improve the accuracy and relevance of the results by understanding a few basic concepts about radon. Because radon infiltrates into homes through the ground, basements are likely to exhibit the highest radon levels. For this reason, if residents want to know the peak concentrations to which they may be exposed, a monitoring device should be located in the basement (or lowest level of the dwelling), placed about 3–6 feet above the floor and away from walls, doors, or windows. However, if occupants spend little time in the basement and want a measurement more representative of the exposure they are receiving, monitors can be placed in living areas of the next highest floor. Another likely spot for monitor placement is near suspected sources of radon entry, such as sump holes or crawl spaces (however, don't use charcoal canisters in humid environments such as bathrooms and kitchens; the charcoal absorbs moisture and test results will not be accurate). Since monitoring devices are relatively inexpensive, it may be advisable to use two or three simultaneously in different areas of the house. Radon concentrations in most states tend to be highest in winter, so this is the best time for using short-term monitoring devices.

Home radon detectors are available for purchase at hardware stores or supermarkets; information regarding companies offering mail-order services for radon monitoring devices can be obtained from local health departments. Although there are as yet no mandatory standards which radon monitoring equipment or testing laboratories are required to meet, manufacturers may voluntarily submit their products or facilities for EPA evaluation. Therefore, it's a good idea for those considering purchase of a radon detection device to check whether the company is listed as "EPA-approved." Similarly, EPA publishes regularly updated lists of radon measurement and abatement firms which meet the agency's voluntary proficiency standards and recommends that anyone planning to hire a contractor for radon-related work first check that person's professional qualifications as determined by the agency's proficiency programs.

Chemical Fumes and Particles

Numerous household products (including furniture polish, hair sprays, air fresheners, oven-cleaners, paints, carpeting, pesticides, disinfectants, solvents, etc.), release chemical fumes and particles that can reach very high levels indoors. While relatively little research has been done on the health impact of inhaling these substances on a regular basis, it is known that several commonly used household chemicals cause cancer in laboratory animals. Paradichlorobenzene, the active ingredient in moth crystals and many air fresheners and room deodorants, as well as limonene, another odorant, present perhaps the highest cancer risk among indoor organic chemicals. Tetrachloroethylene, a solvent used in dry cleaning, is another carcinogen to which household residents may receive significant exposure when wearing freshly dry-cleaned garments or by breathing emissions from closets in which such articles were stored (Smith, 1988).

When used in accordance with instructions, most household chemicals are not known to provoke acute health effects. However, use of pesticides inside homes has occasionally resulted in a wide range of health complaints, including headaches, nausea, vertigo, skin rashes, and emotional disorders. Chlordane, which for almost 40 years was the most widely used insecticide for controlling termites, was taken off the market in 1988 in response to hundreds of complaints about alleged chlordane-induced illnesses among residents following pesticidal applications in homes. Inappropriate pesticide use inside homes can result in long-term exposure to toxic residues and vapors. Chemicals that break down quickly outdoors in the presence of sunlight and bacteria can persist for years in carpets, presenting an on-going threat to residents (Ott et al., 1998).

Biological Pollutants

A diverse group of living organisms, most of them too small to be seen with the naked eye, also can pose serious air quality problems inside homes and public buildings. Bacteria and fungal spores can enter structures via air handling systems and occasionally cause disease outbreaks (the Legionnaires' Disease episode in Philadelphia in 1976 is the classic example of this sort of occurrence). Many allergies are associated with exposure to household dust which may contain fungal spores, bacteria, animal dander, and feces of roaches or mites. Perhaps most significant in stimulating allergic reactions are live dust mites, tiny arthropods less than 1 millimeter in size that are

BOX 12-6

Smoky Kitchens = Sick Cooks

Aside from the occasional finger nicked with a paring knife, meal preparation isn't regarded as a particularly hazardous occupation by those of us living in the industrialized world. Nevertheless, in over 100 countries where firewood, animal dung, charcoal, crop residues, or coal constitute the main domestic fuel source, the simple task of cooking dinner is killing millions of women and their children every year. Indoor air pollution, mostly generated by unvented cookstoves or open fires, is regarded by the World Health Organization (WHO) as one of the four most critical environmental problems in developing countries, responsible for as many as 2.8 million deaths annually. Stoking fires and stirring pots in the close confines of small, poorly ventilated kitchens, housewives throughout the Third World daily work in a smoke-laden environment with direct exposure to toxic emissions. As a result, they and the small children who spend most of their time close to mother are falling ill and often dying from diseases provoked by indoor air pollution.

Of the various ailments associated with cookstove emissions, acute respiratory infections affect the largest number of people, with infants and toddlers the most frequent victims. Studies of Zulu children in South Africa found that youngsters living in homes with wood cookstoves were five times more likely to be hospitalized with severe respiratory infections. In Nepal, a significant correlation was found between the incidence of moderate to severe respiratory infections among 2-year-olds and the number of hours they spent near a fire. In Gambia, researchers found that babies whose mothers carried them on their backs while cooking were 2.5 times more likely to contract life-threatening pneumococcal infections than were children not exposed to wood smoke. Adult women experiencing long-term smoke exposure are themselves at high risk of developing chronic lung diseases such as emphysema, bronchitis, and asthma. A study conducted in Mexico among women who had been exposed to wood smoke for many years found their risk of lung disease was equivalent to that of heavy smokers and 75 times that of women not exposed. Cancer is another health threat associated with this form of indoor air pollution, as are reproductive problems such as stillbirths, low birth weight babies, and difficulties during delivery for women who inhale cookstove emissions during pregnancy.

The types of pollutants emitted from cookstoves vary, depending on the type of fuel burned. Biomass fuels—wood, charcoal, crop residues, animal dung—are the dirtiest. Used by an estimated 2.5–3 billion of the world's poorest people, wood and other biofuels emit levels of particulate matter many times higher than WHO limits and significantly add to the haze of pollution blanketing virtually every developing world city today.

Coal, though considered a step up the energy ladder from biofuels in terms of pollutant emissions, is nevertheless a dirty fuel as well, emitting prodigious amounts of $PM_{2.5}$, the most dangerous form of particulate matter. In China, where close to 400 million people rely on coal as their chief domestic fuel, the problem of indoor air pollution has assumed major proportions in both rural and urban areas. The coal used in Chinese cookstoves is, for the most part, mined from deposits containing excessive traces of toxic elements such as arsenic, mercury, fluorine, and antimony. Used directly without washing, these coals release toxic emissions when burned. The situation is made worse in some parts of China by the practice of drying certain agricultural products, such as chili peppers and corn, directly over coal fires. Doing so results in volatilized toxic metals concentrating in the dried foods. In China's southwestern Guizhou Province, several thousand people suffer from chronic arsenic poisoning due to eating arsenic-contaminated dried chillies (while fresh chili peppers contain less than 1 ppm arsenic, those dried over high-arsenic coal fires have levels that exceed 500 ppm). Many more Chinese—an estimated 10 million—are experiencing bone deformities and dental fluorosis due to fluoride contamination of foods dried over dirty coal fires. Millions of Chinese homemakers are affected by volatile organic compounds released by coal-burning cookstoves. Polycyclic aromatic hydrocarbons (PAHs) from unvented coal stoves are believed to be the main cause for the high incidence of lung cancer in China. In homes where smoky coal is burned, the lung cancer death rate is five times above the national average. Studies conducted in China by EPA researchers found a strong association between lung cancer incidence in women and the length of time they had spent cooking indoors. Blood samples taken from the women, along with indoor air analyses, demonstrated that indoor coal-burning was to blame for the observed cancers.

The solution to these problems is perfectly straightforward: replace wood and coal-burning stoves with those fueled by natural gas or electricity. Even liquid fuels such as kerosene and liquified petroleum gas (LPG) would be far preferable to the dirty fuels so widely used today. Unfortu-nately, a rapid changeover is scarcely conceivable, given the widespread poverty in the countries affected and the sheer numbers of households still dependent on biofuels or coal. In the short term, efforts to improve the health of women and children sickened by poor indoor air quality have focused on designing a better cookstove. Over the past two decades nearly 200 projects have been launched throughout the Third World to develop appropriate cookstove technologies using locally available materials to produce improved stoves at a price poor people can afford. While the main intent of most of these programs has been to enhance the energy efficiency of the stoves rather than improving indoor air quality, many of the newer models that use a flue or chimney to remove smoke from the house have succeeded in substantially reducing pollutants as well (unfortunately, by diverting smoky emissions from inside to outside the house, improved cookstoves have worsened neighborhood air quality problems). Among the more successful cookstove projects has been the Kenya Ceramic Jiko project, which has distributed almost a million energy-efficient, charcoal-burning ceramic-lined stoves since the mid-1980s. Though its $2–5 price tag is still too expensive for many rural villagers, the Jiko has become quite popular in urban Kenyan households, more than half of which now own one. A government-subsidized program in India to promote improved cookstoves has met with only limited success, but efforts in China have been much more fruitful. More than 120 million stoves have been distributed in that country, where nearly 70% of rural families now possess one. Among urban Chinese, access to gas for cooking has substantially increased, with about one-third now utilizing this cleaner fuel. Among those still burning coal, less-polluting, more energy-efficient briquettes are gaining in popularity.

Despite notable progress in some countries to advance the use of cleaner fuels, for many of the world's poorest people, any change in current conditions remains but a distant hope. National governments could, if they desired to do so, help speed up the transition by adopting policies to reduce the cost of new stoves or to subsidize the cost of service connections for electricity. Differential electricity charges could be very beneficial as well; in Thailand, poor urban households that use very little electricity are charged lower rates than better-off consumers who use more. As a result, virtually all urban Thai homes are electrified. Unfortunately, in the developing world, as elsewhere, indoor air pollution—despite its enormous health costs—receives scant attention in comparison with outdoor air quality prob-

lems. The cookstove projects undertaken over the past two decades have operated on shoestring budgets and additional funding has been extremely difficult to obtain. Without a reordering of priorities by national governments and international lending institutions, Third World kitchens are likely to remain smoke-filled, dangerously unhealthy environments.

References
Finkelman, R.B., et al. 1999. "Health Impacts of Domestic Coal Use in China." *Proceedings of the National Academy of Sciences* 96 (March):3427-31.

Kammen, D.M. 1995. "Cookstoves for the Developing World." *Scientific American* (July):72-75.

World Resources Institute. 1998. *World Resources 1998-99: Environmental Change and Human Health.* Oxford University Press.

found in enormous numbers on bedsheets and blankets where they feed on sloughed-off scales of skin. Humid conditions or the presence of stagnant water seem to favor buildup of large populations of these unwanted guests and their dissemination has sometimes been associated with the use of humidifiers or vaporizers which harbored fungal or bacterial growth. Flooding problems or other water damage to homes can result in an indoor air quality problem that was largely unrecognized until the mid-1990s. Growth of the toxic fungus *Stachybotrys chartarum* on damp wallpaper, ceiling tiles, carpeting made of natural fibers, cardboard boxes, bundles of newspapers, and, especially, the paper covering sheetrock can cause serious illness among residents of affected structures. Symptoms can include headaches, respiratory distress, recurring colds, heart palpitations, fatigue, skin rashes, and general malaise. In Cleveland, Ohio, at least 12 infants died during 1993–94 of bleeding lung disease, thought to have been provoked by high levels of mold growing in their water-damaged homes. Detecting the presence of *S. chartarum* requires careful inspection of areas that may not be readily visible—in wall voids, above false ceilings, in basements—any place where leaks, condensation, or sustained flooding could occur. The fungal mass is black in appearance, slightly shiny when fresh and powdery when dry. Although the mold won't continue to grow once it dries out, spores can be sucked up by the furnace fan and spread throughout a dwelling. If mold growth is found in a structure, the situation requires prompt action, first to correct the water problem and then to clean up the mold. The latter step usually requires professional help, since householders are not advised to tackle any mold-contaminated area larger than two square feet. The surface of small areas can be disinfected using 1 cup of chlorine bleach in a gallon of water (rubber gloves and a dust mask should be worn while working). However, the fungal mycelium within the contaminated material often survives surface disinfection and may subsequently resume growth. Thus it is usually advisable to discard and replace fungal-infested materials (Nelson, 1999).

Sick Building Syndrome

Some indoor air pollutants can provoke complaints among building occupants of problems such as chest tightness, muscle aches, cough, fever, and chills. These symptoms of what is now termed **building related illness (BRI)** may persist for an extended time period after affected persons leave the building, but they have clearly identifiable causes and can be clinically diagnosed. By contrast, a somewhat more mysterious malady reported with increased frequency since the mid-1970s is a condition described as **sick building syndrome (SBS).** SBS refers to situations where building occupants experience various forms of acute discomfort—eye irritation, scratchiness in the throat, dry cough, headache, itchy skin, fatigue, difficulty in concentrating, nausea and dizziness—but no causative agent of such symptoms can be found. Furthermore, these symptoms generally vanish soon after sufferers leave the building (sometimes the complaints are associated with only one part of the building or even with a single room). This situation has become so widespread in recent years that a committee of the World Health Organization has suggested that as many as 30% of the world's new and remodeled buildings may be generating complaints. While some of the symptoms reported may, in fact, be caused by illnesses contracted somewhere else, by preexisting allergies, or by job-related stress, in many cases poor indoor air quality is the major culprit. Although some of the reported outbreaks of sick building syndrome are eventually traced to specific pollutants—e.g. microorganisms spread through ventilation systems, vehicle exhausts entering intake vents, ozone emissions from photocopying machines, VOCs outgassing from new carpeting—in most cases these contaminants aren't present in concentrations high enough to provoke the reported symptoms. Synthetic mineral fibers released into the air from acoustical ceiling tile and insulating material have been identified by researchers at Cornell University as the prime cause of many SBS situations. Most often, however, SBS has been traced to inadequate ventilation and its rise in frequency parallels efforts since the 1973 Arab oil embargo to incorporate energy conservation features into building design.

Unlike the situation in homes, most new nonresidential structures are equipped with mechanical heating, ventilation, and air conditioning (HVAC) systems and feature windows tightly sealed to restrict air infiltration from outside. These HVAC systems recirculate air throughout the building, with a significant portion of the air being reused several times prior to being exhausted, the purpose of such reuse being to lessen energy costs for heating or cooling incoming fresh air. Building codes require that a specified minimum amount of outside air be provided in order to establish an acceptable balance

BOX 12-7
Multiple Chemical Sensitivity: Fact or Fantasy?

A new public health problem is being reported with increasing frequency across the nation, its symptoms provoking angry debate among health care providers and toxicologists who have not yet reached consensus on whether the ailment reported by thousands of sufferers is real or simply "in their heads."

Multiple chemical sensitivity (MCS) represents a condition in which some people claim to develop a wide range of potentially debilitating symptoms from exposure to an ever-expanding range of chemical substances at lower and lower levels. Among those most likely to claim chemical sensitivity are Gulf War veterans, people working in "sick buildings," those living near hazardous waste sites, and workers in certain industries. The chemicals blamed for these maladies are ones that most people tolerate without any ill effects whatsoever and the phenomenon itself cannot be explained in terms of any known medical or psychiatric disorder. Development of MCS is a two-step process; exposure to a significant amount of some environmental chemical (e.g. a pesticide, solvent, combustion product, etc.) "sensitizes" the victim, who then begins to experience severe reactions to even minute amounts of other commonplace substances such as perfume or cigarette smoke. Reported symptoms vary widely but include such complaints as muscle aches and pains, headaches, dizziness, fatigue, and nausea. These symptoms develop within a relatively short time after some sort of change in that person's environment. Exposure to vapors from a newly installed carpet, a whiff of a coworker's aftershave lotion, entering a room recently treated with pesticides—all are examples

of typical events capable of triggering an MCS attack. In some cases sufferers are unable to recall any single, obvious high-dose exposure that could have led to the onset of symptoms, causing some researchers to conclude that repeated, cumulative exposure to low levels of certain chemicals may also give rise to MCS symptoms.

Other investigators draw quite a different conclusion from these same facts, regarding MCS as some sort of modern neurasthenia. Indeed, most medical authorities are highly skeptical, if not downright disbelieving, of the existence of MCS as a true physiological ailment. Among the professional health care groups to reject MCS as an established organic disease are the American Medical Association, the American College of Physicians, and the American Academy of Allergy and Immunology. Their lack of acceptance is based not only on the fact that MCS is perhaps the only illness in which the patient defines both the cause and the symptoms of his or her own disease, but also because MCS violates all the fundamental tenets of toxicological science. Critics are troubled by the fact that MCS produces no objective evidence of disease that can be tested and observed in the clinical setting; the major symptoms are subjective ones—stomach pains, poor memory, difficulty concentrating, and "woozy head." The ailment is not associated with any specific chemical nor with any specific effect; in fact, descriptions of MCS include accounts of how symptoms spread from one organ to another over time for no apparent reason. The dose-response relationship so basic to toxicological theory appears foreign to MCS—severity of symptoms appears to be entirely independent of the amount of exposure. Finally, there is no proven mechanism of illness, no generally accepted physiological data to explain how trace amounts of chemicals could produce the adverse health effects being reported. And MCS sufferers generally *look* reasonably healthy, even when they *feel* miserable!

Judging by their own accounts, victims *do* feel miserable as they develop an increasingly broad range of symptoms that can render them partially to totally disabled. Many patients report they can no longer engage in such commonplace activities as shopping, working in conventional office or industrial settings, dining in restaurants—even living in a typically furnished home. One young woman afflicted with MCS felt compelled to move out of her house to live year-round in a tent due to the multiple chemical exposures indoors that rendered her constantly ill.

Regardless of whether or not MCS is a valid medical concern, it definitely has become a social and economic issue high on the activist agenda. Protest groups use MCS as a sympathy-generating weapon against the chemical industry, publishing newsletters and maintaining websites attesting to the sufferings of MCS victims. Multiple chemical sensitivity has been defined as a disability under the Americans with Disabilities Act, enabling those claiming affliction to demand special accommodation at work or school. Some states recognize MCS as a disability under workers' compensation laws, resulting in free medical care and payment for lost wages for eligible workers. Hundreds of personal injury lawsuits alleging harm have been filed against manufacturers of paints, carpets, household cleaning supplies, and a wide variety of other consumer products. Many of these cases are settled out of court or are dismissed, and a 1993 Supreme Court decision *(Daubert vs. Merrell Dow)* has given trial judges the right to exclude unscientific testimony; nevertheless, cases continue to be filed.

More research on chemical sensitivity is sorely needed, particularly in light of its severe social, financial, and emotional repercussions. In 1998 the federal government convened an interagency work group to review the scientific literature on MCS and to develop recommendations on technical and policy issues. The panel, predictably, called for additional research on MCS, with focus on such glaring data gaps as the ailment's mechanism of action. The group also called for an information campaign to raise physicians' awareness and understanding of the problem. Whether additional studies simply confirm the contention of mainstream health practitioners that MCS is not a medical problem remains to be seen. Regardless of the scientific findings, MCS sufferers will continue to regard themselves as "miners' canaries," warning society of the dangers of an increasingly toxic environment.

References

Gist, G.L. 1999. "Multiple Chemical Sensitivity—The Role of Environmental Health Professional." *Journal of Environmental Health* 61, no. 6 (Jan/Feb.).4–5.

Mazell, M.K., and Suruda, A. 1998. "Multiple Chemical Sensitivity Syndrome." *American Family Physician* 58, no. 3 (Sept. 1):721–28.

between oxygen and CO_2 indoors, to dilute odors, and to remove contaminants generated within the structure. Prior to 1973 that specified minimum was approximately 15 cubic feet per minute (cfm) per building occupant; after 1973 the standard was reduced to just 5 cfm, an amount which, in a number of situations, proved inadequate for maintaining healthy, comfortable conditions. In some situations HVAC systems were improperly installed, had defective equipment, or functioned poorly because of improper vent placement. When errors such as these occur, an insufficient amount of ventilation air will be supplied. Once such problems are identified, they can generally be corrected by repairing or adjusting the air handling system to provide additional outside air; in some cases, however, building design itself may be at fault, requiring much more extensive renovations (Turiel, 1985; EPA, 1991; Beek, 1994).

In general, the public has been slow to demand action on this problem because access to information about indoor air pollutants has been very limited and possibly because people don't want to believe that pollution problems have invaded the home. Nevertheless, an increasing awareness of the threat posed by indoor air pollutants has stimulated thinking on new ways of dealing with this problem. Monitoring and enforcing air quality standards inside millions of American homes is obviously impossible. However, standards could be set to control pollutant emissions by modifying product design or manufacture. For example, the United States has set standards regulating emissions of formaldehyde from plywood and is considering regulating emissions from unvented fossil-fuel heating appliances; there have even been proposals to require catalytic converters on wood stoves! In the future, updated building codes which incorporate design features and materials which minimize release and retention of indoor air pollutants could ensure that most new structures have acceptable air quality. In the meantime, efforts must be made to educate homeowners and occupants on the impact personal behavior and consumer choices can have on the quality of the indoor environment. Decisions as to which products we buy, how we use certain appliances, our consideration for the health of others as reflected in personal smoking habits—all have a profound impact on indoor air quality and will ultimately determine the success or failure of any government effort to minimize indoor air pollution (Nero, 1988).

References

Acid Rain: What It Is. 1982. National Wildlife Federation.

Air Pollution Primer. 1969. National Tuberculosis and Respiratory Disease Association.

Beek, Jim. 1994. "Man-Made Minerals Could Be Key to SBS." *Indoor Air Review* 3, no. 11 (Jan).

Boyle, Robert, and R. Alexander Boyle. 1983. *Acid Rain.* Schocken Books/Nick Lyons Books.

Brown, Lester R., Michael Renner, and Christopher Flavin. 1998. *Vital Signs 1998.* W.W. Norton.

———. 1997. *Vital Signs 1997.* W.W. Norton.

Bryner, Gary C. 1993. *Blue Skies, Green Politics: The Clean Air Act of 1990.* CQ Press.

Cobb, Nathaniel, and Ruth A. Etzel. 1991. "Unintentional Carbon Monoxide-Related Deaths in the United States, 1979 through 1988." *Journal of the American Medical Association* 266, no. 5 (Aug).

Cohen, C. J., L. C. Grothaus, and S. C. Perrigan. 1982. "Effects of Simulated Sulfuric and Sulfuric-Nitric Acid Rain on Crop Plants: Results of 1980 Crop Survey." *Special Report* 670, Agricultural Experiment Station, Oregon State University, Corvallis.

Dockery, Douglas W., et al. 1993. "An Association Between Air Pollution and Mortality in Six U.S. Cities." *The New England Journal of Medicine* 329, no. 24 (Dec. 9).

"Easy Guide to the Air Toxics Law." 1993. *The Environmental Manager's Compliance Advisor,* no. 344 (Feb. 1).

Environmental Law Handbook, 12th ed. 1993. Government Institutes, Inc.

Environmental Protection Agency. 1991. *Indoor Air Facts* No. 4 (revised), *Sick Building Syndrome.* ANR-455-W, April.

Evelyn, John. 1661. *Fumifugium.* London National Society for Clean Air, 1969.

Health Effects of Air Pollution. 1978. American Thoracic Society.

Kerr, Richard A. 1998. "Acid Rain Control: Success on the Cheap." *Science* 282 (Nov. 6):1024–1027.

Lawrence, Gregory B., and T.G. Huntington. 1999. *Soil Calcium Depletion Linked to Acid Rain and Forest Growth in the Eastern United States.* U.S. Geological Survey, WRIR 98-4267 (February).

Likens, G.E., C.T. Driscoll, and D.C. Buso. 1996. "Long-Term Effects of Acid Rain: Response and Recovery of a Forest Ecosystem." *Science* 272, no. 5259 (April 16):244–246.

McDonald, Alan. 1999. "Combating Acid Deposition and Climate Change: Priorities for Asia." *Environment* 41, no. 3 (April): 4-11, 34-41.

Munton, Don. 1998. "Dispelling the Myths of the Acid Rain Story." *Environment* 40, no. 6 (July/August):4–7, 27–34.

National Science & Technology Council (NSTC). 1998. *National Acid Precipitation Assessment Program Biennial Report to Congress: An Integrated Assessment* (May).

Nelson, Berlin. 1999. *Stachybotrys chartarum: The Toxic Indoor Mold.* American Phytopathological Society, APSnet Feature (February).

Nero, Anthony V., Jr. 1988. "Controlling Indoor Air Pollution." *Scientific American* 258, no. 5 (May).

Ott, Wayne R., and John W. Roberts. 1998. "Everyday Exposure to Toxic Pollutants." *Scientific American* (February):86–91.

Rhodes, S. L., and P. Middleton. 1983. "The Complex Challenge of Controlling Acid Rain." *Environment* 22, no. 4 (May).

Smith, Kirk R. 1988. "Air Pollution: Assessing Total Exposure in the United States." *Environment* 30, no. 8 (Oct).

Turiel, Isaac. 1985. *Indoor Air Quality and Human Health.* Stanford University Press.

Waldbott, George L. 1978. *Health Effects of Environmental Pollutants.* C. V. Mosby.

Wallace, L. A. 1987. *Total Exposure Assessment Methodology* (TEAM Study: Summary and Analysis), vol. 1, Environmental Protection Agency.

Ware, J. H., et al. 1984. "Passive Smoking, Gas Cooking, and Respiratory Health of Children Living in Six Cities." *American Review of Respiratory Disease* 129:366–74.

Weller, Phil. 1980. *Acid Rain: The Silent Crisis.* Between the Lines & the Waterloo Public Interest Research Group.

World Resources Institute (WRI). 1998. *World Resources 1998-99.* Oxford University Press.

———. 1996. *World Resources 1996-97.* Oxford University Press.

———. 1992. *World Resources 1992-93.* Oxford University Press.

———. 1990. *World Resources 1990-91.* Oxford University Press.

CHAPTER 13

Noise Pollution

Noise, n. A stench in the ear. . . .The chief product and authenticating sign of civilization.

—Devil's Dictionary (1911)

An ever-increasing cacophony of sound is today grudgingly accepted as an inescapable component of the modern urban environment. From the traffic-clogged streets of New York and Paris to the bustling bazaars of Bombay and the crowded sidewalks of Hong Kong, the blessings of "the quiet life," extolled by poets of yesteryear, are increasingly difficult to procure. Unfortunately, public and policymakers alike tend to regard noise as an inevitable by-product of modern life, sometimes unpleasant but largely unavoidable. At the same time, polls taken among urban residents in both the United States and Europe reveal that most city dwellers certainly are bothered by noise. A "quality of life" telephone survey commissioned by New York Mayor Giuliani in the autumn of 1996 registered more complaints about noise than any other irritant, including crime. Similarly, a poll conducted by a research group in the United Kingdom found that one out of every three Britons felt their enjoyment of life was diminished by noisy neighbors or the din of traffic (Bond, 1996). In Greece, reputedly the noisiest nation in Europe, a senior member of the Association for the Quality of Life recently remarked that "noise pollution is becoming the country's greatest health threat. If effective measures are not taken, Greeks will either turn mad or deaf."

Sources of Noise

Most concerns about noise as a pollutant have focused on the occupational environment where high levels of noise associated with machinery, equipment, and general work practices have long been recognized as a serious threat to both the physical and psychological health of workers. However, the sources of noise that torment the general public are far more diverse than

**Figure 13-1 Examples of Outdoor Day-Night Average Sound Levels
in dB Measured at Various Locations**

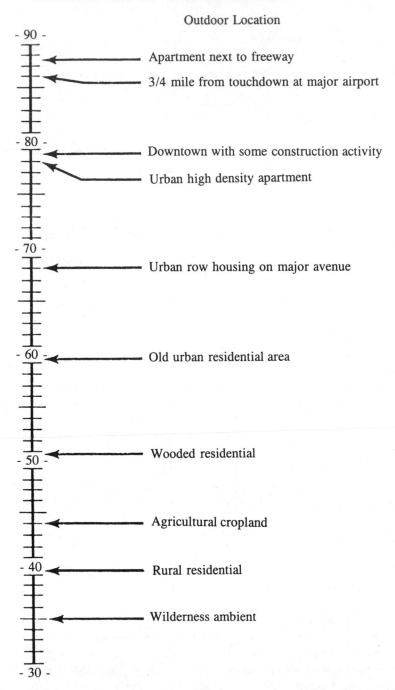

Source: EPA, *Protective Noise Levels,* EPA 550/9–79–100.

those which constitute an occupational hazard. Around the world, rapidly growing numbers of cars, trucks, and motorcycles have been boosting noise levels on crowded streets and highways, while the skies above metropolitan neighborhoods are regularly deafened by the roar of jets taking off or landing at urban airports. Even once-quiet residential areas are losing their tranquility as noise-generating home appliances and motorized yard tools are increasingly regarded as essential components of the good life. While most people perceive community noise as a general din, originating from a multiplicity of sources, vehicular noise—particularly that from motorcycles and large trucks—seems to be regarded as the most annoying by community residents. Unfortunately, overall noise levels are growing steadily worse, in part because modern lifestyles and transportation habits are changing in ways that inevitably result in more noise generation. We are also carrying noise with us to places that formerly were havens of peace and quiet. The advent of snowmobiles, trail bikes, and powerful motorboats have brought noise pollution to once-silent wilderness areas; amplified music now jars city parks when partying crowds forget that not everyone finds loud rock bands pleasurable, and the desert air occasionally reverberates to a similar beat, thanks to "boom car" sound-offs where enthusiasts compete to see whose car stereos are the most ear splitting.

Beyond the technological and lifestyle changes that have made contemporary life noisier than in days gone by, there are simply more of us on the planet, adding to the din. For the most part, levels of outdoor noise are directly related to population density—the more populous the city, the noisier conditions are likely to be. Predicted trends in noise levels are not particularly encouraging. One of the most important sources of excessive community noise, urban traffic, is expected to increase considerably in the years immediately ahead, with the U.S. Department of Transportation estimating that the number of automobiles on the road will increase by 0.6–0.7% annually. Overseas, a study on noise control strategies revealed that efforts taken to reduce traffic noise in several western European countries (e.g. screens along main highways) helped to offset the increase in traffic noise but didn't result in an overall lowering of noise exposure—simply because of the rapid increase in size of the car fleet. In the Netherlands alone, private car ownership is projected to increase from 4.6 million in 1985 to 7.9 million by 2010, during which time passenger traffic on that nation's highways will grow by 70%; truck traffic is expected to increase by an even larger percentage. Europeans have been experimenting with rerouting traffic, prohibiting vehicles entirely in certain areas, and constructing noise screens, a combination of which has resulted in some lowering of noise levels in central cities. However, the spread of residential suburbs into rural areas is resulting in a steady expansion of noise exposure into areas formerly undisturbed by such problems (OECD, 1991).

Noise As a Nuisance

More than 2000 years ago, the Roman Emperor Julius Caesar grappled with the issue of noise as a public nuisance when he attempted to ban chariot racing on the Eternal City's cobblestone streets due to the racket it created. History doesn't record whether or not he was successful, but as the clamor of

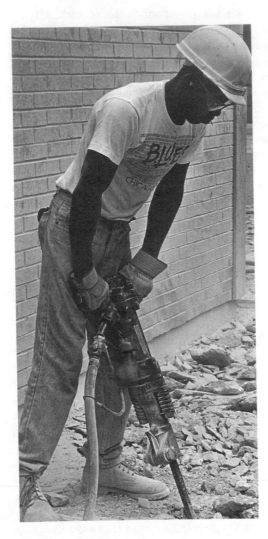

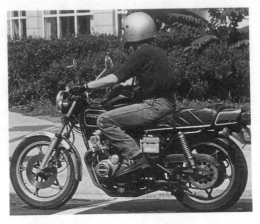

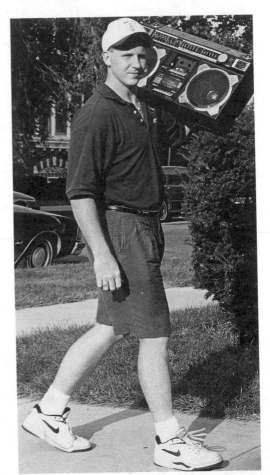

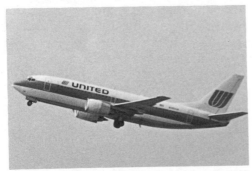

Millions of Americans are dally being exposed to levels of noise that could permanently damage their ability to hear. *[Photos by Nora Byrne]*

urban life continued to increase during the ensuing centuries, the irritant value of noise grew apace and has occasionally caused frayed tempers to snap, sometimes with fatal results. An elderly Greek farmer is currently serving two life sentences in a maximum security prison for shooting two residents of a neighboring apartment who ignored his repeated complaints about the loud music blasting from their residence. When taken into custody, the old man said that all he wanted was to listen to the evening news in peace ("Mad About...," 1998). In Japan a newspaper reported that a woman in densely populated Kawasaki picked up a neighbor's dog and threw it out the window of her apartment, exclaiming that the animal's constant barking was driving her to distraction. The enraged neighbor then retaliated by stabbing the woman to death! Perhaps to avoid just such altercations, more and more Japanese city dwellers are having their canine pets' vocal chords cut or are fitting them with antibarking shock collars to make sure they remain quiet all day in the tiny, yardless living quarters typical of modern Japan (Shapiro, 1989).

Just as beauty is in the eye of the beholder, the perception of a sound as "noise" (arbitrarily defined by some writers as "unwanted sound") depends on the point of view of the individual listener. A case in point was recently reported from South Aukland, New Zealand, where two churches were warned by the Manukau City Council that they would be forced to close if they didn't tone down their hymn-singing, whose loudness had prompted numerous complaints by church neighbors. Unfortunately for those attempting to set standards regulating noise exposure, loudness of a noise and the annoyance it causes are not always directly correlated. As any college student partying near a residential neighborhood well knows, people *generating* loud sounds may frequently enjoy them, while those forced to listen usually find the same noise profoundly objectionable. In general, people most easily tolerate noise when 1) they are causing it, 2) they feel it is necessary or useful to them, or 3) they know where it is coming from. To the extent that other people exposed to the same sounds do not experience equivalent benefits from the noise, conflict between participating and nonparticipating groups is generated (Bugliarello et al., 1976).

While most people are well acquainted with the feelings of annoyance and irritation that unwanted sounds can arouse, it is becoming increasingly evident that noise levels commonly encountered in thousands of cities, factories, places of recreation, and even inside homes represent far more than a simple nuisance. Noise today has become a public health hazard; more insidious than easily-recognized air and water pollution, noise is invisibly undermining the physical and psychological well-being of millions of people around the world. The remainder of this chapter will describe the ways in which noise affects human health, but first it is necessary to take a brief look at the physical nature of sound and how noise levels are measured.

Nature of Sound

Sound is produced by the compression and expansion of air created when an object vibrates. The positive and negative pressure waves thus formed travel outward longitudinally from the vibrating source. Two basic characteristics of sound, **frequency** (or **pitch**) and **amplitude**, are related to how loud and annoying a sound will be perceived.

Frequency describes the rate of vibration—how fast the object is moving back and forth. The more rapid the movement, the higher the frequency of the sound pressure waves created. The standard unit used today for measuring frequency is the **hertz (Hz),** equivalent to one wave per second passing a given point. Most people can hear sounds within a frequency range of 20–20,000 Hz, though there exists a great deal of individual variation in ability to perceive very low or very high frequency sounds. Because low-frequency sounds (e.g. bass sounds from amplified music, traffic noise) are more penetrating than those of high frequency, they are more difficult to control by shielding and thus are often the main source of irritation related to community noise.

Amplitude refers to the intensity of sound—how much energy is behind the sound wave. Sound waves of the same frequency can be heard as very loud or very soft, depending on the force with which they strike the ear. In technical terms, amplitude measures the maximum displacement of a sound wave from its resting, or equilibrium, position, but it is perceived psychologically as **loudness.** The unit for measuring intensity, or amplitude, of sound is the **decibel (dB)**; the decibel scale ranges from 0, which is regarded as the threshold of hearing for normal, healthy ears, to 194, regarded as the threshold for pure tones. Because any increase of 10 dB will result in a doubling of perceived loudness, even a small rise in decibel values can make a significant difference in noise intensity.

A listener's perception of a sound as loud, however, does not depend entirely on its amplitude, being affected to some extent by its frequency as well. Although hearing ability ranges from 20–20,000 Hz, not all of these frequencies sound equally loud to the human ear. Maximum sensitivity to sound occurs in the 1,000–5,000 Hz range. For reference, normal human speech frequencies can vary from 500–2,000 Hz. However, sounds at the very low or very high ends of the full audible range seem much fainter to our ears than do those in the middle frequencies. Thus, for example, an extremely low-pitched sound must have an amplitude many times greater than a sound of medium pitch in order for both to be heard as equally loud. For this reason, decibel values are sometimes weighted to take into account the frequency response of the human ear. When this is done, the unit measurement designation may be written as dB(A). Table 13–1 indicates approximate decibel values for a number of commonly encountered sounds.

Noise and Hearing Loss

...I've shot my hearing; it hurts and it's painful, and it's frustrating when little children talk to you and you can't hear them.

—Pete Townshend

While everyone has experienced irritation due to noise, many people are unaware that the sounds which annoy them may also be affecting their hearing. Pete Townshend's confession during a 1989 press conference that his career as a rock musician had irreversibly damaged his hearing may not have

Table 13-1   Sound Levels and Human Response

Common Sounds	Noise Level (dB)	Effect
Air raid siren	140	Painfully loud
Jet takeoff	130	
Discotheque	120	Maximum vocal effort
Pile driver	110	
Garbage Truck	100	
City Traffic	90	Very annoying, hearing damage
Alarm clock	80	Annoying
Freeway traffic	70	Phone use difficult
Air conditioning	60	Intrusive
Light auto traffic	50	Quiet
Living room	40	
Library	30	Very quiet
Broadcasting studio	20	
	10	Just audible
	0	Hearing begins

Source: U.S. Environmental Protection Agency.

dampened fans' enthusiasm for ear-splitting concerts, but it did serve as a warning to the general public that "feeling the beat" may produce longer-lasting results than the temporary high elicited by good vibrations. Unfortunately, Townshend is but one among the estimated 10 million Americans who have already suffered full or partial hearing loss due to excessive noise exposure; according to EPA, at least 20 million people in the U.S. are daily being exposed to noise levels that will permanently damage their ability to hear.

Most people are familiar with the temporary deafness and ringing in the ears that occurs after sudden exposure to a very loud noise such as a cap gun or firecracker exploding close to one's head. This type of partial hearing loss generally lasts a few hours at the most and is referred to as **temporary threshold shift (TTS)**. In addition to the obvious impact of sudden, high-intensity sounds, noise research has found that TTS can also result from longer-term exposure (16–48 hours) to noise and that recovery to normal hearing may take as long as two days, depending on both the intensity and duration of noise exposure (Melrick, 1991). The type of short-term hearing loss typified by TTS is an accepted fact of life among workers in noisy occupations, performers and patrons at rock concerts, wildly-cheering spectators at sporting events, and many others. However, most people don't realize that regular, prolonged exposure to noise, even at levels commonly encountered in everyday life, can eventually result in permanent hearing impairment. Because damage to the ear is usually painless and seldom visible, few people recognize the injury they are incurring until it is too late. The Occupational Safety and Health Administration (OSHA) has determined that exposure to daily noise levels averaging just 85 decibels (approximately the loudness of an electric shaver or a food processor) will result in irreversible hearing loss. For this reason, OSHA recommends hearing protection for workers whose 8-hour, time-weighted average noise exposure is at or above 85 decibels; for exposure to noise levels of 90 decibels and above, hearing protection is *required*.

The noise of city traffic, subways, power lawnmowers, motorcycles, certain household appliances, babies screaming, and even people shouting all exceed the decibel level considered "safe." Above 85 dB, progressively higher levels of noise exposure exert ever-increasing risk of damage—and the louder the noise, the shorter the exposure time required to wreak lasting harm. With each additional five decibels of loudness the time required to cause permanent injury is cut in half (Jaret, 1990). For revelers rocking with the beat at a nightclub, where the intensity of sound may hit 120 dB, the damage is done in less than 30 minutes.

Mechanism of Hearing Loss

Noise results in hearing loss through its destructive effect on the delicate hair cells in the Organ of Corti within the cochlea of the inner ear. These hair cells convert fluid vibrations in the inner ear into impulses that are carried by the auditory nerve to the brain, resulting in the sensation of sound. The outer hair cells at the base of the cochlea, primarily associated with high-frequency sounds, are the first to be affected, but continued exposure to loud noise will eventually result in damage to hair cells in other areas of the cochlea. Over a period of time, prolonged exposure to excessive noise levels may result in the complete collapse of individual hair cells, thus affecting the transmission of nerve impulses. The average individual is born with approximately 16,000 sensory receptors within the Organ of Corti; while 30–50% of these hair cells can be destroyed before any measurable degree of hearing loss is detectable, losses above this level result inevitably in an impairment of hearing ability. Unfortunately, there is no method at present by which a doctor can diagnose the beginning stages of noise-induced hearing loss. The earliest warning signs—inability to hear high-frequency sounds—are unlikely to be noticed unless the affected individual has his or her hearing tested for some other reason. By the time enough hair cells have been lost to affect perception of lower-frequency sounds, a process that may require many years of excessive noise exposure, the damage has been done.

This type of hearing loss, categorized as **sensorineural,** is irreversible and cannot be restored by the use of a hearing aid since both the auditory nerve and cochlear structures have been affected. By contrast, hearing loss resulting from infections (e.g. "swimmer's ear," mumps, measles, etc.) or by trauma (e.g. a blow to the head that ruptures the eardrum or puncturing the eardrum with a cotton-tipped swab or toothpick) is referred to as **conductive** hearing loss and can often be corrected by surgery or medication (Thurston and Roberts, 1991). To a limited extent the ear can protect itself against loud continuous noise by a tightening of the membrane at the entrance to the inner ear, thereby dampening sound. However, in situations where noise volume increases very rapidly or instantaneously, as when a military jet makes a low-altitude flyover or someone fires a rifle close to the ear, adaptation processes

BOX 13-1

The Not-So-Friendly Skies

Motor vehicles still top the public's noise complaint list, but aircraft din is a rapidly growing contender for first place, as millions of people worldwide suffer the environmental impacts of airport construction and expansion. In the United States, air travel is the fastest-growing form of transportation, increasing at nearly double the pace of automobile travel. To meet the burgeoning demand, airports nationwide are expanding operations—the Federal Aviation Administration (FAA) reports that 60 of the 100 largest U.S. airports propose to build new runways or runway extensions to accommodate a steadily growing number of daily flights.

All of this means a greater noise burden for communities located near these facilities. Of the numerous environmental problems posed by modern airports—air pollution, odorous fumes, toxic releases, contaminated runoff—noise is by far the most frequent complaint voiced by angry airport neighbors. Concerns expressed by affected residents go well beyond mere annoyance and fear of declining property values; studies demonstrate significant health problems among people subjected to the constant roar of planes overhead. Research conducted in the Netherlands near Amsterdam's Schiphol International Airport revealed that incidence of heart disease had doubled and the use of sleeping pills increased 20–50% during a 10-year period after the addition of a new runway. One resident of the area who keeps a decibel meter on his balcony reports regular readings of 100 dB or higher as aircraft roar overhead every 90 seconds during peak hours. Little wonder that the million Dutch citizens living in the vicinity of Schiphol violently oppose a government plan to add yet a fifth runway, due to be in operation by 2003.

The opening of a new international airport in a rural area outside Munich, Germany, provided researchers from Cornell University an opportunity to observe the impact of noise on a group of elementary school children residing within the airport's noise impact zone. By testing the children both before and after operations at the facility commenced, the Cornell scientists demonstrated that exposure to chronic airport noise caused children to exhibit such stress-related responses as increased blood pressure and elevated adrenaline levels. Nor were the children's adverse reactions restricted to physical symptoms; researchers also found that the youngsters' reading skills and long-term memory were impaired as a result of their noisy surroundings. In the United States, similar reports of reading problems among children in a New York school impacted by aircraft noise constitute persuasive evidence of its harmful effects and should bolster efforts by groups pressing for stronger noise pollution controls.

Airport authorities, often prodded by citizen complaints or municipal lawsuits, have attempted to alleviate noise problems by altering flight patterns to avoid nighttime jet overflights of residential areas. In many cases airports can tap federal funds to soundproof nearby homes and schools or even buy out homeowners whose residences are excessively impacted by airport noise. However, the most significant initiative taken to alleviate airport noise, both in the U.S. and abroad, has been the introduction of the quieter planes required by stricter certification standards of the International Civil Aviation Organization. This new generation of jet aircraft has been credited with a slight decline in air traffic noise throughout the 1980s and into the 1990s. Unfortunately, the sharp increase in air traffic witnessed in recent years—and the continued rapid growth projected for the first decade of the 21st century—threatens to reverse the gains achieved through engineering advancements and regulations. After the year 2000, it is anticipated that the land area and numbers of people exposed to unacceptable levels of airport noise will grow significantly, particularly since efforts to prohibit residential development or commercial construction on land near airports have proven largely futile.

References
Evans, Gary W., Monika Bullinger, and Steffan Hygge. 1998. "Chronic Noise Exposure and Physiological Response: A Prospective Study of Children Living Under Environmental Stress." *Psychological Science* 9, no. 1 (Jan):75–77.

Skelton, Renee. 1996. "The Sky's The Limit?" *Amicus Journal* 18, no. 2 (Summer):31–35.

"Mad About the Noise." 1998. *Time International* 150, no. 48 (July 27):38.

and reflex protective mechanisms don't have time to function effectively. In such cases, risk of damage to the inner ear is greater than it would be if the volume of noise were increasing more slowly (Ising et al., 1990).

Many people take it for granted that a gradual loss of hearing is one of the inevitable consequences of growing older, a belief bolstered by statistics which report that by the age of 65, one out of four Americans is experiencing hearing loss significant enough to interfere with communication; by the time they reach their nineties, nine out of ten seniors are so afflicted. Many researchers are convinced, however, that the extent of the problem is considerably greater than it need be. Some years ago, an audiologist traveled to a remote African village near the Sudan-Ethiopian border to test the hearing of tribe members who had never heard the blare of amplified music or the din of urban traffic. He found that 70-year-old Africans, unlike their American peers, could easily hear sounds as soft as a murmur from as far as 300 feet away (Jaret, 1990). While some degree of age-related hearing loss (clinically described as **presbycusis**) may be inevitable, the Sudanese experience provides a meaningful lesson—one of the best ways to preserve lifelong sharpness of hearing is to limit as much as possible one's exposure to a noisy environment.

Effects of Hearing Loss

Hearing disability caused by noise can range in severity from difficulty in comprehending normal conversation to total deafness. In general, the ability to hear high-frequency sounds is the first thing to be affected by noise exposure; for this reason, tests for early detection of hearing loss should pay special attention to hearing ability in the 4,000 Hz range. People affected often have difficulty hearing such sounds as a clock ticking or telephone ringing and cannot distinguish certain consonants, particularly *s, sh, ch, p, m, t, f,* and *th*. Individuals suffering hearing loss not only have trouble with the volume of speech, but also with its clarity. They frequently accuse people with whom they are speaking of mumbling, particularly when talking on the tele-

Figure 13-2   How We Hear

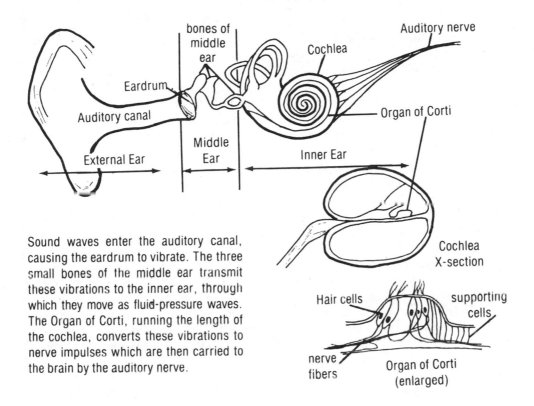

Sound waves enter the auditory canal, causing the eardrum to vibrate. The three small bones of the middle ear transmit these vibrations to the inner ear, through which they move as fluid-pressure waves. The Organ of Corti, running the length of the cochlea, converts these vibrations to nerve impulses which are then carried to the brain by the auditory nerve.

phone or when background noises interfere with conversation; listening to the radio or television may become impossible. The psychological impact of such difficulties—the fear of being laughed at for misunderstanding questions or comments, the frustration of not being able to follow a conversation, the feeling of isolation or alienation experienced as friends unconsciously avoid trying to converse—are frequently as severe as the physical disability. Individuals experiencing hearing loss tend to become suspicious, irritable, and depressed; their careers suffer and their social life becomes severely restricted, sometimes to the point of complete withdrawal (Perham, 1979). Some researchers even suspect that the confusion and unresponsiveness blamed on Alzheimer's disease may actually, in some cases, be due to hearing loss.

In addition to these problems, a person with partial hearing loss may suffer sharp pain in the ears when exposed to very loud noise and may experience repeated bouts of **tinnitus**—a ringing or buzzing sound in the head that can drive the victim to distraction, interfering with sleep, conversation, and normal daily activities. Probably the single most common side effect of noise-induced hearing loss, tinnitus can become a permanent condition, though it is usually only a temporary nuisance. To sufferers, the intensity of the noise in their heads can be maddening, likened by one victim to "holding a vacuum

BOX 13-2

Just Turn It Down!

They seem to be the height of fashion in headgear these days, adorning joggers panting along the roadside, accompanying children walking to school, soothing rush-hour commuters on trains and subways, staving off boredom for those engaged in yard chores, providing background music for college studies. Everyone is wearing them, especially young people who find in these Walkman- or Discman-type portable stereos and headphones a way to carry their music with them wherever they go. The proliferation of these devices and their enormous popularity worldwide has sparked intense debate among noise experts as to the extent to which use of personal stereos has contributed to the documented hearing loss among teenagers and young adults. The question is given urgency by the fact that in the United States alone, more than 20 million personal stereos with headsets have been sold annually in recent years.

While the amount of noise exposure received by a listener obviously varies, depending on the volume setting chosen, most brands are capable of reaching decibel levels of 105 to 126—considerably higher than the 85 dB volume at which damage to hearing begins. Loudness alone, of course, is not the sole determinant of how damaging to the ears personal stereos can be; equally important are the frequency and duration of their use. While the majority of researchers agree that most users select volume settings lower than 90 dB and hence are at minimal risk of long-term hearing damage, a sizable minority turn up the sound levels to more than 100 dB and listen for extended periods of time. Many who misuse their personal stereos in this way report experiencing tinnitus or a sensation of fullness in the ears, indicative of a temporary hearing loss. Unfortunately, incremental hearing loss can't be felt at the time it is occurring unless decibel levels are in excess of 140, the "threshold of pain." To assist listeners in determining when the volume of their Discman is high enough to present a hearing threat, some noise experts urge that manufacturers provide some sort of warning device on stereo units, such as an indicator that lights up when sound intensity exceeds 90 dB or a volume control logo painted red for settings that exceed this noise level. In the absence of such aids, people wishing to safeguard their hearing should keep in mind two simple rules-of-thumb: on a scale of 1–10, any setting above 4 is potentially ear-damaging; and if music from one's headphones is loud enough to be heard by passers-by, it's loud enough to be causing noise-induced hearing loss.

Overall, personal stereos present a minimal auditory hazard, particularly when compared to target-shooting or playing in a rock band. Nevertheless, such devices do have the potential for harm if misused and efforts to educate the public on the importance of protecting their hearing not only from personal stereos but from all sources of excessive environmental noise is sorely needed.

cleaner to your ear" (Murphy, 1989). The pitch of the ringing characterizing tinnitus can sound like a high scream, and volume levels as high as 70 dB have been measured. Among those afflicted with permanent tinnitus, certain medications, diet, or relaxation therapies may ease the symptoms, but the condition at this stage is essentially irreversible (Cohen, 1990).

Other Effects of Noise

Hearing loss is the most obvious health threat posed by noise pollution, but it is by no means the only one. Noise can adversely affect our physical and psychological well-being in a host of other ways.

Stress and Related Health Effects

Exposure to unwanted noise involuntarily induces stress, and stress can lead to a variety of physical ailments including an increase in heart rate, high blood pressure, elevated levels of blood cholesterol, ulcers, headaches, and colitis.

Stressful reaction to loud or sudden noise undoubtedly represents an evolutionary adaptation to warnings signalling approaching danger. Bodily responses to the snarl of a predatory beast or the rumble of a boulder crashing down a mountainside cause a surge of adrenaline, an increase in heart and breathing rates, and the tensing of muscles—all physiological preparations for fight or flight that have important survival value. However, these same metabolic responses are today being triggered repeatedly by the innumerable noises of modern society. As a result, our bodies are subjected to a constant state of stress which, far from being advantageous, is literally making millions of people sick—even though they may not attribute their problems to noise. While many individuals insist that they have "gotten used to noise" and are no longer bothered by it, the truth is that no one can prevent the automatic bio logical changes that noise provokes.

Teratogenic Effects of Noise

The human uterus is not an inner sanctum of peace and quiet. Research has shown that fetal development proceeds amidst constant internal noise generated by the throbbing of maternal arteries and rumbling of bowels. Background noise levels within the pregnant uterus have been variously estimated as ranging anywhere from 56 to 95 dB (as compared with, for example, a typical office environment where decibel levels average about 50). Although the mother's body tissues to some extent attenuate penetration of external noise into the womb, both experimental and anecdotal evidence indicate that outside noise can provoke a physical response in the developing unborn child.

For over half a century, one method used by physicians for determining fetal viability has been to place a sound source near the mother's abdomen and expose the fetus to noise of 120 Hz frequency. Since a fetus' hearing ability is well-developed by the 28th week of pregnancy, such noise exposure causes a noticeable increase in heart rate and kicking among third-trimester fetuses. Less scientific but equally persuasive testimony comes from pregnant

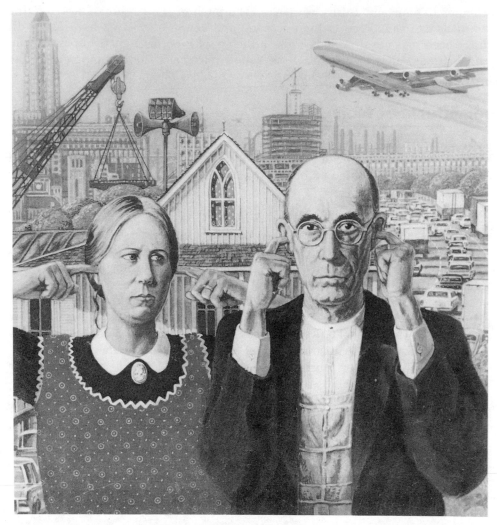

Contemporary American life is much noisier than in days gone by due in part to advanced technology, lifestyle changes, transportation habits, and population density. *[EPA Journal]*

women who have reported that they felt considerably more fetal movement while listening to music in a concert hall, the kicking reaching a peak when the audience began to applaud!

While the fact that noise exposure begins well before birth is undisputable, it is less clear whether such exposure presents any risk of hearing impairment to the unborn child. The question is of some concern because approximately 45% of the U.S. workforce is now female and many of these women will experience one or more pregnancies during their working years. Since occupational noise pollution control frequently is focused on providing ear protection to workers, the question of possible noise-induced hearing damage to the fetuses of pregnant employees is of more than academic interest. While a few epidemiologic studies have reported some degree of hearing impairment among children whose mothers received occupational noise exposures up to 100 dB during pregnancy, most of the limited research done to

Table 13-2 Noise around our Homes

Noise Source	Sound Level for Operator (in dBA)
Refrigerator	40
Floor Fan	38 to 70
Clothes Dryer	55
Washing Machine	47 to 78
Dishwasher	54 to 85
Hair Dryer	59 to 80
Vacuum Cleaner	62 to 85
Sewing Machine	64 to 74
Electric Shaver	75
Food Disposal (Grinder)	87 to 93
Electric Lawn Edger	81
Home Shop Tools	85
Gasoline Power Mower	87 to 92
Gasoline Riding Mower	90 to 95
Chain Saw	100
Stereo	Up to 120

date indicates that hearing loss induced in a fetus by external noise is highly unlikely. The insulating effect of maternal tissues, which limits the amount of outside sound penetrating the uterine environment, renders noise an unlikely teratogenic agent (Thurston and Roberts, 1991).

Much more research is needed to define the extent of the relationship, if any, between noise and birth defects, as well as to establish how high noise levels must be to cause developmental problems. Lacking definitive information, some doctors recommend that pregnant women try to avoid noise exposure to the greatest extent possible, one such expert offering the tongue-in-cheek advice that "any expectant mother should get out of New York."

Effects of Noise on Learning Ability

It has long been recognized that noisy surroundings at school and in the home can adversely affect children's language development and their ability to read. A classic study in the early 1970s, comparing reading ability among children living on different floors of an apartment building located adjacent to a busy highway, revealed that youngsters living on the higher (i.e. quieter) floors had better reading scores than those living on lower (i.e. noisier) floors. It also showed that the longer a child had experienced excessive noise exposure, the poorer was his/her reading ability. Investigators concluded that a noisy home environment has more of an impact on reading skills than do such factors as parents' educational level, number of children in the family, or the child's grade level (Cohen et al., 1973).

More recently, an important study conducted by a Cornell University researcher on first- and second-grade students whose school is located within the flight contour of a major New York metropolitan airport (overflights during school hours averaged one flight every 6.6 minutes) demonstrated convincingly that children constantly exposed to noise have poorer reading skills than children attending school in quiet areas. Investigators concluded that the children's reading difficulties stem, at least in part, from noise-related impairment of their ability to recognize and understand spoken words. In order to cope with the constant noise to which they are subjected, children living and attending school near the airport unconsciously reduce their noise burden by "filtering out" certain sounds, including human speech (Evans et al., 1997). Given the large number of schools worldwide located near airports or busy highways, as well as the increase in residential area noise levels in developed and developing countries alike, the link between noise exposure and children's language development should be a serious cause for concern to educators and parents.

Safety Aspects of Noise

Safety, as well as health, can be in jeopardy when noise levels are high. A tragic case in point involved a Bloomington, Illinois, teenager who was killed when struck from behind by an Amtrack train while walking in the middle of the tracks en route to school. Investigators subsequently concluded that the young man failed to hear the approaching train because he was wearing large earphones while listening to a radio set at high volume. As a police officer at the scene remarked, "The engineer blew the horn, then laid on it to get this person off the tracks. It didn't work. We believe he never heard the train because he had his stereo on" (Simpson, 1997). In the occupational environment as well, high noise levels can pose a safety hazard by preventing workers from hearing shouts of warning or cries for help. Many traffic accidents are thought to be caused by drivers' inability to hear emergency sirens. Both by interfering with shouts for help or by masking warning signals, high levels of background noise pose a very real threat to public safety.

Table 13-3 Permissible Noise Exposures Established by OSHA

Duration per day (hours)	Sound level (dB)
8	90
6	92
4	95
3	97
2	100
1½	102
1	105
½	110
¼ or less	115

Source: OSHA

Sleep Disruption

Sleep is a biological necessity. We need sleep to repair the wearing out of bodily tissues and to rejuvenate them; deprivation or disruption of sleep can thus directly threaten both physical health and mental well-being.

Noise can prevent people from going to sleep, can waken them prematurely, or can cause shifts from deeper to lighter stages of sleep. While individual response to noise in relation to its impact on sleep varies widely, in general adults are wakened by noise more easily than are children; the elderly are more sensitive than the middle-aged; sick persons are more affected than healthy ones; and women are more easily disturbed than men (Bugliarello, 1976). In 1996 the World Health Organization cited noise as a significant health threat and the following year published guidelines that recommended lowering average nighttime noise levels suitable for undisturbed sleep from 35 to 30 decibels, with a peak nighttime maximum of 45 dB(A). Given such recommendations for healthful sleep, it is troubling to note that millions of people currently are subjected to noise levels well above the WHO guidelines. Indeed, a survey of traffic noise in western Europe estimates that 16% of Europeans are subjected to more than 40 decibels in their bedrooms every night (Bond, 1996).

Noise Control Efforts

Historically, noise abatement efforts have consisted primarily of local ordinances directed at specific community nuisances. One of the earliest of such laws was a London ordinance that went into effect in 1829 (Lipscomb, 1974), allowing stagecoach horses to be confiscated if they disrupted church services! Over the years since then, cities have adopted a wide variety of local restrictions on noise sources. A brief sampling of such regulations include: requirements for mufflers on cars; bans on leaf blowers; prohibitions against construction activity, garbage collection, or lawn mowing during early morning or evening hours; bans on roosters or other noisy animals within city limits; restrictions on auto horn-blowing; bans on truck traffic through residential neighborhoods; and prohibitions on "boom cars" or other forms of amplified music outdoors. Overseas, governments are taking legislative action against nuisance noise as well. In Beijing, China, the municipal government recently issued new regulations on car alarms, requiring that they ring for no more than 35 seconds and then only when the engine catches fire, when a door, trunk, or hood is opened, or when the entire car is moved. The new regulations were provoked by a flood of complaints about excessive noise from the city's 300,000 vehicles with anti-theft devices, some of which were so sensitive they began ringing when the car was merely touched or even when exposed to thunder, hail, or rain! In Switzerland, public complaints about truck noise resulted in passage of a nationwide referendum requiring that heavy trucks transiting the country will have to be put on trains when they cross the Swiss border to spare that small Alpine country the pollution and thundering noise that occasionally has been known to cause avalanches and landslides.

The federal government entered the noise control arena in 1972 with passage of the Noise Control Act—the first national law aimed at relieving over-stimulated American ears by regulating certain commercial products considered to be major noise sources. The law called for noise emission limits to be set for products such as medium- and heavy-weight trucks, buses, motorcycles, power lawnmowers, jackhammers, and rock drills. In addition, the

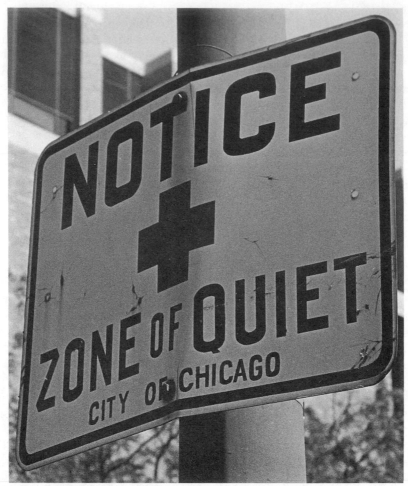

In most urban areas noise-control regulations are nonexistent or are routinely ignored. *[Nora Byrne]*

EPA was to draft noise labeling requirements for noisy products as well as conduct studies on the health impact of noise in order to provide an objective basis for the numerical noise standards yet to be promulgated.

In 1978 the Noise Control Act was amended by the Quiet Communities Act which authorized EPA to work in partnership with state and local governments, helping them to develop anti-noise programs appropriate to their own special needs and abilities. Federal funding provided aid in the form of grants, seminars, and training programs to assist lower levels of government. With the EPA serving as a coordinating agency and providing seed money for local initiatives, hundreds of community noise abatement programs were launched during the 1970s. Noise control efforts suffered a serious setback in the 1980s, however, with the advent of a Reagan Administration committed to an anti-regulatory agenda on environmental issues. In 1982, to the dismay of noise experts, EPA's Office of Noise Abatement and Control (ONAC) was disbanded and has yet to be restored. With the EPA leadership terminated and its technical assistance and funding eliminated, research on the impact of noise on

BOX 13-3

Play Can Be Deafening!

The association between high noise levels and hearing loss in the occupational environment has been recognized—and regulated—for years. The Occupational Safety and Health Administration (OSHA) has set an eight-hour time-weighted average of 90 dB(A) as the maximum permissible noise exposure for the American worker. In recent years, however, it has become increasingly clear that dangerous levels of noise are found not only in factories but also in the home and in association with a wide range of recreational activities. The same individual whose hearing is protected by regulations while on the job may, during off-work hours, incur irreparable damage by engaging in noisy activities where sound levels are totally unregulated and where those exposed seldom wear ear protection.

Perhaps most at risk of nonoccupational noise-induced hearing loss are millions of children and young adults whose ideas of fun are often inseparable from noise: listening to amplified music, playing electronic arcade games, participating in noisy sports events, playing in the school band. Researchers have been surprised to discover that noise-induced hearing loss can begin at 10–20 years of age, much earlier than they previously had thought possible. In 1990 a group of British researchers reported unexpected frustration in their efforts to study hearing damage among youths aged 15–23. Their project was stymied because they couldn't assemble a sufficient number of young people to serve as "controls"—virtually all the candidates had already been exposed to loud music!

Hearing impairment among rock musicians is legendary, as testimony by such notables as Pete Townshend, Ted Nugent, Joey Kramer, and others bears witness. The impact on those whose exposure is limited to *attending* rock concerts or noisy nightclubs is probably less dramatic. Attendees are typically exposed to noise levels of 100 dB or higher (OSHA standards permit no more than 2 hours exposure to noise of this intensity in the workplace). They frequently experience temporary threshold shift (TTS) but generally recover within a few hours to a few days after exposure (Clark, 1991).

The roar of the crowd at athletic events may be endangering fans' hearing, particularly if the event in question happens to be a Minnesota Twins game at the Metrodome. Perhaps because its dome is smaller than average, with a roof configuration that returns noise to the field, the Metrodome may reverberate with noise levels exceeding 100 dB when the stands are full and the home team is winning. As in the situation with rock concerts, spectators who spend a limited amount of time in these raucous surroundings are at minor risk of long-term harm, but Twins players and the concessionaires who spend most of the season amidst the cheering throngs are at serious risk of permanent hearing impairment (Gauthier, 1988).

Many household appliances expose persons of all ages to noise levels that frequently exceed the 85 dB "safe" level; fortunately the duration of exposure to such noises as the whir of a food processor or the drone of a vacuum cleaner is generally quite brief. On the other hand, certain power tools such as chainsaws or leaf blowers could present a risk if used for prolonged periods without hearing protection. Similarly, farm equipment such as tractors can be a significant cause of hearing impairment for rural youngsters. A study conducted in Wisconsin revealed that more than half the children involved in farm work experienced some degree of noise-induced hearing loss, double the rate of children *not* working on farms.

Of all the dangerous forms of recreational noise exposure, however, the greatest toll on young ears (and older ears as well!) is wrought by hunting and target shooting, activities regularly enjoyed by an estimated 13% of the U.S. population. With decibel levels frequently exceeding the threshold of pain, the crack of gunfire, or even cap pistols, can instantly destroy receptor cells in the inner ear and irreversibly damage hearing ability. Among a study group of 94 children or teenagers who were victims of noise-induced hearing loss, an analysis of the noise sources revealed that fully 46% suffered because of guns or fireworks; only 12% had been damaged by exposure to live or amplified music, 8% by power tools, and 4% by recreational vehicles.

Since noise-induced hearing loss is cumulative, growing slowly but steadily worse with continued exposure to a wide variety of high-decibel activities, people of all ages, but especially children, need to become more aware of how to protect themselves. For those young people who shrug off the importance of ear protection, downplaying the impact hearing loss could have on their lives, an analogy by Senator Richard Durbin of Illinois, then a member of the House Committee conducting hearings on noise pollution, seems particularly apt: "if you are color blind you can visit an art museum, but you miss a lot. People who have lost their hearing are missing so much. They hear *something*, but they are missing a lot in the process" (U.S. Congress, 1991).

References

Clark, William W. 1991. "Noise Exposure from Leisure Activities: A Review." *Journal of the Acoustical Society of America* 90, no.1 (July).

Gauthier, Michele M. 1988. "Clamorous Metrodome Hard on Ears and Foes." *The Physician and Sports Medicine* 16, no. 3 (March).

U.S. Congress. House. 1991. *Turn It Down: Effects of Noise on Hearing Loss in Children and Youth.* Hearing before the Select Committee on Children, Youth, and Families, July 22. Washington, DC: U.S. Government Printing Office.

health and hearing has declined sharply since the early 1980s. Most information on noise pollution appearing in current textbooks is still based on studies conducted during the 1970s. The promising proliferation of municipal noise abatement efforts which characterized the late 1970s has suffered a similar reversal. Of the more than 1,100 state and local noise control programs that existed 20 years ago, only about 15 are still functioning. Although the Noise Control Act mandates are still theoretically in effect, they are not being enforced. Regulations that were about to be promulgated at the time ONAC closed were never completed and those that had been finalized have been ignored. Of the wide range of equipment targeted by the Noise Control Act, the only products for which noise emission standards have yet been promulgated are air compressors, motorcycles, trucks, and waste compactors. In 1991 hearing experts testified before a Congressional Committee, urging restoration of EPA leadership in national noise abatement efforts and calling for renewed noise emission information and warning labels on dangerously noisy equipment. Unfortunately, these initiatives were not followed by legislative action and as the decade of the 1990s drew to a close, noise pollution control remained an issue largely neglected by policymakers. Undoubtedly the most serious obstacle to implementing effective programs is the difficulty of convincing both policymakers and the public that noise pollution is really important. As one EPA official remarked, "Noise is something we grow up with, and it is very difficult to believe that such a common pollutant could be doing anything serious to our health or the environment." Until an aroused public insists that excessive noise is a community health hazard that must be controlled, it is unlikely that elected officials will give noise abatement efforts the attention they deserve.

References

Bond, Michael. 1996. "Plagued by Noise." *New Scientist* 152, no. 2056 (Nov. 16):14-15.

Bugliarello, George, Ariel Alexandre, John Barnes, and Charles Wakstein. 1976. *The Impact of Noise Pollution.* Pergamon Press.

Cohen, Peter. 1990. "Drumming: How Risky Is It To Your Hearing?" *Modern Drummer* (October).

Cohen, S., D.C. Glass, and J.E. Singer. 1973. "Apartment Noise Auditory Discrimination and Reading Ability in Children." *Journal of Experimental Social Psychology* 9:407-422.

Evans, Gary W., and Lorraine Maxwell. 1997. "Chronic Noise Exposure and Reading Deficits: The Mediating Effects of Language Acquisition." *Environment and Behavior* 29, no. 5 (Sept.):638.

Ising, Hartmut, Ekkehard Rebentisch, Fritz Poustka, and Immo Curio. 1990. "Annoyance and Health Risk Caused by Military Low-altitude Flight Noise." *International Archives of Occupational and Environmental Health* 62:357–63.

Jaret, Peter. 1990. "The Rock & Roll Syndrome." *In Health* (July/Aug.).

Lipscomb, David M. 1974. *Noise: The Unwanted Sounds.* Nelson-Hall.

"Mad About the Noise." 1998. *Time International* 150, no. 48 (July 27):38.

Melrick, William. 1991. "Human Temporary Threshold Shift (TTS) and Damage Risk." *Journal of the Acoustical Society of America* 90, no. 1 (July).

Murphy, Elliott. 1989. "Townshend, Tinnitus and Rock & Roll." *Rolling Stone,* July 13–27.

OECD. 1991. *Fighting Noise in the 1990s.* Paris: OECD.

Perham, Chris. 1979. "The Sound of Silence." *EPA Journal* 5, no. 9 (Oct.).

Shapiro, Margaret. 1989. "Crowds are Made in Japan Too." *Washington Post,* Feb. 13.

Simpson, Kevin. 1997. "Train Kills Teen in B-N." *The Pantagraph,* Bloomington, IL. (Oct. 18):A-1.

Thurston, Floyd E., M.D., and Stanley L. Roberts, PA-C, M.P.H. "Environmental Noise and Fetal Hearing." *Journal of the Tennessee Medical Association* 84, no. 1 (Jan).

CHAPTER 14

Water Resources

All the rivers run into the sea, yet the sea is not full; to the place from whence the rivers come, thither they return again.

—Ecclesiastes 1:7

Although the ancient writer of Ecclesiastes expressed his scientific observations in poetic form, his statements relating to the cycling of water through the hydrosphere are basically correct, albeit overly simplified. Water moves in what is essentially a closed system, circulating from one part of the earth to another, changing in form from liquid to solid or gas and back to liquid again, yet remaining relatively constant in total amount. Water occurs as vapor in the atmosphere, as rain or snow falling on the earth or oceans, as ice locked in massive glaciers or ice caps, and as rivers, streams, lakes, seas, and subterranean groundwater. The manner by which water moves from place to place, changing from one form to another, is called the hydrologic cycle.

Hydrologic Cycle

The hydrologic cycle, like virtually all other processes on earth, is powered by energy from the sun that causes water to evaporate from the surface of the oceans, rivers, lakes, and from the soil. The movement of this water vapor in the atmosphere is an important factor in the redistribution of heat around the earth. Because heat is absorbed when water evaporates, the atmosphere becomes a reservoir of heat energy. This heat energy then drives the hydrologic cycle which gives rise to the atmospheric forces involved in weather and climate. The principal processes involved in the hydrologic cycle are:

1. Evaporation of water from surface waters and from the soil.

2. Transportation of water by plants; because both evaporation and transpiration produce the same result (i.e. the addition of water vapor to the atmosphere), the two processes are often collectively called evapotranspiration.

3. Transport of atmospheric water from one place to another as water vapor or as liquid water droplets and ice crystals in clouds.

4. Precipitation when atmospheric water vapor condenses and falls as rain, hail, sleet, or snow.

5. Runoff, whereby water that has fallen finds its way back to the oceans, flowing either on or under the surface of the continents.

The amount of time required for the completion of the cycle can vary widely from place to place and from one part of the cycle to another. On the average, a water molecule spends nine days in the atmosphere from the time it evaporates until it falls again as rain or snow (Ehrlich, Ehrlich, and Holdren, 1977). However, if it happens to fall as a snowflake on the Antarctic ice sheet, it may remain there for thousands of years before it breaks off as part of an iceberg and melts into the ocean; conversely, if it falls during a desert thunderstorm, it might evaporate in an hour or two.

Approximately 71% of the earth's surface is covered with water, a resource amounting to almost 1.5 billion km^3 in total volume. Of this amount, however, only a very small percentage is readily available for human use. Most of the water on the planet, about 97.4%, is found in the world's seas and oceans—enormously abundant but too salty for drinking or agricultural use; 2% is fresh water locked up in glaciers and polar ice caps; the, remainder, less than 1% of the total, consists of fresh water in rivers, lakes, groundwater, and water vapor in the atmosphere (World Resources Institute, 1992; Maurits la

Figure 14-1   Hydrologic Cycle

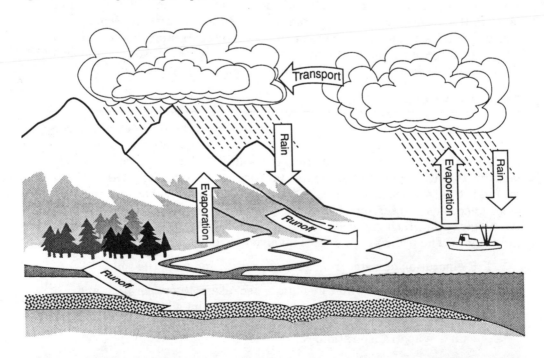

Riviere, 1989). Obviously, for humans this is the portion of greatest significance, since it constitutes the water we drink, bathe in, and use for irrigation and industrial purposes. Of this small percentage of water on which human life depends, only a minuscule portion is found in the rivers, streams, and lakes of the world. Likewise, at any given moment only a tiny amount of the world's water occurs as atmospheric water vapor. By far the greatest amount of all available fresh water, approximately 96.5% of the total, is found beneath the surface of the soil in the form of groundwater.

Water Quantity and Health

The human body's absolute dependence on regular intake of water is second only to its need for oxygen. While an individual can, if necessary, survive for a number of weeks without food, deprivation of water will result in death within a few days at the most. Water makes up approximately 65% of the adult human's body, a somewhat higher percentage in children. Blood consists of 83% water, while bones contain 25%. Water is essential for the body's digestion of food, transport of nutrients and hormones, and removal of wastes. Depending on a person's size, weight, degree of activity, and the prevailing level of temperature and humidity, an individual requires approximately 1–3 liters of water daily just to maintain bodily functions.

To maintain good health and an adequate standard of living, however, 50 liters of water per day are considered the bare minimum essential for drinking, food preparation, cooking, dish washing, and bathing (Simon, 1998). The use of sewer systems for safe removal of human wastes—wastes which present serious problems when mismanaged—also requires considerable amounts of water. In typical urban residential areas, sewers will not transport wastes efficiently if per capita water use is less than 100 liters a day. In industrialized countries and among the more affluent segments of the urban population in developing nations, water quantity is generally more than ample to meet these basic human needs; average daily water consumption in such situations ranges between 200–400 liters per person per day. However, in developing countries almost 1.5 billion people still lack access to adequate supplies of safe water, in spite of impressive gains made during the United Nations-sponsored 1981–1990 International Drinking Water Supply and Sanitation Decade (WRI, 1998). In many rural areas the problem is not the lack of water per se, but rather that the source of such water is far from the point of use. In some countries, women may spend several hours each day hauling water from a distant river, well, or standpipe to their homes, leaving little time for more economically productive tasks such as gardening or trading in the marketplace. The sheer physical effort involved in carrying water long distances also exerts a toll on the health of rural women who, not infrequently, may be malnourished and overworked. In most urban areas of the Third World, water supply systems are in place, but frequently they are in poor condition or are unreliable, functioning perhaps only a few hours each day. While walking distances for the urban poor are less than for their country cousins, such people nevertheless spend hours waiting in long lines for their turn at the standpipe. Among many poor urban residents in the Third World, water is obtained by purchasing it from vendors at a cost many times higher than the cost per unit

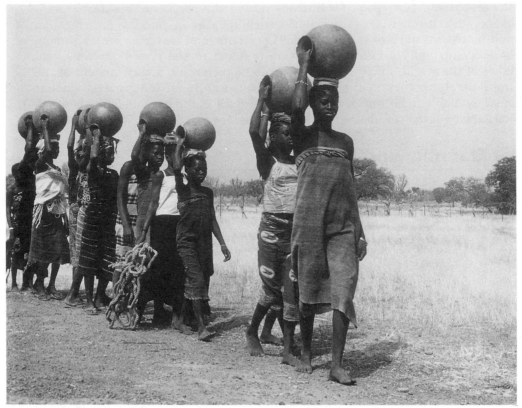

Women and girls from a small village in Burkina Faso walk to a distant well to fetch water. *[UN/ DPI/Ray Witlin]*

of a piped-in municipal supply. The necessity of buying water imposes a heavy financial burden on family incomes; in Port-au-Prince, Haiti, 20% of a typical slum-dweller's household budget is spent on water.

In situations such as these, where safe water is in short supply, difficult or time-consuming to obtain, or exorbitantly expensive, important aspects of personal hygiene and basic sanitation such as washing hands and eating utensils is frequently neglected. In addition, there is a strong temptation to utilize polluted sources of water if higher-quality supplies are not easily accessible. A study published by the World Health Organization demonstrated that improved access to water reduced the incidence of diarrheal cases by 25%, while improvements in both water quality and access reduced such illnesses by fully 37%. Perhaps the most essential prerequisite for improving the health and living standards among the Third World poor is an increase in the quantity of readily available safe water supplies (Briscoe, 1993).

Water Supply: Our Next Crisis?

While water is indeed a renewable resource, the rate at which it is renewed within the global hydrologic cycle is both fixed and slow. Water is also a finite resource—although human technologies can devise means for uti-

BOX 14-1

Water from the Sea:
The Ultimate Solution to Water Scarcity?

Answering a reporter's question as to what scientific progress he would like to see during his term of office, President John F. Kennedy in 1961 replied that if we could perfect technology to convert sea water to fresh water at reasonable cost, such an accomplishment "can do more to raise men and women from lives of poverty than any other scientific advance." Like Kennedy and numerous other visionaries, inhabitants of arid coastal regions have long dreamed of transforming seawater into a potable beverage. Today such schemes no longer seem unrealistic, as pressures on the world's freshwater resources spur developments that make desalination projects both technologically feasible and increasingly common in water-short areas of the world. By the late 1990s, there were approximately 11,000 desalination plants in operation in more than 120 countries around the globe. Of various sizes and types, these facilities produce, collectively, 5.4 billion cubic meters of fresh water from the sea each year (an amount which, nevertheless, represents only 0.25% of total water use). The leading producer of desalted seawater is the oil-rich desert kingdom of Saudi Arabia which boasts 34 desalination plants that yield over 800 million gallons a day of desalted water. A distant runner-up for second place is the United States, with more than 130 small plants in southern Florida and 19 either operating or under construction in California, including the nation's largest desalination facility at Santa Barbara, completed early in 1992. The high costs associated with this plant, as well as a sharp decline in local water demand due to effective water conservation measures, have resulted in its being taken out of regular operation, its use being reserved for periods of drought. The Persian Gulf nations of Kuwait and the United Arab Emirates rank just below the United States in desalination capacity, while numerous other facilities are scattered around the Caribbean, in Australia, Spain, and elsewhere.

The technologies for desalting seawater are straightforward and relatively simple. Large plants, such as the 1 million m^3/day facility at Jubail, Saudi Arabia, and the plant at Key West, Florida, typically employ a multistage flash distillation process, in which water is heated under pressure and then injected into a low pressure chamber where it instantly "flashes" into steam which is captured and condensed into pure water. The fact that pressurized hot water from a single source can be flashed into several chambers simultaneously makes it possible to produce large amounts of water quite dependably by this method. Smaller plants more commonly rely on reverse osmosis, a process by which seawater is forced, under high pressure, through a membrane that permits passage of water molecules but screens out the slightly larger ions of sodium and chlorine.

The problem with both methods—and the main factor limiting their use—is the enormous amount of energy needed to power both processes, a requirement which translates into a high price per unit of water. Currently, desalination of sea water is three to four times more expensive than obtaining the same amount from conventional freshwater sources. Although technology has gradually advanced to the point that the unit cost of desalted water may be feasible for use as drinking water, it is still far too expensive for irrigation or industrial purposes—categories that comprise 85% of all water demand. There is an urgent need for a much greater research commitment on the part of the United States and other governments to develop more economical methods of desalination in order to forestall serious impending water shortages in many arid parts of the world. At a time when global warming threatens increased likelihood of prolonged dry spells and worsening of current water shortages, desalination offers a drought-proof solution to humanity's water supply needs. The fact that many of the regions currently most in need of water border oceans or seas is another reason for aggressive pursuit of the desalination option. Although limited progress has been made in recent years, a greater government commitment to research is needed if desalination is to satisfy more than a small fraction of the world's water needs anytime in the foreseeable future.

References
Gleick, Peter H. 1998. *The World's Water.* Island Press.
Simon, Paul. 1998. *Tapped Out.* Welcome Rain Publishers.
World Resources Institute. 1992. *World Resources 1992-93.* Oxford University Press.

lizing the existing supply more efficiently, science cannot create additional water nor alter the rate at which water is circulated through the biosphere. Faced with these realities, many water resource experts view current water use trends with alarm, warning that the approaching "water crisis" which they foresee could be the first resource constraint to impose serious limits on further world economic growth. Such fears are based on the fact that over the past 300 years worldwide, withdrawals from freshwater resources have increased more than 35-fold and continue to grow rapidly. Since the beginning of the 20th century, water consumption has risen more than twice as fast as the rate of population growth. A continuation of this trend into the 21st century seems inevitable as water demand from growing cities, industry, and irrigated agriculture steadily increases. According to a 1997 United Nations assessment of global freshwater resources, one-third of the world's population lives in regions already experiencing moderate to severe water stress—a number that is expected to reach two-thirds by 2025. The problem is most acute in rapidly growing developing nations, but is an issue in several industrialized countries as well, including the United States (WRI, 1998).

Recent water emergencies, precipitated by drought or water mismanagement, in such diverse areas as California, eastern Africa, southeastern India, and Uzbekistan are, these experts insist, but harbingers of more difficult times to come. At first glance, such gloomy predictions seem at variance with the facts. Although the amount of fresh water readily available for human use constitutes less than 0.01% of all the water on earth, it still represents an abundant supply—theoretically sufficient to satisfy the needs of 20 billion people if equally divided (Maurits la Riviere, 1989). Obviously, however, neither the planet's water resources nor its human population are evenly distributed. Depending on local patterns of annual precipitation and evaporative demand (i.e. the maximum amount of moisture the atmosphere is capable of absorbing), water availability varies widely from one region to another. In the United States, for example, average annual rainfall is approximately 30 inches. This amount is distributed quite unevenly, however; whereas the Pacific Northwest receives about 80 inches of precipitation annually and the states east of the Mississippi River average 40–45 inches, the Great Plains and the Southwest are chronically water short. The driest state, Nevada, receives only 9 inches of rainfall in an average year. Viewing the world as a whole, nations lying between 20–30 degrees of latitude both north and south of the equator (the transition zone between temperate and tropical regions) tend to have the lowest annual rates of precipitation and are also most subject to recurrent droughts. Perhaps not by coincidence, these lands also are home to some of the world's poorest countries and experience some of the highest population growth rates. Even within regions where water supplies are usually adequate, periodic dry spells and increasing industrial and municipal demands may result in localized shortages. Compounding the problem of regional disparities in water supply is the fact that everywhere—both in water-rich and water-poor areas of the world—pollution is rendering much of the available supply unusable without extensive (and expensive) treatment.

Impact of Population Growth on Water Demand

To some extent, water demand within a society is determined by that society's level of affluence and technological development. On a per capita basis, today's largest water consumers are the rich nations of the industrialized world. The average American consumes, directly or indirectly, more than 70 times as much water each year as the average Ghanaian (Maurits la Riviere, 1989). However, in the years ahead the major factor accounting for increased water demand, especially in urban areas, will be the explosive growth of human populations. Within any region, the amount of available water, determined primarily by precipitation, is finite. Thus, the amount available per capita is directly proportional to population size. While more efficient water management can help to ensure more equitable distribution and prevent wastage, unchecked population growth will inevitably result in chronic water shortages. The problem is most acute today for the countries of the Middle East (see Box 14-2), a naturally arid, drought-prone region with some of the world's highest birth rates. In Gaza, Jordan, Syria, and Iraq, populations will double in less than 20 years, yet water availability will remain unchanged. In Africa and southern Asia also, rapid population growth is increasing the stress on water supplies; by 2025 it is expected that more than a billion people throughout this area will be plagued by a scarcity of water (Falkenmark and Widstrand, 1992).

The impact of burgeoning population on water supplies promises to be most sorely felt in Third World cities. Even in countries where national averages indicate adequate water resources, runaway rates of urbanization and industrialization are seriously endangering both the quantity and quality of water supplies within many metropolitan areas. In China, overpumping of groundwater to meet soaring urban water demand has resulted in drastic lowering of the water table in many areas. Since the 1960s, the water table

BOX 14-2
War Over Water?

"Whiskey is for drinking and water is for fighting over." This truism from the 19th century American "Wild West" could be relevant to future struggles simmering just below the surface in many water-short regions of the world today. World population passed the 6 billion mark in 1999 and is expected to increase by another 2.5–3 billion within the next 25 years. Water *demand*, driven by a rising global standard of living, is increasing at twice the rate of population growth, but the world's water *supply* is constant and finite. Already 30 countries, home to 20% of the global population, are experiencing chronic water shortages; by 2025, 50 nations and 30% of humanity will be water-short. Obviously a crisis looms in the not-too-distant future; neither people nor nations can survive without water and when faced with a dangerously dwindling essential resource, governments typically resort to war. As one international law expert warns, a shortage of fresh water is likely to be *"the* national security issue of the 21st century."* Prospects for peaceful resolution are not helped by the fact that there are more than 200 rivers that flow between two or more countries and close to 47% of the world's land area (excluding Antarctica) lies within shared river basins. Yet in spite of the potential for conflict, no enforceable body of international law governs the use or allocation of these waters. As a result, those who pay attention to such matters are bracing for trouble. Klaus Toepfer, Executive Director of the United Nations' Environment Programme, sees future wars over water as a distinct possibility.

A number of potential flashpoints for water wars exist around the world: the Ganges basin in South Asia, where water diversions to boost Indian crop yields are depriving Bangladeshis of their traditional share of the river's flow; the Amu Dar'ya and Syr Dar'ya Rivers, whose waters irrigate central Asian cotton fields to the detriment of communities bordering the fast-disappearing Aral Sea; the Nile, indispensable to the life and economic survival of 68 million Egyptians, yet controlled by upstream Ethiopia and Uganda who have plans of their own for utilizing its waters.

Perhaps nowhere is the looming water supply crisis more acute than in the volatile Middle East, where all major rivers are shared and where several nations are overpumping groundwater from common aquifers. Indeed, when U.S. intelligence services listed the ten places in the world where war was most likely to erupt over dwindling shared water supplies, most of them were in the Middle East. Throughout the region, the nature of each country's water woes is remarkably similar: a naturally arid to semiarid climate, rapidly falling water tables due to overpumping, and exploding population growth.

In the Jordan Valley, Israelis, Palestinians, and Jordanians compete for shrinking water supplies which, even if equitably shared, are insufficient to meet the demand. In Israel, renewable water supplies are being overdrawn by close to 30% annually. Thanks to rapid population increase spurred by unprecedented levels of Jewish immigration from Russia, as well as high birth rates among Israeli Arabs, water demand in Israel has been soaring. Certainly the current water situation is complicating efforts to conclude a lasting peace agreement with Israel's Arab neighbors, who feel Israel is taking more than its fair share of the region's water. Jordanians protest Israeli diversions from the Sea of Galilee into an aqueduct serving Tel Aviv, thereby diminishing the flow of the Jordan River and rendering it too saline for irrigation. Jordanian attempts to stave off impending water shortages by drilling deeper wells, improving the efficiency of irrigation, and reusing wastewater effluent for irrigation constitute little more than stop-gap solutions. For a nation that is 70% desert, has only one small river entirely within its own territory, and a population of 5 million, expected to double within 28 years, Jordan's water supply challenges appear almost insurmountable. In the occupied West Bank, Palestinians chafe under military orders that cut off their access to irrigation water from the Jordan River while simultaneously setting limits on the amount of water they can withdraw from existing wells and prohibiting the digging of new ones. In the meantime, Palestinians charge, Israeli settlers pumping from the same aquifer are under no such restrictions and have withdrawn so much water that many Arab wells have gone dry. In Gaza, whose population growth rate is among the highest in the world, the water situation is even more critical. Completely dependent on a single heavily polluted aquifer, Gazans are pumping water out of the ground at more than twice the rate of natural recharge. As a consequence, the water table is falling rapidly, and saltwater intrusion into the coastal aquifer, added to the chemical and biological contamination, threatens to render Gaza's groundwater reserves undrinkable within the next few years.

While political tensions over water appear most immediate and serious in the Jordan basin, in the Tigris-Euphrates watershed two other nations with rapidly growing populations—Syria and Iraq—nervously speculate on the water-hoard-ing intentions of an upstream neighbor. Turkey, one of the few Middle Eastern countries with an adequate supply of water within its borders, is engaged in a major development project in its arid southeastern Anatolia province. Consisting of a series of irrigation and hydroelectric dams on the Tigris and Euphrates Rivers, including the massive Ataturk Dam 340 miles southeast of Ankara, Turkey's Anatolia Project has neighboring countries seriously worried. While bringing immense benefits to the Turkish people in terms of electrical power and water for irrigation, the project could conceivably reduce the volume of the Euphrates by as much as 60% by the time it reaches Syria. Further downstream, Iraq could experience diminished flows of as much as 90% if water sharing agreements are not worked out among the three countries. Although Turkey has behaved responsibly thus far, Turkish leaders intend to expand their irrigated acreage, a fact that almost certainly means less, more saline water for nations downstream.

As pressures on water resources mount throughout the world, logic suggests that national leaders would set aside the fear, mistrust, and hostility that have poisoned their relations in recent decades and seek common ground in forging cooperative water management agreements. Unfortunately, there are few indications as yet that neither political leaders or the general public are giving the issue of water scarcity the priority it deserves. By the time they do, it may be too late to prevent disaster.

References
Simon, Paul. 1998. *Tapped Out.* Welcome Rain Publishers.

Starr, Joyce R. 1991. "Water Wars." *Foreign Policy,* no. 82 (Spring).

beneath portions of Beijing has dropped more than 110 feet, and by the mid-1990s farmers in the surrounding rural areas were no longer allowed to draw irrigation water from nearby reservoirs because city dwellers' demands for existing water supplies took precedence over the needs of agriculture (Postel, 1996; Brown and Halweil, 1998). Pollution of existing sources further reduces the usable water supply in many cities of the developing world. Bodily wastes generated by soaring numbers of urban poor lacking the most basic sanitation facilities have so polluted many urban water supplies with microbial pathogens that cities from Shanghai to Lima have been forced to divert millions of dollars from other urgently needed projects to finance increased levels of wastewater treatment. Such problems will become even more severe in the years ahead if current population growth trends persist.

Groundwater

Mention "water resources" and most people immediately think of rivers, lakes, and constructed reservoirs—surface water sources that are visible, accessible, and useful not only for direct consumption but for transportation and recreation as well. However, as pointed out earlier, over 96% of all available fresh water supplies occur in the form of groundwater, a resource whose immense importance is often overlooked and little understood by the general public. Approximately half of all Americans and more than 95% of farm families depend on groundwater for their drinking water supplies (EPA, 1998); similarly, in Asia groundwater provides over half the drinking water in most countries, while in Europe the proportion of domestic supplies derived from groundwater is even higher—as much as 98% in Denmark, 96% in Austria, and 88% in Italy (Gleick, 1993). This vast unseen reservoir flows very slowly toward the sea and is a major source of replenishment for most surface water supplies. Estimates indicate that most rivers receive as much of their flow from groundwater seepage as from surface runoff.

Groundwater supplies constitute an invaluable natural resource—one that has long been regarded as having certain inherent advantages over surface water supplies. Groundwater is usually cleaner and purer than most surface water sources. This is true because the soil through which it percolates filters out most of the bacteria, suspended materials, and other contaminants that find easy access to rivers and lakes. In addition, because evaporation is virtually nil and seasonal fluctuations in supply are small, groundwater supplies are dependable year-round. In terms of cost, groundwater has advantages also. The expense of digging a well is generally less than that of piping surface water to its place of use and because of its greater purity it is less expensive to treat prior to consumption.

Until recently, communities relying on groundwater for their municipal supplies tended to take this resource largely for granted. Today, however, a sense of alarm is spreading with the realization that the twin evils of pollution and over-use are threatening the integrity of groundwater supplies. To understand how this situation has come about, it is necessary to take a brief look at the physical characteristics of our groundwater resource.

Figure 14-2 Nature of Groundwater

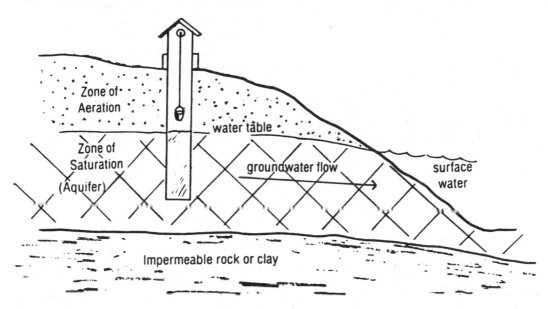

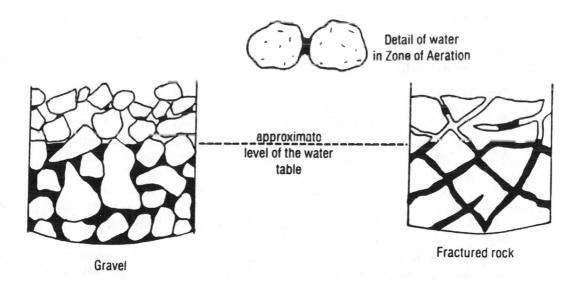

How Water Occurs in the Rock

Source: U. S. Geological Survey, *A Primer on Groundwater.*

Nature of Groundwater

When rain falls upon the earth, that which is not taken up by plant roots or lost as surface runoff percolates downward through the soil until it reaches the water table. Contrary to what some people think, the water table is not a vast underground lake or river, but the upper limit of what hydrologists call the **zone of saturation**—an area where the spaces between rock particles are completely filled with water. Such moisture-laden strata are called **aquifers** (Latin for "water carriers"). Above the zone of saturation lies the **zone of aeration,** where some soil moisture may be found as capillary water—useful for plants but incapable of being pumped out by humans. The zone of saturation extends downward until it is limited by an impermeable layer of rock. Sometimes there are successive layers of groundwater separated by impermeable rock layers. Aquifers may range from a few feet to several hundreds of feet in thickness and they may underlie a couple of acres or many square miles. They may occur just below the soil surface or thousands of feet below the earth, though seldom deeper than two miles.

The amount of water that any given aquifer can hold depends on its **porosity**—the ratio of the spaces between the rock particles to the total volume of rock. Sand and gravel aquifers are examples of rocks with high porosity. Additionally, if water is going to move through an aquifer, its pores must be interconnected. To qualify as a good aquifer, a rock layer must contain many pores, cracks, or both. The rate of water movement through an aquifer varies, not surprisingly, with the type of rock: through gravel it may travel tens or hundreds of feet per day; in fine sand only a few inches or less per day. When hydrologists measure the flow of surface streams, they do so in terms of feet per second; when measuring groundwater flow, figures in feet *per year* are the rule.

Groundwater Pollution

The inherent superiority of groundwater over surface water due to its supposed freedom from contamination can no longer be taken for granted. In recent decades, chemical, biological, and radiological contaminants from a wide variety of sources have been identified in groundwater deposits throughout the world. Although estimates by the National Research Council suggest the total geographic extent of groundwater pollution in the United States remains quite limited, such cases tend to occur in populated areas where the aquifer in question may be the principal or only source of local drinking water. Such findings have raised legitimate concerns among the public regarding both acute and chronic health effects and have resulted in the closure of hundreds of wells, affecting the water supplies of millions of Americans. In numerous cases involving synthetic organic chemicals, levels of contamination have been many times higher than those found in the most heavily polluted surface waters. Within affected communities the discovery that wells are contaminated frequently has come as an unwelcome surprise since, contrary to the situation in lakes and rivers, groundwater pollution is in a sense hidden, out of sight and difficult to detect without sophisticated chemical analyses. Since many pollutants in groundwater are colorless, odorless, and tasteless,

Figure 14-3   Sources of Groundwater Contamination

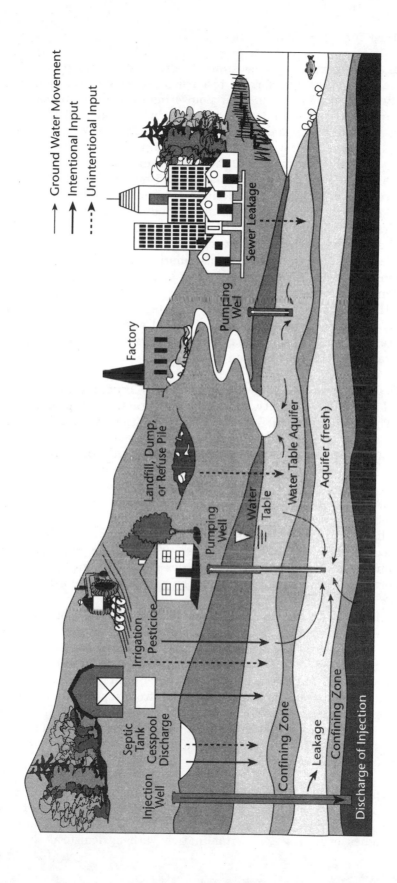

Source: EPA, 1998. "National Water Quality Inventory 1996 Report to Congress." EPA Office of Water, 841-R-97-008 (April).

citizens may unknowingly consume health-threatening poisons for years. Because routine tests performed to ensure drinking water safety have only recently been expanded to include monitoring for toxic chemicals, well water pollution in the past was often detected only when noticeable numbers of people began to fall ill. Amendments to the Safe Drinking Water Act in 1986 significantly expanded the number of contaminants for which public water systems must monitor in both surface and groundwaters. However, these regulations do not cover the approximately 10.5 million private wells, mostly in rural areas, which frequently are shallower and thus even more vulnerable to pollution than municipal wells (Sanford and Oosterhaut, 1991). Since well water traditionally has been regarded as pure enough to drink untreated, only about half of the public water systems in the U.S. that utilize groundwater sources disinfect the water prior to distribution. Likewise, very few of the noncommunity systems disinfect well water and a negligible number of private well owners chlorinate their supplies. Given the extent of microbial contamination that has been identified in groundwater in recent years and the failure of many suppliers to treat such water, it's not surprising that over half (58%) of the reported waterborne disease outbreaks in the U.S. between 1971–1994 were traced to the consumption of microbially-tainted groundwater (NRC, 1999).

Degradation of groundwater supplies by human-generated pollutants occurs largely due to faulty waste disposal practices or poor land management. The most significant sources of contamination include:

Waste Storage, Treatment, or Disposal Facilities. Unplanned seepage from open dumps, landfills, waste ponds, underground storage tanks, tailings piles—even graveyards!—constitute a well-recognized and severe groundwater pollution threat if such facilities are improperly sited. In the U.S., petroleum products leaking from underground storage tanks constitute the leading source of groundwater pollution in most states, with landfill seepage close behind in second place (EPA, 1998). Design requirements for the development of new land disposal facilities emphasize incorporation of barriers to prevent leachate migration, thereby protecting groundwater quality.

Septic Systems. On-site sewage disposal facilities constitute the third most commonly reported source of groundwater contamination in the United States. Such systems feature the deliberate discharge of wastewater effluent directly into the ground. If such facilities are properly sited, waste discharges pose little hazard, but if located adjacent to or uphill from an aquifer or well, a potential for pollution exists. Contamination from septic systems, which serve approximately 30% of U.S. households, can be either microbial or chemical. A number of outbreaks of waterborne diarrheal diseases such as salmonellosis, hepatitis A, and typhoid fever have been traced to well water contaminated by sewage from septic tanks.

Pipes, Materials Transport, Transfer Operations. Unintentional leakage from sewers or oil pipelines or accidental spills during transport or transfer of hazardous substances can be another source of groundwater pollution. Studies of well water contamination with agricultural chemicals conducted by the Illinois EPA revealed that the majority of problems—and all those involving high concentrations of pollutants—could be traced to locations where pesticidal formulations were routinely prepared (and routinely spilled on the ground!) prior to field application.

Nonpoint Sources of Pollution. Many instances of groundwater contamination can be traced to substances discharged as a result of other activities: irrigation practices, mine drainage, field application of farm chemicals or manures, de-icing of highways, and urban street runoff, among the most notable examples. Sources such as these are responsible for a host of water quality problems, among them the elevated nitrate levels found in numerous private wells in farming areas and the high chloride content in wells in some northern states where large quantities of road salts are applied during the winter months.

The most disturbing aspect of groundwater pollution is the fact that by the time the problem is discovered, it is generally too late to do anything about it. Because of the very slow rate of groundwater flow, chemical pollutants will not be flushed out of an aquifer for many years after the source of contamination is cut off (conversely, and for the same reason, contamination of one part of an aquifer does not necessarily affect the use of other parts). Unlike the situation in surface waters, where naturally occurring microbes gradually break down organic pollutants, groundwater is largely devoid of the oxygen needed by the bacteria and other decomposer organisms that endow streams and lakes with their capacity for self-purification. Cleanup of a polluted aquifer, while theoretically possible, is so expensive and time-consuming that it is usually not feasible. The process generally involves drilling numerous wells, pumping out enormous quantities of water, treating the water to remove the contaminants, and then reinjecting the water into the aquifer (Rail, 1989). For all practical purposes, a community that finds its groundwater seriously contaminated has little choice but to close the affected wells and seek a new water supply. Groundwater protection strategies, therefore, logically focus on preventing pollution in the first place rather than on efforts to clean up an aquifer after the damage is done.

Groundwater Depletion

With water demand and per capita water consumption increasing steadily in recent decades, many groundwater-dependent regions of the world have experienced an alarming decline in the water table, a direct result of overpumping. Periodic fluctuations in the level of the water table are normal, with levels rising during wet periods and falling during dry spells (generally the water table is highest in the late spring, sinks in summer, rises somewhat during the fall, and reaches its lowest point just before the spring thaw). However, when the water table lowers persistently it means that more water is being taken out of the groundwater reservoir than is being returned to it through precipitation or stream flow. Such a situation is akin to mining an aquifer, and if continued over an extended time period it can permanently deplete the groundwater supply or render it uneconomical to exploit due to

Figure 14-4   Groundwater Use As a Percentage of Total Withdrawals, U.S.

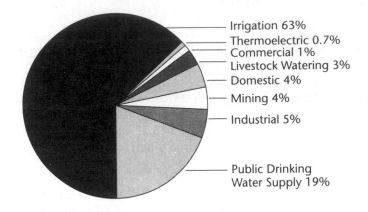

- Irrigation 63%
- Thermoelectric 0.7%
- Commercial 1%
- Livestock Watering 3%
- Domestic 4%
- Mining 4%
- Industrial 5%
- Public Drinking Water Supply 19%

Source: EPA, 1998. "National Water Quality Inventory 1996 Report to Congress." EPA Office of Water, 841-R-97-008 (April).

excessive pumping costs. Groundwater depletion problems have assumed major proportions in parts of the Middle East, North Africa, India, China, Thailand, Mexico, and the western United States (Postel, 1992).

Instances of groundwater "mining" can occur even in well-watered areas when demand generated by rapid population growth, along with residential and commercial development, result in a sharp decline in groundwater reserves. In the United States, however, depletion is most acute in arid regions such as the Great Plains and Southwest where the insatiable demand for irrigation water and the water needs of homes and industries in the booming cities of the Sunbelt have resulted in serious groundwater overdrafts.

A classic case of groundwater depletion in the American West is exemplified by the exploitation of the Ogallala Aquifer, the world's largest underground water reserve. Underlying portions of six states in the High Plains, the Ogallala supplies almost one-third of all the groundwater used for irrigation in the United States. This enormous sand and gravel formation was deposited millions of years ago as the eastern front of the Rocky Mountains eroded. The plentiful rains of Pleistocene times saturated the formation with water, but due to subsequent changes in the geology and climate of the region, replenishment of the aquifer by natural recharge ceased long ago. Consequently, the Ogallala in a very real sense represents **"fossil" water**—a nonrenewable resource much like coal or oil which, once gone, is gone forever. Thus the heavy rates of groundwater withdrawal which, beginning in the early 1940s, transformed 11 million acres of shortgrass prairie into lush expanses of corn, cotton, and alfalfa raised serious concerns about the region's long-term economic viability as the water table plummeted. Overpumping has been most pronounced in the Texas Panhandle where, by 1990, 24% of that state's portion of the aquifer had been depleted. Rates of extraction during the peak years of the early 1970s led same experts to project that the Ogallala's

BOX 14-3

Three Gorges Dam:
Economic Boon or Eco-Disaster?

Construction of a gigantic dam to tame the mighty Yangtze River has been a dream of Chinese policymakers since the idea was first conceived by Sun Yat-sen in 1919. Decades of social and economic upheaval postponed implementation of the grandiose scheme until 1994, when work began to excavate and prepare the dam's foundations. In November 1997, Chinese engineers diverted the Yangtze out of its riverbed and building of the main dam commenced. The wisdom or folly of such a gargantuan undertaking has prompted an intense, on-going debate in China and abroad over the virtues and drawbacks of massive water management projects.

The practice of obstructing the flow of rivers with earthen barriers, thereby creating a reservoir of stored water, is at least 5,000 years old. Throughout history, humans have engaged in dam building to ensure an adequate supply of water for irrigating crops or to control flooding. By the 20th century, dam construction was also being promoted as a means of providing cheap, clean power, while the reservoirs created by hydroelectric dams offered opportunities for water-based recreation. Until the early 1900s, all dams were relatively small, but improvements in engineering technology and building skills ushered in a new era of megadam construction, with approximately 35,000 large dams now in existence worldwide. The United States was at the forefront of this trend; by 1945, the five largest dams on earth (Hoover, Bonneville, Fort Peck, Shasta, and Grand Coulee) were all in the western U.S. Today, reservoirs behind the thousands of American dams store roughly 60% of the entire average river flow in this country.

In recent decades, however, the allure of megadams has been fading in the United States and other industrialized nations and few, if any, are expected to be built in the years ahead. Lack of suitable sites, high up-front costs, and mounting opposition due to a realization of the serious environmental and social impacts of large dams are constraining future dam construction. In fact, there are now signs, at least in the U.S., that some dams may be dismantled, allowing their rivers to resume normal flow. In 1997, for the first time ever, the U.S. government refused to relicense a small hydroelectric dam on Maine's Kennebec River and ordered its destruction because it was preventing migratory fish from returning to their spawning grounds upstream. Two other dams in Washington State face demolition for the same reason. Licenses for approximately 550 U.S. dams are due to expire within the next 10–15 years and it is expected that a number of them will not be renewed because their ecological costs outweigh their power production benefits.

In the developing world, by contrast, the outlook for megadam construction is far different. Hundreds are now being built or planned in China, India, the Philippines, Nepal, Malaysia, Russia, Brazil, Mexico, and elsewhere. Third World leaders view large dams as symbols of modernity and a highly visible source of national pride. The current dam construction boom is fueled by rapidly growing demand for irrigation water and electricity, both of which additional dams are expected to provide. Nowhere are the plans as ambitious—or the stakes as high—as in China, where the Three Gorges project has provoked intense controversy among hydrologists, engineers, environmentalists, and social scientists worldwide.

The scope of the undertaking is awe-inspiring. Three Gorges is indisputably the largest engineering project the world has ever seen. At the time of scheduled completion in 2009, the main dam will tower 575 feet (185 meters) above the Yangtze River, spanning a distance of approximately one mile. The reservoir formed behind the dam will extend over 350 miles (600 km) upstream and have a storage capacity of approximately 40 billion cubic meters. Project boosters boast that, once operational, Three Gorges will have a hydroelectric capacity close to 18,000 megawatts and will supply one-ninth of China's electrical power. This shift to hydropower, they emphasize, will reduce the country's near-total dependence on coal, lowering Chinese emissions of air pollutants and greenhouse gases. Justification for the Three Gorges project also focuses on the dam's ability to prevent the periodic floods that have historically devastated the Yangtze Valley, thereby protecting the 300 million people and valuable agricultural lands downstream. Since the reservoir created by the dam will increase the Yangtze's upstream water depth, ocean-going vessels for the first time will be able to sail 1,500 miles inland from the Pacific to Chongqing, now China's largest city and destined to become the world's largest seaport.

Groups opposed to the project are concerned that these benefits are more than offset by the dam's environmental and social costs. Construction at Three Gorges will irreversibly alter the ecology of the Yangtze River basin. Dam-induced changes in water chemistry and tempera-ture are expected to have a seriously adverse effect on the river's now-abundant fish species, some of which are unique to the region where the reservoir will form. Observers fear that many commercial fish stocks are likely to disappear as a result. The dam itself will block upstream migration of at least 172 different fish species, preventing spawning. Periodic releases of water from the reservoir will scour the riverbed downstream, washing away small islands that constitute critical habitat for endangered species. Of most concern to local ecologists is the fate of the Chinese River Dolphin (*Lipotes vexillifer*), a "living fossil" descended from a 30-million-year-old species found only in the middle and lower reaches of the Yangtze. With fewer than a hundred individuals left, the dolphins' survival is severely threatened by loss of habitat, decline in food supply, and the potential for accidental collisions with increasing ship traffic. Efforts to relocate the dolphins to nature reserve areas elsewhere on the Yangtze have proven unsuccessful and Chinese naturalists hold out little hope that these unique aquatic mammals can be saved from extinction. Stressing the importance of the Yangtze as a genetic reservoir of freshwater species, Chinese ecologists are racing against the clock to identify and move to safer territory as many threatened fish and plant species as possible before they vanish forever.

Loss of high-quality agricultural land is another unavoidable consequence. Approximately 14,000 hectares of farmland will be inundated and more than 150 towns and hundreds of small villages will be flooded as well. Over 100 archeological sites, some more than 12,000 years old, will be lost to the rising waters, as will some of the world's most spectacular scenery.

Most problematic, however, will be the resettlement of an estimated 1.2 to 1.9 million people, half peasants and half townspeople, living in areas soon to be flooded. Although the Chinese government solemnly promised to give these people land and homes as good as or better than those they were forced to evacuate, such lands simply don't exist in that already overpopulated country. Observers fear that displaced farmers will be squeezed onto marginal lands high on the mountainsides. Recent Chinese government mandates forbidding further deforestation in the Yangtze Valley and prohibiting the construction of terraces on slopes steeper than 25 degrees further reduces the amount of land available for resettlement. Difficulties in relocating more than a half million urban residents will likely prove even more complicated and expensive than resettling farmers. Reports are rife of massive corruption among local officials responsible for resettlement, shoddy construction practices, and lack of employment opportunities for those displaced. As dissatisfaction with the pace of resettlement grows, the potential for social unrest and outbreaks of violence looms.

Because the Three Gorges Dam project is so much larger than any previous undertaking, other impacts are more difficult to predict. Rates of siltation in the world's fourth-muddiest river remain a source of controversy among hydrological engineers but will have a major impact on the water storage capacity of the reservoir. Most experts agree that more than 70% of the sediment carried by the river will be trapped behind the dam each year, gradually reducing its hydropower potential. Below the dam, loss of nutrients traditionally supplied by riverborne sediments could, over time, diminish the fertility of farmlands downstream. Sedimentation

may also interfere with navigation above the dam, causing blockage of the harbor at Chongqing and reducing the project's anticipated financial benefits. Public health impacts of the dam have received little attention. China's Ministry of Health is evaluating the potential for increased rates of schistosomiasis, a serious parasitic disease that still persists in several areas along the Yangtze. Other health risks—malaria, epidemic hantaanvirus hemorrhagic fever, leptospirosis, encephalitis, enterovirus infections, and so forth—have thus far been ignored. Relatively poor health conditions among the present population of the area are likely to be aggravated by project-induced overcrowding, substandard living conditions, and contaminated water supplies.

Concerns about all the adverse consequences of the Three Gorges project prompted a number of important outside financiers and builders to withold funding and support for China's $30 billion undertaking. The World Bank proclaimed the current design of the project "not an economically viable proposition"; the U.S. Bureau of Reclamation declared Three Gorges not to be "environmentally or economically feasible." Several Canadian utilities were instructed not to bid on the project. The U.S. Export-Import Bank has advised companies seeking contracts for the Three Gorges Dam that it would not guarantee their loans, due to serious questions about the dam's environmental, social, and economic sustainability. Several other countries, most notably Germany and Japan, have, however, provided export credits and loans to China for the project.

Within China, opposition to the project has been voiced by a number of prominent intellectuals, scientists, and journalists, but their views have not been widely reported within the country. The editor of a collection of essays (*Yangtze! Yangtze!*) critical of the project was imprisoned for a year without trial and threatened with execution, so it's not surprising that outspoken dissenters are few and far between.

Construction on the dam is now proceeding "full steam ahead," with electrical production scheduled to begin in 2003. The project has given an unexpected boost to tourism, as both Chinese and foreign visitors rush to get a last look at the picturesque beauty of mist-shrouded limestone canyons before they are irretrievably lost. Whether Three Gorges turns out to be the economic panacea envisioned by China's political leaders or the "Chernobyl of hydropower" remains to be seen.

References
Gleick, Peter H. 1998. *The World's Water*. Island Press.

Sleigh, A., and S. Jackson, 1998. "Public Health and Public Choice: Dammed Off at China's Three Gorges?" *The Lancet* 351, no. 9114 (May 16):449–50.

reserves would last only 40 more years and predicted that production of corn, the crop with the highest water demand, would cease entirely within a few years. In fact, irrigated acreage in the High Plains of West Texas declined by 26% between 1979 and 1989. These cutbacks, along with more efficient irrigation techniques, have substantially reduced the rate of groundwater withdrawal in the region, but depletion is still estimated at 12 billion cubic meters annually (Postel, 1996).

Elsewhere in the world, several governments are repeating the mistakes made on the American High Plains. Both Saudi Arabia and Libya have embarked on short-sighted efforts to irrigate desert fields with prodigious amounts of fossil groundwater reserves. Although food self-sufficiency is the stated objective of these undertakings, many experts question the economic wisdom of depleting a nonrenewable resource for agricultural commodities that could be purchased with petrodollars at a much lower price than they are currently spending to encourage domestic production. At current rates of pumping, experts predict Saudi water reserves could be exhausted by 2007, while Libya's aquifer may be pumped dry sometime around 2050.

The impact of groundwater overdrafts extends well beyond constraints on irrigated agriculture. In arid western states, aquifer depletion can precipitate serious environmental problems, the most visible of which is the drying up of many surface streams (recall that many rivers, particularly in dry climates, receive the bulk of their flow from underground sources with which they are in hydrologic contact). In coastal areas around the world, excessive pumping of groundwater to meet the demands of growing urban populations has resulted in migration of seawater into depleted aquifers, contaminating existing freshwater supplies. Saltwater intrusion is now a serious problem in such far-flung cities as Jacksonville, Florida; Dakar, Senegal; Jakarta, Indonesia; and Lima, Peru. Along Israel's Mediterranean shoreline, 20% of the important coastal aquifer is now polluted and officials fear that one out of five coastal wells may have to be abandoned within the next few years. In the United States, saltwater intrusion is endangering water supplies in southern

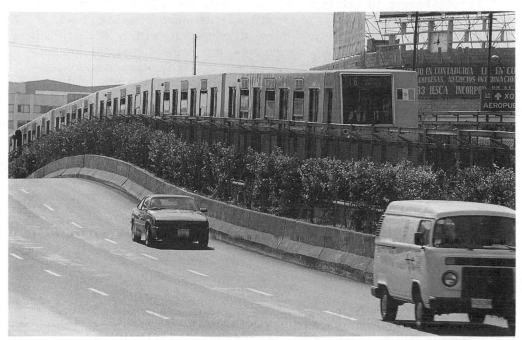

Mexico City's "roller-coaster" highway—the product of overpumping of groundwater and the resulting land subsidence. *[Gerardo Magallon/NYT Pictures]*

California, south Florida, and in portions of Long Island and New Jersey (World Resources Institute, 1992; Postel, 1992; Ashworth, 1982). In addition, as groundwater reserves are depleted, land subsidence is occurring, accompanied by the formation of fissures and faults that disrupt irrigation canals and highways, as well as endangering buildings. In Mexico City, where the pumping of groundwater to supply the needs of 18 million people greatly exceeds the rate of natural recharge, the 16th century Metropolitan Cathedral dominating the city's historic plaza is one of many structures now sagging precariously, and a main thoroughfare has assumed a roller-coaster configuration, both victims of land subsidence. Around Orlando, Florida, overexploitation of groundwater reserves has created huge sinkholes that virtually overnight swallow up chunks of roads, yards, and, occasionally, homes. Falling water tables are also resulting in the abandonment of hundreds of thousands of acres of irrigated lands, as energy costs render pumping too expensive to make such farming economically feasible.

Natural Recharge

Under natural conditions aquifers are recharged by moisture filtering downward from the surface or by seepage from a lake or stream. The area of land which, because of its permeable soils, is the main source of the groundwater inflow is called the **recharge area** of the aquifer. This recharge zone may be many miles from the point at which the water is pumped out of the ground; and because groundwater flows so slowly, the natural refilling of an aquifer may be a very slow process, requiring many centuries in some cases.

In recent years it has become increasingly apparent that a major threat to both the quality and quantity of our groundwater supplies is the growth of industrial, commercial, and residential development within the critical recharge areas of an aquifer. When such areas are stripped of vegetation and covered with buildings and asphalt, the amount of precipitation that can penetrate the soil is greatly reduced. Even in rural areas, land degradation due to deforestation or overgrazing can have an adverse impact on groundwater recharge by reducing the absorptive capacity of soils and increasing the rate of surface runoff. Such factors assume heightened significance in regions where most of the annual precipitation falls during a distinct "rainy season." In some parts of India, for example, where 80% of the rainfall occurs during the summer monsoon, degraded soils can no longer capture as much of the deluge as in previous years and hence even high-rainfall areas now find themselves short of water during the nine dry months of the year.

Development within the recharge area can affect the quality as well as the quantity of groundwater. As human activities within such areas intensify, the potential for infiltration into aquifers of contaminants from waste facilities, leaky sewage pipes, chemical spills, or street runoff increases. A growing realization of the importance of protecting groundwater resources has prompted many state governments in recent years to enact laws regulating the types of development and activities permitted within the critical recharge area of aquifers. In some areas land acquisition plans, funded by either state or local governments, have been instrumental in preserving sensitive recharge areas from potentially harmful development and local citizens' groups have been extremely effective in generating the public support necessary for developing and implementing such programs.

Water Management: Increasing Supply versus Reducing Demand

In the past, as population increase and industrial development boosted urban water demand, cities typically sought to quench their growing thirst by searching for new sources to augment dwindling local supplies. Frequently their reach extended far beyond municipal borders to exploit previously untapped resources in the rural hinterlands. Doing so seemed an obvious solution for a number of reasons: the potential supply appeared limitless and, therefore, relatively cheap; such water generally was of high quality and required little expenditure for treatment; and legal rights to the watershed lands could usually be obtained easily, especially since rural residents seldom had the political savvy necessary to outmaneuver the urban interests which frequently dominated state legislatures. Thus today in places like southern California, where local sources supply only a third of the demand generated by a burgeoning population, the water that maintains lawns, fills swimming pools, and makes life pleasant in the Golden State is imported from the Colorado River, 170 miles to the east, and from sources in northern California as far as 400 miles distant. Similarly, when New Yorkers turn on the tap in Manhattan, the liquid that flows out could have originated from one of a thousand streams in the Catskills, Hudson, or Delaware River valleys. Hetch Hetchy

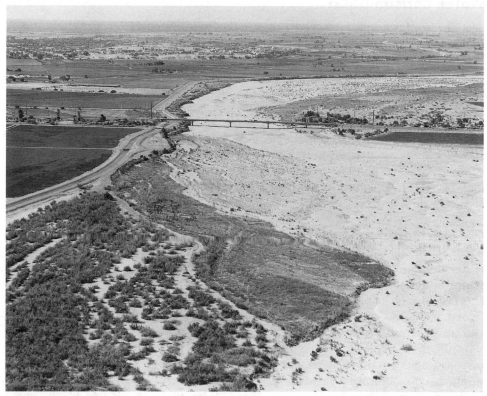

By the time the Colorado River reaches the Southern International Border, there is nothing but dry riverbed. The last of the river's water was diverted 20 miles upstream at the Morelos Dam during the 1950s. *[U.S. Department of the Interior, Bureau of Reclamation]*

Valley in Yosemite National Park provides much of the water supply for San Francisco; Denver taps the headwaters of the Colorado on the opposite side of the Rocky Mountains; and Oklahoma City pipes its supplies from reservoirs in the northeastern Oklahoma hill country more than 100 miles away (Ashworth, 1982).

Since the 1970s, however, city planners have tempered their once-automatic response of pursuing supply-side solutions. Such modern realities as the scarcity of new untapped sources; the sharply escalating costs of building dams and reduced federal funding for the same; competition between urban and agricultural interests for existing supplies; growing opposition to such projects on environmental grounds; plus organized legal resistance by groups in areas targeted for water development have basically brought to a close the era in which city planners attempted to solve water problems through a supply augmentation approach. Today, in metropolitan areas as diverse as Los Angeles and Boston, the emphasis for ensuring adequate water resources has shifted decisively from increasing *supply* to managing *demand*.

Demand management, more commonly referred to by environmentalists as **water conservation,** can include several components: reducing overall use of water, reducing wastage of water, and recycling used water so it can be made available for other purposes.

Water Consumption

To understand how demand management strategies can help meet increased water needs, it is necessary to examine current water use patterns. Worldwide, irrigated agriculture accounts for the lion's share of water consumption—almost 69% of the total. (In Asia, farmers account for fully 82% of all water use; in the United States, 41%; and in Europe, just 30%.) Industries constitute the second largest consumers of water at 23% (more in heavily industrialized areas, less in others), while household use averages about 8% worldwide (obviously, in regions devoid of irrigated agriculture, the percentage of water use attributed to household and industrial use are considerably greater than world averages indicate). Focusing on these three major categories of water consumers, what opportunities do water managers have for reducing demand?

Agriculture. As the largest user—and the largest waster—of water, agriculture also offers the greatest potential for substantial reductions in water demand, in most cases without reducing crop yields. Because irrigation water is almost everywhere priced far below its true value, farmers are given the impression that the supply is plentiful and thus have little incentive to invest in more efficient irrigation technologies. As a result, in most parts of the world irrigators continue to channel or flood water across their fields in a manner that would have looked entirely familiar to their ancestors thousands of years ago. Such practices waste, on average, more than 60% of the water applied, as evaporation or seepage from unlined channels robs thirsty plant roots of the moisture intended for them. More widespread use of advanced techniques such as the automated "drip irrigation" method developed by Israeli scientists can cut water loss to 5% and reduce energy expenses in the bargain. Since the 1980s, farmers in West Texas have achieved dramatic savings by adopting techniques of "surge irrigation" or by installing low-energy

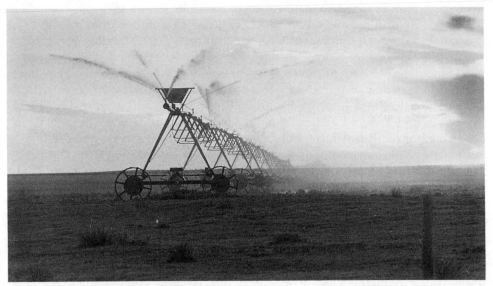

Agricultural irrigation is the largest user—and waster—of water. *[U.S. Department of Agriculture]*

precision application (LEPA) sprinklers that can achieve water use efficiencies as high as 95%. Experts estimate that if the world's farmers could reduce water losses due to inefficient irrigation practices by as little as 10%, the amount saved would be enough to double current domestic use (Postel, 1992). Unfortunately, even though the use of water-saving irrigation methods has grown impressively since the mid-1970s, it is still used on less than 1% of the world's irrigated croplands (WRI, 1998).

Industry. The huge amount of water needed by factories and power plants for processing, cooling, or generating steam accounts for a sizeable portion of total water use in Europe (54%), North America (42%), and other highly developed areas of the world (World Resources Institute, 1992). Since water used by industry is not "consumed" in the traditional sense (i.e. it may become heated or polluted but isn't used up), industrial water use can be substantially reduced by recycling. Within the past decade or so, increasingly stringent federal mandates requiring treatment of industrial wastewater prior to discharge, coupled with the escalating costs of waste treatment and disposal, have given industry a strong incentive to embark on waste minimization strategies that entail recycling and reuse of process waters. Such efforts have resulted in sharp declines in water withdrawals in many industries. Further savings are likely in the years ahead as more and more industries recognize the advantages of climbing aboard the pollution prevention bandwagon.

Households. Although domestic water consumption averages far less than that used for agricultural and industrial purposes, societal norms and public health considerations require that such water be of very high quality, necessitating expensive treatment and distribution systems. In past years, municipal efforts in some areas to restrict residential water consumption were launched as a temporary reaction to drought conditions, largely abandoned when the rains returned or new supplies were tapped. Today urban planners are urging that water conservation become a way of life, even in areas of adequate rainfall, as a means of enhancing water availability and containing rising water costs. Contrary to popular belief, a call for water conservation is not a demand for citizens to change their lifestyle radically, nor does it necessarily imply deprivation. Rather, water conservation means making more efficient use of the resource available.

A number of years ago when a lengthy drought in the Northeast had dangerously lowered the levels of reservoirs supplying water to New York City, officials of the Big Apple sponsored a contest for the best water conservation slogan. One of the catchiest advocated, "Save water: take a bath with a friend!" Those who value their privacy can take heart from the fact that today's options for stretching scarce water supplies are far more sophisticated and entail considerably less personal sacrifice than the old Saturday night frontier practice of everyone bathing in the same progressively dirtier tub!

Water Conservation

Some of the major elements in an effective water conservation program include the following.

Rational Water Pricing. Pricing water to reflect its true cost is fundamental to the success of all other water conservation efforts. Ironically, in many cities current price structures reward profligate users through a system of declining block rates, whereby the cost of additional water units above a certain point is lower than the cost of the initial units. An opposite approach, now used in 15% of the major U.S. metropolitan areas, imposes *higher* unit costs on water use above a specified level, thereby encouraging conservation. Peak demand pricing (e.g. summer: winter price ratio of 3:1) can also help curtail profligate use of water for nonessential purposes. Studies conducted in the United States and elsewhere have shown that when water prices increase by 10%, household water consumption drops 3 to 7% (Bhatra and Falkenmark, 1992). Of course household water use can't be priced appropriately if it isn't metered. The failure of cities in many parts of the world to meter home water use actively discourages water conservation efforts, since consumers see no connection between the amount of water they use and the price they pay. Cities such as New York, Buffalo, Denver, and Sacramento witnessed declines in water use ranging from 10–30% after they installed residential water meters.

Leak Detection/Correction Programs. Both at the household and municipal level, leaky plumbing can waste enormous volumes of water. In homes, leakage accounts for 5–10% of all residential water consumption. A faucet that loses 1 drop per second due to a worn out washer is wasting 7 gallons of water each day; that figure rises to 20 gallons per day with a steady drip. A leaky toilet tank can waste fully 200 gallons per day without making a sound. (To check for toilet tank leakage, simply pour a small amount of food coloring into the tank; if color appears in the toilet bowl before it is flushed, leakage is occurring, probably caused by a worn-out or defective flush ball.) Correcting these leaks is the easiest and cheapest way to reduce home water consumption.

Cities as well as households may be plagued by leaky plumbing. The problem is particularly acute in many developing world cities. Plagued by chronic water scarcity, Amman, Jordan, loses 59% of the water flowing from its water purification plant to homes and institutions, thanks to leaky distribution pipes; in Manila, capital of the Philippines, the figure is 58%; in Mexico City, about one-third (Simon, 1999). Municipalities in the industrialized world are certainly not immune to such problems; it's estimated that cities in the United Kingdom may waste as much as 25% of all treated water due to leakage. In many older U.S. communities the pipes that carry water from a central treatment plant to thousands of homes, institutions, and businesses were installed during the 1800s or early 1900s and have for decades been in serious need of replacement. The current fiscal plight of many urban areas has resulted in short-sighted postponement of these urgently needed renovations. In those cities that have made the necessary investment, however, results have been striking. Prior to a major leak repair program, Boston was losing an estimated 20% of the water entering its distribution system each day; following recent completion of that program, officials credit leak repair with saving the city 35 million gallons daily.

Figure 14-5   Major Water Users in Typical U.S. Home

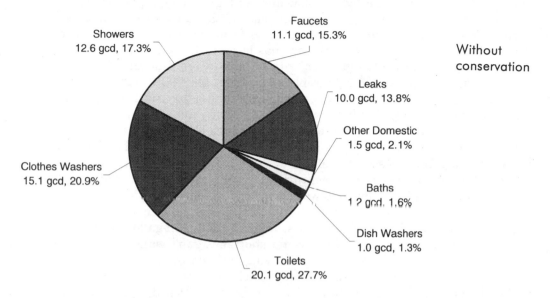

Showers
12.6 gcd, 17.3%

Faucets
11.1 gcd, 15.3%

Without
conservation

Leaks
10.0 gcd, 13.8%

Other Domestic
1.5 gcd, 2.1%

Clothes Washers
15.1 gcd, 20.9%

Baths
1.2 gcd, 1.6%

Dish Washers
1.0 gcd, 1.3%

Toilets
20.1 gcd, 27.7%

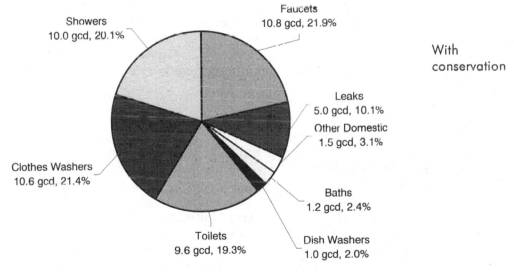

Showers
10.0 gcd, 20.1%

Faucets
10.8 gcd, 21.9%

With
conservation

Leaks
5.0 gcd, 10.1%

Other Domestic
1.5 gcd, 3.1%

Clothes Washers
10.6 gcd, 21.4%

Baths
1.2 gcd, 2.4%

Toilets
9.6 gcd, 19.3%

Dish Washers
1.0 gcd, 2.0%

Source: American Waterworks Association.

Installation of Water-Saving Plumbing Devices. Technology now exists to cut household water use by close to one-half, with no loss of comfort or convenience. Since more water is used in the bathroom than any other room in the house, the focus of home water conservation efforts has been the installation of water-efficient toilets, showerheads, and faucet aerators. The prime candidate for replacement is the water-hogging conventional toilet which, at

5–7 gallons per flush (gpf), is the single largest water user in a typical American home. By the early 1980s, new low-flush (3.5 gpf) toilets became available, followed several years later by ultra-low flush (1.6 gpf) models offering significant water savings. Although early versions of the ultra-low flush toilets encountered customer complaints of poor performance (mainly the need to double-flush), re-engineering of the bowl has largely eliminated this problem. Recent surveys indicate the vast majority of purchasers find ultra-low flush toilets as good or better than the replaced models. In 1992 Congress passed the federal **Energy Policy Act**, establishing mandatory nationwide standards for water-saving plumbing fixtures and specific flush volumes and flow rates for plumbing products. These standards, which took effect on January 1, 1994, include the requirement that any new or replacement toilets sold or installed in the U.S. must be the ultra-low flush 1.6 gallon type. Since approximately 8 million new or replacement toilets are installed in the country each year, it is estimated that by 2025 water-conserving toilets will have replaced most of the pre-1994 stock currently in use. When complete, this transition is expected to result in nationwide water savings of 6.5 billion gallons per day.

Some cities plagued by chronic water shortages don't want to wait until 2025 to enjoy the full benefits of water savings offered by the new plumbing fixtures. As a result, they are providing financial inducements for citizens to replace older models now. Santa Monica, California, imposed a $2 per month "conservation incentive" fee for all single-family homes that hadn't installed low-volume toilets and showerheads. As a result, the city has now completed its toilet replacement program and achieved a permanent 15% reduction in average total water demand and a 20% decrease in total wastewater flow. Santa Rosa, California, requires that whenever new toilets are installed, all old showerheads and faucets must be upgraded also. To make the switchover more palatable, the city offers free water-efficient fixtures in exchange for the older models.

Altered Landscape Practices. Americans' deeply-held conviction that a broad, verdant expanse of weed-free, neatly manicured grass is an essential component of any respectable residence constitutes a major obstacle to meeting urban water conservation goals. Across the United States, approximately 25 million acres are covered with cultivated lawns that annually consume prodigious amounts of fertilizers, pesticides, and high-quality treated water. In some communities in the western United States, fully 40–50% of household water use is devoted to maintaining lawns and gardens.

In an effort to discourage water wastage associated with landscaping practices, a number of communities have initiated some innovative programs aimed at changing American attitudes toward yard maintenance and design. In southern California, where a six-year drought (1987–1992) prompted major changes in water supply planning, the Metropolitan Water District has implemented landscape water conservation regulations for commercial, industrial, institutional, and multifamily properties; MWD is also encouraging similar practices for single-family residences and urging homeowners to select plantings that can thrive with minimal watering. Elsewhere, some communities have enacted legislation restricting the amount of yard space property owners can devote to grass. On Long Island, the town of Southampton, concerned

BOX 14-4
Water Conservation in Your Own Back Yard

Since lawn and garden maintenance typically account for as much as half of all household water use during the warmer months of the year, it is not surprising that the first action taken by many drought-stricken communities is to impose limitations—or an outright ban—on the use of sprinkler systems or hoses for landscape irrigation. Such mandates certainly are effective in terms of water savings but they can exert a heavy economic and aesthetic burden on areas targeted by the restrictions. Expensive horticultural plantings may shrivel up and die, while whole neighborhoods assume a parched yellow-brown appearance. Landscaping firms, nurseries, and lawn-care companies see their profits evaporate as potential customers postpone purchase of water-thirsty sod or shrubs. Are community efforts to ensure their water security through effective water conservation programs incompatible with the desire of property owners to surround themselves with natural beauty? Not for those familiar with the principles of Xeriscape landscaping, a concept that has been spreading rapidly in recent years.

The term Xeriscape™ (derived from the Greek *xeros*, meaning "dry"), was coined and trademarked in 1981 by a group in Colorado searching for a creative new approach to landscaping that would be compatible with and, indeed, enhance water conservation strategies. Convinced that the effects of future droughts could be lessened by water-saving landscaping practices without any sacrifice in landscape beauty, the task force developed and publicized guidelines for Xeriscape landscaping that, if widely adopted, could significantly reduce urban water demand, save home gardeners long hours wielding a hose, and ensure that the periodic dry spells which virtually every region experiences at one time or another (or the long-term climate change many fear is coming) can be weathered with minimal effect on natural surroundings.

Contrary to popular misconceptions, Xeriscape landscaping does not mean a yard composed of pebbles sprayed with green paint nor does it limit one's choice of plants to cactus and yucca. Xeriscaping means designing an outdoor environment that minimizes the need for water input and selecting those plant varieties that can thrive on the amount of natural precipitation characteristic of the region in question. This amount can vary from 8 inches per year in parts of the Southwest, to 30–50 inches in the New England states, to nearly 100 inches per year in the Pacific Northwest. It should be kept in mind that while certain regions of the country may appear to be abundantly well-watered in terms of annual rainfall statistics, many experience prolonged periods of the year during which there is little or no precipitation. Thus in places like proverbially damp Seattle, xeriscaping can be a boon to gardeners during the summer when, in an average year, only 6–10 inches of rain fall from May until October. In such places, Xeriscape landscaping is being actively promoted as "drought insurance."

Just as a xeriscaping approach to landscape design is appropriate in every region of the country, it is also adaptable to virtually any style of landscaping, from the most formal to the most natural. Similarly, there are varying degrees of stringency for executing a xeriscape approach; practitioners may find that they need to water on occasion, but by following certain guidelines they can still achieve considerable reduction in water use (depending on the specific situation, xeriscaping can result in residential water savings of 20–80%). Best of all, when properly carried out, xeriscaping can greatly enhance the visual appeal of one's surroundings. By using a variety of plants appropriate to and reflective of the natural environment of the local area, one can create surroundings far more pleasing aesthetically than the sterile monoscapes of generic grass and shrubs so often the standard choice of homeowners across the country. As proponents of the concept insist, "if it isn't beautiful, then it isn't a Xeriscape landscape."

While "xeriscaping" is not yet a household word, the concept has been gaining adherents rapidly through the combined efforts of gardeners and water managers, both of whom share a common goal: conserving water resources and enhancing the beauty of urban landscapes.

Reference

Ellefson, Connie Lockhart, Thomas L. Stephens, and Doug Welsh. 1992. *Xeriscape™ Gardening*. MacMillan.

about groundwater pollution by lawn chemicals, mandates that no more than 15% of a residential lot be devoted to fertilizer-requiring lawns or vegetables, while a minimum of 80% must be retained in its natural wooded condition; in Tucson, Arizona, an ordinance passed in 1991 prohibits planting grass on any more than 10% of the landscaped area in new developments (Dziegielewski and Baumann, 1992).

Methods of managing water demand such as those just described, accompanied by intensive public information and conservation education programs, will play a major role in meeting future water needs. Encouraging results are already evident from recently launched programs in such disparate regions as southern California and metropolitan Boston, providing convincing evidence that water conservation not only will provide our largest single source of additional water within the next 20 years but will become an accepted way of life. Provided with appropriate technologies and a cost incentive, citizens, farmers, and industrialists alike will validate the assertion of water managers that the cheapest, quickest, most environmentally benign way to meet future water needs is to use existing supplies more efficiently.

References

Ashworth, William. 1982. *Nor Any Drop to Drink*. Summit Books.

Bhatra, Ramesh, and Malin Falkenmark. 1992. "Water Resource Policies and the Urban Poor: Innovative Approaches and Policy Imperatives." *International Conference on Water and the Environment: Development Issues for the 21st Century*. Dublin, Ireland (January 26-31).

Briscoe, John. 1993. "When the Cup is Half Full: Improving Water and Sanitation Services in the Developing World." *Environment* 35, no. 4 (May).

Brown, Lester R., and Brian Halweil, 1998. "China's Water Shortage Could Shake World Food Security," *World Watch* 11, no. 4 (July/August):10-21.

Dziegielewski, Benedykt, and Duane D. Baumann. 1992. "The Benefits of

Managing Urban Water Demands." *Environment* 34, no. 9 (Nov).

Ehrlich, Paul, Anne Ehrlich, and John Holdren. 1977. *Ecoscience*. W. H. Freeman and Co.

Environmental Protection Agency (EPA). 1998. *National Water Quality Inventory: 1996 Report to Congress*. EPA 841-R-97-008 (April).

Falkenmark, Malin, and Carl Widstrand. 1992. "Population and Water Resources: A Delicate Balance." *Population Bulletin* 47, no. 3 (Nov).

Gleick, Peter, ed. 1993. *Water in Crisis: A Guide to the World's Fresh Water Resources*. Oxford University Press.

Maurits la Riviere, J. W. 1989. "Threats to the World's Water." *Scientific American* (Sept).

National Research Council (NRC). 1999. *Setting Priorities for Drinking Water Contaminants*. National Academy Press.

Postel, Sandra. 1996. *Dividing the Waters: Food Security, Ecosystem Health, and the New Politics of Scarcity*. Worldwatch Paper 132 (September).

———. 1992. *Last Oasis: Facing Water Scarcity*. W. W. Norton & Co.

Rail, Chester D. 1989. *Groundwater Contamination: Sources, Control, and Preventive Measures*. Technomic Publishing Co.

Sanford, Cynthia, and Joe Oosterhout. 1991. "Protecting Groundwater: The Unseen Resource." *The National Voter* 40, no. 5 (June/July).

Simon, Paul. 1998. *Tapped Out*. Welcome Rain Publishers.

U.S. Water Resources Council. 1978. *The Nation's Water Resources, 1975–2000*. U.S. Government Printing Office.

Vickers, Amy. 1993. "The Energy Policy Act: Assessing Its Impact on Utilities." *Journal of the American Waterworks Association* (August).

World Bank. *The World Development Report 1992: Development and Environment*. Washington, D.C.

World Resources Institute (WRI). 1998. *World Resources 1998–99*. Oxford University Press.

———. 1992. *World Resources 1992-93*. Oxford University Press.

CHAPTER 15

Water Pollution

Water, water everywhere
Nor any drop to drink…

—Samuel Taylor Coleridge
(*The Rime of the Ancient Mariner*)

Back in the days when human settlements were relatively small and far apart, the issue of water contamination seldom occupied much attention on the part of the general public. Prevailing sentiment insisted that "the solution to pollution is dilution," and popular wisdom held that "a stream purifies itself every ten miles." While such statements have a certain amount of validity, they lost their relevance as villages mushroomed into crowded cities and as the expanse of countryside between towns steadily contracted under the impact of urban sprawl. The rapid growth of human population and of industrial output has resulted in a corresponding decline in water quality, as both municipalities and industry regarded the nation's waterways as free, convenient dumping grounds for the waste products of civilized society. During the 19th century our careless waste management practices turned most rivers into open sewers and many once-healthy lakes into algae-covered cesspools. It is estimated that most of the world's water drainage basins are polluted with such contaminants as toxic chemicals, human and animal excrement, heavy metals, pesticides, silt, and fertilizers. These contaminants are carried downstream where they are discharged into coastal waters that have become increasingly degraded over the past two decades. The problems posed by such pollutants involve far more than unpleasant sights and odors. Waterborne disease outbreaks, massive fish kills, long-lasting changes in aquatic ecosystems, and severe economic loss to sports and recreation-based industries are all directly related to degradation of water quality by human activities.

Controlling Water Pollution: The Clean Water Act

Although water pollution had been recognized as a major environmental problem in the United States for many decades, it was not until 1972 that a tough, comprehensive federal program to deal with this issue was enacted by Congress. Known originally as the Federal Water Pollution Control Act Amendments (Public Law 92-500), this landmark piece of legislation underwent some "mid-course corrections" in 1977, at which time its name was changed to the Clean Water Act. Prior to passage of this law, our nation's water pollution control strategy, such as it was, focused on attempts to clean up waterways to the point that they could be used for whatever purpose state governments had determined their function should be (e.g. drinking water, swimming, fishing, navigation, etc.). Thus each stream or portion of a stream might have a different water quality standard, and if that standard was not being met, it was up to the state water pollution control agency to determine which discharger was responsible for the violation and to seek enforcement action. This system was totally ineffective for a number of reasons: designations of desired stream use were frequently modified to retain or attract industrial development; insufficient information was available on how pollutant discharges were affecting water quality; blame for violation was difficult, if not impossible, to assess when more than one source was discharging into a waterway; little attention was paid to the effects of pollution on the aquatic environment as a whole; and only contaminants entering a waterway through pipe discharges were given much attention. Undoubtedly the most serious drawback of the pre-1972 water pollution control strategy was the lack of enforcement power. State agencies had to negotiate with all the polluters along a given waterway, trying to persuade each individual source to reduce its discharges to the point at which water quality standards for the particular river or lake in question could be met. Not uncommonly, when industries disliked what they were being told, they would threaten to close down and move to a less demanding state. Also, due to the nature of river basins, many states discovered that in order to improve their own water quality, they had to persuade states upstream to pollute less.

Passage of the Clean Water Act radically altered this approach to water pollution control and took a new philosophical stance toward the problem, reflected in the 1972 Senate Committee's statement that "no one has the right to pollute . . . and that pollution continues because of technological limits, not because of any inherent right to use the Nation's waterways for the purpose of disposing of wastes." Stressing the need to "restore and maintain the chemical, physical, and biological integrity of the Nation's waters," Congress declared as national goals the attainment, wherever possible, of water quality "that provides for recreation in and on the water" (popularly referred to as the "fishable-swimmable waters" goal) by July 1, 1983, and the elimination of all pollutant discharges into the nation's waterways by 1985 ("zero discharge" goal). These goals are not the same as legal requirements—they cannot be enforced and certainly were not attained by the dates indicated; nevertheless, they have been useful in providing objectives toward which to strive and against which progress in improving water quality can be measured.

Progress in moving toward the goals set forth by Congress is difficult to assess on a comprehensive national basis because budgetary constraints, both at the federal and state levels, preclude the possibility of continuously monitoring the quality of all U.S. waterways. In addition, water quality at any one location changes from season to season and year to year. Even determining long-term trends for specific pollutants is somewhat problematic because of the lack of historical records and inconsistencies in the data that has been collected. Also, since the various states and organizations that survey water quality utilize different monitoring strategies, it is often impossible to combine or compare survey results. Active efforts are currently underway to improve nationwide monitoring efforts and to establish an effective, uniform means of collecting, interpreting, and presenting water quality information. In the meantime, policymakers must rely on the EPA's biennial *National Water Quality Inventory: Report to Congress*—a compilation of data submitted to the EPA by individual states, territories, Indian tribes, Interstate Water Commissions, and the District of Columbia. Important information on water quality conditions and trends in 60 representative river basins and aquifers is also provided by the U.S. Geological Survey's National Water Quality Assessment Program (NAWQA). A compilation of information from these and several other government agency sources is provided by the Index of Watershed Indicators (IWI), first released in 1997 and scheduled to be updated periodically. According to the IWI, 16% of the nation's watersheds are characterized by water of good quality, 36% had moderate water quality problems, and 21% had more serious problems; for 27% of the watersheds sufficient data for characterization was lacking. Assuming these figures are reliable, they indicate commendable progress in the years since passage of the Clean Water Act, when fully 95% of all U.S. watersheds were regarded as polluted. During several decades when both the economy and population size have grown substantially, the fact that overall surface water quality hasn't deteriorated gives evidence that the billions of dollars spent on water cleanup efforts have had a positive impact. Nevertheless, EPA's most recent water quality assessment reported that 40% of the rivers, lakes, and estuaries surveyed are too polluted for fishing and swimming, indicating we have a long way to go before the goals of the Clean Water Act are fully met. While many of the conventional sources and types of water pollution are now being dealt with fairly adequately, newer problems such as toxic chemical pollutants and difficult to control runoff from farms, construction sites, and city streets have stymied pollution abatement efforts (EPA, 1998).

Elsewhere in the world, water quality issues rank high on the list of international environmental concerns. Not surprisingly, progress in controlling water pollution varies widely from one country to another. Most developed nations have imposed controls on industrial dischargers similar to those in the United States and the majority have helped finance the construction of sewage treatment plants. As a result, at least two-thirds of all western Europeans and North Americans are served by wastewater treatment facilities (Switzerland, Denmark, Netherlands, Sweden, and western Germany provide such services to nearly all their citizens). By contrast, in the nations of southern and eastern Europe, half or more of the population live in municipalities where sewage is discharged untreated into waterways. The percentage of the population served by wastewater treatment plants in some representative

European countries include: Greece, 11%; Portugal, 21%; Hungary, 31%; Poland, 37%; Czech Republic, 50%. In Asia, Japan and South Korea have made notable progress in expanding access to sewage treatment which, by 1990, served 50% and 43%, respectively, of their populations (WRI, 1996). Unfortunately, in the developing nations and most of the former Soviet republics the situation is bad and getting worse. Rapid industrial growth has given rise to numerous toxic "hotspots" of pollution, as industrial dischargers dump poisonous effluent into nearby waterways, unhindered by nonexistent or seldom-enforced water pollution laws. In China, for example, industrial discharges containing both toxic and carcinogenic compounds are fouling rivers that provide the main source of drinking water. Though many people attempt to protect themselves by boiling water before using it for human consumption, doing so has no effect on most toxic contaminants. Throughout the developing world untreated sewage, as well as salt- and fertilizer-laden irrigation return flows further contaminate lakes, rivers, and coastal waters. In South Asia, the South and Southeast Pacific, and in Africa modern sewage treatment is virtually nonexistent; of India's 3,119 towns and cities, only 8 provide full treatment of municipal wastewaters. In developing countries as a whole, 95% of urban sewage is discharged untreated (Pimentel et al., 1998). Even in Latin America, where sanitary standards are generally better than in other developing regions, by the early 1990s only 41% of city dwellers were served by sewer systems and over 90% of the wastewater collected flowed directly into surface waters without receiving any treatment whatsoever (WRI, 1992).

To understand the worldwide impact of water pollution on the health of both ecosystems and their human inhabitants requires a look at the major sources and types of pollution and the problems posed by each. The remainder of this chapter will examine these issues and will describe the pollution control policies developed by the U.S. Congress and regulatory agencies as they strive to protect public health through improving water quality.

Sources of Water Pollution

Pollutants can enter waterways by a number of different routes. Strategies for preventing water contamination must take into consideration the nature of the pollutant source and must devise appropriate methods of control for each source category. Congress has coined two terms—**point source** and **nonpoint source**—to refer to the two general types of water pollution, and pollution control regulations adopted within recent years have by necessity been tailored according to source.

Point Sources

Pollutants that enter waterways at well-defined locations (e.g. through a pipe, ditch, or sewer outfall) are referred to as point source pollutants. Characterized by discharges that are relatively even and continuous, typical point sources of water pollution include factories, sewage treatment plants, and storm sewer outfalls. Point sources have been the most conspicuous violators of water quality standards, but because effluent from such sources is relatively easy to collect and treat, considerable progress has been made during

BOX 15-1

"The Cell From Hell"

Pfiesteria piscicida, dubbed "the cell from hell" by various commentators, is blamed for numerous massive fish kills along America's eastern seaboard during the 1990s. From the brackish riverine waters of the North Carolina coast to Chesapeake Bay and Maryland's Pocomoke River, "*Pfiesteria* hysteria" has provoked fear, dismay, and a determination among researchers to find out what's amiss in the nation's coastal waters.

The subject of all this attention is a single-celled, toxic dinoflagellate alga, unknown to science until 1988 when it was discovered by Dr. Joan Burkholder, an aquatic ecologist at North Carolina State University. Although most dinoflagellates function like typical plants, obtaining energy through the process of photosynthesis, *Pfiesteria* behaves quite differently. Lacking chlorophyll and hence incapable of photosynthesizing, *P. piscicida* thrives by eating other organisms, primarily algae and fragments of organic matter. Research has revealed an extremely complex life cycle, parts of which are still not completely understood. *P. piscicida* can assume at least 24 different morphological forms, at various times amoeboid, flagellated, encysted, and so forth. Several of these forms are capable of producing a powerful toxin as yet unidentified, reported to be 1,000 times more poisonous than cyanide. Factors triggering the transformation of *Pfiesteria* from its normally benign state into a killer are still being investigated; some researchers suggest that the presence of large schools of fish, particularly Atlantic menhaden, may somehow cause *P. piscicida* to assume a lethal form. When this happens, *Pfiesteria* begins to release a toxin that stuns the fish and causes them to become lethargic. Other toxins subsequently emitted by *Pfi-* *esteria* destroy the fishes' skin, producing open lesions that often prove fatal. *Pfiesteria* then feeds on exposed fish tissues and blood.

Aside from the ecological and economic concerns raised by large-scale fish kills, human health problems associated with exposure to *Pfiesteria* toxins have generated concern. A number of individuals who were fishing or swimming in waters where *Pfiesteria* toxin was present report developing skin rashes, memory loss, and a feeling of light-headedness. More dramatic were the symptoms experienced by Dr. Burkholder and a graduate student who, working with *P. piscicida* in an inadequately ventilated laboratory, were stricken with headaches, nausea, vomiting, respiratory problems, mood changes, burning eyes, memory loss, and open sores on their hands and arms. The Centers for Disease Control and Prevention (CDC) has established a multi-state surveillance system and is evaluating potential public health risks of *P. piscicida*. Referring to the condition as **possible estuary associated syndrome (PEAS)**, CDC in 1999 announced it was not yet able to establish a definitive link between PEAS and *Pfiesteria* because the toxin itself had not yet been identified. Anecdotal reports suggest that people experience the described effects when the toxins come into contact with the skin or when toxins are inhaled; risk also is associated with the length and intensity of exposure. Fortunately, the adverse effects provoked by *P. piscicida* toxin are reversible—all the individuals recovered completely within six months. Another health concern expressed by coastal community residents—the safety of eating fish from waters where *Pfiesteria* toxin is present—appears to be groundless; there is no evidence as yet that exposed fish present any food poisoning risk to local residents.

While much has been learned about *P. piscicida* over the last decade, the big question of what triggers toxic blooms remains unanswered. Many environmentalists and Dr. Burkholder herself strongly suspect that the mammoth hog- and poultry-raising operations proliferating along the mid-Atlantic coastal plain since the early 1990s are largely to blame. Nutrient-laden runoff from fields heavily fertilized with animal manures is believed to be stimulating the growth of algae, which are *Pfiesteria*'s prime food source during its nontoxic stage; *P. piscicida* populations then explode as an indirect result of the algal blooms. Some research also suggests that phosphorus, a major component of agricultural runoff, can directly stimulate growth and reproduction of *P. piscicida*, though conclusive proof of this is still lacking. To some residents along North Carolina's Neuse River, the fact that *Pfiesteria* problems began soon after megahog farms moved into the area seems more than coincidental. In North Carolina, which was the fastest-growing pork producing state in the country until a moratorium on new and expanded factory hog farms was imposed in 1998, manure spills from waste impoundments and runoff from fields fertilized with hog manure have been identified as the source of serious water pollution problems. In Maryland's Pocomoke watershed, the most likely culprits endangering water quality are 600 million chickens. Maryland's eastern shore now boasts a $1.5 billion/year poultry industry and chicken wastes, minimally regulated, are routinely land-applied to nearby cornfields.

It's long been known that nitrogen and phosphorus runoff from animal feedlots or manure-fertilized fields can cause algal blooms in waterways. Although spreading manure on cropland is a time-honored method of recycling nutrients, the enormous amounts of waste generated by factory-scale livestock production facilities overwhelm the assimilative capacity of adjacent fields. For many years governments have decreed that sanitary wastes from human communities be treated prior to discharge, but regulations setting comparable standards for concentrated livestock operations have yet to be issued. As a result, factory farms whose animals produce amounts of waste with a BOD (see Box 15-3) equivalent to that of a medium-sized town are disposing these materials without any treatment whatsoever. Because the amount of land that would be necessary to distribute manure at agronomic rates is so much greater than what is usually available, factory farm managers typically apply excessive quantities to a given land area. Not surprisingly, the excess nutrients run off into streams or infiltrate underlying aquifers and pollute groundwater supplies.

Fears of offending powerful agri-business interests or, conversely, endangering the livelihood of small farmers under contract to large corporations, have until recently deterred state legislators from enacting strict controls on factory farming. *Pfiesteria*'s sudden notoriety may have altered the equation. Regulatory controls are gradually being toughened and state agencies in North Carolina, Maryland, Virginia, Delaware, and Florida are now working closely with university researchers to address issues posed by harmful algal blooms. Several agencies of the federal government, including EPA, the USDA, CDC, the National Oceanic and Atmospheric Administration, the U.S. Geological Survey, the FDA, and the National Institute of Environmental Health Sciences, are joining in the effort to learn more about *Pfiesteria* and to determine the causes of *P. piscicida* outbreaks, particularly the role played by nutrient runoff. A federal program to reduce runoff from 450,000 livestock confinement facilities across the country was unveiled in the spring of 1999 and efforts were launched to secure additional funding for states to control polluted runoff. For such a tiny creature, *Pfiesteria* has created quite a stir!

References

Environmental Protection Agency. 1999. *Pfiesteria piscicida Fact Sheet.* Office of Water.

Ecological Society of America. "Nonpoint Pollution of Surface Waters with Phosphorus and Nitrogen." *Issues in Ecology,* no. 3, Summer.

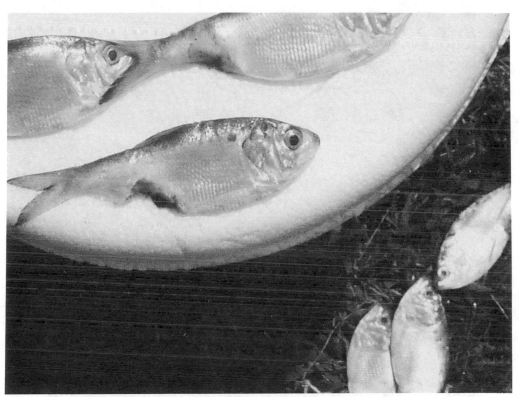

Gaping raw sores are the classic symptom of fish attacked by *Pfiesteria piscicida.* [Marty Katz/ NYT Pictures]

the past decade in reducing this type of pollutant discharge. The two major categories of point source pollution are sewage treatment plants and industrial discharges. Each will be discussed in greater detail later in this chapter.

Nonpoint Sources

Until the 1980s, nonpoint source (NPS) pollutants—those which run off or seep into waterways from broad areas of land rather than entering the water through a discreet pipe or conduit—were largely overlooked as significant contributors to water contamination. However, when stringent effluent

Approximately half of our water quality violations can be traced to stormwater runoff from broad land areas. Controlling pollution from these diverse sources is proving far more difficult than reducing pollutants from point sources.

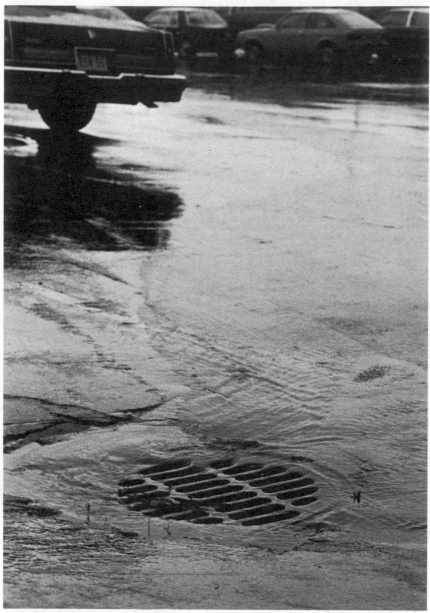

Nonpoint source of water pollution: urban street runoff. *[Illinois Environmental Protection Agency]*

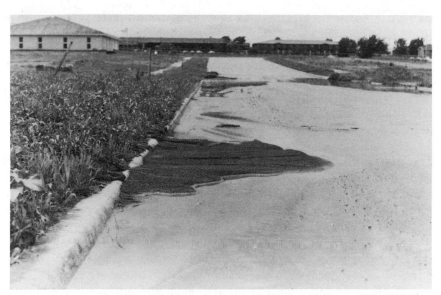

Nonpoint source of water pollution: construction site runoff. *[Gary Fak, Soil Conservation Service]*

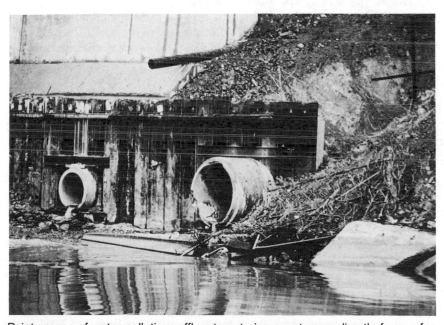

Point source of water pollution: effluents entering a waterway directly from a factory outfall, pipe, ditch, or sewage treatment plant outlet are the most visible source of water pollution. *[Illinois Environmental Protection Agency]*

limitations on point sources failed to result in dramatic improvements in water quality, it became increasingly evident that in many waterways the largest pollutant contribution was coming from nonpoint sources. Today the majority of states identify pollutants coming from nonpoint sources as the main reason they have been unable to attain their water quality goals. Nonpoint source pollution (really just new terminology for old-fashioned runoff and sedimentation) results primarily from a variety of human land-use practices and includes the following.

Agriculture. In the United States as a whole, agriculture is the leading source of water pollution, adversely affecting the quality of 50–70% of the nation's surface waters. Among the various contaminants present in farmland runoff, the single most abundant is soil. While most people tend to think of erosion largely in terms of its adverse impact on agricultural productivity, soil entering streams or lakes can severely damage aquatic habitats as well. By increasing the turbidity of the water, sediment sharply reduces light penetration and thereby decreases photosynthetic rates of producer organisms; it buries bottom-dwelling animals, suffocating fish eggs and aquatic invertebrates. Stormwater runoff from fields and pastures carries more than just sediment into waterways, however. Manures from grazing lands or from large livestock management facilities (i.e. "megahog" farms) located adjacent to streams or lakes can contribute five or six times as many nutrients to waterways as do point sources. Manure spread on fields can cause similar problems unless it is applied at rates moderate enough to permit complete uptake of nutrients by plants (i.e. at agronomic rates of uptake). In the same way, chemical fertilizers and pesticides, when applied immediately prior to a storm or in amounts exceeding the assimilative capacity of the crop in question, can be carried by runoff water from fields into adjacent lakes or streams. Upon entering a waterway, farm chemicals can poison fish or promote algal growth; if runoff seeps through the soil into shallow aquifers, chemical contamination of drinking water wells can occur. Since these toxic pollutants generally enter waterways attached to soil particles, they can best be controlled by the same strategies used to prevent soil erosion—conservation tillage, terracing, contour plowing, etc.—which aim to keep soil on the land and out of the water. Additional management strategies include: applying pesticides when there is little wind and the potential for heavy rain is low; using nonpersistent, low-toxicity pesticides; disposing of containers properly; applying fertilizers or manures only when they can be incorporated into the soil (i.e. not when the ground is frozen); and using any type of chemical in the proper amount and only when field checks indicate they are needed. Controlling runoff from pasturelands can be managed relatively easily by maintaining a buffer zone of vegetation along waterways and using fences to prevent livestock from walking into streams.

Construction Activities. Acre for acre, runoff from sites where homes, shopping centers, factories, or highways are under construction can contribute more sediment to waterways than any other activity—typically 10–20 times more than the amounts from agricultural lands. More than 500 tons of sediment per acre per year can wash off such sites into streams during the construction period, frequently carrying with them cement wash, asphalt, paint and cleaning solvents, oil and tar, and pesticides. These contaminants from construction sites have impaired an estimated 5% of U.S. surface waters. Fortunately the actual construction time during which land surfaces are unprotected is relatively short and the amount of land exposed is small in comparison with farm acreage. Nevertheless, damage to water quality due to construction site runoff can be severe and long-lasting. Many municipalities are now mandating the use of readily available erosion control techniques on construction sites, the basic approach being to expose the smallest area of land possible for the shortest period of time and scheduling construction activities so that the minimum amount of land is disturbed during the peak runoff period in the spring. Using mulches and fast-growing cover vegetation, retaining as many existing trees and shrubs on the site as possible, roughening the soil surface or constructing berms to slow the velocity of runoff, and building retention basins to detain runoff water long enough to promote settling out of suspended sediment are all well-established management practices for reducing pollutant runoff from construction sites.

Urban Street Runoff. Although people seldom consider city streets and sidewalks as important sources of water pollution, studies have shown that during storm episodes, particularly storms that terminate a long dry spell, very large amounts of sediment and other pollutants are carried by runoff water into adjacent rivers, streams, or lakes. In many cities, the total pollutant load from urban runoff exceeds that from industrial discharges. Contaminants commonly found in urban runoff include sand, dirt, road salt, oil, grease, and heavy metal particles (lead, zinc, copper, chromium, etc.) from paved surfaces; pesticides and fertilizers from lawns; leaves, seeds, bark, and grass clippings; animal and bird droppings; and other substances too numerous to mention. The EPA has documented discharge of suspended solids from storm sewers in amounts far exceeding those entering waterways from sewage treatment plants. EPA also cited urban runoff as a major contributor of oil to surface waters and a prime source of the pollutants that impair the nation's estuaries (EPA, 1998).

Reducing pollution from this source requires broad-based cooperation and effort on the part of both municipal officials and citizens: more frequent street-sweeping to prevent sediment accumulation on streets; proper disposal of pet wastes; careful and limited application of lawn and garden fertilizers and pesticides; litter control on both public and private property; judicious use of road salt and sand; application of organic mulches to reduce erosion on bare ground; incorporating more green space within the urban areas and along waterways to allow runoff to filter into the ground; use of surface ponds, holding tanks, rooftop catchments, subsurface tunnels, or similar structures to hold, retain, and gradually release stormwater.

Acid Mine Drainage. When the iron pyrite found in association with coal deposits is exposed to air and water during mining operations, a series of chemical reactions is initiated, culminating in the formation of a copper-colored precipitate (iron hydroxide) and sulfuric acid. The precipitate frequently covers the bottom of streams in mining regions, smothering bottom life and

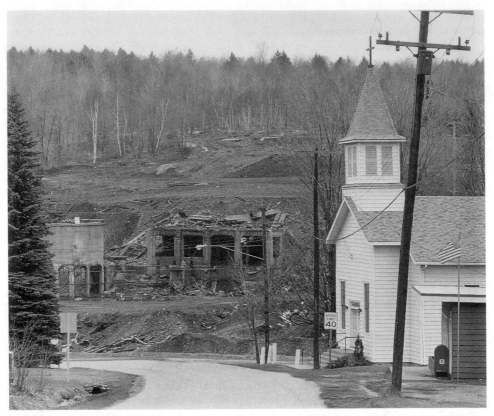

Acidified water flowing out of abandoned mines such as the one in the center of this photo constitutes an important nonpoint source of water pollution. *[U.S. Department of Agriculture]*

giving such streams a characteristic rusty appearance. The sulfuric acid lowers the pH of the water, eliminating many aquatic species that cannot survive or reproduce in the acidified water. Both operating and abandoned coal mines of either the underground or surface type are characterized by acid drainage, although only *abandoned* mines are termed nonpoint sources (*active* mines are classified as point source polluters). In West Virginia, the third largest coal-producing state in the United States and home to thousands of inactive mines, acid mine drainage constitutes the leading nonpoint pollution source—a problem shared by many other mining areas as well. Acids, however, are not the only water quality problem posed by abandoned mines. Under the low pH conditions prevailing in such regions, metals such as iron, aluminum, copper, zinc, manganese, magnesium, and calcium are leached from soil and rock, contaminating streams. Large amounts of silt and sediment from slag heaps or refuse piles erode into waterways, clogging streams and burying bottom-dwellers under a thick layer of silt. Legislatively mandated regrading and revegetation of abandoned strip mines have been helpful in reducing runoff of sediment from abandoned mine sites, but have had minimal impact on acid drainage. Sealing openings to abandoned underground mines, thereby cutting off the supply of oxygen and water that permit acid formation, has been the chief means of combatting acid mine drainage. Although this practice signifi-

BOX 15-2

Hypoxia in the Gulf of Mexico

Journalists call it the "dead zone"—a huge underwater expanse on Louisiana's continental shelf that each summer becomes so oxygen-deficient that any creatures in the vicinity flee elsewhere or die. Extending over approximately 6,000 to 7,000 square miles (18,000 km^2) from the mouth of the Mississippi River almost to the Texas coast, this **hypoxic zone**, as it is properly termed, is characterized by waters with dissolved oxygen concentrations below 2 parts per million—the minimal amount required for survival of most species of marine organisms. Hypoxia is not a situation unique to the Gulf of Mexico. Several major water bodies—the Black Sea, Baltic Sea, and Chesapeake Bay, to name a few—have always experienced periodic bouts of hypoxia, as do many smaller lakes and ponds. The Gulf "dead zone" is generating unusual concern, however, because of its considerable increase in size during the 1990s and due to its location in the midst of one of the United States' most important commercial and recreational fishing areas. There is also a growing conviction among scientists studying the phenomenon that a better understanding of the "dead zone" will be invaluable for tackling similar problems in many areas around the world.

Gulf hypoxia—to the extent it occurs today—is unquestionably a human-made problem. While a small hypoxic area probably always existed near the mouth of the Mississippi, there is general agreement that today's "dead zone" was gradually created since the 1950s by increasing amounts of nutrients, primarily nitrates and phosphates, discharged into the Gulf by the Mississippi and Atchafalaya Rivers. The impact of pollutants draining from the Mississippi watershed into the Gulf was never more dramatic than during the summer of 1993, when record flooding throughout the region caused the hypoxic zone to expand suddenly from 3,500 to nearly 8,000 square miles. To the puzzlement of Gulf ecologists, the area of oxygen depletion has decreased only slightly since 1993, averaging a bit less than 7,000 square miles during the peak months of June-July-August before breaking up in late autumn. In July 1999 it broke all previous records, extending over an area the size of New Jersey.

The biological chain of events that gives rise to hypoxic conditions in the Gulf is a phenomenon frequently observed in freshwater lakes and ponds during warm summer months—a process known as **eutrophication**. A term meaning "well fed," eutrophication is initiated when dissolved nutrients enter a body of water where they stimulate the growth and proliferation of algae. These algal "blooms" cause several problems. Because some species produce powerful toxins, their sudden appearance may result in massive fish kills. These so-called "red tides" seem to be increasing in frequency in coastal waters worldwide. Equally important, as algal numbers increase exponentially, large numbers die and drift to the bottom where they constitute an unexpected feast for decomposer organisms, primarily bacteria. As bacterial populations explode in response to the increased food supply, their high rate of metabolic activity causes levels of dissolved oxygen in the water to plummet. The drop in oxygen content is particularly rapid in summer because high temperatures promote more rapid metabolism and because warm water holds less dissolved oxygen than does colder water.

The ultimate effect of oxygen depletion is the loss of fish and other organisms requiring high levels of dissolved oxygen and their replacement by species more tolerant of hypoxic conditions.

The source of the nutrients that set this whole process in motion in the Gulf remains the subject of acrimonious debate. Early contentions that Gulf hypoxia simply reflects naturally occurring fluctuations in dissolved oxygen have been put to rest by research results demonstrating a clear association between Mississippi River flow, abundant amounts of riverborne nitrates and phosphates, increased algal growth in the Gulf, and bottom water hypoxia. Although the nutrients discharged to the Mississippi watershed obviously come from a multitude of sources—sewage treatment plant effluent, urban stormwater runoff, atmospheric deposition—the general consensus is that Midwestern farmers bear most of the blame for the approximately 1 to 1.5 million tons of nitrogen flowing into the Gulf each year. Using radioisotopes to date animal remains in sediment cores taken from the dead zone, scientists have demonstrated a sharp decline in the numbers of high oxygen-demanding species and a corresponding increase in low oxygen tolerant species during the same years that chemical fertilizer applications were soaring in the Corn Belt. As an economist at the University of Minnesota remarked, "The gulf has become the end of the pipe for American agriculture."

Analyzing the cause of the problem is relatively straightforward; reversing the situation promises to be much more difficult, although scientists are optimistic that recovery is possible. A significant reduction (20% or more is regarded as essential) in nitrogen loadings to the Mississippi watershed—a vast area draining over 40% of the land area of the lower 48 states—is key to solving the problem.

Phosphorus is usually the limiting nutrient whose over-abundance causes eutrophication in freshwater bodies, but in marine environments like the Gulf nitrogen concentrations are more critical. Since industrial and municipal point sources combined are estimated to contribute a mere 3–5% of all the nitrogen carried down the Mississippi, agriculture will bear the brunt of control measures, should they be imposed. Scientists are convinced that only a change in farming practices, particularly in the Corn Belt states of the upper Midwest, can reduce Gulf nitrogen loadings enough to ease hypoxic conditions in the dead zone. Dr. Keith Kelling, a soil scientist at the University of Wisconsin, believes significant reductions are feasible because, he contends, half to three-fourths of the corn acreage in Illinois, Indiana, Iowa, Nebraska, and Minnesota is currently receiving nitrogen fertilizer applications 25% above recommended rates. Dr. Otto Doering, an agricultural economics professor at Purdue, argues that farmers can use a variety of methods, such as not applying fertilizers in the fall, to cut nitrogen runoff by 20–25% without having a detrimental effect on food prices or farm exports. Another proposed approach is the restoration of major wetlands along the Mississippi watershed—an undertaking that would provide significant flood control benefits as well. Suggestions that farmers be paid to create wetlands reserves along river banks to capture and contain farmland runoff are now receiving serious consideration by federal and state agencies.

As policymakers discuss the thorny issue of how the burden of resurrecting the dead zone should be shared, researchers continue efforts to expand their understanding of the diverse factors controlling algal blooms and hypoxia. A cooperative venture linking government agencies, private industry, and citizens' groups—The Gulf of Mexico Program—has been studying the hypoxia problem and is assisting with efforts to examine all aspects of the situation. Meanwhile, as the talk and investigations continue, Gulf Coast fishers and shrimpers bypass the dead zone, knowing any nets or lines cast into the bright blue waters will come up empty.

References

National Oceanic and Atmospheric Administration. 1998. *Gulf of Mexico Hypoxia Assessment Plan.* Committee on Environment and Natural Resources Hypoxia Work Group (March).

Rabalais, N.N., et al. 1996. "Nutrient Changes in the Mississippi River and System Responses on the Adjacent Continental Shelf." *Estuaries* 19:286-407.

Warrick, Joby. 1999. "Death in the Gulf of Mexico." *National Wildlife* 37, no. 4 (June/July):48-52.

cantly reduces acid loadings, it doesn't eliminate them and efforts to find better ways of dealing with the problem continue. In recent years, the use of engineered wetlands to remove toxic chemicals from mine leachate have yielded promising results, as have alkaline recharge zones incorporated into more advanced artificial wetlands designed to neutralize acids. These and other innovative approaches to abating acid mine drainage are undergoing active investigation and offer hope that a solution to this challenge will eventually be found (Bennett, 1991).

Fallout of Airborne Pollutants. The situation represented by acid rainfall (see chapter 12) is but one example of pollution from the sky causing water quality problems. A great many of the particles released into the atmosphere through human activities eventually return to earth and enter rivers,

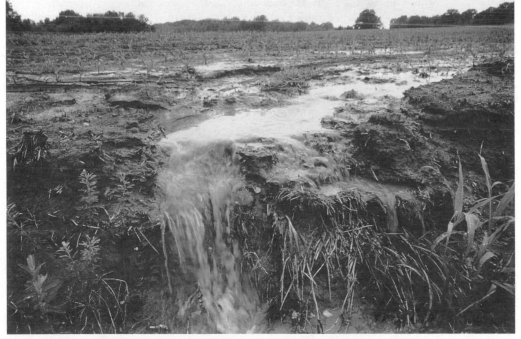

Farm runoff is the leading source of water pollution in the U.S. today. *[USDA]*

Figure 15-1   How Excess Nutrients Degrade Water Quality

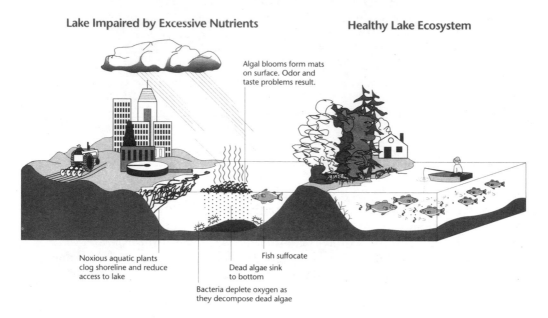

Source: EPA, *National Water Quality Inventory 1996 Report ot Congress,* April 1998.

lakes, or oceans either directly or in runoff. These airborne particles include many hazardous chemicals such as lead, asbestos, PCBs, mercury, fluorides, and various pesticides. The contribution to water pollution by synthetic chemical fallout is surprisingly large—the major portion of PCBs and other toxic chemicals in the Great Lakes and a substantial amount of the hydrocarbons found in the oceans entered these waters through airborne deposition.

As point source pollutants decline in importance, thanks to improved pollution control technology and enforcement of effluent limitations, nonpoint sources such as those just described present the greatest single challenge to attaining our nation's clean water goals. The "top down" strategy, whereby federal and state governments promulgate regulations with which individual polluters must comply under threat of civil or criminal penalties, has served us well in reducing pollution from point sources but is entirely inappropriate for controlling poison runoff from broad land areas. Recognizing the near-impossibility of requiring discharge permits for every farm field or parking lot, regulators striving to control NPS pollution thus far have focused their efforts on altering harmful land use practices. In 1987 Congress required states to conduct surveys and develop "assessment reports" describing the nature and extent of NPS pollution within their jurisdictions. Subsequently they were to implement management programs to combat the problems identified. Control strategies to deal with NPS pollution fall into one of two possible categories:

- increasing the land's capacity to retain water, thereby reducing runoff (e.g. a wide variety of erosion control measures), or

- minimizing the amount of pollutants available for runoff during storms (e.g. keeping manure piles away from streams, judicious application of farm chemicals, regular street sweeping, capturing potential air pollutants before they become airborne and subject to fallout).

Controlling nonpoint pollution unfortunately demands more than just a technological "fix"; it requires instead the cooperation of farmers, ranchers, municipal officials, developers, homeowners, and others in implementing better land management practices to prevent these diverse pollutants from running off the land and into the water.

Past regulatory efforts to deal with NPS pollution were not very successful. State runoff control programs varied widely in their focus, but few emphasized the watershed protection approach so critical to an effective program. Most even today continue to rely on *voluntary* compliance with recommended land management practices—a politically popular stance but not a particularly effective one. Insufficient monitoring data and a perennial lack of adequate funding to implement needed programs have further hindered progress to deal with NPS pollution in a meaningful way.

In an effort to rectify this situation and to improve national water quality management strategies, the federal government in 1998 launched a new initiative, the **Clean Water Action Plan**. Encompassing a wide range of water quality issues, the Action Plan addresses the problem of polluted runoff by encouraging states and tribes to adopt enforceable controls on nonpoint sources. It also has increased incentives and provided new funding to help farmers control polluted runoff from agricultural lands. Most significant for the long term, however, is that the Clean Water Action Plan finally emphasizes the importance of a watershed approach as the most effective means for further improving the quality of our rivers, lakes, and estuaries.

Municipal Sewage Treatment

In 1854 the city of London was reeling under a severe epidemic of Asiatic cholera, a disease characterized by the sudden onset of profuse watery diarrhea and vomiting, resulting in rapid dehydration and death of approximately half of those afflicted. Not all parts of the city were equally affected, however. Within a district called St. James Parish, the cholera death rate hit 200 per 10,000 population, while in neighboring Charing Cross and Hanover Square districts fatalities were considerably lower. Dr. John Snow, a member of the commission of inquiry appointed to investigate the outbreak, noted that the vast majority of individuals who had died of cholera obtained their drinking water from a well on Broad Street; in other respects there seemed to be no fundamental difference between conditions in St. James Parish and nearby districts where cholera rates were low. Although the cholera bacillus and its method of transmission had not yet been discovered, Snow recommended that the handle of the Broad Street pump be removed to prevent further consumption of water from the well. Shortly thereafter, the cholera epidemic subsided.

Subsequent investigations disclosed that prior to the outbreak, residents of one house on Broad Street had been ill with an unidentified disease. Their fecal wastes had been dumped into an open cesspool near the well, a common method for disposing of human wastewater in those years. Unfortunately, the brick lining of the cesspool had deteriorated to the point that the liquid wastes could readily seep through the ground and contaminate the well water with still viable pathogenic organisms. The connection between poorly managed human wastes and serious human disease was clearly demonstrated (Cholera Inquiry Committee, 1855).

London's use of open cesspools as a method of sewage disposal was a well-established practice in many parts of the world until the late 19th and early 20th centuries. These pits in the ground simply collect wastes which are then stabilized by bacterial action. Seepage of liquids into the soil from such holes was common, and since no disinfection was used, contamination of wells and aquifers with human fecal pathogens frequently occurred. During the 19th century the growing popularity of flush toilets in urban areas resulted in greatly increased volumes of wastewater requiring disposal. This additional influx produced frequent overflowing of public cesspools and caused a further spread of filth and waterborne disease, particularly cholera and typhoid fever. Installation of sewer systems which carried wastes directly from homes into nearby rivers helped to alleviate problems of well contamination but caused severe degradation of surface water quality, resulting in the elimination of many forms of aquatic life and enhancing the risk of waterborne disease in communities downstream which used surface water supplies for drinking.

By the end of the 19th century rapid urban growth convinced city planners that sewage treatment facilities were needed to alleviate the health and aesthetic problems created by dumping raw sewage into waterways. Today in the United States approximately 70% of the population live in areas where domestic wastes pass through a sewage treatment plant before being discharged. The remainder, for the most part, rely on on-site wastewater disposal systems—usually a septic tank and soil absorption field or sand filter. Provision of adequate methods of sewage treatment, along with the chlorination of drinking water, has done far more to reduce the incidence of epidemic disease and to upgrade standards of public health than has the more widely acclaimed introduction of modern medicines and vaccines.

The aim of sewage treatment is to improve the quality of wastewater to the point that it can be discharged into a waterway without seriously disrupting the aquatic environment or causing human health problems. Achieving these goals requires killing pathogenic organisms present in human wastes (within any human population there will always be some individuals suffering from various gastrointestinal diseases and releasing the causative bacteria, protozoans, etc., in their excreta; it is assumed, therefore, that domestic sewage entering the treatment facility is contaminated with pathogens capable of causing disease outbreaks) and, to the greatest possible extent, removing organic wastes or converting them to inorganic forms so that after discharge they will not deplete the oxygen content of the receiving waters as they decompose. To accomplish these ends, several levels of sewage treatment are necessary.

Primary Treatment

The used water supply of a community, averaging about 100 gallons/person/day in cities having separate storm and sanitary sewers, flows from homes and institutions into the municipal sewer system which carries the wastes to a treatment plant (in regulatory jargon a "**POTW**"—publicly owned treatment works). At this point sewage consists not only of human feces and urine, but also of wastes from laundry, bathing, garbage grinding, and dishwashing, as well as all the miscellaneous articles that find their way into the sewer system—sand, gravel, rubber balls, leaves, sticks, dead rats, etc. Primary sewage treatment consists of several mechanical processes designed to remove the larger suspended solids through screening and sedimentation. Though there may be minor variations in the methods used by different treatment plants, in general the incoming flow first passes through one or more screens to remove large floating objects. After the waste-laden water has passed the screens, it enters a grit chamber where the reduced velocity of flow permits sand, gravel, and other inorganic material to settle out. Air is sometimes injected into the tank to maintain aerobic conditions and to remove trapped gases. Following several hours in an additional sedimentation tank (a "primary clarifier"), the wastewater enters the secondary treatment system or, in those POTWs having only a primary level of treatment, is chlorinated and discharged into the receiving waters. The solid material (sludge) that settles out in the sedimentation tank is regularly removed, dried, and disposed of by one of several methods.

While primary treatment is unquestionably better than no treatment at all, it does not result in an effluent of sufficiently high quality to prevent degradation of the receiving waters. During primary treatment approximately 50–65% of suspended solids are removed and the BOD (see Box 15-3) is reduced by about 25–40%. Because the pollution potential of such wastewater is still quite high, the Environmental Protection Agency does not consider primary treatment by itself an adequate level of sewage treatment.

Secondary Treatment

Whereas primary treatment is based upon physical and mechanical methods of removing suspended solids from wastewater, secondary treatment depends on biological processes, similar to naturally occurring decomposition but greatly accelerated, to digest organic wastes. Microorganisms, predominantly aerobic bacteria, are utilized in the presence of an abundant oxygen supply to break down organic materials into inorganic carbon dioxide, water, and minerals. This can be accomplished by means of **trickling filters**—beds of crushed stone whose surfaces are covered with a microbial slime consisting of bacteria, protozoans, nematodes, etc., which absorb the organic material as the wastewater is sprayed over the surface of the rocks—or by the more modern **activated sludge process.** This involves "seeding" a tank of sewage with bacteria-laden sludge, pumping compressed air into the mixture and agitating it for 4–10 hours. During this time the microbes adsorb most of the colloidal and suspended solids onto the surfaces of the sludge particles and oxidize the organic material. After the process is complete, the sludge is separated from the remaining liquid by settling ("secondary clarification"). Most of this

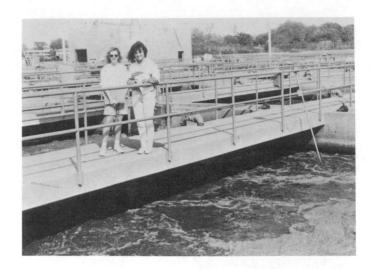

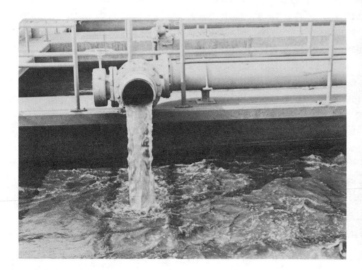

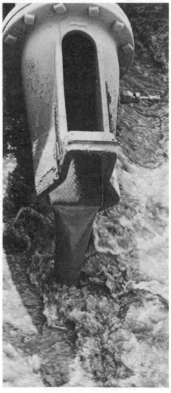

Activated sludge method: (top) a form of secondary sewage treatment in which wastewater effluent from primary treatment is mixed in aerated tanks with large numbers of bacteria ("activated
sludge"). These bacteria feed on the organic nutrients, converting them to simpler inorganic substances. This process is energy-intensive, due to power requirements for running the pumps, but
can achieve a very high degre of pollutant removal; (bottom left) wastewater entering tank; (bottom right) introduction of activated sludge. *[Author's Photos]*

sludge, consisting primarily of masses of bacteria, is removed, but some must be retained and fed back into the incoming sewage to perpetuate the process.

After wastewater has passed through both primary and secondary treatment, the level of suspended solids and of BOD has been reduced by about 90–95% (however, cold weather can reduce the efficiency of pollutant reduction because it slows the metabolic rate of the microorganisms on which secondary treatment depends). Secondary treatment is not effective in removing viruses, heavy metals, dissolved minerals, and certain other chemicals (Koren, 1980). In the United States, a federally-imposed mandate requiring that all POTWs provide at least secondary wastewater treatment took effect in July 1988.

Advanced Wastewater Treatment (Tertiary Treatment)

A third level of sewage treatment may be required in situations where effluent from the secondary treatment process still contains substances that are causing water quality problems; when the sheer volume of effluent is large enough that the remaining 10% of suspended solids and BOD are sufficient to initiate eutrophication; or if the treated wastewater is to be used for purposes of drinking, irrigation, or recreation. Advanced waste water treatment

---

BOX 15-3

BOD

The most commonly used measurement of the amount of pollutant organic material in water is a parameter referred to as biochemical oxygen demand or BOD. When bacteria act upon the organic matter in sewage or certain industrial wastes discharged into waterways, large amounts of dissolved oxygen are rapidly used up; this can result in fish kills and drastic alterations in the aquatic environment. Biochemical oxygen demand basically is an indication of how much putrescible organic material is present in the water or wastewater, with a low BOD indicating good water quality and a high BOD reflecting polluted conditions.

BOD is calculated by taking a sample of water, diluting it with fully-oxygenated water, and determining the amount of oxygen present at that time. The sample is then incubated in the dark at 20°C (68°F) for five days, after which the oxygen content is again measured. The difference between the initial and final readings, expressed in milligrams per liter (mg/L), is the BOD. Some representative BOD values are:

Pollutant	5-day BOD (in mg/L)
raw sewage	150–250
cannery wastes	5,000–6,000
discharges from pulp mills	10,000–15,000
wastewater from wool scouring	>20,000
treatment plant effluent (EFA standard-maximum average	30

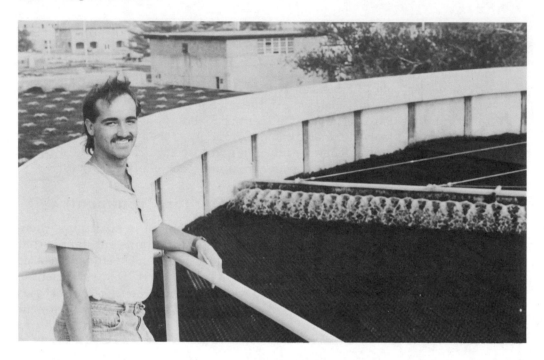

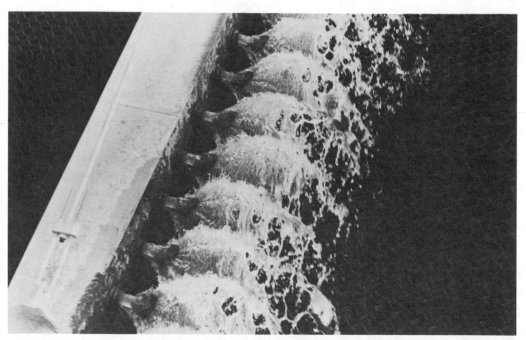

Nitrification tower: a method of advanced wastewater treatment for reducing the ammonia content of wastewater; (top) rotating bars distribute treated wastewater over the upper surface of a 40–50 inch high honeycomb-like plastic grid; as water trickles downward, aerobic nitrifying bacteria on the surfaces of the grid convert ammonia to nitrate; (bottom) closeup of nitrification tower grid surface. *[Author's Photos]*

Table 15-1   Tertiary Treatment Processes

Tertiary Treatment Method	Pollutant Removed
Chemical coagulation, followed by filtration or sedimentation	phosphates, tertiary suspended solids, and BOD
Activated carbon adsorption	synthetic organic chemicals, tastes, odors
Nitrifying towers	ammonia
Air stripping	ammonia
Oxidation ponds and aerated lagoons	BOD, phosphates
Reverse osmosis	BOD, nitrates, phosphates, dissolved solids
Electrodialysis	dissolved minerals
Oxidation	organic material
Foam separation	organic chemicals
Land application	phosphates, nitrates, BOD, suspended solids

involves either one or a combination of several biological, chemical, or physical processes designed to remove such pollutants as phosphates, nitrates, ammonia, and organic chemicals. It also further reduces the concentration of remaining suspended solids and BOD to about 1% of that present in raw sewage. Some examples of tertiary treatment processes can be seen in Table 15-1.

Disinfection

Since the most common waterborne diseases are caused by pathogenic bacteria, viruses, or protozoans present in human excrement, one of the primary purposes of sewage treatment is to kill such organisms before they can infect new victims. Simple exposure to the hostile environment outside the human intestine is sufficient to reduce the number of bacteria appreciably as they pass through the treatment process. However, because a substantial number of live organisms still remain in the wastewater after primary and secondary treatment are complete, it was standard procedure for many years to disinfect treated effluent by adding chlorine prior to discharge in order to eliminate any remaining disease-causing organisms. More recently, the policy of chlorinating all sewage treatment plant discharges has met with increasing resistance and today more than half of all states no longer require chlorination of wastewaters. There are several reasons for this change in accepted practice.

1. Chlorine is effective in killing bacteria, but less so in relation to viruses and parasites (e.g. *Giardia, Cryptosporidium*), many of which survive this treatment.

Figure 15-2   Schematic Municipal Wastewater Treatment Process

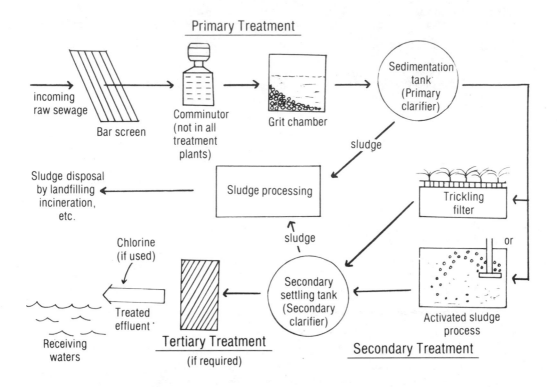

2. Chlorine is very destructive of fish and other forms of aquatic life, many of which are eliminated for a considerable distance downstream from sewage treatment plants due to the presence of this chemical in the water.

3. Chlorine treatment is expensive and poses safety problems at the treatment plant in the eventuality of cylinder leaks or system disruption.

4. Chlorine disinfects only a fraction of the wastes in streams because bacteria-laden runoff from farmland and urban areas enters waterways untreated.

Proponents of chlorinating POTW discharges correctly point out, however, that this practice helps reduce outbreaks of disease that have been associated with swimming in sewage-polluted water or with consuming shellfish taken from contaminated waterways. Although disinfecting such effluent with chlorine does not sterilize the water, in the sense of killing every last microbe, it reduces their numbers significantly and thereby enhances the self-purifying capacity of natural waterways. As the controversy between wastewater chlorination opponents and proponents continues to rage, a compromise solution has been reached in some states where disinfection of discharge waters is required only during the summer bathing season, with the practice being discontinued during the winter when recreational contact with water is unlikely (Shertzer, 1986). In certain other states, requirements for disinfecting POTW effluent have been dropped altogether, except in those situations where a drinking water intake point or a bathing beach is located a short distance downstream.

Unfortunately, as population density increases and the distance between POTW effluent discharge points and public drinking water intake pipes shrinks, fewer treatment plants may have the option of bypassing disinfection. This is especially relevant in states like Texas and California, where serious consideration is being given to proposals for discharging treated effluent directly into drinking water reservoirs as a means of augmenting water supplies. As a result, there is growing interest in non-chlorine methods of killing microbes. While some POTWs now employ membrane filtration or ozonation as their method of disinfection, the most popular nontraditional disinfectant is ultraviolet light. Currently about 1,500 POTWs nationwide are utilizing UV systems and the rapid pace at which this technology is being improved suggests it will be an even more widely adopted disinfection choice in the years ahead (Marshall, 1999).

Biosolids Management

Ironically, the high degree of pollutant removal achieved at modern sewage treatment plants has created a new challenge for POTW operators—how to manage the steadily growing volumes of sludge (the term applied to untreated biosolids) which our increasingly efficient sewage treatment technologies are producing. The quantity of biosolids produced annually by U.S. municipal treatment plants has approximately doubled since passage of the Clean Water Act, thanks to continued population growth, further gains in the efficiency of wastewater treatment, and more widespread compliance with Clean Water Act requirements. Because sewage sludge itself can be a pollutant if improperly managed, its treatment, ultimate disposal, and potential use must be handled in ways that will not endanger public health or the environment.

Routinely removed at each step in the sewage treatment process, the watery sludge (before treatment, sludge consists of 93–99% water) generally is first thickened through the use of coagulant chemicals or dissolved air flotation. It is then stabilized through a two-step anaerobic digestion process in order to reduce problems associated with odors and the presence of pathogenic organisms—a process that takes approximately 60 days to complete. To reduce its volume for ease in handling, the sludge is then dewatered, either by mechanical processes or by drying on sand beds. At this point sludge has the appearance of rich black dirt and is largely odor-free. A number of POTWs subsequently compost, heat-dry, or otherwise treat their sludge to kill remaining pathogens. Contrary to the negative public image of anything pertaining to sewage, the treated biosolids at this point represent a valuable resource rather than an objectionable waste. Indeed, the nitrates, phosphates, and organic matter present in sludge make it useful as a fertilizer and as a soil conditioner. Biosolids have a long history of use for improving marginal lands, increasing forest productivity (studies have shown that the rate of tree growth doubles on sludge-enriched soil), boosting home garden yields, and reclaiming lands devastated by strip-mining.

Since sewage treatment plants, particularly those in the larger metropolitan areas, generate enormous amounts of sludge during their normal course of operations, finding a place in which to dispose of this material poses major dilemmas for many such facilities. Incineration can present problems of air pollution and in many communities where landfill space is at a premium, burying sludge is increasingly controversial—and increasingly expensive. In fact, so expensive has biosolids management become that, whatever the disposal option chosen, treatment and disposal of biosolids now account for over 50% of the operating costs of a typical POTW providing secondary sewage treatment.

Since the mid-1990s, EPA regulations have encouraged a marked trend toward **"beneficial reuse"** of biosolids, particularly forms of land application. The 1987 Clean Water Act amendments established a comprehensive program for reducing potential environmental risks posed by sludge through requirements that EPA 1) identify toxic substances that may be present in sludge at potentially dangerous levels, and 2) promulgate regulations that specify acceptable management practices and numerical limitations for sludge containing those pollutants. These regulations, referred to as the **Part 503** standards, were issued in February of 1993 and have now been implemented nationwide. The main concern that has limited beneficial reuse of biosolids in the past is the fact that sewage sludge often contains toxic chemicals and pathogens as well as desirable nutrients such as phosphates and nitrates. In particular, sludge from POTWs receiving industrial wastewater discharges in addition to residential sewage may contain potentially dangerous concentrations of heavy metals and other toxics—cadmium and lead are of special concern, but copper, zinc, nickel, PCBs, and a number of other contaminants may also be present. EPA addressed this issue by setting maximum loading rates on soils for biosolids containing these contaminants, advising POTWs to police industrial discharges in their communities in an effort to eliminate toxic pollutants at the source. While some fears have been expressed regarding the possible presence of pathogens, the number of organisms in *digested* sludge is relatively low and can be further reduced by such management practices as composting or heat drying. Such treatment is required for biosolids to be designated "Exceptional Quality," permitting its application to land without any restrictions. To ensure the highest degree of public health protection, EPA has ruled that only biosolids categorized as exceptional quality may be applied to home lawns and gardens. Although some environmental groups continue to harbor misgivings about the use of biosolids on crop lands, the results of more than 30 years of research and practical experience have shown that food crops grown on lands fertilized with biosolids are perfectly safe for human consumption. Perhaps the most definitive statement on the matter was a 1996 report published by the National Research Council of the National Academy of Sciences which concluded that, if used according to existing federal guidelines and regulations, biosolids present a negligible risk to consumers, to crop production, and to the environment. As confidence grows that biosolids can be used safely and profitably to increase production on farm fields, forests, and pasturelands, beneficial reuse practices will inevitably grow in popularity among municipal water reclamation districts as the most environmentally acceptable, cost-efficient method for disposing of their sludge. New York City eagerly seized upon this option in 1992 when, ordered to cease ocean dumping, it began shipping its biosolids 2,065 miles across country to the Sierra Blanca Ranch in Hudspeth County, Texas. There the anaerobically digested biosolids are spread over native desert grasslands at a rate of 3 dry tons/acre/year. Scientists from Texas Tech and Texas A&M Universities monitoring the site report an increase in the density and biomass of grasses and in the number of desirable species. They also report decreased rates of erosion and no buildup of heavy metals (Carlile, 1995).

Although agricultural lands are currently the destination for most of the biosolids being land applied, farmers are not the only ones interested in taking advantage of this "black gold." While some municipalities are giving biosolids away to anyone who will take it, the majority are selling the stuff to home gardeners, nurseries, or landscaping firms at prices ranging from $1.00–$22.00/cubic foot! Milwaukee and Madison, Wisconsin, and Austin, Texas, have employed imaginative marketing skills in promoting their products, selling biosolids under such catchy tradenames as *Milorganite, Metrogro,* or *Dillo Dirt* (EPA, 1993; Tenenbaum, 1992).

New Approaches to Wastewater Treatment

Financing the improvements in municipal sewage treatment required by the 1972 Clean Water Act would have been impossible had Congress not included, in that same piece of legislation, the creation of a massive **Construction Grant Program.** This fund provided federal monetary assistance to communities which could not otherwise have afforded the multimillion dollar expenditures necessary to construct new or upgraded POTWs capable of providing the mandatory secondary level of sewage treatment. Under the Construction Grant Program, the second-largest public works project in U.S. history (exceeded only by construction of the interstate highway system), the federal government agreed to provide fully 75% of the cost of such projects, an amount that was subsequently reduced to 55% by the Reagan Administration in 1981. Over nearly two decades Washington contributed $57 *billion* for sewage treatment plant construction (state and local expenditures during the same period exceeded an additional $70 billion); as a result, by the late 1980s, 58% of the U.S. population was served by POTWs providing either secondary or secondary and advanced wastewater treatment. Since POTWs cumulatively serve about 70% of the American population (most of the remainder utilizing on-site wastewater disposal systems), it is obvious that domestic wastewaters in the majority of sewered communities now receive a commendably high level of treatment prior to discharge.

Nevertheless, remaining sewage treatment needs are considerable. In the late 1980s, approximately one out of every ten Americans lived in communities providing less than secondary treatment—and some small towns still had no sewage treatment at all, discharging raw wastewaters directly into streams. In 1990, EPA estimated the total cost of bringing all municipal dischargers into compliance with CWA water quality requirements could exceed $110 billion—yet by 1990 the federal well had run dry (Adler et al., 1993). Amendments to the Clean Water Act passed by Congress in 1987 called for a phaseout of the federal Construction Grant Program by 1994, replacing it with a **State Revolving Fund** providing low-interest *loans* (no more free gifts from Uncle Sam!) to municipalities with unmet sewage treatment needs. Unfortunately, the demand for such loans exceeds the supply—but federal deadline dates for compliance with CWA requirements remain unchanged and potential penalties for violation of such standards can be severe. Thus the fiscal and legal realities of the 1990s provided a major incentive to develop new, less costly, yet equally effective methods of treating sewage—alternatives to the highly engineered, energy-consuming, sludge-producing, exorbitantly expensive POTWs which offered a convenient "technological fix" during the era of free-flowing federal dollars but which constitute an unrealistic option for communities of limited means.

Fortunately, the old adage, "Necessity is the mother of invention," is as valid in relation to emerging wastewater management technologies as it is in other spheres of life. In recent decades a variety of innovative approaches to solving wastewater problems have attracted considerable interest and a number are now in the pilot-project stage, undergoing extensive field studies; several are in full-scale use, having proven their ability to produce good quality effluent at a fraction of the cost of conventional sewage treatment. The majority of new systems are based on the concept that wastewater effluent, like biosolids, should be viewed as a nutrient-laden resource to be utilized rather than as a pollutant to be discarded.

One of the earliest and most widely adopted approaches to alternative treatment was land application of wastewater. This method involves spraying effluent from secondary treatment onto forest, pastures, or crop lands. Land application not only helps to prevent stream pollution by keeping nutrients out of the water, it also utilizes those same nutrients as fertilizer for the plants on which it is applied. A further advantage of this method is that the wastewater is largely purified as it percolates through the soil to recharge the groundwater supply. Early health concerns that dissolved metals or pathogens in the effluent might contaminate soils or vegetation have been dispelled by many years of problem-free experience with land application at Pennsylvania State University; in communities in Texas, Michigan, California, and New York; and in Germany, France, Israel, and Australia.

In the 1980s, emphasis shifted to the potential for artificial wetlands ("designer swamps"), duckweed systems *(Lemna spp.)*, and water-purifying hydroponics-type systems inside greenhouses. In the United States, the Tennessee Valley Authority (TVA) has been at the forefront of research and development efforts focused on wetlands treatment. TVA views such systems as a viable wastewater treatment option for small communities that lack the expertise, as well as the financial resources, to operate highly sophisticated mechanical plants. Since the mid-1980s, TVA has designed and constructed engineered wetlands for a number of small towns in southern Appalachia, enabling such communities to comply with federal water quality standards at a fraction of the cost of conventional facilities. Although the sizeable land requirements for engineered wetlands have deterred many communities from giving such systems serious consideration, some larger cities such as Orlando,

Figure 15-3   Types of Constructed Wetlands

SURFACE FLOW SYSTEMS

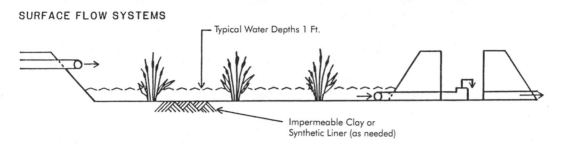

SUBSURFACE FLOW SYSTEMS

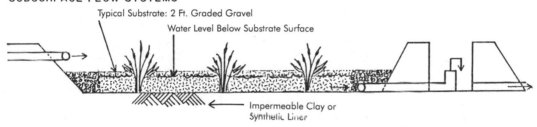

Source: Tennessee Valley Authority.

Florida, and Columbia, Missouri, have opted to utilize wetlands as one element in their treatment process.

Of the municipalities nationwide currently employing wetlands systems to treat sewage, the most renowned is Arcata, California, a community of 16,000 located on the north shore of Humboldt Bay. In the early 1980s, Arcata faced a serious fiscal dilemma: effluent from the town's POTW consistently violated discharge permit limitations and Arcata was being pressured by the state environmental agency to close the plant and join with neighboring municipalities in constructing a large regional facility. Wary of the exorbitant costs such an undertaking would entail, Arcata opted for a radically different solution to its problem. Assisted by faculty at Humboldt State University, the town proceeded to develop a series of ponds and marshes to remove the troublesome pollutants remaining in its effluent following primary treatment at the POTW. Today Arcata's wastewater receives secondary treatment in a 50-acre stabilization pond where suspended solids settle to the bottom, while dissolved organic materials are broken down through a symbiotic association between bacteria and algae. From here the effluent flows into a three-celled, five-acre "treatment marsh" where rooted aquatic plants such as cattails (*Typha latifolia*) and bulrushes (*Scirpus acutis*) flourish. The submerged stems of these plants harbor countless numbers of microorganisms that further metabolize dissolved organic nitrates and phosphates. Passage through the marsh also effectively breaks down pesticides, industrial solvents, and most of the heavy metals in wastewater. After passing through the treatment marsh, the effluent is pumped to a chlorine contact tank for disinfection and is subsequently discharged into an "enhancement marsh" for additional wetlands treatment. This enhancement marsh, open to the public, is interlaced with jogging and hiking trails, picnic areas, and a nature center; it also serves as a wildlife sanctuary, annually attracting more than 150,000 visitors and 160 species of birds and other wildlife—living proof that the imperatives of providing for society's urgent wastewater management needs and restoring valuable ecosystems are mutually compatible.

After treatment in the enhancement marsh, the effluent is chlorinated once again and finally discharged into Humboldt Bay (source of 60–70% of California's oyster crop), its levels of suspended solids and BOD by now well below the NPDES limits of 30 mg/L.

Completed in 1986, Arcata's wetland system has been both an environmental and financial success. Once a polluter of Humboldt Bay, Arcata's wastewater treatment process produces an effluent which not only exceeds water quality standards but is even cleaner than the seawater into which it flows—and it has managed to do so at a cost far lower than that of a standard treatment facility. Residents of neighboring Eureka, faced with similar sewage treatment imperatives, opted for the more familiar conventional technology and are now paying wastewater treatment bills more than double those in Arcata. By the late 1990s, the obvious advantages of Arcata's natural approach to wastewater treatment had persuaded city officials in Davis and Pacifica, California, to construct their own wetlands treatment systems.

Why haven't more communities followed Arcata's example? The major limitation to such systems is the amount of land they require—about 20 acres for a town of 10,000 people. Unless a community already owns land on its outskirts, being able to afford, or even find, this much land may present serious difficulties. Perhaps the biggest obstacle is sheer ignorance and inertia. Only recently have adequate design guidelines become available for engineers and regulators; municipal officials frequently are unaware of the advantages such systems offer; conventionally trained engineers are frequently reluctant to embark on new, little-tried technologies and often lack the understanding of environmental conditions needed to factor these into their designs. Cynics might also wonder if engineers' general lack of enthusiasm might stem from the fact that cheaper artificial marshes translate into lower fees for engineering firms, since payment is typically calculated as a percentage of total project cost ("Small Community...", 1993). Despite these obstacles, the idea is gradually winning converts, and not only in small towns. The city of Phoenix, Arizona, is in the process of creating a wetlands system to treat a portion of its wastewater flow because doing so is a much more economical way of meeting effluent standards than upgrading its conventional treatment plant (Brown et al., 1999).

A more futuristic approach to meeting community wastewater treatment needs in an economical and environmentally benign manner is "The Living Machine," developed by Burlington, Vermont-based Living Technologies. Designed to treat both human wastewaters and high-strength industrial organic wastes, the Living Machine relies on a series of tanks and biofilters containing a wide spectrum of microorganisms, algae, snails, plants, and fish

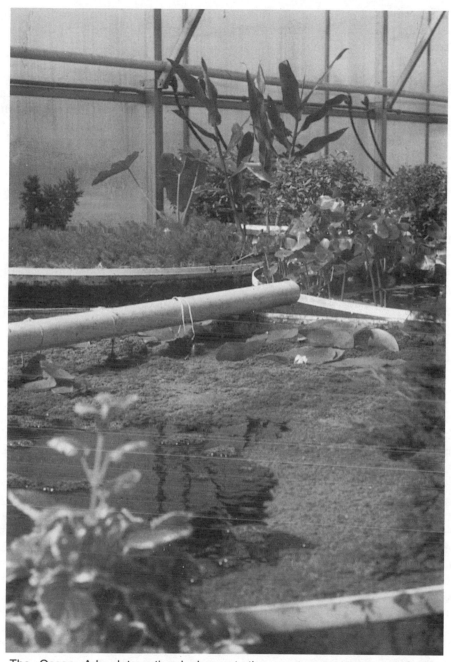

The Ocean Arks International demonstration wastewater treatment facility employs "Living Machine" type technology to treat wastewater in an environmentally benign manner. *[Author's photo]*

inside a greenhouse-like structure. After passing through this natural treatment system, the resulting effluent is clean enough to be discharged directly into a waterway or to be recycled. By 1999, fifteen Living Machines were operating worldwide, providing a low-cost, sustainable alternative to high-tech conventional wastewater treatment (Riggle and Gray, 1999). As communities

struggle to avoid stringent penalties for noncompliance with mandated effluent requirements in the absence of federal funding, it's likely that alternative
natural systems will receive much wider and more serious attention in the
years ahead.

Elsewhere in the world, a variant on wetlands treatment is the use of
fish ponds for treating sewage while simultaneously supporting aquaculture.
In Lima, Peru, a portion of the city's sewage is directed to stabilization ponds
where solids settle out and bacteria decompose the organic wastes. After three
or four weeks the water is sufficiently cleansed of pollutants to use for irrigation and for fish culture. Similar systems are currently in operation in Hungary, Germany, Israel, and a number of countries in South and Southeast
Asia. The largest of these can be found in Calcutta, India, where human
wastewaters nourish algae in two large lakes. Herbivorous fish such as carp
and tilapia feed upon these algae and are subsequently harvested to provide
Calcutta markets with approximately 7,000 metric tons of fish each year.
Obvious concerns about the potential for contamination of fish with human
gastrointestinal pathogens can be allayed by retaining sewage in the stabilization lagoons for at least 20 days before allowing it to enter the fish ponds or
by transferring the fish to clean waters for a period of time prior to harvesting
(World Resources Institute, 1992).

Septic Systems

Approximately 30% of all Americans live in unsewered areas where they
must utilize on-site septic systems for the disposal of wastewaters from bathrooms, kitchens, and laundries. Most on-site wastewater disposal systems
consist of two basic parts: 1) a septic tank, buried in the ground at some distance from the house, to which it is connected by a pipe, and 2) a soil absorption field or sand filter.

The septic tank itself is a watertight container made of concrete or fiber-
glass with a minimum capacity of 750 gallons. Sewage entering the septic
tank is partially decomposed by bacteria under anaerobic conditions. During
this process, sludge settles to the bottom of the tank, while lighter solids and
grease, as well as gases from the decomposing sludge, rise to the top to form a
floating scum. The partially clarified liquid then passes through an outlet and
the effluent is evenly dispersed among several perforated pipes in a carefully
designed absorption field, which must be of adequate size and proper soil
porosity to ensure that the effluent seeping out of the perforated pipe moves
quickly enough to prevent ponding, but not so rapidly as to infiltrate aquifers,
wells, or surface water supplies before contaminants in the effluent have been
filtered out or oxidized.

Since more than half of the solids in the wastewater settle out during the
retention period in the septic tank, the accumulation of sludge at the bottom,
as well as the scum layer at the top, must be removed periodically (usually
every 3–5 years). If this is not done, the sludge build-up reaches the point that
solids are discharged into the absorption field, resulting in clogging and ponding. This accumulation of particulates and scum in the pores of the soil prevents proper drainage of the effluent and eventually results in failure of the
system. In addition to improper maintenance of the septic tank, other reasons

BOX 15-4

"Deep Tunnel"
Chicago's Response to Combined Sewer Overflows

Deep under the streets of Chicago the 31-mile Mainstream Tunnel System constitutes a visionary—and highly successful—effort to solve a major water pollution problem facing many of our older cities: how to manage combined sewer overflows during periods of heavy rainfall. While most sewer systems installed in recent decades feature separate sanitary and stormwater conduits, the older sections of many urban areas still have combined sewers which carry not only sewage from households, but also stormwater runoff from city streets, rooftops, and lawns—all the water which isn't absorbed into the ground when it rains. Most sewage treatment plants are designed to accommodate the usual domestic wastewater flow (referred to as "dry weather flow"), usually with some built-in excess capacity. During storm episodes, however, water volume in combined sewers may be as much as 100 times greater than usual. Because the excess water would overwhelm the treatment capacity of the sewage plant, it is diverted past the facility and enters the receiving stream untreated. Laden not only with human wastes but also with the wide variety of contaminants characteristic of urban runoff, combined sewer overflows seriously degrade the aquatic environment and are a common cause of water quality violations in older cities.

Beset by approximately 100 storm episodes per year that discharged raw sewage and stormwater into Chicagoland waterways and frequently caused flooding of streets and residential areas as well, the Windy City began looking for a long-term solution to its problem. Efforts to deal with this challenge in other com-

munities suggested several alternative approaches: 1) separation of sewer systems in areas with combined sewers—a massive construction project presenting almost insurmountable difficulties in highly developed urban areas; 2) enlargement of POTW capacity to permit treatment of entire stormwater plus sanitary sewage flow—technically possible but not cost-efficient, since this approach would require enormous capital investments for excess capacity that would sit idle most of the time; 3) construction of retention basins to hold stormwater runoff, gradually releasing it to the treatment plant in volumes which can be accommodated.

Chicago eventually settled upon one of the most ambitious and innovative public works projects ever undertaken. In 1975 the city began construction on its Tunnel and Reservoir Plan (TARP), the key segment of which is the Mainstream Tunnel, completed in 1985 and chosen by the American Society of Civil Engineers as the Outstanding Civil Engineering Achievement for 1986 (technologies developed for TARP facilitated construction of the "Chunnel" connecting France and England). The "Deep Tunnel," as it was promptly dubbed by the media, captures sewage-polluted stormwater from a 204-square mile urban area and stores it temporarily in 31 miles of tunnels at depths ranging from 240–300 feet below ground. After a storm has ended, this water is pumped back to the surface and sent at a controlled rate to sewage treatment plants prior to subsequent discharge into a waterway. Since the Mainstream Tunnel came on line, the frequency of combined sewer overflows and flooding throughout most of Chicago and 15 neighboring communities dropped dramatically—down 80% in its first year of operation.

When the tunnel construction phase of TARP is complete, about 85% of the pollution caused by combined sewer overflows will be captured. A second phase of the project, designed to control flooding, is underway; the first of three huge reservoirs designed to store combined sewer overflows captured by the tunnel system is now under construction. When finished, these reservoirs will increase TARP's water storage capacity by 41 billion gallons. Upon completion, TARP will make it possible for Chicago to capture and contain entire storms, eliminating forever fears of flooding and pollution whenever skies darken over Chicagoland. No longer do engineers from around the world come to the Windy City just to view its skyline—now they come to admire its sewer system as well!

Reference
Metropolitan Water Reclamation District of Greater Chicago.

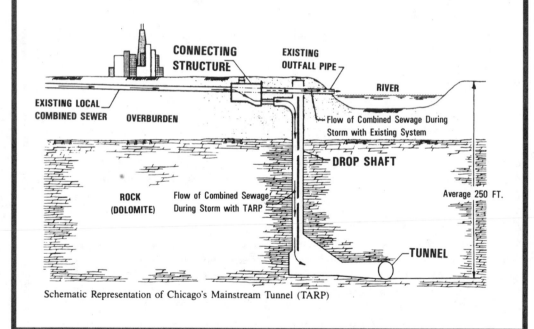

Schematic Representation of Chicago's Mainstream Tunnel (TARP)

for septic system failure may be: use of a septic tank that is too small for the householders' needs, excessive household water use (large parties in homes on septic systems can be disastrous; repair men jokingly comment that they routinely notice garbage containers overflowing with beer cans when on a call to deal with sewage backups!), insufficient size of the absorption field, soil too impervious to receive effluent, or tree roots clogging the effluent distribution lines.

Although a well-located, carefully constructed, and properly maintained septic system can be a perfectly adequate method of sanitary wastewater disposal (and is the only feasible option in most rural areas), malfunctioning septic systems frequently give rise to serious nonpoint source water pollution, as leachates containing pathogenic organisms and nutrients seep from absorption fields into water supplies. The rapid growth of rural subdivisions, many of which rely on septic systems installed on lots too small to provide adequate waste dispersal, ensures that pollution problems related to septic systems will continue to plague public health officials.

Industrial Discharges

Effluent discharges from industry comprise the second major category of point source water pollution and consist of a wide range of pollutants which, for regulatory purposes, have been subdivided into three major groups:

1. *Conventional Pollutants*—These include organic wastes high in BOD, suspended solids, acids, oil and grease, etc. Such pollutants originate from food processing plants, pulp and paper mills, steel mills, oil tanker spills and cleaning operations, accidents involving offshore oil drilling, and so forth

2. *Toxic Pollutants*—A list of 129 priority toxic pollutants was developed by EPA in 1976 (3 subsequently have been delisted); substances listed include heavy metals such as cadmium, mercury, and lead, PCBs, benzene, chloroform, cyanide, arsenic, 2,4-D, and a number of other pesticides. The electroplating and metal-processing industries, plastics manufacturers, and chemical companies are but a few of the industries discharging toxic effluents.

3. *Nonconventional Pollutants*—All the other pollutants not classified by EPA as either conventional or toxic are grouped into this third category—substances such as nitrogen and phosphorus, iron, tin, aluminum, chloride, and ammonia. As in the preceding categories, the sources of such pollutants can be traced to a wide variety of industrial processes.

The Clean Water Act requires EPA to develop technology-based national treatment standards for each category of industrial discharger (e.g. petroleum refiners, textile mills, iron and steel, leather tanning, etc.), directing that standards be reviewed periodically and made increasingly stringent as pollution control technologies advance. Industries discharging directly into the nation's waterways must obtain an NPDES permit, specifying the allowable amounts and constituents of pollutants in their effluent. Dischargers are required to monitor their effluent on a routine basis and violations of permit limitations can result in serious civil or criminal penalties.

For the most part, industry has a better record of compliance with existing water pollution control regulations than do municipal dischargers (i.e. POTWs); EPA estimates that the use of best available pollution control technologies in 22 targeted industrial categories has reduced releases of certain toxic organic chemicals by 99% and heavy metals by 98% since passage of the Clean Water Act in 1972. Altogether, controls imposed on toxic industrial discharges have, according to EPA estimates, prevented the release of more than a billion pounds of toxics yearly into U.S. surface waters; even larger amounts of conventional pollutants have been controlled. However, industrial point sources remain one of the major contributors of pollutants degrading estuaries in urbanized coastal areas (EPA, 1998). Overall, stream monitoring data and self-reporting by industry both indicate a steady downward trend for industrial discharges in recent years—slow but encouraging progress toward the elusive goal of "zero discharge."

Direct Versus Indirect Discharges

Current water pollution laws distinguish two categories of industrial waste discharges: **direct discharges** which flow directly into a receiving stream or lake and **indirect discharges** which go into the sewer system, where they first pass through the municipal sewage treatment plant before entering a waterway along with sanitary wastewater effluent. When citizens think about industrial pollutant discharges, they generally envision the direct type—pipes from a factory leading straight to the water's edge, pouring a poisonous brew onto the back of some hapless fish. In point of fact, however, the majority of industrial dischargers, some 270,000 in the United States, are of the indirect type, discharging huge volumes of industrial wastewaters into sewer systems every year. In cases where indirect industrial discharges consist primarily of biodegradable organic wastes, sending them to the sewage treatment plant is appropriate, since the same processes that decompose human excreta are effective on other organic materials as well. In situations involving toxic substances, however, indirect discharges via the sewer system have caused a number of very serious problems.

Structural Damage to Sewer System and Treatment Plant. Industrial discharges of strong acids or alkalis can corrode both sewer pipes and equipment at the POTW. Some chemicals react to produce toxic fumes which can present a serious health threat to workers at the treatment plant, and certain volatile substances can generate a build-up of gas in the sewers, occasionally resulting in explosions. An event of this type occurred in Louisville, Kentucky, in February of 1981 when an industrial discharge of hexane exploded in the sewers, injuring four people and causing over $10 million worth of damage (Banks and Dubrowski, 1982). A similar situation took place the same year in Cincinnati when wastewater containing both hydrochloric acid and volatile organic solvents was discharged into city sewers by a large paint factory. The acid corroded the concrete sewer pipe, causing it to collapse and leaving a hole in the street 24 feet in diameter. When workers entered the sewer three days later to try to repair the damage, several were overcome suddenly by nausea, dizziness, vomiting, and eye and nose irritation due to exposure to chemical vapors. All work had to be stopped until the discharges were halted and fumes had dissipated ("Sewer Collapse," 1981).

Interference with Biological Treatment Processes. When toxic chemicals such as the synthetic organic pesticides pass through a sewage treatment plant, they have the same effect on the microbes responsible for the secondary treatment process as they do on the target pests—they kill them, and in so doing render the sewage treatment plant ineffective. In 1977, again at the ill-fated Louisville POTW, pesticide wastes illegally dumped into a city sewer caused a total breakdown in treatment at the huge plant. As a result, for nearly two years until the cleanup was completed, 100 million gallons of untreated sewage were discharged into the Ohio River every day and taxpayers were confronted with a repair bill amounting to millions of dollars.

Biosolids Contamination. Certain toxics such as cadmium, mercury, lead, and arsenic may pass through the sewage treatment plant without damaging equipment or interfering with biological treatment. Nevertheless, they pose major problems because they can be assimilated by the bacteria that provide secondary treatment and subsequently accumulate in the sludge, seriously limiting disposal options for biosolids. Sludge containing excessive concentrations of heavy metals cannot be land-applied due to concerns that toxics may be taken up by plants or leach into groundwater. Similarly, there are restrictions on incineration of metals-contaminated sludge (Banks and Dubrowski, 1982).

Violation of POTW Effluent Limitations. Because sewage treatment plants, like industries, must comply with the terms of their NPDES permit, toxic chemicals which pass through the treatment plant and pollute the receiving waters make it necessary for the POTW to install methods of advanced wastewater treatment to prevent such violations from occurring. This, of course, is a costly undertaking, the expense of which will be borne by the taxpaying public.

Need for Pretreatment of Indirect Discharges

Problems such as those just described led Congress to legislate a national **pretreatment program** that would require indirect dischargers of industrial wastes to detoxify their effluent before it entered the sewage system. EPA has been charged with setting categorical pretreatment standards for groups of industries, comparable to the effluent limitations requiring best available technology for controlling pollution from direct dischargers. The work of developing, implementing, and enforcing the program has been assigned to approximately 1,600 local POTWs (those treating five million gallons of wastewater or more on a daily basis) which also have authority to set additional discharge requirements above and beyond the federal standards if such action is deemed necessary. Although originally mandated in 1972, the pretreatment program was extremely slow in getting started, in part because EPA did not formulate basic rules for the program until 1980. Implementation of the program by local sanitary districts moved into high gear by the mid-1980s and today most industries discharging wastewaters to municipal sewers have some form of pretreatment program in place. This program is having a significant impact in reducing problems caused by indirect discharges, but it hasn't yet eliminated toxic woes at treatment plants. Problems persist not only because some industrial dischargers are in significant noncompliance with pretreatment program requirements but, more importantly, because many categorical standards have not yet been promulgated by EPA. The agency reports that only about 10% of all industries discharging toxics to POTWs are covered under national pretreatment standards (they may, however, be subject to locally imposed requirements). Certain as-yet unregulated commercial establishments such as car washes and photo-processing plants also contribute a significant percentage of certain toxics to a treatment plant's incoming flow. Finally, not all of the hazardous chemicals flowing into sewage treatment plants are of industrial origin. Of the regulated toxics entering POTWs, about 15% come from residences—all those bleaches, toilet bowl cleaners, paint thinners, outdated medications, etc., that we flush down the drain don't simply disappear but merge with the myriad of other substances moving through the sewers and eventually arrive at a sewage treatment plant. We all contribute to the problem.

Industrial Accidents, Spills, and Stormwater Runoff

In addition to direct and indirect effluent discharges, some industrial pollutants enter waterways due to transportation accidents, leaks in chemical containers, tanker spills or oil rig blow-outs, or chemical runoff from industrial waste sites during storm episodes. Of these various events, the dramatic visual impact of oil spills at sea attract the most public attention. Fortunately, experience from numerous such events indicate their long-term ecological impact is frequently less serious than many fear. Studies of past marine spills show that while petroleum is toxic to many organisms, there is no strong evidence that oil spills have done any permanent damage to the world's ocean resources. Such spills, in fact, comprise a relatively small portion of the oil entering the seas each year. Routine tanker operations such as tank cleaning and ballasting contribute almost twice as many petro-pollutants to the ocean on an annual basis as do spills, even though they attract much less attention. While tanker accidents or offshore rig blowouts can have a catastrophic short-term impact on biotic communities, recovery begins within a matter of months and many such communities have returned to their pre-spill appearance within a year or two.

A different and more worrisome type of water contamination due to massive chemical discharge is that done deliberately as an act of terrorism or revenge. During the Persian Gulf War in 1991, the firing of 788 Kuwaiti oil wells by retreating Iraqi troops resulted in the release of enormous amounts of petroleum which formed 246 oil "lakes," fouled 1500 km of Persian Gulf coast, and contaminated the Gulf itself with an amount of oil equivalent to 10 million barrels (by comparison, the 1978 wreck of the Amoco Cadiz off the French coast—the largest tanker spill on record—resulted in the release of less than one-sixth this amount of oil). Although 95% of the oil spilled on land has now been cleaned up, the remaining 5% has penetrated the desert soil and has contaminated 40% of Kuwaiti groundwater reserves. Intertidal areas along the Kuwaiti coast also have been severely damaged (DeSena, 1999).

In 1987 mounting concerns about the adverse environmental impact of urban stormwater runoff prompted Congress to mandate a far-reaching new program to control stormwater discharges. Implementation of the first phase of the program began in 1995, with regulations imposed on more than 170 cities (those with populations of 100,000 or more), 47 counties, approximately 100,000 industrial facilities, and sites of construction activity disturbing five or more acres of land. Affected parties must identify the sources and types of pollutants which could be present in stormwater runoff from their premises and subsequently implement controls to prevent potential contaminants from washing into storm sewers. For municipalities, required preventive measures will include programs to detect and remove illegal connections, ending the improper dumping of used oil and other wastes into storm sewers, preventing and controlling spills, and adopting street de-icing methods less environmentally damaging than the use of road salt. Affected industries, which include those engaged in activities as diverse as manufacturing, airport operations, recycling, mining, wood treating, landfilling—virtually any facility where stormwater could come into contact with raw materials or wastes—must devise improved methods for handling and storing materials and for preventing spills. All potential contributors to stormwater contamination, municipalities and industries alike, are required to obtain discharge permits stipulating exactly how they intend to minimize polluted runoff by developing and implementing comprehensive management programs. The second phase of the program, expected to get underway by 2001–2002, will extend the requirement for stormwater discharge permits to small, municipal storm sewer systems located in urban areas (approximately 3,500) and to construction activities disturbing 1–5 acres of land (about 110,000 per year). Due to the protracted schedule for filing permit applications and extended timetables for achieving compliance, it will likely be years before all sources of urban stormwater are regulated. Nevertheless, after years of handwringing over urban water quality problems caused by stormwater runoff, meaningful steps to tackle this problem are finally underway (EPA, 1999; Goldberg, 1993).

Water Pollution and Health

If a pollster were to conduct sidewalk interviews on what major concerns the average man or woman might have regarding water pollution, it's a safe bet that eutrophication of Chesapeake Bay, fish kills in the Mississippi, or New York City's sludge disposal headaches would rank far down on the list. Among the vast majority of respondents, the number one water quality priority undoubtedly would be assurance that the water flowing from their kitchen or bathroom faucet was safe to drink. Such public concerns stem from the recognition that human health is directly threatened by impure drinking water. There exists today a growing realization that the quality of drinking water is inextricably linked to the quality of our environment as a whole, inasmuch as air pollutants, agricultural chemicals, leachates from landfills, sewage, and industrial effluents all can invade public water supplies. While the nature of drinking water contamination problems differs somewhat in the developing nations versus more industrialized societies, the extent to which polluted water adversely affects health and well-being is a worldwide source of concern.

Microbial Waterborne Disease

Prior to the late 19th century, outbreaks of epidemic waterborne disease in every part of the world claimed a heavy toll in human lives and suffering. As late as the 1880s, typhoid killed 75–100 people per 100,000 population in the United States each year. A major outbreak of the disease in Chicago in 1885 claimed 90,000 victims and persuaded city officials to divert the flow of

BOX 15-5
Environmental Change and Waterborne Disease

Algal blooms, global warming, urban slums, and El Niño on the surface appear to be totally unrelated phenomena. However, a growing body of evidence suggests that a fatal convergence of all these factors may be responsible for a deadly cholera epidemic that raged along the coast of South America from 1991 to 1995, killing 11,000 people and sickening more than a million.

The outbreak caught health officials by surprise, since cholera, one of the most feared 19th century killers, had been absent from the Americas for nearly a century. Subsequent outbreaks in Africa, also in 1991, and in Russia in 1994 led those who study infectious diseases to question whether something new and ominous could be causing a nearly banished disease to return with a vengeance.

Typically an ailment associated with poverty and unhygienic living conditions, cholera is caused by the bacterium *Vibrio cholerae*. Lodging in the human intestines, *V. cholerae* produces a toxin that causes rapid onset of severe watery diarrhea, vomiting, and cramps. The sudden loss of huge amounts of body fluids and salts results in complete dehydration and collapse of the vascular system, frequently killing its victims in less than a day unless treatment is promptly initiated. Exclusively a human pathogen, the cholera bacterium is transmitted from one person to another via food or drinking water contaminated with human fecal material. However, in spite of the sewage connection, *V. cholerae*'s optimal habitat is the moderately salty waters of coastal estuaries, and the organism is capable of surviving in waters of the open ocean. In fact, *V. cholerae* can survive in freshwater

bodies only when they are highly polluted with sewage.

The fact that most cholera epidemics, including the recent South American outbreak, first appear in coastal communities is not surprising, given the pathogen's ecological preferences. However, health authorities were at a loss to explain what precipitated the event and how it happened to occur almost simultaneously in coastal cities of Peru, Ecuador, Colombia, and Chile hundreds of miles apart. Certainly the unsanitary conditions typically associated with cholera were present in all these places. In the Peruvian capital of Lima, for example, where the epidemic struck first and hardest, 70% of the city's drinking water is drawn from the sewage-choked River Rimac. Thanks to rapid population growth and a failure of city services to keep pace, 5 to 6 million Limeños lack decent latrines. Raw wastewater is carried to coastal discharge points by sewers that pour their fetid contents onto beaches adjacent to densely populated settlements where children regularly bathe and play in the contaminated water. Although Lima has a modern water purification plant and a good water distribution system, 40% of its residents have no access to the water it provides. Many slum dwellers must rely on the river or on house-to-house delivery by government tank trucks, which collect their cargo from polluted surface and groundwater sources. In addition to the obvious potential for waterborne spread of cholera, contaminated food was also an issue. In Peru at least, most cases in the 1991 outbreak seemed to be associated with consumption of fish or shellfish harvested from sewage-tainted coastal waters. *Ceviche,* a local dish of raw fish, marinated in lemon juice and onions, was targeted for special blame. Since *V. cholerae,* like most bacteria, is sensitive to heat, well-cooked fish would not have transmitted the infection.

Nevertheless, these factors—which had existed long before the cholera outbreak and which are daily facts of life in many cholera-free areas today—don't fully explain the pathogen's sudden re-emergence. A search for more complete answers has yielded some provocative possibilities. The discovery in the mid-1990s that certain species of marine zooplankton can serve as hosts for *V. cholerae* led researchers to speculate that the pathogen may persist for years in a dormant state in coastal waters, suddenly reappearing with algal blooms. Observations that cholera outbreaks in Bangladesh frequently coincide with algal blooms in the Bay of Bengal provide anecdotal support for this hypothesis. The cholera-plankton association would also explain how the pathogen could travel long distances along a coastline or across oceans, spreading infection from Asia to South America to Africa, simply by riding along inside planktonic cells drifting with the ocean currents. The weather phenomenon, El Niño, may play a role as well; by heating ocean surface waters, El Niño encourages massive phytoplankton blooms, quickly followed by blooms of zooplankton, especially in shallow coastal waters

fertilized by nutrient-rich sewage and fertilizer runoff. These blooms seem to activate *V. cholerae* "hitchhikers," causing the pathogen to revert to its infectious state. The fact that the South American cholera epidemic occurred in tandem with the most prolonged El Niño episode yet recorded may thus be more than coincidence.

These findings have prompted a new look at the ecology of infectious disease outbreaks and suggest that humanity could be in for some unwelcome surprises in the years ahead. If global climate change produces more sea surface warming, algal blooms are likely to increase in size and frequency—particularly along the coasts of developing-world cities where urban slums and inadequate or nonexistent sewage treatment facilities daily discharge enormous quantities of nutrients into waterways. Such environmental conditions are made to order for a resurgence of cholera and suggest that governments and international lending institutions need to redouble efforts to expand access to safe drinking water, upgrade wastewater treatment, and alleviate urban poverty.

References

Colwell, Rita R., 1996. "Global Climate and Infectious Disease: The Cholera Paradigm." *Science* 274 (Dec. 20):2025-2031.

World Resources Institute. 1998. *World Resources 1998-99.* Oxford University Press.

Chicago's sewage from Lake Michigan, also the source of municipal drinking water supplies, into the Sanitary and Ship Canal (completed in 1900) and ultimately to the Illinois River and the Mississippi—a policy decision that had the unintended side effect of seriously degrading the quality and attractiveness of the Illinois River. Cholera also was a feared disease in 19th century America; a major outbreak in the Mississippi Valley during the 1870s claimed many lives and large numbers of westward-bound settlers died of cholera along the wagon trails.

In the Third World, contamination of waterways with a wide range of microbial pathogens found in human body wastes constitutes the most pressing environmental health problem. The World Health Organization estimates that fully 7% of all deaths and disease worldwide can be attributed to fecally-contaminated drinking water. Each year approximately 2.5 million young children die of waterborne diarrheal diseases, a problem directly stemming from lack of adequate sewage disposal facilities. The gastrointestinal infections which occur when such pathogens are ingested are the leading cause of illness and death in most developing countries. Reducing the incidence of such disease requires not only the installation of water purification technologies, but also provision of sanitary wastewater disposal and public education regarding personal and household hygiene. During the 1980s, designated by the U.N. as the "International Drinking Water Supply and Sanitation Decade," significant gains were made in expanding access to safe water supplies, particularly in rural areas where the number of people served increased by 240% worldwide (150% increase among city dwellers). Access to sanitation facilities improved as well, but these gains were largely offset by the continued rapid rate of population growth and urbanization in nations throughout the developing world. In spite of these herculean efforts, by the late 1990s there were still 1.4 billion people lacking safe drinking water and 2.9 billion without adequate sanitary facilities—largely a reflection of the inability of public works projects to keep pace with burgeoning human numbers (WRI, 1998).

In industrialized countries, disease caused by fecal pollution of waterways is much less common now than it was several generations ago. Nevertheless, outbreaks of gastroenteritis traced to microbial contamination of drinking water do occur from time to time, occasionally in headline-provoking magnitude. In the United States, despite the impression that waterborne disease is a thing of the past, the Centers for Disease Control and Prevention has documented 684 waterborne disease outbreaks affecting more than 164,000 people between 1971–1992, for an average of 31 outbreaks per year (NRC, 1999). Although most such occurrences in recent years have been associated with small water systems where financial resources preclude the sophisticated equipment and highly trained personnel generally found in larger communities, a 1993 outbreak in Milwaukee, Wisconsin, sickened almost 400,000 people. These numbers, of course, represent only those illnesses which are reported to public health authorities. EPA estimates that for every case of waterborne disease identified, 25 more never appear in the statistics because of haphazard reporting.

Diarrheal illness may be caused by any of a large number of microbial species associated with sewage-tainted drinking water and fall roughly into one of the following groups.

Bacteria. Typhoid fever and cholera are the most notorious of the bacterial enteric diseases and over the centuries have been responsible for millions of human deaths and illnesses worldwide. Other bacterial waterborne ailments include dysentery *(Shigella),* paratyphoid, salmonellosis, *Campylobacter,* and some forms of *E. coli*—ailments which, like typhoid and cholera, can also be contracted by eating food harboring pathogens of fecal origin. Whereas typhoid and paratyphoid are characterized by headache, muscle

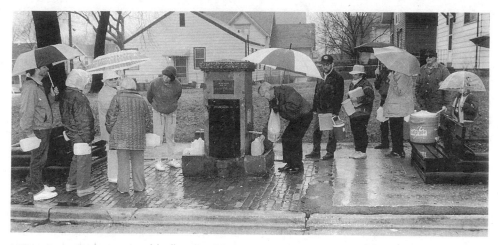

Milwaukee residents stand in line to obtain fresh water after protozoa in the public water supply caused a massive disease outbreak in 1993. *[Milwaukee Sentinel Photo]*

pains, high fever, and constipation alternating with diarrhea (all symptoms being less severe in paratyphoid), cholera, dysentery, and salmonellosis are all typified by severe diarrhea (bloody in the case of dysentery) and vomiting.

Viruses. Hepatitis A, poliomyelitis, and Rotavirus are among the most common of the several hundred species of enteric viruses associated with waterborne diarrheal illness. Many health authorities suspect that most waterborne ailments caused by unidentified pathogens are, in fact, viral diseases. Viruses are much more resistant to disinfection with chlorine than are bacteria, a fact which explains why outbreaks of hepatitis A have occasionally occurred in communities where drinking water was chlorinated and presumably was safe. While it was once thought that viral pathogens present a concern only in surface waters, it is now known that viruses also contaminate 20–30% of U.S. groundwaters, where they can survive for many months (NRC, 1999).

Protozoans. While more than 30 species of parasites may infect the human gut, only a few present a serious disease threat. Of these, the most common is giardiasis, caused by the flagellated protozoan *Giardia lamblia,* an inhabitant of the intestines of a wide variety of vertebrate animals. Over the past 25 years *Giardia* has been blamed for close to 100 reported outbreaks in the United States, some of them in remote areas where the source of the problem was traced to infected beavers or deer which were polluting the water with feces containing protozoan cysts. Since *Giardia* is largely resistant to chlorination, filtration of drinking water supplies is important in forestalling outbreaks of giardiasis. Another chlorine-resistant protozoan parasite causing serious concern is *Cryptosporidium*, the culprit responsible for the massive disease outbreak in Milwaukee in April 1993, as well as for two other major outbreaks a few years earlier in Georgia and Oregon. Finally, amoebiasis (amoebic dysentery) is another widespread parasitic infection afflicting an estimated half billion people worldwide. Amoebic dysentery constitutes a

BOX 15-6

Water Woes

Milwaukee pharmacists were the first to notice that something was very much amiss in the city that beer made famous. Already for several days in early April 1993, there had been a run on anti-diarrheal medicine all over town and the drugstore shelves were bare. Hospital emergency rooms were also doing a brisk business; from across the city, Milwaukeeans suffering from watery diarrhea, abdominal cramping, fever, and nausea flocked in seeking relief. On April 6th officials from the Public Health and Water Departments met to compare notes and confer as to the nature of the widening outbreak. They soon decided the problem wasn't foodborne and suspected "something in the water" but were baffled as to what it could be. Results of bacteriological testing were negative, but one hospital reported that several patients had tested positive for *Cryptosporidium*, a protozoan parasite which, until 1976, was not even recognized as a human pathogen. On April 7th a citywide "boil order" was announced and the following day the Howard Avenue water treatment plant, serving the area of Milwaukee where the largest number of illnesses had been reported, was closed, leaving one other plant in operation to meet the city's needs. On April 10th the presence of *Cryptosporidium* in water from both plants was confirmed, although there was still no solid evidence on the origin of the problem. Several days later, by April 14th, tests for the parasite registered negative for the second consecutive day and the boil order was lifted, leaving Milwaukee officials with the daunting task of assessing the damage and figuring out how things had gone so wrong.

The toll was staggering—contaminated water had sickened almost 400,000 people and had hastened the deaths of several AIDS patients whose immuno-compromised status made them especially vulnerable to the ravages of cryptosporidiosis. Milwaukeeans took a crash course on parasitology, learning that the protozoan responsible for their misery is a pathogen that infects many different species (the first reported incident of *Cryptosporidium* as a disease agent came in 1955 when the parasite was blamed for an outbreak of fatal enteritis in turkeys) and is now the cause of serious gastrointestinal disease worldwide. Characterized by a fecal-oral route of transmission, *Cryptosporidium* can readily infect humans when drinking water supplies are polluted with sewage or animal manures. The protozoa multiply inside the host organism and resistant oocysts are then passed in the feces, ready to infect a new host. Virtually all communities which obtain their water from surface supplies are at risk of having their drinking water contaminated with *Cryptosporidium* (as well as with *Giardia*, for that matter). While watershed protection—prohibiting the sort of activities likely to generate polluted runoff—offers the best safeguard for minimizing outbreaks of waterborne pathogens, good filtration practices can remove the protozoan cysts responsible for most outbreaks. For those cities not practicing filtration, chlorination constitutes the sole line of defense against infectious organisms, but chlorine is of questionable value in combatting *Cryptosporidium*. While chlorine quickly kills bacteria and most viruses, it is not as effective at destroying protozoan cysts. *Giardia* frequently survives disinfection with chlorine; *Cryptosporidium* is even tougher, requiring doses of chlorine 100 times stronger than those needed to kill *Giardia*. If the water is clouded with tiny soil particles, as is often the case in waters contaminated with runoff, chlorination frequently is ineffective. By combining filtration with disinfection, a much higher level of water safety can be achieved. In general, those communities which rely solely on disinfection experience waterborne disease outbreaks eight times more often as do communities employing both disinfection and filtration. Even these measures are not foolproof, however. Milwaukee, ironically, *did* filter its water, as did three other cities subsequently experiencing outbreaks, yet *Cryptosporidium* still managed to wreak havoc. Although the cause of Milwaukee's outbreak has never been conclusively established, officials suspect that runoff due to heavy spring rains throughout the watershed area washed large quantities of animal manures into reservoirs, increasing turbidity levels (oocysts

can survive in moist soil for 2–6 months, enhancing the danger posed by erosion into waterways). The appropriateness of certain procedures at the city's filtration plant have also been questioned. Since the outbreak, Milwaukee has taken several steps to ensure against any repetition of the 1993 debacle, setting stringent new effluent goals for turbidity; discharging, rather than recycling, filter backwash waters; and testing raw water for the presence of *Cryptosporidium* on a bimonthly basis. Other communities are less well prepared and officials at the Centers for Disease Control and Prevention worry that what happened in Milwaukee could be repeated elsewhere. As a CDC epidemiologist remarked, "There's nothing in the present system as I see it that would prevent future outbreaks."

Reference

King, Jonathan. 1993. "Something in the Water." *Amicus Journal* 15, no. 3 (Fall).

major health problem in Mexico, eastern South America, western and southern Africa, China, and throughout Southeast Asia (Nash, 1993).

Water Purification

At the beginning of the 20th century, a growing awareness of the link between waterborne pathogens and disease outbreaks prompted municipal officials in North America and Europe to institute various methods of drinking water treatment which largely succeeded in eliminating the serious water-related epidemic diseases of the past. The most important new treatment method introduced at this time was chlorination, first used as a water disinfectant in Belgium in 1903. Introduced to the United States five years later, chlorine disinfection made its American debut in Chicago in 1908 and was swiftly adopted by larger communities nationwide. Such advances in water treatment quickly effected a precipitous decline in deaths due to gastrointestinal waterborne disease and immeasurably improved public health. Nevertheless, the organisms that cause typhoid, cholera, dysentery, and other gastrointestinal ailments are still in our midst, ready to make their presence known whenever a breakdown in water treatment processes affords opportunity for such pathogens to penetrate our technological lines of defense.

Unlike sewage treatment, which is intended to reduce levels of wastewater contamination to the point where the effluent can be returned to a stream without provoking serious health or ecological damage, drinking water treatment theoretically should entirely remove all contaminants in the water, or at least reduce them to acceptable levels. All drinking water, regardless of its source, should be treated prior to consumption, since it can never be safely assumed that such water is totally free from contamination.

Although the precise details of drinking water treatment vary from plant to plant, depending largely on the quality of the local raw water supply (i.e. water from polluted surface sources will require more extensive treatment than does well water drawn from a high quality uncontaminated aquifer), the basic steps in the process can be described as follows:

1. *Sedimentation*—Incoming raw water is detained in a quiet pond or tank for at least 24 hours to allow heavy suspended material to settle out.

2. *Coagulation*—Alum (hydrated aluminum sulfate) is added to the water to cause smaller suspended solids to form flocs which then precipitate to the bottom of the tank.

3. *Filtration*—Filtration through beds of sand, crushed anthracite coal, or diatomaceous earth further reduces the concentration of remaining suspended solids, including many bacterial cells and protozoans.

4. *Disinfection*—Most commonly accomplished with chlorine (ozone, bromine, iodine, or ultraviolet light can also be used for disinfection), disinfection is the most important method utilized for killing pathogens in water. An important advantage enjoyed by chlorine over other disinfectants is that it leaves a residual in the water that continues to provide germ-killing potential as the water travels through the distribution system to its point of use. Thus in the event of cross-contamination due to faulty plumbing or a break in water lines, some disinfectant is still present to kill intruding bacteria. However, disinfection in the absence of the preceding steps is not highly effective because organic materials and suspended solids in the water interfere with the germicidal action of the chlorine. In addition, occasional outbreaks of hepatitis, giardiasis, and cryptosporidiosis in cities where water has been disinfected indicate that chlorine is not as effective in killing viruses and protozoa as it is against other disease organisms.

In many water treatment plants, particularly those utilizing well water, preliminary treatment also includes aerating the water to remove iron and dissolved gases such as hydrogen sulfide which impart objectionable tastes and odor to the water. In parts of the country where water contains excess amounts of dissolved calcium or magnesium (i.e. where the water is "hard"), lime and soda ash are added to precipitate these minerals out of solution, thereby "softening" the water. Ion exchange is an alternative method which can be used for this purpose. Finally, many treatment plants today add fluoride to the finished water to reduce the incidence of tooth decay (Koren, 1980).

To ensure that the water treatment process is working efficiently, laboratory tests of finished water samples are carried out on a regular basis. Historically, the presence of appreciable numbers of coliform bacteria in a water sample has been used as an indication that the water is unsafe to drink. In fact, coliforms themselves rarely cause disease; however, because they are common inhabitants of the intestines of warm-blooded animals, present in greater numbers than the pathogenic bacteria, and because they can survive for longer periods of time in water than do the latter, coliforms serve as indicators that the water is contaminated with fecal material and hence potentially hazardous. In other words, the presence of fecal coliform bacteria in a water sample warns health officials that less abundant, but more harmful organisms such as the dysentery bacillus or hepatitis virus might also be present, since all of these organisms live in the intestinal tract and are expelled with fecal material. The predictive value of the coliform test for establishing the safety of a given water supply is not absolute, however. As outbreaks of hepatitis A and cryptosporidiosis have demonstrated, disinfection that kills coliform bacteria may not always eliminate pathogenic viruses and protozoa.

Chemical Contaminants in Drinking Water

Standard water treatment processes, designed primarily to remove bacteria, hardness, and odors from water supplies, have been outstandingly successful in reducing the incidence of acute waterborne disease throughout the industrialized world. However, in spite of the considerable improvement in drinking water quality from a bacteriological perspective, the public today is justifiably alarmed about the safety of water supplies due to recent revelations of toxic chemicals in drinking water. With purification processes aimed at preventing the microbial diseases of the past, few water treatment plants are equipped to remove—or even to detect—the 100,000 or more synthetic organic chemicals now in use, many of which are known to be present in drinking water supplies across the country. Although these substances may be present in concentrations measured in parts per million (ppm) or even parts per billion (ppb), the fact that many of them are known to be mutagenic or carcinogenic raises unanswered questions concerning the long-term health effects of ingesting small amounts of poison on a daily basis. Indeed, the fact that some organic chemicals can be harmful to human health and to aquatic organisms at levels well below those currently detectable by standard analytical methods makes the issue particularly worrisome. A direct cause-and-effect relationship between toxic chemicals in drinking water and human health damage has not yet been conclusively demonstrated, but circumstantial evidence and the testimony of people who, unknowingly, consumed high levels of toxic chemicals with their water for a number of years, indicate no reason to be complacent about the situation.

Synthetic Organic Pollutants. The kinds of synthetic organic chemicals (SOCs, as they are now called) contaminating surface waters and aquifers worldwide consist of a vast array of pesticides, industrial solvents and cleaning fluids, polychlorinated biphenyls, and disinfection byproducts. They originate from a wide range of activities such as chemical manufacturing,

BOX 15-7

Poison at the Pump

Good intentions sometimes produce tragic results. In the South Asian nation of Bangladesh and the neighboring Indian state of West Bengal, thousands of people are slowly dying of arsenic poisoning and health experts predict tens of millions more will be similarly afflicted in the years immediately ahead. Ironically, the tragedy unfolding is the unintended outcome of a well-meaning development effort launched years ago by the United Nations' Children's Fund (UNICEF), working with the enthusiastic support of the government of Bangladesh.

For centuries, waterborne diarrheal diseases had been the leading cause of death and disease in the lush delta lands adjacent to the Bay of Bengal. Rural villagers who comprise the bulk of the population traditionally drew their drinking water from hand-dug wells or ponds polluted with both human and animal wastes. In the 1970s, UNICEF embarked on an ambitious effort to improve the deplorable health conditions by drilling tubewells into the aquifers underlying the region. The intent was to provide an abundant, pathogen-free supply of water for drinking and irrigation. Over the following 25 years, an estimated 3.5 to 4 million tubewells with hand-operated pumps were sunk throughout Bangladesh, about one million of these drilled by the UNICEF-Bangladeshi government partnership, the remainder by private groups or individuals, often financed by loans from aid agencies. Laboratory analysis of groundwater samples for possible contamination was regarded as unnecessary, since the water was being drawn from supposedly pollution-free deep aquifers. A similar tubewell project was launched in West Bengal by the Indian government in the 1950s, again with the aim of improving access to safe drinking water and providing a reliable water supply for irrigated agriculture. Extensive educational efforts were undertaken to persuade initially hesitant villagers to abandon traditional surface water sources for the new tubewell supplies. The success of these programs was soon evident from health data showing a dramatic decline in deaths due to cholera and other water-related illness, and UNICEF could boast that 97% of Bangladeshis were at last within a short walking distance of safe water. This self-congratulation unfortunately proved premature, as what initially appeared to be a resoundingly successful international development project turned out to be an unmitigated human disaster.

The first reports of arsenic poisoning surfaced during the 1980s, but attracted little notice. By the mid-1990s, however, as thousands of villagers in both Bangladesh and West Bengal began exhibiting symptoms of chronic arsenicosis, the problem could no longer be ignored. Studies launched by a number of both national and international groups in Bangladesh and India subsequently revealed that in many localities where groundwater reserves were assumed to be clean enough to drink without treatment, well water contains dangerously high levels of naturally occurring arsenic. While soil scientists still can't explain exactly what caused these arsenic compounds to dissolve into solution and contaminate groundwater, the problem is extremely widespread. Of some 80,000 Bangladeshi wells sampled, approximately 40% contain excessive levels of arsenic contamination, far above the 10 parts per billion (ppb) limit for arsenic set by the World Health Organization. Similar surveys in West Bengal demonstrated that a large number of tubewells there contain arsenic levels 5–50 times greater than WHO permissible limits. Wherever sampling showed well water contamination, signs of chronic arsenic poisoning among unsuspecting villagers were apparent, with many individuals already seriously ill. As a rule, chronic arsenic poisoning takes ten to twenty years to be manifested as outward symptoms of disease; thus people drinking from tubewells drilled in the late 1970s or 1980s are only now beginning to show evidence of arsenicosis. The poison accumulates in the hair, nails, skin, and urine, from which it slowly passes out of the body. As arsenic body burdens gradually increase, affected persons begin to experience a variety of health problems, including liver and kidney damage, nervous system disorders, hair loss, and general weakness. Most characteristic, however, is a mottling of the skin and, in more advanced cases, the development of warts and open sores on the palms of the hands and soles of feet. These symptoms constitute a sure sign of the arsenic-induced skin cancers that health authorities fear will become a leading cause of death in the decade ahead.

By the time the extent of groundwater contamination was recognized, the number of victims seeking medical care was already in the thousands and climbing; undoubtedly thousands more are ill but not sufficiently aware of the nature of their problems to seek help. The social implications of the situation are nearly as tragic as the health consequences. All over Bangladesh young women disfigured with skin lesions and blotchy appearance are unable to attract husbands, and young men find it impossible

to obtain employment. Health experts say that, if caught early, arsenic poisoning can be reversed by removing the source of exposure and eating a nutritious diet, but in the poverty-ridden villages of Bangladesh and West Bengal, neither of these requirements is easily achievable.

By the late 1990s the plight of arsenic poisoning victims belatedly caught the attention of world health experts who, along with their Bangladeshi and Indian counterparts, have launched a number of initiatives in both countries to assess the extent of the problem and attempt to alleviate the mass catastrophe looming on the horizon. Most urgent is the need to sample all of the millions of wells in the region to determine which are polluted. Due to quirks in the area's geology, a dangerously polluted well may lie within a few hundred feet of a well whose water is uncontaminated. Thus, if informed, villagers could restrict pumping to safe wells only. Informing villagers about the hazards of drinking arsenic-polluted water is another major challenge. The majority of people still know nothing about the situation and when told that using tubewells may not be safe after all, many are outraged. Some are fatalistic about the situation while others are simply puzzled.

In the meantime, aid agencies and government officials are scrambling to find alternative safe water sources to replace contaminated tubewells. Some have suggested reserving one pond in each of Bangladesh's 68,000 villages to use exclusively for drinking water and providing purification facilities for those surface supplies. However, local treatment requires a certain level of expertise in operation and maintenance practices which may not always be available. An abortive attempt to supply villagers with chlorine tablets to disinfect surface waters was terminated by the discovery that the chlorine concentrations used were too high, rendering them more of a health hazard than the arsenic. Suggestions that villagers could remove pathogens from pond water simply by boiling it before drinking foundered on the reality that the cost of fuel for doing so was unafford-able for most families. There are now reasons to suspect that surface waters, even if treated, might not be a safe alter-native to contaminated groundwater. In 1999, hydrologists at Duke University found that many ponds and reservoirs in Bangladesh also contain elevated con-centrations of arsenic, a result of their hydrologic connection with groundwater or due to contamination of surface impoundments with irrigation return water, originally derived from polluted tubewells. Some surface waters sampled by the Duke team contained arsenic con-centrations as high as 176 ppb (the peak groundwater level measured was 2,000 ppb!). Catchment basins for rainwater are another proposed alternative, though their adequacy during dry spells might be problematic. Inventors from several countries have offered innovative water purification devices which they believe could remove arsenic from well water cheaply and efficiently, but commercial-ization of such equipment is still several years in the future.

In 1997 the World Bank allocated $32.4 million in credit to Bangladesh to develop an arsenic control project, but two years later few concrete accomplish-ments were apparent. Within Bang-ladesh, anger is mounting against international aid agencies, with UNICEF the most prominent target. In July 1999, a group calling itself The Forum for Arsenic Patients accused the U.N. agency of provoking what may be the largest mass poisoning in human history. The Forum threatened a lawsuit to win com-pensation for the millions of unsuspecting arsenic poisoning victims now slowly dying. Government officials in Bang-ladesh are becoming resentful as well. Citing numerous international meetings and seminars on the problem, but little concrete action, a Health Ministry official quipped, "The only beneficiaries in the whole issue have been the national and international consultants."

References

Nath, K.J. 1998. "Weighing Risks in West Bengal." *World Resources 1998-99*. Oxford University Press.

West Bengal, India and Bangladesh Arsenic Crisis Information Centre.

petroleum refining, iron and steel production, coal mining, wood pulp process-ing, textile manufacturing, and agriculture. They enter surface waters through direct and indirect discharges, by surface runoff, or by volatilization and subsequent fallout during precipitation episodes. Wellwaters can concen-trate high levels of SOCs as a result of poor waste disposal practices or down-ward percolation of farm chemicals after heavy rains. The presence of SOCs in drinking water supplies has been a steadily growing source of public concern since the mid-1970s when several epidemiologic studies suggestively, though not conclusively, linked the presence of these chemicals with an elevated inci-dence of various types of cancer among exposed populations. Certain disinfec-tion by-products called **trihalomethanes (THMs)** attracted the most attention and initiated a controversy over drinking water disinfection that persists in muted form even today. THMs, which include the carcinogen chlo-roform, are formed at the water treatment plant itself when chlorine is added to water containing the naturally occurring humic substances found in virtually any lake or river. The fact that traces of chloroform have been detected in almost every water system tested for this chemical led some people to call for the discontinuation of drinking water chlorination. However, since THMs usually are present only in minute amounts, many water experts argue that they pose a minimal health risk. More importantly, they contend that abandoning chlorination would result in a return of the microbial waterborne diseases that pose a much more immediate health threat than do THMs. Nevertheless, the controversy has spurred a more serious look at possible alternatives to chlorine for drinking water disinfection.

While a number of the more than 100,000 SOCs currently in use (e.g. chloroform, benzene) are known or suspected carcinogens, establishing a direct causal relationship between polluted drinking water and cancer has been problematic. At present, the human health impact of exposure to organic chemicals in water supplies is thought to be relatively minor. Results of a U.S. Geological Survey study of 20 major U.S. river basins revealed that two or more pesticides were present in every stream sample taken and in half the well water samples. Fortunately, the amounts detected were almost always well below EPA's maximum contaminant levels for drinking water. However, over half the stream samples from both urban and agricultural areas contained at least one pesticide at concentrations that exceeded guidelines for the protection of aquatic life (some of the pesticides most frequently detected are suspected endocrine disruptors). Although public health does not appear to be seriously at risk from the low concentrations of pesticides detected, the survey raises some concerns. Health criteria and guidelines are still lacking for a number of the chemicals detected, nor do standards exist for their breakdown products—some of which are more toxic than the original pesticide. In addition, established guidelines fail to consider possible synergistic effects among the various chemicals present in the waterways sampled nor do they take seasonal pulses of higher-than-average concentrations into account. While not a cause for panic, the USGS report highlights some major challenges for improving protection of our nation's water resources (USGS, 1999).

Lead. That ingestion or inhalation of lead can cause human poisoning resulting in a wide range of health problems has been known for many years (see chapter 7). Government initiatives to lower the lead content of housepaint and to phase out the use of leaded gasoline were prompted specifically by the desire to reduce human exposure to this toxic metal. However, recent scientific findings have identified a hitherto-unrecognized source of environmental lead—water from our own kitchen or bathroom sinks. Indeed, in many areas of the country, household drinking water is the major route of lead exposure. EPA estimates that more than 40 million Americans are drinking water containing more than the legally permissible level of lead (50 ppb) and that 10–20% of children's total lead exposure comes from drinking water.

This situation does not mean that municipal water treatment plants are doing a poor job, for in almost all cases lead enters drinking water after it leaves the purification plant or private well. The problem arises within the home plumbing system as a result of corrosion when water passes through lead pipes or through pipes soldered with lead, when brass fixtures are used, or in situations where the water itself is corrosive (i.e. low pH). This type of reaction is particularly likely with "soft" water; corrosion is also increased by the common practice of using water pipes for the grounding of electrical equipment, since electrical current traveling through the ground wire hastens the corrosion of lead in the pipes.

The age of a home's plumbing system is a major determinant of whether or not a lead problem exists. In older structures—those built prior to the 1930s—lead was commonly used for interior piping as well as for the service connections that joined the house to a public water supply. Obviously if a home has lead plumbing, a potential problem exists. After 1930, copper piping largely replaced lead for residential plumbing, but such pipes were typically joined with lead solder; it is this solder that many authorities consider the main contributor to drinking water contamination with lead. Over time, the amount of lead leaching into water from plumbing decreases because mineral deposits gradually form a deposit on the inside of the pipes, preventing water from coming into direct contact with the solder. For this reason, homes with the greatest likelihood of having high lead levels are those less than five years old (unless the plumbing is made of plastic, in which case there's no problem).

Although telltale signs of corrosion (rust-colored water, stained dishwasher or laundry, frequent leaks) or recognition that the house falls into one of the high-risk age categories mentioned above can alert residents to a potential problem, the only way to make a definite determination of excess lead levels is to have the water tested at a certified laboratory (unfortunately, this is not a cheap procedure).

If lab analysis confirms high lead levels, abatement options short of total replacement of the plumbing system are somewhat limited. Reverse osmosis devices, cartridge filters, and distillation units can be installed at the faucet but are quite expensive and of variable effectiveness. Lead exposure can be minimized by two simple actions that should be taken by anyone who has, or suspects, a lead problem:

1. Don't drink water that has been in contact with pipes for more than six hours. The longer water has been standing, the greater the amount of lead likely to be present. Before using such water for drinking or cooking, flush out the pipes by allowing water to run for several minutes or until it is as cold as it will get (this water can be used for washing, watering plants, etc.).

2. Don't consume or cook with hot tap water, since lead dissolves more readily in hot water than in cold. If you need hot water, draw it cold from the tap and use the stove to heat it.

In response to this health hazard, Congress has prohibited the use of solder containing more than 0.2% lead (formerly, solder was 50% lead) and has banned any pipe or fittings containing more than 8% lead in new installations or for repair of public water systems. In addition, a number of states have now banned all use of lead materials in drinking water systems (EPA, 1987).

The realization that lead in drinking water presents a health hazard in many homes has prompted regulators to take a look at the school environment as well. In 1988, under the Lead Contamination Control Act, Congress urged both schools and day care centers to test water from electric water coolers (some models of which were believed to have lead-lined tanks or other components made of lead) to ensure that children attending those facilities were not receiving excessive lead exposure. While the recommendations for testing and remediation were purely advisory and thus not legally enforceable, many schools complied with the government's request. Unfortunately, other potential sources of lead-contaminated water such as ice machines, non-cooled water fountains, and classroom and kitchen sinks were not mentioned in the advisory.

Continuing concerns about lead in drinking water have led to further EPA actions to reduce this hazard. In May of 1991 the agency promulgated the Lead and Copper Rule, setting an "action level" (not the same as an enforceable standard) of *15 ppb* lead at the water's point of use. In cases where that level is exceeded, the new rule calls for the water treatment plant to take steps to reduce the corrosivity of the water—an action designed to reduce the leachability of lead within the plumbing system (Gnaedinger, 1993). New alarms were sounded in the spring of 1994 when EPA issued a warning to millions of private well owners, advising them to have their drinking water tested for possible high levels of lead contamination after research carried out by environmental groups at the University of North Carolina-Asheville revealed that the toxic metal was leaching into wellwater from lead-based brass and bronze alloys in submersible pumps, particularly from those recently installed (of the 11.8 million U.S. homes with private wells, approximately half feature submersible pumps, though not all such pumps have brass components). Environmental groups promptly urged pump manufacturers to recall all pumps containing lead components and replace them with safe, readily available lead-free models made of stainless steel.

Nitrates

Contamination of drinking water supplies with inorganic nitrates from fertilizer or feedlot runoff, seepage from septic systems, or airborne fallout of nitrogen compounds emitted by industry or motor vehicles has been a concern since the 1940s. At that time a mysterious ailment called "blue baby disease" caused 39 deaths and several hundred illnesses among infants in rural areas. By 1945 the condition, more accurately referred to as **methemoglobinemia**, had been linked to the use of nitrate-polluted water from shallow farm wells to prepare infant formula. Bacteria in the babies' intestinal tract convert nitrates to toxic nitrites which bind to hemoglobin, displacing oxygen and producing a bluish discoloration of the skin; in extreme cases, death by asphyxiation can result. Although all members of a household typically drink from the same contaminated water supply, only infants under six months of age are at risk of developing methemoglobinemia because their stomach juices are less acid than those of older children and adults, and hence support a larger bacterial population. Better understanding of the disease and regular monitoring of public drinking water supplies for nitrate content have greatly reduced the incidence of methemoglobinemia in recent decades. Nevertheless, risk of the disease still persists, particularly in agricultural areas of the Midwest where heavy use of nitrogen fertilizers is standard practice and where shallow aquifers supply much of the drinking water used by rural families (surface waters seldom contain concentrations of nitrates high enough to pose serious concerns). Monitoring of private wells for water quality is not a routine practice, but a 1994 national survey revealed that 22% of private farm wells contain nitrate levels in excess of the 10 mg/L EPA standard for public water supplies (unpolluted water supplies contain an average of 2 mg/L nitrogen). Because nitrates can persist in aquifers for many years, becoming increasingly concentrated as more nitrogen is applied to the land surface season after season, nitrates in drinking water will remain an on-going health concern (EPA, 1995).

Safe Drinking Water Act

The federal program to protect drinking water quality in the United States is governed by the provisions of the Safe Drinking Water Act (SDWA), first passed by Congress in 1974 and subsequently amended in 1986 and again in 1996. Prior to 1974, regulation of drinking water supplies was the prerogative of the individual states, with federal involvement limited to developing advisory standards (which the states, for the most part, ignored) and to ensuring that interstate carriers such as railroads and airlines provided safe water to their passengers. Even the latter authority was limited to a focus on microbial pathogens only; not until passage of the SDWA were any enforceable provisions dealing with hazardous chemicals in drinking water incorporated into law. Today the situation is quite different. The SDWA has established a federal-state partnership to ensure compliance with federal standards aimed at protecting U.S. residents from a wide range of contaminants potentially present in drinking water supplies. Under the act, EPA establishes **maximum contaminant levels (MCLs)** for more than 80 biological, chemical, and radioactive pollutants. These MCLs must be met by water supplied by every community water system (defined as one having at least 15 service connections used by year-round residents or regularly serving 25 or more people). Concerns about the hundreds of additional unregulated pollutants known to be present in various water supplies around the country prompted Congress to amend the SDWA in 1996. These most recent provisions require EPA to compile a list every 5 years of currently unregulated drinking water contaminants that may pose health risks. The agency must then decide whether to develop standards for at least five of those contaminants, ensuring that the list of regulated drinking water pollutants will continue to expand in the decades ahead. In addition to its requirements for setting MCLs, the Safe Drinking Water Act sets uniform guidelines for drinking water treatment and mandates that public water systems follow a prescribed schedule for monitoring and testing the quality of their treated water and report the results to the appropriate state agency. For regulation of some types of drinking water contaminants, specifically microbes, stipulating treatment techniques rather than focusing on maximum allowable concentrations has been the traditional basis for control. Demands that more be done to protect the public from such waterborne pathogens as *Giardia* and *Cryptosporidium* have resulted in amendments to SDWA requiring water suppliers to employ filtration in addition to the standard practice of disinfection. Permis-

Table 15-2 National Primary Drinking Water Standards

Contaminant	MCL (mg/L)	Contaminant	MCL (mg/L)
Acrylamide	*	Glyphosate	0.7
Alachlor (Lasso)	0.002	Gross Alpha Particle Activity	15 pCi/L
Aldicarb (3)	0.003	Heptachlor (H-34, Heptox)	0.0004
Aldicarb Sulfone (3)	0.002	Heptachlor Epoxide	0.0002
Aldicarb Sulfoxide (3)	0.004	Heterotrophic Plate Count	**
Antimony	0.006	Hexachlorobenzene	0.001
Asbestos	7 MFL†	Hexachlorocyclopentadiene	0.05
Atrazine (Atranex, Crisazina)	0.003	Lead	††
Arsenic	0.05	Legionella	**
Barium	2	Lindane	0.0002
Benzene	0.005	Methoxychlor (DMDT, Marlate)	0.04
Benzo [a] Pyrene (PAH)	0.0002	Monochlorobenzene	0.1
Beryllium	0.004	Mercury	0.002
Beta Particle & Photon Emitters	4 mrem/yr	Nickel	—
Cadmium	0.005	Nitrate (as nitrogen)	10
Carbofuran (Furadan 4F)	0.04	Nitrite (as nitrogen)	1
Carbon Tetrachloride	0.005	Total Nitrate/Nitrite	10
Chlordane	0.002	Oxamyl (Vydate)	0.2
Chromium	0.1	Pentachlorophenol	0.001
Copper	††	Picloram	0.5
Cyanide	0.2	Polychlorinated Biphenyls (PCBs)	0.0005
2, 4-D (Formula 40, Weeder 64)	0.07	Radium 226 & Radium 228	5 pCi/L
Dalapon	0.2	Selenium	0.05
Di (2-ethylhexyl) adipate	0.4	Simazine	0.004
Di (2-ethylhexyl) phthalate	0.006	Styrene	0.1
Dibromochloropropane (DBCP)	0.0002	Sulfate	500 mg/L
o-Dichlorobenzene	0.6		(proposed)
p-Dichlorobenzene	0.075	2, 3, 7, 8-TCDD (Dioxin)	0.00000003
1, 2-Dichloroethane	0.005	Tetrachloroethylene	0.005
1, 1-Dichloroethylene	0.007	Thallium	0.002
cis-1, 2-Dichloroethylene	0.07	Toluene	1.0
trans-1, 2-Dichloroethylene	0.1	Total Coliforms	none
Dichloromethane	0.005	Total Trihalomethanes	0.10
1, 2-Dichloropropane	0.005	Toxaphene	0.003
Dinoseb	0.007	2, 4, 5-TP (Silvex)	0.05
Diquat	0.02	1, 2, 4-Trichlorobenzene	0.07
Endothall	0.1	1, 1, 1-Trichloroethane	0.2
Endrin	0.002	1, 1, 2-Trichloroethane	0.005
Epichlorohydrin	*	Trichloroethylene	0.005
Ethylbenzene	0.7	Turbidity	**
Ethylene dibromide	0.00005	Vinyl Chloride	0.002
Flouride	4.0	Viruses	**
Giardia Lamblia	**	Xylenes	10.0

* Each Public Water System must certify annually in writing to the state that when acrylamide and epichlorohydrin are used in drinking water systems, the combination (or product) of dose and monomer level does not exceed the levels specified.
† MFL is million fibers per liter.
†† The lead and copper rule is a treatment technique which requires water systems to take tap water samples from homes with lead pipes or copper pipes with lead solder and/or with lead service lines. If more than 10 percent of these samples exceed an action level of 1.3 mg/L for copper or 0.015 mg/L for lead, the system is triggered into additional treatment.
** These contaminants are regulated under the Surface Water Treatment Rule.

BOX 15-8

Safer from the Bottle?—Not Really

Worried about tap water quality, Americans by the millions have been turning to bottled water to quench their thirst. Surveys reveal that 54% of U.S. residents use bottled water at least occasionally, while over one-third drink it more than once a week. Average yearly consumption reached 12.7 gallons per person in 1997, nearly tripling from 4.5 gallons per person a decade earlier. With over 700 brands from which to choose, American consumers collectively spend $4 billion each year for a beverage whose labels evoke such back-to-the wild imagery as "natural alpine spring water," "glacier water," "pristine," or "prepared by Nature." Demand is greatest in the Southwest, with trendy Californians buying three times the national average.

Why the rush to the supermarket for a product much more cheaply available from public water supplies? Primarily because many consumers perceive bottled water as safer and tastier than tap water—and because skillful marketing, particularly of expensive imported brands, has made consumption of bottled water fashionable. The bottled water industry has been quick to take advantage of public fears raised by well-publicized events such as Milwaukee's *Cryptosporidium* outbreak. Advertisements promote their product as 100% contaminant-free and hence a safer, healthier alternative to tap water—well worth its premium price. When compared with the cost of an equivalent volume of water from public supplies, bottled water may be hundreds or even thousands of times more expensive, depending on brand. Whereas a gallon of tap water costs, on average, about

one-tenth of a cent, a half-liter bottle of imported "designer water" may carry a price tag of $1.50—a 10,000-fold differential. Ironically, the actual cost of the water itself in bottled brands ranges from a fraction of a cent to a few cents; buyers are paying mostly for bottling, packaging, shipping, advertising, retailing, and profits as high as 25–30% in some cases.

That health and aesthetic factors are important determinants of bottled water's appeal is obvious from the fact that demand is highest in those localities where taste and odor problems are prevalent or where reports of water contamination have prompted consumer worries about waterborne disease. But can health-conscious buyers really be sure that the bottled water they're purchasing is any safer than the tap water they spurn? Results from a four-year study published by the Natural Resources Defense Council (NRDC), a prominent environmental advocacy group, demonstrate that industry claims of bottled water's superiority are simply untrue. NRDC found that nearly one-fourth of the 103 bottled water brands tested for the presence of chemical or biological contaminants had at least one sample that violated California's water quality regulations, with arsenic or synthetic organic compounds being the contaminants most frequently detected. (*Note:* California has standards considerably more protective than federal EPA maximum contaminant levels for drinking water.) Seventeen percent of the brands tested contained, in one or more samples, bacterial contamination and many contained traces of nitrates or other inorganic contaminants. While the concentrations of these pollutants were not high enough, in most cases, to render the water unsafe, advertising claims of absolute purity are obviously misleading. From a taste standpoint, many municipal supplies are as good or better than bottled water. The public water supply in cities such as New York and Los Angeles, for example, consistently rank among the best-tasting waters in the nation, commercial brands included. However, it is true that bottled waters are free of the taint of chlorine detectable in some publicly-supplied waters. This is because most bottling companies disinfect their product with ozone, a chemical that leaves no residual.

The bottling industry emphasizes that its product, like publicly supplied water, is heavily regulated by the federal government, in this case by the Food and Drug Administration (FDA), which classifies bottled water as a "food." FDA regulations require that water be bottled in facilities that follow food plant regulations, that they be processed under federally approved manufacturing processes, and that they be delivered to customers in sanitized containers. In addition to FDA imposed requirements, domestic bottled water must meet EPA's drinking water standards and must comply with any state-imposed regulations. Like any food processing facility, all U.S. bottled water plants are required to be inspected by federal officials at least once a year. Inspection of foreign bottling plants is beyond FDA jurisdiction, though imported brands are supposed to meet the same regulations as domestically produced water. While these requirements at first glance appear to be sufficiently protective, NRDC points out that the 60–70% of bottled water brands that are packaged and sold within one state are not subject to FDA regulation. While the states in which they operate may reg-

ulate them (about 40 states do so), about one out of five do not. In addition, FDA has exempted seltzer water and carbonated water from meeting bottled water standards, and less than half the states require that they do so. Regulatory programs for bottled water at both the federal and state level are seriously underfunded and understaffed, raising concerns about the quality of enforcement and oversight activities to ensure that bottled water complies with mandated standards.

A "truth in advertising" issue raised in recent years concerns the source of bottled water. Brand names and logos alike suggest that water on the supermarket shelves arrived direct from a wilderness mountain stream or Elysian spring. Many consumers are thus shocked to discover that an estimated 25–30% of the bottled water sold in the United States is obtained directly from municipal sources, sometimes given additional treatment, sometimes not. Bottling companies selling these brands simply fill their containers with public tap water, apply a fancy label, boost the price, and put them on the supermarket shelf. Pepsico's *Aquafina®* brand is a case in point, drawn from eleven different municipal supplies across the country. While such water is perfectly safe, it's not the specialty product its purchasers were led to believe. A more egregious example of misleading labeling was a product being sold in Massachusetts as "spring water," featuring a picturesque lake and towering mountains on the label. Investigators discovered that the contents were actually being pumped from a well located at an industrial warehouse facility next to a hazardous waste site! When the State of Massachusetts petitioned the FDA to take action against the company for misuse of the term "spring water," FDA dismissed the complaint. The agency argued that, under their definition of the term the source could legally be called a "spring" because water sometimes rose to the ground surface in an unpaved area of the industrial parking lot where the well was located. Although the FDA had issued new labeling rules in 1995 in an effort to prohibit misleading claims by less-than-honest bottlers, it's obvious from the example just cited that, while an improvement, the new rules haven't totally eliminated the problem.

Public water supplies provide American consumers with a bargain product—inexpensive and in most communities of such good quality as to make bottled water a nonessential status symbol. Nevertheless, the industry fills an important role as a provider of an alternative source of safe drinking water when emergency situations render a public supply unsafe, when special health or dietary requirements necessitate low sodium or low nitrate water, or when consumers' demands that water taste good and look clean are not met by their municipal source of supply.

Reference

Natural Resources Defense Council. 1999. *Bottled Water: Pure Drink or Pure Hype?* NRDC, New York (March).

sion to forego the enormous expense of installing filtration technologies can be obtained only when suppliers can prove that effective watershed protection programs are in place to prevent pathogen-contaminated runoff from entering drinking water reservoirs (NRC, 1999). They also must be able to demonstrate that their disinfection controls are stringent enough to remove 99.9% of all viruses and *Giardia* cysts. These are difficult parameters to meet; EPA estimates that only 12% of the approximately 125,000 unfiltered public water systems serving populations over 10,000 will be able to meet these criteria.

The gradually evolving framework of state and federal drinking water legislation—beginning with simple disinfection requirements and culminating in the highly complex mandates embodied in the SDWA—has given Americans a high degree of assurance that the water they drink won't make them sick. Indeed, the provision of safe water supplies to the vast majority of the U.S. population has been one of the great public health success stories of the 20th century. Nevertheless, continued sporadic outbreaks of waterborne disease remind us that vigilance can never be relaxed. A survey of U.S. community public water systems revealed that nearly one out of four treatment plants violated SDWA microbial standards at least once between October 1992 and January 1995; 1.3% violated chemical standards during this time period (NRC, 1999). Not surprisingly, conditions are most worrisome in impoverished rural areas where the U.S. Department of Agriculture (USDA) estimates that at least 2 million people are experiencing critical problems of drinking water quality and availability. Types of rural water-related difficulties include lack of running water, water contaminated by animal wastes running into streams, chemicals leaching into water supplies from waste disposal sites, inadequate sewage treatment, and water sources that are unprotected or inadequate to meet demand. Because a number of states exempt operators of water purification plants serving fewer than 500 people from certification requirements, employees in these small treatment plants frequently have minimal training and qualifications. This fact, plus local financial constraints that limit the ability to upgrade facilities and equipment, may explain why a disproportionate share of U.S. waterborne disease outbreaks are associated with small public water systems.

Looking Ahead

As a new century dawns, enormous water quality challenges confront societies worldwide. In the United States, despite significant improvement over the past 25 years, 40% of our rivers, lakes, and estuaries have yet to attain the "fishable, swimmable" goal set forth in the Clean Water Act. Policymakers increasingly acknowledge the need to do far more to reduce the poison runoff largely responsible for the continued degradation of American waterways. The need to address nutrient reduction, currently exempt from CWA regulation, is particularly urgent. A consensus is emerging among researchers, policymakers, and the general public that discharges of persistent toxics which bioaccumulate in aquatic organisms must be prohibited altogether, that more federal dollars must be allocated for State Revolving Funds; that enforcement actions be strengthened; that technological innovation and market-based approaches to pollution control should be encouraged; and that our regulatory emphasis must shift from its past focus on "end-of-pipe" controls to a broad-based comprehensive watershed approach, using in-stream biological indicators as a yardstick for measuring progress in cleaning up the nation's surface waters.

In Europe, Japan, Canada, and most other industrialized regions of the world, water quality challenges parallel those in the United States. All have relied heavily in the past on expensive treatment technologies which deal with pollution problems after the fact and all need to refocus efforts on pollution prevention strategies and regional watershed management.

In the developing world the problems are far more daunting. Water quality is steadily deteriorating under the combined assault of human population increase, rapid urbanization, and growing volumes of toxic pollutant discharges. Simply quantifying water quality problems in Third World countries is difficult, since monitoring is virtually nonexistent and little data has been collected even on such basic concerns as sewage contamination and the frequency of microbial waterborne disease. Virtually nothing is known about the extent of toxic chemical pollution beyond anecdotal accounts of sickness and death wherever Third World residents are forced to utilize waters tainted with industrial effluents. For the immediate future, data collection and interpretation will be high on the priority list. At the same time, however, existing knowledge must be used to protect as-yet undegraded waters since widescale construction of expensive treatment facilities to deal with pollution problems after damage has occurred is beyond the means of most Third World nations (Nash, 1993).

Around the globe, in developed and developing countries alike, unrelenting human pressures on the environment have created unprecedented water quality challenges. Confronting these challenges will be expensive and will require some fundamental changes in our traditional approach to environmental protection. Nevertheless, the importance of clean water to human well-being—indeed, to our very survival—is so great that we have no choice but to make the effort. A generation ago the U.S. Senate's leading environmentalist, Senator Ed Muskie of Maine, urged his legislative colleagues to override then-President Nixon's veto of the Clean Water Act. His stirring appeal rings as prophetic today as it did in the autumn of 1972:

> Our planet is beset with a cancer which threatens our very existence and which will not respond to the kind of treatment that has been prescribed for it in the past. The cancer of water pollution was engendered by our abuse of our lakes, streams, rivers, and oceans; it has thrived on our half-hearted attempts to control it; and like any other disease, it can kill us.

References

Banks, James T., and Frances Dubrowski. 1982. "Pretreat or Retreat?" *The Amicus Journal* (Spring). Natural Resources Defense Council.

Bennett, Lyle. 1991. "Abandoned Mines: Report from West Virginia." *EPA Journal* 17, no. 5 (Nov/Dec).

Brown, Lester R., Christopher Flavin, and Hillary French. *State of the World 1999*. Worldwatch Institute. W.W. Norton.

Carlile, B.L. 1995. "Yankee Biosolids Benefit West Texas Rangeland." *Water Environment & Technology* 7, no. 5 (May):37-38.

Cholera Inquiry Committee. 1855. *Report on the Cholera Outbreak in the Parish of St. James, Westminster, During the Autumn of 1854*. J. Churchill, London.

DeSena, Mary. 1999. "Green Cross Report on Kuwait Stresses Need to Address Environmental Effects of Warfare." *Water Environment & Technology* 11, no. 6 (June):29.

Environmental Protection Agency. 1993. "Standards for the Use or Disposal of Sewage Sludge; Final Rules." *Federal Register 40 CFR Part 25 7 et al.* (Feb. 19).

Environmental Protection Agency (EPA). 1999. *Proposed NPDES Storm Water Regulations for Phase II and the "No Exposure" Incentive of Phase I*. Office of Wastewater Management, Washington, DC.

———. 1998. *National Water Quality Inventory: 1996 Report to Congress*. Office of Water, Washington, DC.

———. 1995. *National Water Quality Inventory: 1994 Report to Congress*. EPA 841-R-95-005. Washington, DC.

———. 1987. *Lead and Your Drinking Water*. OPA-87-006 (April).

Gnaedinger, Richard H. 1993. "Lead in School Drinking Water." *Journal of Environmental Health* 55, no. 6 (April).

Goldberg, Rob. 1993. "EPA Expands Stormwater Control Permitting." *Water Environment & Technology* 5, no. 7 (July).

Griffin, Robert, Jr. 1991. "Introducing NPS Water Pollution." *EPA Journal* 17, no. 5 (Nov/Dec).

Koren, Herman. 1980. *Handbook of Environmental Health and Safety: Principles and Practices*. Pergamon Press.

Marshall, Tom. 1999. "Deadly Pulses." *Water Environment & Technology* 11, no. 4 (April): 37-41.

Nash, Linda. 1993. "Water Quality and Health." In *Water in Crisis: A Guide to* the World's Fresh Water Resources, edited by Peter H. Gleick. Oxford University Press.

National Research Council (NRC). 1999. Setting Priorities for Drinking Water Contaminants. National Academy Press.

Pimentel, David, et al. 1998. "Ecology of Increasing Disease: Population Growth and Environmental Degradation." Bioscience 48, no. 10 (October):817-826.

Riggle, David, and Kevin Gray. 1999. "Using Plants to Purify Wastewater." Biocycle 40, no. 1 (January):40-41.

"Sewer Collapse and Toxic Illness in Sewer Repairmen—Ohio." 1981. Morbidity and Mortality Weekly Report 30, no. 8 (March 6). U. S. Department of Health and Human Services/Public Health Service.

Sheiman, Deborah A. 1982. Blueprint for Clean Water. League of Women Voters Educational Fund, Pub. 639.

Shertzer, Richard H. 1986. "Wastewater Disinfection—Time for a Change?" Journal of the Water Pollution Control Federation 58, no. 0 (March).

"Small Community Benefits from Constructed Wetlands." 1993. Water Environment & Technology 5, no. 8 (August).

Tenenbaum, David. 1992. "Sludge." Garbage 4, no. 5 (Oct/Nov).

United States Geological Survey (USGS). 1999. Many Contaminants Found in Nation's Streams, But Few Drinking Water Standards Exceeded, USGS Report Shows. News release, USGS Water Resources Division.

Wolman, M. Gordon. 1988. "Changing Water Quality Priorities." Journal of the Water Pollution Control Federation 60, no. 10 (Oct).

World Resources Institute (WRI). 1998. World Resources 1998–99. Oxford University Press.

———. 1996. World Resources 1996–97. Oxford University Press.

———. 1992. World Resources 1992–93. Oxford University Press.

CHAPTER 16

Solid and Hazardous Wastes

Everyone wants you to pick up the garbage and no one wants you to put
it down!

—William Ruckleshaus (1990)

Throughout the modern world, the "waste not, want not" ethic of past
generations has long since been replaced by the consumerist lifestyle of a
"throwaway society." The inevitable result of our proclivity to "use once and
throw away" has been an ever-increasing volume of refuse which, for both sanitary and aesthetic reasons, must be regularly collected and disposed of in a
manner that will not degrade the environment or threaten public health. As
pointed out by former EPA Administrator William Ruckleshaus in the statement quoted above, doing so presents major challenges to waste managers
because of public opposition to the siting of waste management facilities. The
sometimes explosive "politics of garbage" will only be resolved through a
deeper public understanding of the issues involved in waste management, and
by a societal shift in attitudes and behavior regarding the materials we use
and discard.

Waste Disposal—A Brief History

Human generation of wastes is, of course, as old as humanity itself.
Anthropologists and archaeologists have gleaned illuminating information
about the everyday lives of our primitive ancestors by excavating the rubbish
heaps outside early cave dwellings and other ancient settlements. Among
rural or nomadic peoples, however, discarded wastes seldom accumulated to
an extent great enough to threaten human well-being. The advent of the first
cities after the Agricultural Revolution of approximately 10,000 years ago presented humankind with its first serious problems of refuse disposal. The poor
sanitary conditions and frequent epidemics which characterized city life from
ancient times until the late 19th century derived primarily from the perpetua-

tion of country habits in a crowded urban environment. Human body wastes, garbage, and discarded material items were typically left on the floors of homes or thrown into the streets. A rudimentary awareness of the link between refuse and disease led to the establishment in Athens, Greece, of what was perhaps the first "city dump" in the Western world around 500 B.C.; this innovation was accompanied by what is believed to be the world's first ban against throwing garbage into the streets, as well as by a regulation requiring scavengers to dump wastes no closer than a mile from the city walls. The Athenian example regarding waste management was not widely emulated, however. Throughout the Roman period and the Middle Ages in Europe, open dumping of wastes in streets or ditches remained the prevailing method of urban waste disposal. An ancient Roman signpost warning citizens to "Take your refuse elsewhere or you will be fined" suggests that governmental anti-littering efforts in those days had a very limited focus!

Attempts by municipal authorities to cope with their citizens' slovenly habits were limited and sporadic. In 1388 the English Parliament prohibited dumping of wastes in public waterways; after the 13th century Parisians were no longer permitted to throw garbage out their windows (they obviously pitched it elsewhere, however, for by A.D. 1400 the mounds of garbage outside the city gates of Paris were so high that they obstructed efforts by the military to defend the city). As medieval towns gradually developed into modern cities, and particularly after the onset of the Industrial Revolution in Europe at the end of the 18th century, the solid waste problem became even more acute. Urban areas became grossly overcrowded, polluted, noisy, and dirtier than ever. Rising levels of affluence among some segments of society, as well as sheer growth in population size, resulted in the generation of increasing amounts of waste. It gradually became apparent to civic leaders that the accumulation of filth and refuse in urban centers was directly related to disease outbreaks. Thus by the late 19th century, city-sponsored efforts at improving urban sanitation were launched both in Europe and North America. Refuse, previously regarded simply as a nuisance, was finally perceived as a major pollution problem which posed a serious human health threat—a problem so massive that it could be effectively tackled only by municipal governments, not simply by private individuals acting on their own initiative (Melosi, 1981).

Throughout the 20th century the "garbage problem" continued to mount at a rate several times higher than the rate of population growth. In contrast to the situation in centuries past, the major forces determining waste output since the 1950s have been an affluent lifestyle and changes in marketing techniques (e.g. multiple packaging), which result in more waste materials. While tossing garbage into the streets is no longer considered socially acceptable, modern methods of waste disposal, for the most part, are not a great deal more advanced than they were at the end of the 19th century. Today the enormous volume of refuse generated by homes, businesses, and industry, coupled with the realization that many of these wastes are of a toxic or otherwise hazardous nature, has prompted a concerted effort on the part of both government and the private sector to develop safer, more effective methods for managing the unwanted by-products of modern society.

Municipal Solid Wastes (MSW)

The tragi-comic voyage of the Islip, New York, "garbage barge" during the spring and summer of 1987 did more than any other single event to focus national attention on America's rapidly mounting problems of urban waste disposal. Loaded with over 3,000 tons of commercial trash banned from a local landfill reserved for residential refuse, the "Mobro" cruised the Atlantic and Gulf coasts for five months, searching for a disposal facility that would accept the odorous cargo. Its odyssey well-chronicled by a bemused national media, the barge's load was angrily rejected in North Carolina, Florida, Alabama, Mississippi, Louisiana, Texas, Mexico, Belize, and the Bahamas. This modern-day version of the "Flying Dutchman" finally returned to New York (festooned with an enormous Greenpeace banner advising, "Next Time Try Recycling!") where its overripe cargo was ultimately burned in a Brooklyn incinerator. The public interest generated by this spectacle raised hopes among beleaguered municipal administrators that perhaps at last citizens would begin to heed their warnings about an impending garbage crisis in our nation's cities.

Every sector of the national economy—farms, mines, and factories as well as businesses, institutions, and households—contributes to the mounting mass of unwanted materials requiring disposal. Nevertheless, municipal wastes, although proportionally far smaller in amount than agricultural and mining wastes, arguably represent our greatest waste management challenge (with the possible exception of industrial hazardous wastes). This is because urban wastes are generated where people live and must be quickly removed and properly disposed of in order to prevent serious environmental health problems. Municipal wastes are also much more heterogeneous than are the wastes produced by agriculture, mining, or specific industries. Paper and paper products constitute the single largest portion of household rejects, but an examination of a typical garbage container would also reveal glass, metal,

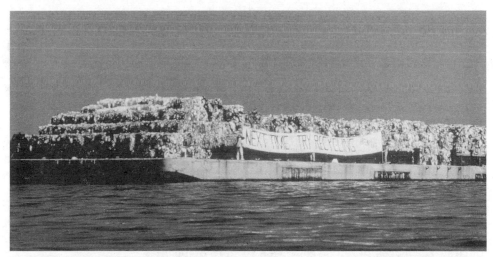

The infamous "garbage barge" from Islip, New York, cruised the Atlantic and Gulf coasts for five months in 1987 searching for a disposal facility for its overripe cargo. It ultimately returned to New York, by which time it sported a Greenpeace banner urging recycling. *[© Dennis Capolongo, Greenpeace 1987]*

Figure 16-1 What's in Our Trash?

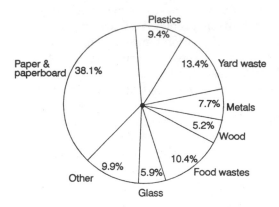

(As of 1996)
Source: EPA, 1998.

and plastic containers; rubber, leather, and cloth items; food wastes; grass clippings, tree trimmings, discarded appliances, and numerous other items.

The quantity of these discards steadily increased from 1960 until the peak year of 1994, after which volumes declined slightly. In 1999, U.S. municipalities generated 375 million tons of nonhazardous solid waste, including construction and demolition debris (Glenn, 1999). Wastes from households and businesses alone accounted for almost 210 million tons—equivalent to 4.3 pounds of refuse tossed away daily by every man, woman, and child in the United States (EPA, 1998). Since the late 19th century, Americans have regarded the collection and disposal of urban wastes as a primary responsibility of municipal governments. Today many cities rely on private haulers to collect wastes, and the majority of disposal facilities are privately owned and operated. Nevertheless, municipal officials bear the ultimate responsibility for seeing that waste management services are provided to the satisfaction of their constituents and in compliance with increasingly stringent state and federal environmental regulations.

Municipal Waste Collection and Disposal

The piles of refuse and unsightly, unsanitary conditions that quickly accumulate during the garbage workers' strikes that occasionally plague some cities provide a dramatic illustration of the importance to public health of regular, frequent urban refuse collection. Any breakdown in this essential service, particularly during the warmer months of the year, can result in odor and litter problems or in the rapid growth of fly and rat populations. To prevent such problems, the Public Health Service recommends that refuse be collected twice weekly in residential areas and daily from restaurants, hotels, and large apartment complexes. This is particularly important during the peak of the summer fly-breeding season when eggs may hatch in less than a day and larval stages can be completed in three to four days. Historically, because the public has been far more concerned that refuse be regularly removed than with what happens to it once the garbage truck rounds the nearest corner (the "out of sight, out of mind" philosophy), municipal solid waste budgets have traditionally allocated a significantly greater proportion of their resources to refuse collection than to disposal.

From a public health and environmental quality standpoint, proper disposal of urban refuse is just as important as regular collection. Until the 1970s this aspect of solid waste management was given scant attention, resulting in cities utilizing the cheapest method available, with little or no consideration given to the often severe pollution problems thereby created. A new ecological awareness on the part of both the public and policymakers gradually led to the legal prohibition of many long-established practices, such as feeding municipal refuse to hogs or dumping it into waterways. Recognition that garbage-fed hogs frequently were infected with the parasite that causes trichinosis in persons who consume undercooked pork diminished the popularity of this waste disposal option. Outbreaks of such diseases as hog cholera among herds of swine fed on raw garbage also provoked second thoughts. By the late 1950s, the U.S. Public Health Service and a number of state health departments passed regulations prohibiting the feeding of uncooked garbage to hogs. Since cooking the wastes made the practice uneconomical, this method of urban refuse disposal has now virtually disappeared. Dumping of municipal wastes into the nearest body of water—a disposal method relied upon for many years by cities such as New York, Chicago, and New Orleans—was halted many decades ago. In 1934 the U.S. Supreme Court banned the dumping of municipal wastes at sea, though certain industrial and commercial wastes were exempted from this ruling. The Marine Protection, Research, and Sanctuaries Act, passed in 1972 and subsequently strengthened by a series of amendments, gradually imposed increasingly strict limitations and now prohibits ocean dumping of industrial waste, sewage sludge, radioactive wastes, and all radiological, chemical, and biological warfare agents.

Until the 1970s, the most common method of urban refuse disposal was **open dumping**, a practice that simply involved hauling collected garbage to a location at the edge of town (usually on "the wrong side of the tracks") and dumping it on the ground. Regarded today as environmentally unacceptable, open dumping epitomizes the problems that can arise when solid wastes are mismanaged. Employed primarily because they are cheap and convenient, open dumps support large populations of rats, flies, and cockroaches that frequently invade nearby dwellings. They contaminate adjacent surface or groundwater supplies when **leachates** (liquids resulting from the interaction of water with wastes) containing dissolved pollutants run off or seep downward through the soil from the dumpsite. If burned over to prevent litter from blowing about or to reduce the volume of wastes, open dumps can pose air quality problems. They are odorous, unsightly, and have a negative impact on property values of adjacent lands. Open dumping as a method for disposing of municipal refuse was outlawed by the federal government in 1976 (earlier by some state governments), and there has been a concerted effort, largely successful, to phase out all open dumping in the United States. In many less-developed areas of the world, however, open dumping remains the most prevalent form of urban waste disposal.

Current Waste Disposal Alternatives

Sanitary Landfilling

In recent decades, most municipalities seeking an economically feasible yet environmentally acceptable alternative to open dumping have opted for sanitary landfills. A sanitary landfill differs from an open dump in that collected refuse is spread in thin layers and compacted by bulldozers. When the compacted layers are 8–10 feet deep, they are covered with about 6 inches of dirt, which is again compacted. At the end of each working day another thin layer of soil is placed over the fill to prevent litter from blowing about, to keep away insect and rodent pests, and to minimize odor problems. When the landfill has reached its ultimate capacity, a final earth cover two feet deep is placed over the entire area and the land can then be used for a park, golf course, or other kinds of recreational facilities.

When properly sited, well designed, and efficiently operated, a sanitary landfill can be a perfectly adequate means of urban refuse disposal, free from offensive odors, vermin, or pollution problems. Unfortunately, in the past most so-called "sanitary" landfills were not well sited, properly designed, or well run. As a result, many landfills caused environmental contamination problems little different from those of open dumps and made sanitary landfills unwelcome neighbors wherever they were located. In the mid-1970s it was reported that of 17,000 land disposal sites surveyed, 94% failed to meet the minimum requirements of a sanitary landfill—requirements which in the 1970s were far less stringent than those prevailing today.

Nevertheless, landfills became the overwhelming waste disposal method

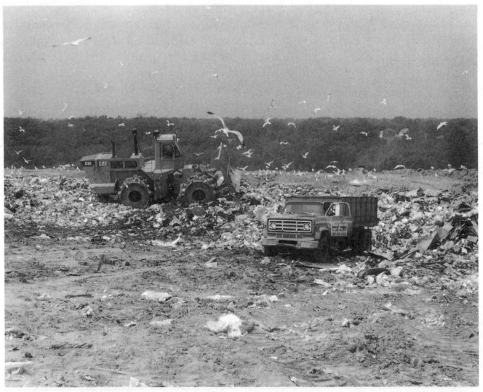

About 61% of solid wastes generated in the United States are disposed of in sanitary landfills. Rapidly dwindling capacity at existing facilities, the difficulty in siting new landfills, and increasing public disfavor have caused many municipalities to explore alternative disposal methods [Author's Photo]

Figure 16-2 Where Does Our Trash Go?

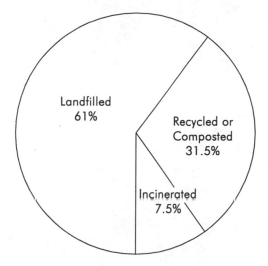

Landfilled
61%

Recycled or
Composted
31.5%

Incinerated
7.5%

Total weight 375 million tons.

of choice nationwide, largely because they were (and still are in most places) the most economical of the legal options. In 1999 the average cost for burying a ton of MSW at a U.S. sanitary landfill (i.e. the **"tipping fee"**) was $33, considerably cheaper than the cost of other management methods (in states such as New Jersey, New York, Vermont, and Connecticut, significantly higher-than-average landfill tipping fees make other alternatives economically attractive). Landfills also appealed to municipal officials because they were capable of receiving any type of waste and could, after completion, be used for facilities popular with the public such as parks, ski slopes, or golf courses. Landfills, of course, are not trouble-free: uneven settling of the land may occur, making them unsuitable as sites for constructing buildings after operations have ceased; anaerobic decomposition of landfilled materials may result in the accumulation of dangerous amounts of methane, which can cause explosions or fires if the gas migrates into nearby structures; perhaps the most serious environmental impact associated with landfills is their potential for polluting nearby surface streams or underlying aquifers with leachates. This problem can be minimized by careful site selection, choosing locations underlaid by impervious clay formations and far removed from any bodies of surface water. In the past such considerations were frequently neglected, with siting decisions typically based on the price of the land. Unfortunately, in many communities wetland areas, once considered "worthless" because of the cost of developing them for residential or commercial purposes, have been utilized as cheap landfill sites. Aside from the fact that wetlands have intrinsic value for their biologic productivity and flood control attributes, the fact that they are usually in hydrologic contact with groundwater makes wetland areas the *least* appropriate siting choice for a sanitary landfill.

Although landfills have been regarded with increasing public disfavor in recent years, largely due to the long-term environmental liability they represent (343 federal "Superfund" sites slated for multimillion dollar cleanup efforts are former municipal landfills), sanitary landfilling remains the most prevalent method of MSW disposal in the United States. According to the most recent estimates published by *BioCycle* magazine, based on surveys of state waste management programs, 61% of the solid waste generated in this country is landfilled (Glenn, 1999). In the mid-1980s, anxious talk about a so-called national "garbage crisis" dominated discussion of MSW issues in the

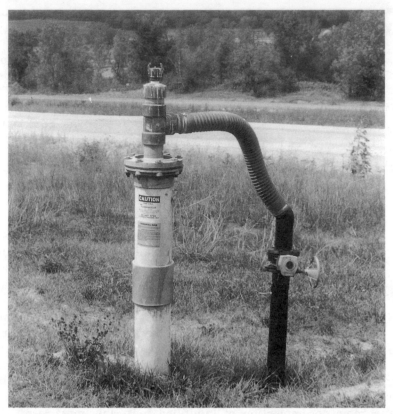

A methane recovery well at a sanitary landfill prevents the gas (a by-product of anaerobic decomposition) from accumulating in dangerous amounts [*Author's photo*]

United States. Commentators cited worrisome statistics indicating a rapidly dwindling number of landfills in many states and sharply escalating tipping fees at those facilities still in operation. Pointing to still-rising rates of waste generation, they warned that half of all American cities would soon have no place to send their garbage. Compounding the problem—indeed, the essence of the dilemma in a country where open spaces still abound—was the political reality of intense public opposition to landfill siting, a situation which time and again has stymied efforts by local government officials or private waste management firms to develop needed replacement facilities.

The new public focus on MSW concerns sparked intensive efforts by local and state officials to develop new, more sustainable waste management strategies for the decades ahead—and to insist that new and existing landfills be better designed and operated than the earlier facilities responsible for so many environmental horror stories. A major step toward the latter objective was EPA's promulgation of its new **RCRA Subtitle D** landfill requirements, now in effect nationwide. Mandating that all landfills install groundwater monitoring wells and methane detection systems, Subtitle D has sharply increased the cost of landfill operations but has also ensured that leachates or potentially explosive gases migrating from the fill don't go unnoticed and neglected. Require-

Figure 16-3 Groundwater Contamination as a Result of Unlined Landfill Disposal

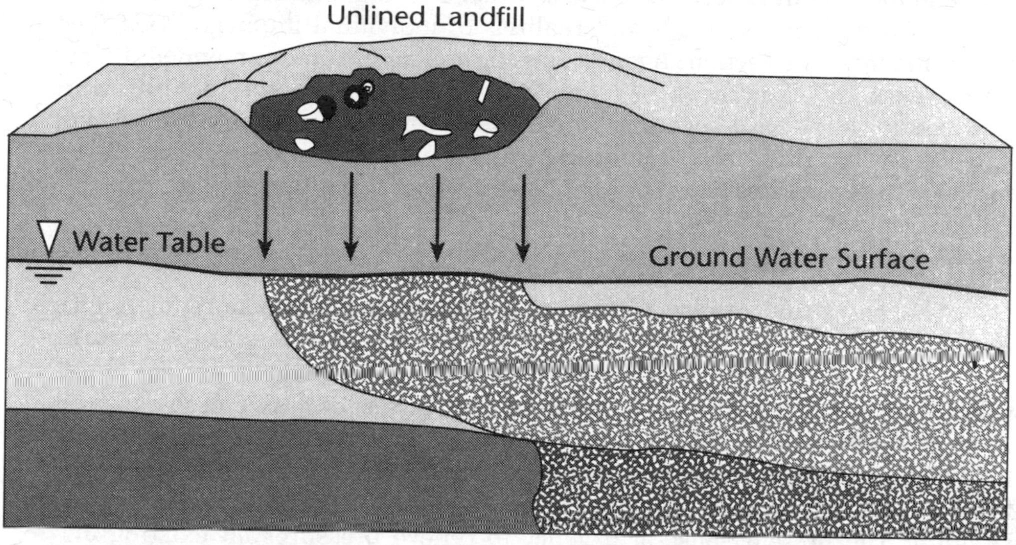

Unlined Landfill

ments that new cells within a landfill be constructed with double liners and a leachate collection system to remove standing water means that new MSW landfills will be virtually indistinguishable in design from land disposal facilities licensed to accept hazardous wastes. Compliance with such requirements, of course, is expensive and owners of many smaller landfills opted to go out of business rather than invest the sums necessary to continue operations under the new regulations. As a result, after the federal rules went into effect in October 1993, the number of operating U.S. landfills dropped from 5,386 to just 2,314 in 1999 (compared to approximately 8,000 in 1988). The sharp decline is much less of a problem than the statistics might suggest, however, for while the *number* of landfills has fallen, remaining landfill *capacity* has not taken a similar nosedive. In fact, of 26 states providing data on remaining landfill space in 1999, only seven reported having less than ten years of remaining capacity. Of those, Vermont and North Carolina are experiencing the most serious space crunch, with existing landfill capacity at just five years. Other states, particularly those in the western U.S., have adequate landfill space well into the 21st century; Wyoming reports its landfills won't be full for at least 100 years! Overall, landfill capacity in the United States at the dawn of a new century is at its highest level in two decades and earlier apocalyptic predictions of garbage piling up in the streets have now largely been discredited. Current trends indicate that for the foreseeable future, MSW will be transported longer distances to fewer, large regional facilities designed and operated in a manner that provides a considerably higher level of environmental protection than the leaky landfills of the past (Glenn, 1999).

In the meantime, waste planners are broadening their perspective, searching for more environmentally friendly MSW management approaches and striving to bring about a paradigm shift in societal attitudes toward the materials we use and throw away. Rather than focusing on one "technological fix" or single disposal alternative to solve every community's problems, most waste management experts view the solution as a combination of approaches, tailored to the specific needs and realities of individual municipalities. The Environmental Protection Agency has formulated a recommended three-tiered hierarchy of methods for managing wastes, ranking **waste reduction and reuse** as the most desirable option, **recycling and composting** second, and **waste combustion** and **landfilling** as methods of last resort, to be replaced to the greatest extent possible by the first two alternatives.

Source Reduction

The best—and cheapest—way of managing wastes is not to produce them in the first place. Accordingly, policies of reducing wastes at their source are top-ranked in every priority listing of waste management options. First raised as a possible approach for dealing with U.S. solid waste problems at a 1975 EPA-sponsored Conference on Waste Reduction, the goal of conserving materials and energy through waste prevention or by reducing the volume or toxicity of wastes generated was given little more than lip service until recently. The present sense of urgency to relieve pressures on existing disposal facilities has prompted a more serious look at the potential for source reduction strategies, which most advocates estimate could cut present urban waste streams by about 5%. Approaches to source reduction variously target consumers, manufacturers, or government and can include either voluntary or mandatory components.

Appealing to consumers to use their considerable purchasing power in a more environmentally aware manner has been a key component of source reduction efforts for years. By shopping selectively—buying only the amount of a product that will be used, choosing items without excessive amounts of packaging, buying products that have fewer toxic ingredients than comparable items used for the same purpose, avoiding single-serve disposable packages, or participating in waste exchanges (yard- or garage-sales might be regarded as an effective source reduction strategy!) are all ways of reducing the garbage we throw away. Another approach involves substituting reusable consumer items for single-use throwaway products—cloth napkins and terry towels instead of paper ones; china or plastic dishes instead of paper plates; handkerchiefs instead of Kleenex; cloth diapers in lieu of Pampers (the 3 million tons of dirty disposable diapers thrown away in the U.S. each year make up 1.4% by volume of the entire MSW stream). Backyard composting of kitchen scraps and garden debris, as well as "grasscycling"—allowing grass clippings to fall and decompose on the lawn or using them for mulch—are other examples of waste reduction that can easily be practiced by individuals.

Opportunities for source reduction of wastes in business or institutional settings are similarly plentiful. Simply by asking employees to use their own coffee mugs rather than the ubiquitous styrofoam cup, daily waste volume can be noticeably reduced. Copy-machines designed to print on both sides of a sheet of paper can save thousands of dollars in business expenditures on paper supplies—as well as on reduced waste disposal fees. Using e-mail rather than paper for interoffice memos, or simply circulating one document rather than making multiple copies, are practices being adopted by thousands of waste-conscious firms.

Manufacturers must play a pivotal role in any national source reduction effort, since their decisions regarding product composition, design, packaging, and durability have such far-reaching implications. Already industry's efforts to reduce packaging and transportation costs through "lightweighting" have had a positive impact on waste reduction trends. When General Mills reduced the thickness of the plastic liners in its cereal boxes, it simultaneously cut the amount of plastic used—and thrown away—each year by half a million pounds. Similarly, since the early 1970s, lightweighting has reduced the weight of a steel can by 43% and decreased that of a one-gallon plastic milk container from 95 grams to under 60 grams today. Many observers feel that manufacturers could do much more, however, by substituting less hazardous components for toxic ones (e.g. Apple Computer several years ago began using brown cardboard packaging containers to replace chlorine-bleached white boxes) and by designing products for easier repair and increased durability, thereby moving away from a corporate policy of "planned obsolescence."

Finally, there are a number of options government could pursue, should it choose to do so, to advance source reduction goals. Aside from efforts at public education—providing citizens with the information they need to make wise purchasing decisions—governments could employ a mix of economic incentives and disincentives, fees, taxes, subsidies, or outright bans to influence consumer choice or manufacturers' behavior. For example, more than 4,000 U.S. municipalities have adopted unit-based pricing (commonly known as "pay-as-you-throw") rather than the traditional flat fee for residential garbage pickup. Essentially a user fee based on the amount of waste discarded, this approach to funding waste management services provides a financial incentive to householders to reduce waste generation and simultaneously encourages recycling and composting. EPA reports an average 14–27% drop in the amounts of MSW discarded in communities that have adopted pay-as-you-throw programs, as well as a 32–59% increase in recycling. Although most unit-based pricing schemes are volume-based (i.e. per-container fees), a few communities have adopted weight-based systems. While a number of municipalities have hesitated to opt for unit-based pricing for fear it would encourage illicit dumping, experience in the communities that have chosen this approach indicates minimal or short-lived problems in this regard. Taxes at the time of purchase on certain hard-to-dispose-of items may not deter their purchase, but can at least provide funds to help offset recycling or disposal costs. At least 18 states now impose such a tax on tires; motor oil, automobiles, lead-acid batteries, antifreeze, and major appliances are additional products upon which certain states levy taxes which reflect their environmental impact. Outright bans on the use of certain troublesome items have been more difficult to impose due to possible conflict of such mandates with laws governing regional or interstate commerce. Nevertheless, a few have been successfully implemented, most notably the nationwide prohibition against flip-top openers on beverage containers.

The ultimate success of fledgling national source reduction efforts hinges upon a fundamental shift in society's basic approach to waste management—a refocusing of attention toward ways to *prevent* wastes from being generated in the first place rather than trying to deal with our discards after-the-fact. Source reduction, if wholeheartedly pursued, would also necessitate a different national lifestyle, though not necessarily a less satisfying one. While the concept has yet to capture the hearts and minds of most Americans and has encountered resistance from certain industries that would be directly affected by such policies, the benefits of source reduction programs in reducing waste management costs, saving natural resources, and easing humanity's impact on the environment guarantee a growing commitment in the years ahead to the *practice,* not just the *promise,* of source reduction (League of Women Voters, 1993).

Recycling

More broadly referred to as **resource recovery**—any productive use of what would otherwise be a waste material requiring disposal—recycling and composting are ranked in second place, after source reduction and reuse, on the EPA's list of most environmentally desirable strategies for municipal solid waste management. Perceived by many environmentally aware citizens as "the right thing to do" and by local officials as a way of extending the remaining lifespan of existing land disposal facilities (thereby postponing politically prickly decisions regarding the siting of new landfills or incinerators), recycling of MSW has made impressive gains since the late 1980s. In its 1999 report on "The State of Garbage in America," *BioCycle* magazine reported that recycling rates, including composting, reached their highest levels ever—31.5% of all MSW generated in the U.S., nearly four times the level attained in 1990.

Recycling, of course, is not a new phenomenon. An earlier generation of Americans diligently recycled during World War II, when saving valuable resources to aid in the war effort was widely regarded as a patriotic duty. However, interest in resource conservation waned during the prosperous 1950s and 1960s and only revived with the emergence of the ecology movement and the energy "crisis" of the 1970s. At that time increased emphasis on recycling was promoted primarily for its very real ecological benefits:

1. *Resource conservation*—recycling reduces pressure on forest resources and extends the nation's supply of nonrenewable mineral ores.

2. *Energy conservation*—recycling consumes 50–90% less energy than manufacturing the same item from virgin materials.

3. *Pollution abatement*—manufacturing products from secondary rather than virgin materials significantly reduces levels of pollutant emissions. For example, recycling scrap metal, as opposed to processing iron ore in a coke oven, reduces particulate emissions by 11 kg/metric ton and eliminates the mining wastes generated in extracting iron ore and coal. Recycling aluminum has an even greater environmental impact—both air pollution and energy use are thereby cut by 95%.

Table 16-1 Statewide Solid Waste Recycling/Reduction Goals

State	% Recycling Goal	% Current Rate[1]	Target Date
Alabama	25	23	—
Arkansas	40	36	2000
California	50	30	2000
Colorado	50[2]	18	2000
Connecticut	40	23	2000
Delaware	25	31	2000
Dist. of Columbia	45	8	1994
Florida	30	40	1995
Georgia	25	33	1996[3]
Hawaii	50	25	2000
Idaho	25	—	1995
Illinois	25	28	2001
Indiana	50	23	2000
Iowa	50	32	2000
Kentucky	25	28	1997
Louisiana	25	14	1992
Maine	50	41	1998
Maryland	20	29	1994
Massachusetts	46[4]	33	2000
Michigan	50[5]	25	2005
Minnesota	50[6]	42	1996
Mississippi	25	13	1996
Missouri	40	33	1998
Montana	25	5	1996
Nebraska	50	27	2002
Nevada	25	15	1995
New Hampshire	40	25	2000
New Jersey	65	45	2000
New Mexico	50	12	2000
New York	50	39	2000
North Carolina	40	26	2001
North Dakota	40	21	2000
Ohio	25/50[7]	19	2000
Oregon	50	28	2000
Pennsylvania	35	26	2002
Rhode Island	70[8]	23	—
South Carolina	30	34	1997
South Dakota	50	42	2001
Tennessee	25	40	1995
Texas	40	—	1994
Vermont	40	30	2000
Virginia	25	35	1995
Washington[9]	50	48	1995
West Virginia	30/50[10]	20	2010
Wyoming	25/35[11]	5	2005

[1]Recycling rates reported in the "State of Garbage in America," BioCycle, April, 1998; [2]Goal announced by governor in 1993, not legislated; [3]Goal expired 7/1/96; [4]Source reduction is planned to offset any growth in per capita generation of MSW; [5]25% recycling, 10% composting 10% source reduction, 5% reuse; [6]50% goal in seven county, Twin Cities area; 35% in greater Minnesota; [7]25% for residential/commercial, 50% for industrial; 50% statewide goal by 2000; [8]Processing for recycling; [9]Goal is still on books although legislation sunset in 1995—no plans for revision; [10]30% by 2000, 50% by 2010; [11]25% without composting, 35% with composting.

Source: *BioCycle*, May 1998. Reprinted with permission.

In recent years, while acknowledging the environmental advantages of resource recovery, advocates point to a more direct impact municipal recycling efforts could have in their own communities. Not only do such programs have the potential to reduce dependence on landfills and incinerators, they also promote individual responsibility for waste-generating behavior and may eventually help to forge a new public ethic regarding consumerism and sustainable lifestyles.

To encourage more aggressive development and implementation of municipal recycling programs, 45 states, as well as a few cities, have set recycling goals, with deadline dates for achievement (so-called **"rates and dates"**). Many have also enacted legislation requiring that local units of government develop long-range comprehensive waste management plans, detailing how they intend to comply with state-mandated recycling goals. These planning requirements have forced local officials and citizen advisory groups to look much more closely at waste management problems and solutions in their own communities, leading to a number of innovative approaches for reducing the amount of refuse destined for landfill burial or incineration.

To attain these admittedly ambitious goals, waste managers must devise innovative strategies for eliciting greater participation in recycling efforts by householders, businesses, and institutions. One of the most successful approaches to increasing rates of residential recycling in recent years has been the introduction of curbside collection programs which make household recycling as easy as setting out the weekly garbage. From just 1,000 programs nationwide in 1988, curbside collection was provided by 9,349 U.S. municipalities in 1999, serving nearly 140 million people—more than half of all Americans. New York currently is the curbside champion, with 1,472 programs (Pennsylvania is in second place with 879), but fully 23 states can boast 100 or more such programs, while only Hawaii lacks any. In terms of percentage of the population served by curbside programs, no state can top Connecticut, where every resident of the state has access to curbside recycling services. Because many cities (e.g. New York, Houston, Philadelphia, Los Angeles) are expanding existing programs to cover additional neighborhoods, growth in curbside service is even greater than the number of new cities participating would suggest.

Once materials are collected through **source separation** programs (which can include curbside collection, neighborhood recycling centers, community drop-boxes, or periodic recycling drives), they must be sorted and baled prior to being shipped to buyers for reprocessing. These tasks are carried out by **materials recovery facilities (MRFs**—referred to in recycling jargon as "murfs") where mixed recyclables are prepared for marketing.

In some regions of the country, municipal leaders have opted for an alternative approach to source separation as a means of complying with state-mandated recycling goals. Since even curbside programs, convenient though they are, almost never achieve 100% public participation, some cities don't even make an attempt to involve citizens in recycling efforts. Instead, they simply collect the mixed residential wastes jumbled together in the garbage can—food scraps, old newspapers, dirty diapers, junk mail, empty milk cartons, and so on—and truck them off to a mixed waste processing facility (not-so-affectionately known in recycling circles as a **"dirty MRF"**). There the recyclable

BOX 16-1
Germany and 'Green Dot': A Recycling Success Story

Among Europeans, Germans lead the pack in waste generation. Now, thanks to a 1991 law which some describe as "the world's most ambitious solid waste policy," they also have become the world's champion recyclers. Confronted with a population density of more than 600 per square mile (compared to just 74 in the U.S.), the German government realized that space for land disposal of refuse was in short supply. With resource constraints in mind and with the active support of an already environmentally aware citizenry, German lawmakers enacted the "Ordinance on the Avoidance of Packaging Waste," mandating that manufacturers, distributors, and retailers collect and recycle all 7–8 million tons of packaging wastes they generate annually. Since packaging materials comprise fully half the volume of all residential waste in Germany (one-third by weight), requiring those who create the waste to be responsible for its ultimate recovery has had a revolutionary impact on waste management practices in that country—an impact that is being closely monitored by Germany's European neighbors and followed with interest by recycling advocates in the United States.

The German law has a 3-pronged focus:

1. *Transport packaging*—shipping containers, pallets, corrugated cardboard or any other containers used to deliver products to stores must be taken back by the manufacturer of those products; alternatively, the manufacturer or distributor can arrange for a third party to pick up the material or pay the retailer to have it recycled. Faced with this imperative, some manufacturers have developed new forms of reusable packaging; a pat-ented shipping container designed for a leading German supermarket chain promises to save a million metric tons of waste annually and could become the standard container of its type across Europe.

2. *Secondary packaging*—the extra cardboard, plastic wrap, blisterpacks, and so on, which help the product "sell itself" or prevent pilfering becomes the responsibility of the retailer, who must either remove these materials prior to sale or provide specially marked bins near the checkout counter so that customers may discard such packaging themselves if they so choose (and, avid recyclers that they are, many German shoppers do just that, leaving piles of cellophane and other wrapping materials as a not-so-subtle hint to store managers that they would prefer less useless packaging with their purchases!). A number of retailers have responded with such sensible waste-minimization tactics as stocking supermarket shelves with toothpaste tubes standing upended on their flat caps, minus their boxes. Though a small decrease in the sales of isolated products and a slight increase in thefts have been reported, retailers solved such problems by changing the location of such items within their stores. The sharp reduction in secondary packaging waste achieved through this program has had a relatively minor overall impact on Germany's total waste stream because, even prior to diversion, these materials constituted less than 0.5% of MSW in Germany. Nevertheless, it is symbolic of consumers' commitment to the ideal of a more environmentally sustainable economy.

3. *Primary packaging*—the myriad cans, bottles, boxes, tubes, and other

types of containers which constitute two-thirds of all packaging wastes pose by far the largest collection and recycling challenges. The most controversial aspect of Germany's 1991 ordinance was its requirement that retail stores take back primary packaging wastes unless German industry met stringent recycling targets, phased in over a several-year period. Under the law, product *manufacturers* must cover all costs of collecting and recycling used packaging material.

The prospect of having to cope with mountains of paper, plastic, and foil spurred nearly 600 German companies to form a not-for-profit consortium, **Duales System Deutschland (DSD)**, and to implement Germany's acclaimed **"Green Dot" (Grüne Punkt)** system. Under this arrangement, officially initiated on January 1, 1993, DSD collects used packaging materials bearing the Green Dot logo which Germans deposit for collection in color-coded containers (this system can cause confusion, however, because colors of the bins for various recyclable items differ from one region to another). This system relieves German retailers of the responsibility for pickup and recycling of used packaging, a task which is assumed by DSD.

In order for their packages to carry the Green Dot symbol, manufacturers must pay a variable licensing fee, dependent on the type and recycling costs of the packaging material in question (highest fees are for plastic, the lowest for glass). Signing on with DSD guarantees manufacturers a recycling market for their packaging; as a result, by 1993 approximately 12,000 companies had purchased licenses and today over 90% of the packages on German store shelves are emblazoned with a Green Dot. Licensing costs paid by manufacturers are, predictably, passed on to consumers in the form of higher product prices.

The program, not surprisingly, suffered some growing pains during its early years of implementation, most notably the collection of a much greater volume of materials than DSD had anticipated. Since prevailing fees for residential waste collection services are quite high in Germany, householders enthusiastically utilized the "free" services provided by DSD bins to deposit mountains of recyclables, including many which didn't bear the "Grüne Punkt" and hence were theoretically ineligible for collection. Plastics were a particularly vexing problem, since DSD was collecting four times more than expected—an amount far exceeding Germany's plastics recycling capacity. To the chagrin of Germany's neighbors, much of this excess was dumped on world markets (some was found illegally stockpiled in French quarries!), depressing secondary materials prices as far away as Pakistan, China, and Indonesia. Much of it ended up in incinerators and some, according to Greenpeace, was even dumped into the ocean.

Inevitable start-up problems have now largely been resolved as steady gains are made in the program's processing capacity for recyclables and in its cost-effectiveness. By the late 1990s, the recycling and recovery quotas mandated by the Packaging Ordinance were being achieved for all the designated material streams. Public enthusiasm for the separate collection of recyclables remains strong, in spite of the higher consumer prices that must be charged to cover costs of the program. Results of a study published in 1999 revealed that 77% of Germans interviewed expressed support for collection and recycling as the best option for MSW management.

Although ostensibly intended to boost recycling rates and thus ease pressure on landfills and incinerators, Germany's innovative ordinance may be most significant in its impact on waste reduction. The mandate has prompted the majority of German manufacturers to switch to lighter-weight packages, make drastic cuts in hard-to-recycle packaging materials such as polyvinyl chloride and blister packs, and in some cases—as with large appliances—to avoid the use of packages altogether. Within the first four years of program implementation, amounts of packaging materials used annually dropped by 900,000 metric tons. By "internalizing" the environmental costs of packaging in the price of the product, Germany has provided manufacturers with a marketplace incentive to incorporate pollution prevention concepts into the design of their products.

The success of the German model has inspired several neighboring countries to adopt elements of the program. The Netherlands has decreed that, after 1999, no packaging waste can be landfilled and is striving to cut total weight of packaging materials on the market to 10% of 1986 levels. France has adopted Germany's Green Dot logo and is promoting "shared responsibility" between government and the private sector for reducing that nation's waste burden. Finland has ordered packaging manufacturers to reuse 82% by weight of all postconsumer packaging. Italy has a total ban on secondary and tertiary packaging in the MSW stream and imposes fines on firms that fail to achieve established recycling and recovery targets.

The Green Dot program has captured the imagination of U.S. recycling advocates, but few harbor any hope that the system will be adopted here. Ample landfill capacity and vigorous opposition by the American packaging industry has stymied fledgling attempts by environmental advocates in Congress to push "polluter pays" legislation. However, several far-sighted industries and corporations are voluntarily assuming responsibility for their discarded products. Most notable in this regard are battery manufacturers, whose trade organization, the Rechargeable Battery Association, has set a 2001 goal for recycling 70% of all used nickel-cadmium batteries at their own expense. Xerox Corporation is similarly proactive with its company-wide Comprehensive Lifestyle Program that provides plans for disassembly and reuse of its products. Auto manufacturers in Detroit have set up the Vehicle Recycling Partnership, striving to increase the percentage of recyclable materials in new cars while eliminating toxic components such as the mercury in switches. Such initiatives are commendable, but piecemeal undertakings of this sort are unlikely to produce the dramatic reductions in waste achieved by Germany's comprehensive program.

Whether American consumers, focused on price and function, will accord recycling and environmental protection a priority on the level of the Green Dot program remains to be seen. Nevertheless, Germany's ongoing experience with the Green Dot system has shown that when financial incentives or disincentives are built into the cost of a product, consumers and manufacturers alike respond in ways that noticeably alter the composition of the municipal waste stream.

References

Bücker, C. 1997. Personal correspondence.

Duales System Deutschland. GmbH, D-51170. Cologne, Germany.

Fishbein, Bette. 1994. *Germany, Garbage, and Green Dot: Challenging the Throwaway Society*. Inform, Inc.

Rembert, Tracy C. 1997. "The Producer Pays." *E Magazine* 8, no. 3 (May/June):36-41.

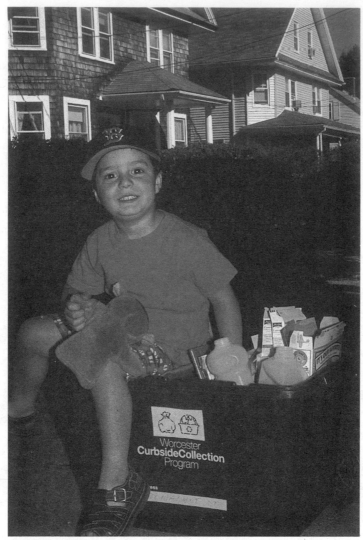

Curbside collection programs have increased the rates of residential recycling in many communities. *[Author's photo]*

components are pulled out of the waste stream and diverted for processing, while the remainder is either landfilled or made into pellets for burning in an incinerator. Proponents of "dirty MRFs" admit that the facilities are expensive to construct and operate, but point out that, in comparison with source separation programs (i.e. separation by the person who generates the waste, as in curbside collection or neighborhood drop-boxes), mixed waste recovery facilities are theoretically capable of diverting a much higher percentage of recyclables from the waste stream. This is because all of a community's refuse is delivered to them, not just that portion removed voluntarily by households. Some local officials favor such facilities because they don't require any public education efforts to persuade or coerce residents into altering long-established waste-generating behavior. Conversely, opponents contend that, aside from their high cost, "dirty MRFs" are environmentally unsound because the *quality* of potentially recyclable materials pulled from the mixed waste stream is so poor as to have little or no value to a secondary materials industry which demands as clean and homogeneous a waste stream as possible (i.e. who would want to buy paper for recycling once it's smeared with tomato sauce from discarded pizza? How could glass be recovered for shipment to a processor when scattered in small fragments among banana peels, dirty facial tissue, and used tea bags?). By the end of the 1990s, "dirty MRFs" comprised less than 15% of all recycling processing projects, numbering 66 nationwide, as compared to 407 materials recovery facilities that process recyclables only (Berenyi, 1999).

Although public response to the concept of resource recovery has generally been enthusiastic, several obstacles have prevented Americans from realizing the full potential of "turning garbage into gold." While increasing the percentage of households actually participating in recycling programs is one challenge, an even greater one is developing strong, reliable markets for secondary materials. Unfortunately, collection is not synonymous with recycling—it's not recycled until it's reused! If the tons of paper, glass, and metal brought to a drop-off center or set out for curbside pickup have no market, or if the prevailing price for such items is less than the cost of transporting materials to the buyer, resource recovery efforts are doomed to fail. In recent years the oversupply of recyclable materials—a surfeit of riches brought about largely due to the proliferation of curbside collection programs—has caused a precipitous decline in market prices for scrap over the past several years, imperiling the economic viability of recycling efforts. Global economic conditions can also have a major impact on the market price of recyclables because overseas buyers purchase a significant percentage of U.S. secondary materials. The Asian financial crisis of the late 1990s drastically reduced international demand for recycled materials, resulting in plummeting market prices of virtually all secondary products. Such economic facts of life mean that for many communities the cost of collecting and processing recyclables far exceeds their resale value. Even taking the avoided costs of disposal into consideration, most municipal recycling programs operate at a substantial loss. Reversing this situation requires stimulation of market demand, or "closing the loop" in a cyclic process in which products are used, collected, fabricated into new products, purchased, and used again.

In an effort to promote recycling, governments at the federal, state, and local levels are pursuing a number of options to boost the supply of high-quality recyclables or to stimulate market demand. Among the legislative approaches to increase the amounts of material diverted through source separation efforts are the setting of "rates and dates" as previously described, as well as the passage of **"Bottle Bills,"** laws currently in effect in ten states (Oregon, Vermont, Maine, Michigan, Iowa, Connecticut, Massachusetts, Delaware, California, and New York) which require consumers to pay a refundable deposit on beer and soft drink containers. First adopted by Oregon in 1972, bottle bills were originally intended to combat littering, a task at which they were resoundingly successful. Surveys performed a few years after bottle bills took effect documented a 75–86% drop in the number of beverage containers discarded along roadsides in comparison with predeposit days (although some

BOX 16-2

Eco-Consumer Quandary

"Paper or plastic?" This constantly repeated query greeting shoppers every time they approach a supermarket checkout counter poses a troublesome dilemma for the environmentally conscious consumer. For the truly committed, of course, the "greenest" response would be to emulate Europeans by whipping out one's own cloth or fiber tote bag. However, for once-a-week American shoppers, this option lacks practical appeal, thus bringing one back to the vexing choice between paper or plastic.

It's obvious which type of bag retailers prefer (the leading question, "Is plastic OK?" is a dead give-away). The once-ubiquitous Kraft paper bag now comprises just 25% of the estimated 40 billion grocery bags used in the United States each year. Supermarket executives have been aggressively pushing the transition to plastic for straightforward economic reasons: 1) they take up considerably less storage space (one truckload of plastic bags contains the same number as seven truckloads of paper bags); 2) they weigh much less than paper bags (15 pounds/1000 bags versus 140 pounds/1000 bags for paper); and 3) their unit cost is approximately half that of paper. Many customers opt for plastic bags because their convenient handles provide ease of carrying, a fact that gave added impetus to the market shift from paper to plastic over the past 20 years. Many recycling-oriented consumers view this trend with dismay, however. True, plastic bags can be recycled and many supermarket chains provide collection bins for customers to return used bags (though the number who actually remember to do so is questionable). Their average market price of about 3 cents per pound has

held relatively steady in recent years, with the collected bags sold to processing plants which convert them into plastic lumber or recycle them into new bags. In the early years of plastic bag recycling, contamination was a problem (some returns contained such nonrecyclable items as dirty diapers or used hypodermic needles!) but is seldom an issue today.

Nevertheless, paper bags remain the dedicated recycler's container of choice. A high-value commodity on the secondary materials market when baled alone or with corrugated cardboard, paper bags are also widely used as curbside collection containers. Many community programs request householders to place old newspapers and mixed paper in bags to keep them separate from glass, metal, or plastic items which might cause problems of contamination. Environmentally aware consumers also point to the biodegradability of paper versus plastic, noting that if bags are thoughtlessly discarded rather than collected and recycled, paper eventually breaks down whereas plastic does not. From a waste reduction perspective, paper bags have an edge as well, since they can hold four times the volume of plastic bags when filled to capacity.

Opinion polls reveal that the average consumer, environmentalist or not, tends to prefer paper. A 1997 survey conducted by Willard Bishop Consulting of Chicago found that 58% of those questioned said they prefer paper bags. However, 78% of these same respondents said they want a grocery bag with handles. As a result, the Paper Bag Council of the American Forest & Paper Association has begun vigorous promotion of a handled paper bag, the benefits of which the Council is now touting to supermarket chains and consumers. Though the handled bag costs four cents more than traditional bags, customer satisfaction may supply the incentive store managers need to make the switch. A poll taken by an Indianapolis-based supermarket chain revealed that 38% of customers would be willing to drive five minutes out of their way to shop at a store that provides handled paper bags. If this latest innovation wins widespread acceptance among grocery retailers, eco-shoppers may no longer equivocate over the "paper or plastic?" question and be able to indulge in guilt-free convenience.

Reference

Barber, Bethany. 1999. "Paper or Plastic?" *Waste Age* 30, no. 2 (February):86-87.

slovenly individuals persist in tossing cans and bottles away even in bottle bill states, there is now financial motivation for others to retrieve them). Bottle bills have subsequently proven themselves equally effective at boosting recycling rates for aluminum, glass, and PET plastic. Data from bottle bill states indicate that over 80% of the beverage containers sold in these states are ultimately recycled—a considerably higher proportion than prevails in states without bottle bills. Florida pioneered a slightly different concept in fee legislation targeted at container packaging. In 1993 the state implemented its **advance disposal fee (ADF)** which assesses one cent (collected at the wholesale, rather than the retail, level) on bottles, cans, jars, and beverage containers ranging from five ounces to one gallon in size—*if* that form of packaging is not being recycled at a minimum rate of 50% (since aluminum and steel containers already feature recovery rates in excess of 50%, they are not affected by Florida's mandate).

Another popular legislative trend in recent years has been the prohibition of landfill disposal of such materials as yard wastes, lead-acid batteries, whole tires, white goods (large appliances), and used motor oil. While the main purpose of these bans has been to conserve landfill space or to prevent the formation of toxic leachates, their enactment has greatly enhanced the amount of these materials diverted to recycling centers or composting facilities since there's now nowhere else for them to go!

Minimum recycled content mandates have become an increasingly popular method of creating market demand for old newspaper, glass, and plastic—even telephone directories! Such laws require that targeted products contain a certain percentage of recycled material. For example, by 1998 twenty-seven states had enacted voluntary or mandatory requirements that newspapers sold in those states contain specified percentages of recycled fiber (Miller, 1998). While unpopular within the newspaper industry, these mandates were adopted in an attempt to ease the glut of old newsprint, caused by an oversupply and too little demand. Florida has opted for a somewhat different solution to the same problem by imposing a 50-cent per ton tax on newsprint containing less than 50% recycled fiber. The impact of these initiatives is evident in figures showing that by the late 1990s, 28% of the fiber in American newspapers originated from recycled newsprint.

Government procurement policies which require government agencies, state universities, and public schools to purchase supplies that are recyclable or contain recycled material have long been advocated as a means to promote market demand for recyclables. Since the purchases of goods and services by federal, state, and local governments in the United States cumulatively amount to 20% of the GNP, use of government purchasing power in favor of secondary materials could provide an important boost to the recycling industry. Accordingly, by the early 1990s, 16 states were allocating a portion of their procurement budget to buy recycled products, while 27 permitted government offices to pay somewhat more for recycled products than for comparable items made of virgin material (League of Women Voters, 1993). In a move widely praised by recycling advocates, President Clinton in 1993 signed an executive order requiring that all agencies of the federal government purchase paper containing a minimum 20% recycled content by 1995, a figure slated to rise to 25% by the year 2000. Since the federal government currently uses 300,000 tons of paper annually (about 2% of all the printing and writing paper produced in the U.S. each year), this requirement will generate significant new market demand for recycled fiber—a demand that will be further enhanced if states opt to follow the federal lead.

Whether such active government support for "demand-side" recycling efforts is economically justified remains a matter of intense controversy. Recycling advocates contend that the environmental and resource conservation benefits of recycling, along with avoided costs of disposal (i.e. the money saved by avoiding landfill or incinerator tipping fees), make recycling a better deal than a comparison of costs and revenue would suggest at first glance. Critics respond that recycling can benefit society in many ways, but only when programs are carried out in an economically efficient manner. They argue that government policymakers should not try to skew marketplace decisions through such demand-side measures as minimum recycled content legislation, but rather should pursue whichever waste management method is most efficient and cost-effective, even if this means reverting to landfill disposal or incineration of those materials for which the cost of collection and processing far outstrips their market value (Boerner and Chilton, 1994).

Composting

Since the late 1980s, proliferation of state mandates prohibiting the landfilling of yard wastes has led to an explosive increase in municipal composting facilities in the United States. By 1999, 21 states had enacted such bans and over 3,800 yard waste composting facilities were operating in every U.S. state except Alaska (bans on the landfilling of yard wastes have also contributed to booming sales of mulching mowers; results from a four-year demonstration project conducted by the Rodale Institute concluded that use of mulching mowers produces healthier lawns with fewer weeds and no thatch buildup). While a number of European countries have long recognized that composting of organic household waste can reduce the amount of refuse requiring disposal, consideration of composting as a viable waste management alternative in the United States is a much more recent phenomenon. Even though readily decomposable food and yard wastes make up nearly 25% of the U.S. urban waste stream (considerably more during the warmer months of the year, less during the winter), perceived lack of demand for the finished prod-

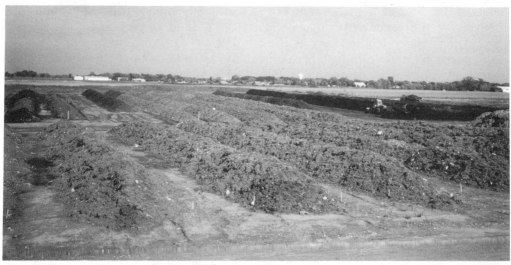

Windrow technique: long rows of composting wastes are piled outdoors and periodically aerated. *[Illinois Department of Energy and Natural Resources]*

uct, plus the ease and low cost of landfilling, led city officials to dismiss composting as an impractical venture. That attitude has now been transformed by the realization that it makes little sense to devote valuable landfill space to grass clippings and autumn leaves when such materials could be converted into a useful and environmentally beneficial product. Nor are yard wastes the only potentially compostable materials in MSW. By 1999, nineteen cities hosted mixed waste composting plants that process the entire organic portion of residential and commercial wastes—food scraps, soiled paper, etc.—removing only noncompostable (but still recyclable) glass, metal, and plastics, as well as any hazardous materials. Though questions have been raised about the quality of mixed waste compost and thus its acceptability to end-users, efforts to educate citizens on the importance of source separation have helped to prevent contamination of the final product and to avoid the loss of potentially compostable materials.

A form of resource recovery, composting utilizes natural biochemical decay processes to convert organic wastes into a humus-like material, suitable for use as a soil conditioner. Although its nutrient content is too low to consider it a fertilizer, compost greatly improves soil structure and porosity, aids in water infiltration and retention, increases soil aeration, and slows erosion. Co-composting of yard wastes with municipal sewage sludge (another increasingly difficult-to-dispose-of waste product), now being practiced in a number of communities, enhances the nitrogen content of the finished product and makes it more valuable for agricultural uses.

A variety of methods for converting wastes to compost are currently in use, ranging from the low-tech, relatively inexpensive **windrow** technique, where long rows of wastes are piled outdoors and mechanically turned periodically to aerate the mass, to highly sophisticated, expensive **in-vessel** operations or processes in which pumps mechanically aerate windrows (**"aerated static pile"**), hastening decay and eliminating the need for frequent turning.

Choice of the most appropriate composting method depends on the needs and resources of the community in question: if land is abundant and funding scarce, the windrow method may be the best option—though it often requires two or three years for complete breakdown of wastes to occur if the piles are turned only once or twice annually. If available space is at a premium and rapid turnover of wastes desirable, a community might be wise to choose a more high-tech method, provided it can afford the considerably higher price tag associated with such facilities. Whatever the technology, the composting process consists of four basic steps:

1. *Preparation*—incoming wastes are shredded to a relatively uniform size; in most composting operations, nonbiodegradable materials such as glass, metal, plastics, tires, and so on are separated from the compostable wastes. In some composting operations, sewage sludge or animal manures are added to the refuse at this point.

2. *Digestion*—microbes naturally present in the waste materials or special bacterial inoculants sprayed on the refuse are utilized to break down organic waste materials. While digestion may be either aerobic or anaerobic, aerobic systems are generally preferred due to shorter time periods required and fewer odor problems. In aerobic decomposition, heat given off by microbial respiration raises the temperature in the windrows well above the 140°F necessary to kill fly eggs, weed seeds, or pathogenic organisms.

3. *Curing*—after digestion of simpler carbonaceous materials is complete, additional curing time is allowed to permit microbes to break down cellulose and lignin in the waste.

4. *Finishing*—to produce an acceptable finished product, compost may be put through screens and grinders to remove non-digested materials and create a uniform appearance. Some composting facilities bag or package the finished product to facilitate marketing or distribution.

While the public rightly regards composting as an environmentally desirable method of organic waste management, composting facilities do not always make good neighbors. Some have been forced to close due to problems with objectionable odors—problems that are gradually being solved as operators compare notes and learn techniques for managing trouble-free facilities. Another public health issue related to composting operations is their potential to emit **bioaerosols**, tiny airborne particles of microorganisms whose inhalation has been blamed for ailments ranging from a runny nose and watery eyes to flu-like symptoms. Bioaerosols, such as spores of the ubiquitous fungus *Aspergillus fumigatus*, were first cited as a potential environmental health concern in 1992 when a New Jersey epidemiologist testified before Congress about potential health risks to persons living within a two-mile radius of composting sites. Since that time bioaerosols have attracted intensive scrutiny and have prompted organized community opposition to siting of compost facilities in several localities. Representatives of the composting industry argue that any fears are vastly exaggerated, stating that public exposure to *Aspergillus* emissions from composting are negligible when the process is performed correctly. A report jointly sponsored by the EPA, USDA, NIOSH, and the Composting Council tends to support industry's contention. Conceding that exposure to bioaerosols could be life-threatening if inhaled by individuals with suppressed immune systems, the report nevertheless points out that the level of such particles is no higher in the vicinity of composting operations than in the general environment. A person is just as likely to inhale *A. fumigatus* spores while mowing the lawn, raking leaves, or cleaning the attic as by living near a composting facility. Experts report that *Aspergillus* at composting sites originates primarily from the storage of bulking agents such as wood chips, with airborne spores being released at the time of initial mixing (the steam rising off the top of windrows does *not* appear to be a major source). Operational considerations such as moisture and dust control and minimization of handling can significantly mitigate bioaerosol emissions. While authorities agree that more research is needed, the general consensus at present is that bioaerosols *do not* present concerns serious enough to warrant a reconsideration of municipal composting operations (Greczyn, 1994).

In the past, the difficulty of finding outlets for municipal compost was a major stumbling block in convincing local officials to consider composting as a waste management strategy. In recent years, however, cities' marketing efforts and increased public awareness of compost's desirability as a soil conditioner have created sufficient demand among landscaping firms, nurseries, parks departments, and home gardeners to provide a ready outlet. This growing willingness to use compost, coupled with improvements in composting technology and a national need to curtail the flood of urban refuse destined for landfill space, suggests that municipal composting will constitute an increasingly significant waste management alternative in the years ahead.

Waste Combustion

Prior to passage of the 1970 Clean Air Act, burning of urban refuse at large municipal incinerators was the waste disposal method of choice in a number of communities where the high cost of land, unavailability of suitable sites, or neighborhood opposition to siting made landfilling unfeasible. By the 1960s, almost 300 municipal incinerators were operating in the United States. As the decade of the 1970s ushered in an era of strict air quality control regulations, however, most of these incinerators closed down, unable to comply with the new emission standards. Studies indicated that in some large cities, close to 20% of all particulate pollutants were coming from municipal incinerators (Melosi, 1981).

By the end of the 1990s, incineration was the management option for only 7.5% of U.S. municipal solid wastes, a figure considerably lower than predicted just a few years earlier. During the 1980s, as the nation's mounting garbage woes assumed center stage in the environmental policy debate, interest in burning as an attractive waste management option was revived by the advent of a new generation of incinerators: **waste-to-energy (WTE)** plants. These facilities not only burn refuse, thereby reducing its volume by 80–90%, but also capture the heat of combustion in the form of salable electricity or process steam. Many communities, particularly in the northeastern U.S. where landfill tipping fees were skyrocketing, committed themselves to this new technology as the most feasible alternative to disappearing landfill space. By the mid-1990s, however, increasing landfill capacity and a drop in tipping fees shifted the economics in favor of landfilling. As a result, some municipalities that had been considering construction of combustion incinerators decided to forego that option; elsewhere small, economically marginal incinerators were shut down. By 1999, just 119 municipal solid waste incinerators were operating nationwide, most of them in New England, the Middle Atlantic states, and Florida. Among states, Connecticut is the most reliant on incineration for MSW disposal, burning 64% of the wastes generated. The District of Columbia is even more combustion-dependent, incinerating fully 92% of the wastes produced in the nation's capital (Glenn, 1999).

From an environmental standpoint, the euphoria that in the 1980s welcomed WTE incinerators as the ideal solution to our disposal dilemmas is now giving way to a more cautious appraisal, as concerns are raised about possible toxic air emissions, especially dioxins, furans, and heavy metals (e.g. lead, cadmium, and mercury). Proponents of the technology insist such problems can be minimized through good emission controls and proper plant operation; in 1991 tighter emissions limitations required by Clean Air Act Amendments for municipal incinerators were approved by EPA, requiring that facilities install state-of-the-art equipment to control acid gases, metal particulates, and organic products of incomplete combustion, such as dioxin. Smokestacks are now being fitted with acid gas scrubbers, baghouse filters for trapping metal particulates, and activated carbon injection systems for capturing mercury vapors. By utilizing advanced combustion controls, plant operators can maintain furnace temperatures high enough to prevent dioxin formation and to ensure a more complete burn.

Disposal of the considerable volumes of incinerator ash generated by large WTE facilities has been another contentious issue. Incineration is not a complete waste management method; in general, for every three tons of refuse burned, a ton of ash remains, requiring disposal. Until recently the most prevalent method for managing incinerator ash was to bury it in ordinary sanitary landfills or in "monofills"—facilities which accepted only incinerator ash for disposal. However, concerns that this material frequently contains dangerous levels of heavy metals (particularly the fly ash captured by pollution control equipment), have led to demands that incinerator ash be classified as "hazardous waste," thereby necessitating its disposal at a hazardous waste landfill—at an anticipated 10-fold rise in tipping fees. In May 1994, the U.S. Supreme Court settled the dispute by ruling that ash from municipal incinerators must be tested, using specified laboratory procedures, and if results indicate that the waste is indeed toxic, it must be managed as hazardous waste. This ruling, while greeted initially with dismay by municipalities currently relying on incinerators, should give a major impetus to resource recovery programs aimed at removing toxics-containing components of the MSW stream—items such as batteries, paint cans, and electrical equipment. Also, by halting the standard practice of combining the often-toxic fly ash with the far more voluminous but much less dangerous bottom ash, incinerator operators can greatly reduce the amount of ash requiring disposal as "hazardous." Pointing out that the Court decision may have provided the stimulus needed to force incinerator operators to do what they should have been doing already, an attorney for the Environmental Defense Fund remarked, "This is not brain surgery. This decision gives municipalities pollution-prevention incentives

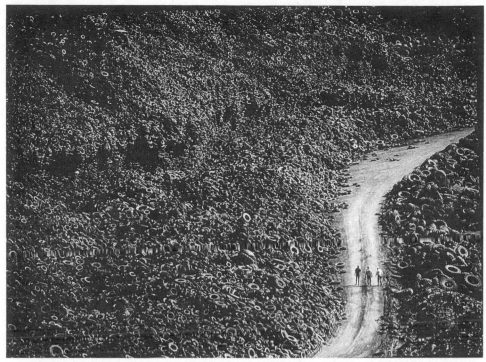

Discarded tires pose one of our more difficult solid waste disposal problems. Currently, incineration for energy recovery is the leading method of tire disposal in the U.S. *[Jose Azel/Aurora]*

that are realistically available" (Greenhouse, 1994).

Nevertheless, opponents remain wary, fearing that cities opting for incineration are going to find they've simply traded one set of environmental problems for another. Perhaps the major question regarding the future of WTE incineration, however, is financing their construction and operation. To remain economically viable, incinerators need a steady supply of trash and a dependable market for the energy they produce—but recent developments make both difficult to guarantee. Competing demands from recycling programs for high-BTU trash and recent court invalidation of local **"flow-control" ordinances** (which communities have imposed to ensure incinerators a predictable daily volume of waste) have resulted in a number of municipal incinerators operating considerably below their design capacity—a money-losing proposition. WTE incinerators are exorbitantly expensive to construct and operate (as a rough rule-of-thumb, WTE projects average $100,000–$125,000 per ton of daily waste capacity; a city contemplating construction of a typical 1,000 ton-per-day facility can thus count on investing well over $100 million). Costs are recovered (hopefully!) through tipping fees (which a *BioCycle* survey of 16 states found averaged $53 per ton in 1999) paid by haulers bringing wastes to the facility and through sales of electricity or process steam produced by the plant. Since prevailing regional rates for electricity determine what this amount will be, low power demand reflected in falling prices has caused some communities to cancel plans for incinerator construction, since anticipated revenues from energy sales turned out to be less than originally projected.

The future role of WTE incineration in a comprehensive waste management strategy thus depends on a number of economic and political considerations, including trends in landfill tipping fees (increases make incineration more cost-competitive and vice-versa); demand for energy (high demand equals brighter future for WTE combustion); congressional initiatives (will Congress impose a legislative moratorium on incinerator construction?); and EPA decisions (will the Agency further tighten emissions requirements or mandate that communities achieve specified recycling goals before building new incinerators?). WTE combustion remains the most important MSW management method in Japan and a number of European countries. However, given the current abundance of landfill capacity in the U.S. and the large discrepancy between per unit disposal charges at landfills versus incinerators, it is unlikely that the percentage of MSW managed by combustion will increase significantly in the years immediately ahead.

Hazardous Wastes

Late in the summer of 1978 the name of a small residential subdivision in the city of Niagara Falls, New York, entered the American vocabulary and became a household word almost overnight, symbolizing the dangers of our chemical age. The tragic sequence of events which unfolded at Love Canal epitomizes the dangers facing millions of citizens in thousands of communities across the nation as a result of our indiscriminate use and careless disposal of hazardous chemicals.

The Love Canal Story

The origin of the chemical dumpsite which became the focus of worldwide attention in the late 1970s can be traced to the mid-1890s when William T. Love began construction of a canal intended to serve as a navigable power channel, connecting the Upper Niagara to the Niagara Escarpment about seven miles downstream, thereby bypassing the Falls. At the point where Mr. Love's canal was intended to reenter the river, the intention was to construct a model industrial city which would be provided with cheap, abundant hydroelectric power. Unfortunately for Mr. Love, his development company went bankrupt shortly after construction of the canal had begun; the project was abandoned, leaving a waterway approximately 3,000 feet long, 10 feet deep, and 60 feet wide. For many years, residents of this area on the outskirts of town used the canal for recreational fishing and swimming; in 1927 the land was annexed by the city. In 1942 Hooker Chemical Company (now a subsidiary of Occidental Petroleum), one of several major chemical industries located in Niagara Falls, received permission to dump chemical wastes into the canal, which it proceeded to do from that time until 1952 (in 1947 Hooker purchased the canal, along with two 70-feet-wide strips of land adjacent to the canal on each side). During this time more than 21,000 tons of chemical wastes—acids, alkalis, solvents, chlorinated hydrocarbons, etc.—were disposed of at this site. Only a few homes were present in the area at that time, but old-time residents recall the offensive odors, noxious vapors, and frequent fires which accompanied the dumping.

By 1953 the canal was full and so was topped with soil and eventually acquired a covering of grass and weeds. Hooker then offered to sell the land to the Niagara Falls School Board for the token fee of $1. At the same time company officials pointedly advised school and city administrators that although the site was suitable for a school, parking lot, or playground, any construction activities involving excavation of the area should be avoided to prevent rupturing the dumpsite's clay lining, thereby allowing escape of the impounded chemicals. In 1955 an elementary school and playground were constructed on the site; in 1957 the city began laying storm sewers, roads, and utility lines through the area, disregarding the warnings received a few years earlier. In the years that followed, several hundred modest homes were built in the neighborhood parallel to the banks of the now-invisible canal. Most of the newer residents had no knowledge of the site's past history and, in spite of occasional chemical odors (not considered unusual in a city where chemical manufacturing was a leading industry), few outward signs of trouble were apparent. Unusually heavy precipitation in the mid-1970s, however, was accompanied by some alarming phenomena. Strange-looking, viscous chemicals began oozing through basement walls, floors, and sump holes. Vegetation in yards withered and appeared scorched. Large puddles became permanent backyard features. Holes began to open up in the field that had once been a dumpsite and the tops of corroded 55-gallon drums leaking chemicals could be seen in places protruding from the soil surface. Complaints and fears expressed by citizens were generally downplayed by local authorities who assured them there was nothing about which to be concerned.

By early 1978 pressure from a local congressman and regular critical coverage of events in the Niagara Gazette prompted the U.S. Environmental Protection Agency to undertake a program of air sampling in the basements of Love Canal homes. New York State authorities also began conducting soil analyses and taking samples of residues in sump pumps and storm sewers. The results of these studies indicated that the area was extremely contaminated with more than 200 different chemicals, including 12 known or suspected carcinogens. Benzene, known to be a potent human cancer-causing agent, was readily detected in the air inside many of the houses sampled. Dioxin was subsequently found in high concentrations in some of the soil samples analyzed. State officials in New York estimate that as many as 10% of the chemicals buried at Love Canal may be mutagens, teratogens, or carcinogens. On August 2, 1978, the Health Commissioner of New York publicly proclaimed "the existence of a great and imminent peril to the health of the general public" at Love Canal and advised all pregnant women and families with children under the age of two to leave the area if they could do so. Five days later, President Carter officially declared Love Canal a national emergency.

The months that followed witnessed mass relocation at public expense of residents living closest to the dumpsite, as well as openly expressed fears by those left behind on adjacent streets that their health was similarly endangered. A number of health studies, whose methodology and conclusions remain highly controversial, suggest that Love Canal residents have experienced statistically significant elevated rates of miscarriage, birth defects, and chromosomal abnormalities. Ultimately 1,004 families were evacuated from Love Canal, their homes purchased by the state. Over 300 of the residences closest to the canal were demolished and the area covered with a protective layer of clay and a synthetic liner to exclude rainwater. Most of the remaining homes were boarded up, awaiting a pending EPA assessment of whether they could ever again be inhabited. Trenches were dug around the old canal site to capture contaminated groundwater which was then pumped to a treatment center for detoxification. Nearby creeks where high levels of dioxin seepage were detected have been fenced off to protect children and animals. Combined federal and state expenditures for relocating residents, investigating environmental damage, and halting chemical seepage from the site total $150 million, and an additional $32 million has been spent to clean up contaminated creeks and sewers and to determine the future habitability of the neighborhood. The Congressional Office of Technology Assessment estimated that if Hooker had employed current disposal standards and practices, its wastes could have been safely managed for about $2 million in 1979 dollars (Levine, 1982).

Occidental Chemical, which acquired Hooker in a 1968 buy-out, has paid $20 million in out-of-court settlements to affected residents; a federal district court ruling in 1988 held Occidental liable for the cost of previous, ongoing, and future cleanup of the Love Canal site—a figure approximating $250 million. Two years later, the State of New York sued Occidental for an additional $250 million in punitive damages, claiming that its subsidiary Hooker had "displayed reckless disregard for the safety of others." In the spring of 1994, a federal judge ruled against the plaintiff, saying the evidence in the state's case was insufficient; this decision, however, did not alter Occidental's liability for cleanup costs. In the fall of 1988, after reviewing a five-year habitability study of the affected area, New York State Health Commissioner David Axelrod declared that most of the Love Canal neighborhood could be safely resettled by former residents. While the decision was controversial, with some environmentalists warning that "Love Canal is a ticking time bomb," by the summer of 1990 over 200 people had expressed interest in renovated homes selling for 20% less than the prevailing market price. Reassured by government claims that the area no longer presents any threat, new residents have reoccupied several dozen homes in the Love Canal neighborhood, now renamed "Black Creek Village" (Newton and Dillingham, 1994). The final chapter in this saga concluded with the December 1995 agreement by Occidental Chemical to pay the federal government $129 million to cover costs for the pollution cleanup at Love Canal. Hailing the final agreement concluded by the U.S. Department of Justice, EPA Administrator Carol Browner remarked that it represented "this administration's firm commitment to ensuring that polluters, not the American people, pick up the tab for cleaning up toxic waste dumps."

The events which transpired at Love Canal cannot be shrugged off as a unique tragedy which unfortunately victimized a few thousand people in western New York State but left the rest of the nation unscathed. Health authorities and environmental agency officials regard Love Canal as but the "tip of the iceberg" in alerting society to the widespread nature of the hazardous waste problem. EPA is currently aware of more than 16,000 hazardous waste dumps scattered across the United States and fear that many of these may be exposing citizens to dangers as serious as those which surfaced at Love Canal.

Little wonder that public opinion polls show citizens ranking hazardous waste management issues among their top environmental quality concerns.

What Is "Hazardous" Waste?

In the 1976 Resource Conservation and Recovery Act (RCRA), Congress legally defined hazardous waste as "any discarded material that may pose a substantial threat or potential danger to human health or the environment when improperly handled." EPA has established a two-tier system for determining whether a specific waste is subject to regulation under current hazardous waste management laws:

1. If the substance in question is among the more than 500 wastes or waste streams itemized in Parts 261.31–33 of the Code of Federal Regulations, it will automatically be subject to regulation as a hazardous waste. Wastes may be placed on the list because of their ability to induce cancer, mutations, or birth defects; because of their toxicity to plants; or because even low doses are fatal to humans. However, the Administrator of EPA can exercise a wide measure of discretion in deciding whether to list a particular waste, so a number of potential carcinogens, mutagens, and teratogens are not yet listed as officially "hazardous."

2. In addition to the wastes listed in the federal code, any waste which exhibits one or more of the following characteristics is defined as hazardous and subject to regulation:

Toxic—wastes such as arsenic, heavy metals, or certain synthetic pesticides are capable of causing either acute or chronic health problems.

Ignitable—organic solvents, oils, plasticizers, and paint wastes are examples of wastes that are hazardous because they have a flashpoint less than 60 °C (140 °F) or because they tend to undergo spontaneous combustion. The resultant fires are dangerous not only because of heat and smoke, but also because they can disseminate toxic particles over a wide area.

Corrosive—substances with a pH of 2 or less or 12.5 and above can eat away at standard container materials or living tissues through chemical action and are termed corrosive. Such wastes, which include acids, alkaline cleaning agents, and battery manufacturing residues, present a special threat to waste haulers who come into bodily contact with leaking containers.

Reactive—obsolete munitions, wastes from the manufacturing of dynamite or firecrackers, and certain chemical wastes such as picric acid are hazardous because of their tendency to react vigorously with air or water or to explode and generate toxic fumes.

Two other categories of wastes which might logically be considered hazardous—radioactive wastes and potentially infectious medical wastes from

BOX 16-3

Environmental Justice

In 1982 when civil rights demonstrators in predominantly African-American Warren County, North Carolina, rallied to protest the proposed siting of a PCB landfill in their midst, they may not have realized they were leading the vanguard of a new social movement in the United States. They *did* know they were angry that, once again, a small, poor, politically powerless community of color was being targeted as the location for a locally unwanted waste disposal facility.

On this occasion, however, the voices of Warren County carried all the way to Congress where Delegate Walter Fauntroy (D.C.) asked the General Accounting Office (GAO) to look into allegations of racial discrimination in the siting of waste facilities. Thus was launched the quest for **environmental equity**—an effort to ensure that environmental risks, where they exist, are fairly distributed across population groups rather than falling disproportionately on those who are already disadvantaged through minority status, low income, or geographic location.

A major contribution to the struggle against environmental racism was the publication in 1987 of a seminal study by the United Church of Christ Commission for Racial Justice, *Toxic Waste and Race in the United States*, detailing for the first time interrelating issues of race, class, and environment across the nation. This work contended that pollution is anything but an "equal opportunity" affliction, blighting and shortening the lives of African Americans, Latinos, and Native Americans to a far greater extent than white Americans. The Commission for Racial Justice study, as well as subsequent reports on the same topic by several other authors, cited statistics showing that the majority of U.S. landfills

and incinerators are located in predominantly African-American or Hispanic communities. Furthermore, 60% of all African-Americans live in communities with one or more abandoned toxic waste sites (highly segregated southeast Chicago, pockmarked by over 100 such abandoned dumps, is a classic example). To environmental justice advocates, these facts suggest deliberate discrimination, "dumping on the poor" by locating a disproportionate number of undesirable facilities in minority communities.

Federal agencies themselves have been accused of perpetuating environmental injustices. Staff writers at the *National Law Journal* in 1992 charged that EPA was guilty of environmental racism in its implementation of Superfund cleanups, citing evidence of faster action, more thorough remediation, and stricter enforcement of hazwaste regulations in white communities than in minority communities. These inequities prevailed, they asserted, regardless of community income levels—race, and race alone, was the determining factor.

Issues of environmental equity provided the impetus for a "Conference on Race and the Incidence of Environmental Hazards" held at the University of Michigan in 1990. Following that event, a group of participants wrote to then-EPA Administrator William Reilly, requesting that the agency take action to deal with environmental risks in minority and low-income communities. Reilly responded by forming an Environmental Equity Workgroup, and the agency recently has begun actively investigating environmental discrimination charges under the 1964 Civil Rights Act.

Proponents of environmental justice gained a most important ally in President

Clinton who, on February 11, 1994, signed Executive Order 12898 prohibiting discriminatory practices in any programs receiving federal financial assistance. For the first time, federal agencies were required to consider the racial and socioeconomic characteristics of a community prior to launching a new project or issuing new environmental rules. EPA now has an active program in place to guarantee that its rulings don't unfairly impact the poor and powerless.

In the late 1990s, however, new studies raised questions regarding the basic premise of the environmental justice movement—namely, that the disparities in waste facility siting documented in the Commission for Racial Justice report were the result of deliberate, discriminatory targeting of minority communities. Skeptics pointed out that the original studies focused solely on the present racial composition of communities where disposal facilities are located, ignoring historical records of the demographic makeup of such areas at the time siting decisions were made. Pursuing that line of research, these investigators have found that in many, if not most, cases, waste facilities were developed originally in areas that were uninhabited or in areas where people of color did not constitute the majority population. Far from maliciously choosing to locate in minority communities, developers selected the sites based on such criteria as access to roads, railways, or water transportation. Over time, however, the declining residential property values in such areas prompted an influx of lower-income and minority residents who were attracted by the cheap housing. As a case in point, the southeast Chicago area, cited earlier, had a negligible African-American population in the early 1900s when the industries whose toxic dumpsites now threaten nearby residents located there. Almost all the minority residents who now live near Superfund sites in south Chicago moved into that area long after the troublesome facilities were well established.

Environmental justice advocates have been increasingly successful in recent years in thwarting development of waste facilities in minority communities on the basis of their discriminatory impact. However, if theories regarding the pivotal role played by market dynamics prove correct, then the strategy of restricting where new facilities are located is unlikely to be effective in protecting minorities over the long term. Wherever such facilities are developed, so the reasoning goes, the same economic forces responsible for today's observed disparities will come into play again. Rather than placing minority communities "off limits" to such development (and thereby depriving them of badly-needed jobs, patronage of local businesses, and tax revenue), some voices now advocate a policy of encouraging facility developers to give compensation to communities agreeing to host them. Such an approach would empower local people to weigh the pros and cons of a proposed development and to base their ultimate decision on an objective assessment of what is in their best interests. Ethical objections that question the morality of allowing people to assume greater risk in return for economic benefit are moot because strict federal and state regulations for new waste management facilities, wherever they are located, ensure that citizens will not be subjected to serious health risks.

Whatever the ultimate resolution of the environmental equity debate, it has had the positive effect of heightening awareness and sensitivity to the unequal burden of pollution and poor health suffered by minority and low-income populations. It has also sparked a broad-based effort by people of color to redefine and reshape the modern environmental movement, expanding the concept to include issues of social and economic justice and the right of *all* people to be protected from environmental degradation.

References

Dorsey, Michael K. 1998. "Toward the Idea of International Environmental Justice." *World Resources 1998-99*. Oxford University Press.

Huebner, Stephen B. 1998. *Are Storm Clouds Brewing on the Environmental Justice Horizon?* Center for the Study of American Business, Policy Study No. 145 (April).

hospitals and clinics—are not presently regulated under the same laws as the groups listed above. Radioactive wastes are managed according to regulations adopted by the Nuclear Regulatory Commission under the Atomic Energy Act, while biomedical waste disposal laws vary from state to state. In 1988, public outrage over incidents of used syringes and other medical wastes washing up on East Coast beaches led to passage of the Medical Waste Tracking Act, which set up a two-year pilot project to attempt regulation of biomedical wastes through a procedure similar in nature to the manifest system currently required for off-site shipments of hazardous wastes. With the expiration of that program, individual states have, for the most part, adopted medical waste management programs of their own involving the manifesting of such wastes shipped off-site and, in several states, requiring that infectious wastes be "rendered innocuous" in specially licensed high-temperature incinerators—a form of disposal considerably more expensive than sanitary landfilling. Many authorities deplore what they regard as exaggerated public fears about the threats posed by medical wastes. Pointing out that wastes generated by hospitals are no more dangerous than many of the items tossed into the trash by householders (e.g. used syringes from home insulin injections, bloody bandages, outdated medications, etc.) and that not a single case of human illness has been traced to contact with infectious medical waste, they question the public health benefit of strict new regulations which significantly increase national costs for health care. Ironically, the highly sensationalized beach littering incidents that provoked the federal legislation, initially attributed to illegal ocean dumping by waste haulers, were subsequently traced to sewer discharges of discarded medical devices from private residences.

Generation of Hazardous Wastes

By the mid-1990s, according to EPA estimates, approximately 20,000 generators in the U.S. were producing 279 million tons of regulated hazardous wastes each year, a figure that does not take into account those wastes which are managed illegally. Production of these wastes is not evenly distributed among industries, however. More than 85% of all hazardous wastes are produced by just three major categories of generators: chemicals and allied products, metal-related industries, and petroleum and coal products. Geographic location of these industries, as well as population density, are major determinants of which states are the leading hazardous waste generators.

At the time when new federal waste management regulations went into effect in November 1980, EPA estimated that fully 90% of all hazardous wastes were being disposed of by methods that would not meet government standards. Thanks to what is widely regarded as the most stringent hazardous waste management program in the world, that situation has now markedly improved.

Threats Posed by Careless Disposal

Mismanagement of hazardous wastes can adversely affect human health and environmental quality in a number of ways.

Direct Contact. Direct contact with wastes can result in skin irritation, the initiation of serious chronic illness, or acute poisoning—as in the case of two 9-year-old Tampa boys who were killed in June 1992, while playing inside a municipal waste bin. Subsequent investigations revealed that the bin, located behind an industrial firm, contained toluene- and acetone-contaminated waste, leading officials to conclude the boys had died due to inhalation of toxic chemical fumes.

Fire and/or Explosions. In April 1980, a spectacular blaze destroyed a riverside warehouse complex in Elizabeth, New Jersey, where 50,000 chemical-containing drums had been sitting for almost 10 years. Such accidents are a constant threat when hazardous wastes are in transit, carelessly stored, or roughly handled. Explosions are a particular threat to workers at landfills accepting hazardous wastes. In Edison, New Jersey, a bulldozer operator who inadvertently crushed a container of flammable phosphorus was burned so quickly that his corpse was discovered with his hand still on the gearshift.

Poison via the Foodchain. Biomagnification of toxic wastes discharged into the environment can result in the poisoning of animals or humans who consume the toxin indirectly. The tragic outbreak of methyl mercury poisoning at Minamata, Japan, typifies this sort of situation.

Air Pollution. When toxic wastes are burned at temperatures insufficiently high to completely destroy them, serious air pollution problems can result. Only specialized types of equipment are licensed for the incineration of hazardous wastes, and even these must be carefully monitored while operating to ensure a complete burn.

Surface Water Contamination. Accidental spills or deliberate dumping of hazardous wastes can easily pollute waterways. The extent and duration of environmental damage to surface waters varies widely, depending on the size of the water body in question and the rate of flow, but short-term damage to aquatic ecosystems can be severe. In Butte, Montana, location of the largest Superfund complex in the nation, several hundred snow geese died in 1995 soon after landing on a lake of toxic wastewater that had formed at an open-pit mine. Post-mortem analyses of the birds revealed acid-burned esophagi, indicating they died from drinking the highly polluted water. Public drinking water supplies can also be endangered by hazardous waste dis-

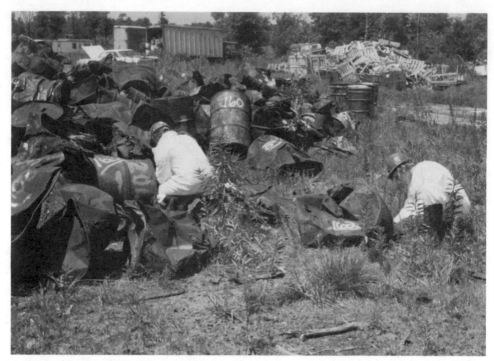

Abandoned hazardous waste dump site where hundreds of corroding drums leak their toxic contents onto the ground, endangering drinking water aquifers below the surface. *[Illinois Environmental Protection Agency]*

charges; municipal water intake points occasionally must be closed until the plume of pollution from an accidental spill flows past.

Groundwater Contamination. The most common problem associated with poor hazardous waste management is the pollution of aquifers with toxic leachates percolating downward through the soil from landfills or surface impoundments. This type of pollution is particularly insidious because it is seldom discovered until it is too late to do anything about it. Citizens in numerous communities around the nation have discovered to their horror that they had unknowingly been consuming well water contaminated with a variety of toxic chemicals which entered the groundwater supply via seepage from disposal sites.

Methods of Hazardous Waste Disposal

Historically, the largest percentage of hazardous wastes have been disposed of on land, primarily because land disposal, particularly prior to government regulation of hazardous waste management, was by far the cheapest disposal option. During the mid-1970s, for example, almost half of all hazardous wastes, the majority of which were in the form of liquids or sludges, were simply dumped into unlined surface impoundments, technically referred to as "pits, ponds, or lagoons," located on the generators' property (even today, approximately 96% of all hazardous wastes generated in this country are treated or disposed of at the site where they are generated; only 4% of all hazardous wastes are sent off-site for management). These wastes eventually evaporated or percolated into the soil, often resulting in groundwater contamination. Other wastes, about 30% of the total, were buried in sanitary landfills, easily subject to leaching, and another 10% were burned in an uncontrolled manner. None of these methods would be in compliance with current regulations.

Although many citizens are convinced that no methods exist for the safe disposal of hazardous wastes, a number of new technologies have been developed which avoid most of the shortcomings inherent in past hazardous waste management practices. All such methods, not surprisingly, are considerably more expensive than simply dumping wastes in a pit or a municipal landfill, and thus were not widely utilized until strict regulatory action was taken by Congress. A listing of legal hazardous waste disposal options would include the following.

Secure Chemical Landfill. Generally, the cheapest method of hazardous waste disposal is the so-called "secure" chemical landfill, a specially designed earthen excavation constructed in such a way as to contain dangerous chemicals and to prevent them from escaping into the environment through leaching or vaporization. In the past, secure landfills frequently differed from sanitary landfills only in that they were topped with a layer of clay to keep water out of the trenches in which chemical drums had been placed. This of course did not prevent chemical seepage from contaminating water supplies. Under current RCRA standards, a secure chemical landfill must be located above the 100-year floodplain and away from fault zones; it must contain double liners of clay or synthetic materials to keep leaching to a mini-

Figure 16-4 A Secure Landfill

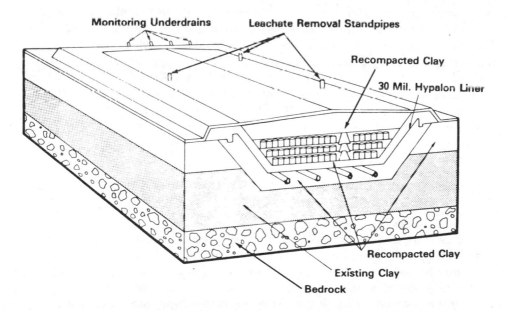

mum; a network of pipes must be laid to collect and control polluted rainwater and leachate accumulating in the landfill; and monitoring wells must be installed to check the quality of any groundwater deposits in the area (surface water supplies must also be monitored by the landfill operator). In spite of these precautions, most experts agree that there is no way to guarantee that sometime in the future contaminants will not migrate from the landfill site. Liners eventually crack; soil can shift or settle. Since many chemical wastes remain hazardous more or less indefinitely, serious pollution problems can occur many years after a secure chemical landfill has been closed and forgotten. Many authorities feel that although chemical landfills are legal, they are the least acceptable method of managing hazardous wastes.

Since 1984 when more stringent requirements for groundwater monitoring, minimum technology standards, and financial guarantees for post-closure activities took effect, the number of operating facilities has dropped substantially. Today there are just 18 commercial hazardous waste landfills operating in the United States and 3 in Canada, compared to more than 1,000 during the 1970s. Within the past few years, the list of wastes for which disposal in landfills is prohibited has been steadily growing; federal legislation enacted in 1984 and fully implemented by 1990 imposed a ban on the landfilling of virtually all hazardous wastes, unless such materials undergo prior treatment to minimize their toxicity and ability to migrate. The explicit intent of such legislation is to reduce reliance on land disposal and to encourage the use of alternative technologies to the greatest extent possible.

Deep Well Injection. The use of deep wells for waste disposal dates back to the late 19th century when the petroleum industry employed this method to get rid of salt brine, but its use for liquid hazardous waste disposal began only during the 1940s. A number of industries, most notably petroleum refineries and petrochemical plants, now utilize this disposal method. Commercial deep well injection currently is practiced only in the Midwest and in Texas and neighboring states, although many other injection wells operated by private firms solely for the disposal of their own wastes are widely scattered across the United States. The process involves pumping liquid wastes through lined wells into porous rock formations deep underground, well below any drinking water aquifers. Some critics point out that cracks in the well casing or undetected faults in the earth which intersect the disposal zone could result in outward migration of wastes. EPA contends that deep wells are safe, provided that they are constructed, operated and maintained in accordance with agency regulations.

Various Chemical, Physical, or Biological Treatment Processes. Processes that render wastes nonhazardous or significantly reduce their volume or toxicity have assumed major importance in recent years, particularly as more and more **"land bans"** have been implemented, prohibiting the landfilling of untreated wastes. With economic motivation spurring invention, a number of promising new technologies are now in the pilot project phase or fully operational, promising safer, more effective ways of cleaning up past mistakes and ensuring that wastes currently being generated are properly managed.

Figure 16-5   Injection Wells and Underground Sources of Drinking Water

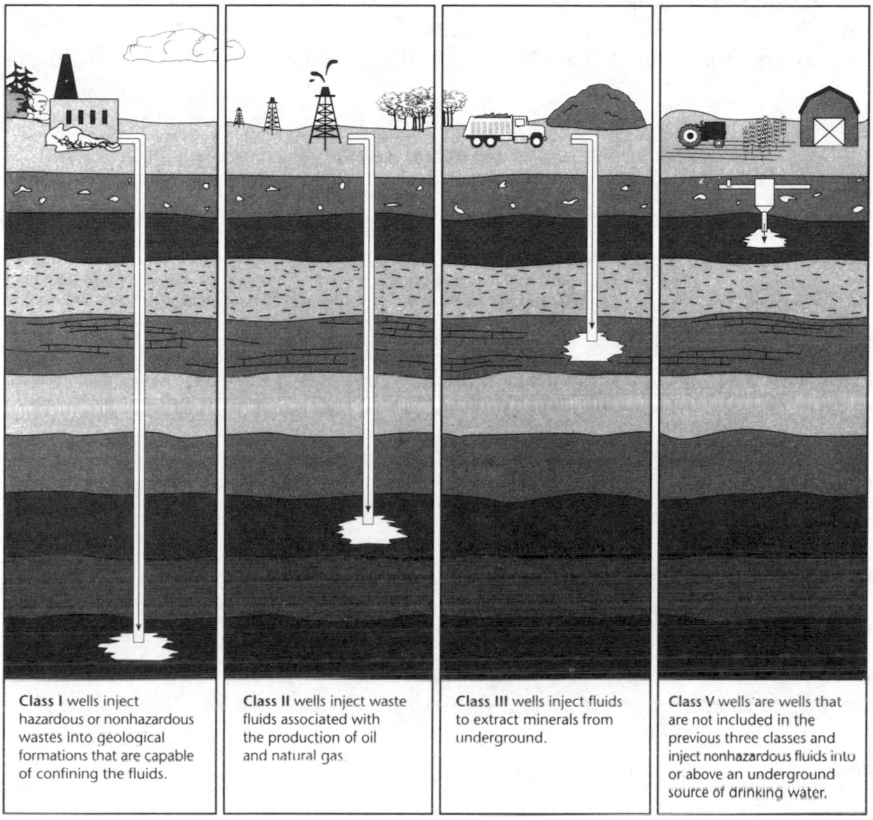

Class I wells inject hazardous or nonhazardous wastes into geological formations that are capable of confining the fluids.

Class II wells inject waste fluids associated with the production of oil and natural gas.

Class III wells inject fluids to extract minerals from underground.

Class V wells are wells that are not included in the previous three classes and inject nonhazardous fluids into or above an underground source of drinking water.

Source: EPA, *National Water Quality Inventory: 1996 Report to Congress.* April, 1998.

Physical methods include **evaporation** to concentrate corrosive brines, **sedimentation** to separate solids from liquid wastes, **carbon adsorption** to remove certain soluble organic wastes, and **air stripping** to remove volatile organic compounds from groundwater.

Chemical techniques involve processes such as **neutralization** to render wastes harmless, sulfide **precipitation** to extract certain toxic metals, **oxidation-reduction** processes to convert some metals from a hazardous to a nonhazardous state, and **stabilization/solidification,** in which the waste material is detoxified and then combined with a cement-like material, encapsulated in plastic, blended with organic polymers, or combined with silica to form a solid, inert substance which can be disposed of safely in a landfill or incorporated into road beds. Another innovative technology is **in-situ vitrification (ISV),** a process which relies on large amounts of electricity (about 750 kilowatt-hours per ton of soil) delivered by giant electrodes fixed at several locations in the soil surrounding the area undergoing cleanup. Suitable for detoxifying soils contaminated with toxic organics (e.g. chlorinated pesticides), heavy metals, or radioactive wastes, ISV actually melts the soil as the electricity flows through it, fusing the toxics into a solid block of glassified material, similar to natural obsidian. The solidified material can simply be left in place, no longer posing any environmental threat (but perhaps causing immense puzzlement among archaeologists five thousand years hence, trying to figure out what kind of cultural artifact that huge chunk of glass could possibly be!).

Bioremediation, based on the ability of microbes, fungi, or plants to break down or absorb organic pollutants or toxic metals, is increasingly used for cleanup of oil spills and remediation of contaminated soil and groundwater. The largest number of projects utilize various species of naturally occurring bacteria. By far the most widely used method of bioremediation is **biostimulation**, in which oxygen and/or nutrients are added to contaminated material to promote more rapid growth of indigenous microbes, resulting in faster, more efficient metabolism of wastes than would have occurred without human intervention. In situations where resident bacteria are too few in number, even with biostimulation, to degrade wastes effectively or when the microbes naturally present are genetically incapable of breaking down a particular waste, it may be necessary to utilize **bioaugmentation**. In such situations, non-indigenous species are added to "lend a hand," working in concert with the local microbes to accomplish pollutant removal more rapidly and completely. In a quest to create new bacterial stains better able to degrade chemicals under specific environmental conditions, scientists have been working to develop genetically-engineered microbes (GEMs) to destroy pollutants which have proven resistant to breakdown by naturally occurring species. In order to avoid any possible risk to human health or the environment, the use of GEMs is strictly regulated under the Toxic Substances Control Act, which requires that they undergo a rigorous safety review prior to approval for field use.

Controlled Incineration. Because burning at very high temperatures actually destroys hazardous wastes (as opposed to storing them out of sight underground as is essentially the case with various land disposal methods), most hazardous waste management experts regard controlled incineration as the best and, in some cases, the only environmentally acceptable means of disposal. In spite of its relatively high cost compared to other hazwaste management options, controlled incineration is assuming increased importance as land disposal regulations grow more restrictive. Waste generators, fearful of legal liability if their wastes migrate from a land disposal site, are increasingly likely to choose a management method that ensures total waste destruction. A controlled incinerator burns at temperatures ranging from 750–3000 °F, with wastes, air, and fuel being thoroughly mixed to ensure complete combustion. Afterburners, which are part of the incineration system, destroy any gaseous hydrocarbons which may have survived the initial incineration process, while scrubbers and electrostatic precipitators remove pollutant emissions from the stack gases. In 1999, EPA further tightened nationwide standards for air emissions from hazwaste combustors. The 20 commercial incinerators, 18 cement kilns, and 134 other facilities throughout the country which burn hazardous wastes were required to achieve a 70% reduction in dioxins and furans as well as reductions in mercury and lead emissions up to 86% by 2002. The technologies employed to lower concentrations of these pollutants will also

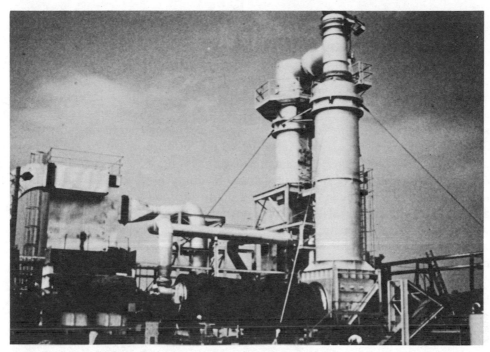

A "mobile" incinerator for destroying hazardous wastes. This equipment can be disassembled and moved from site to site on flatbed trucks. Use of such incinerators is becoming more common as a result of SARA requirements to minimize off-site transport of hazardous wastes from Superfund cleanup projects. *[Author's Photo]*

reduce emissions of particulates, carbon monoxide, hydrocarbons, hydrochloric acid, and other toxic metals. The stringent requirements were justified as necessary to protect the health and environment of the 37 million U.S. residents living in the vicinity of hazardous waste combustors.

Waste Exchanges. The ideal way to manage hazardous materials would be to recycle them, thus preventing their entry into the waste stream and eliminating the disposal problem. This is the idea which prompted the establishment of waste exchanges, which act as helpful third parties in establishing contact between waste generators and potential waste users. For example, a paint manufacturer, faced with the problem of how to dispose of hazardous sludges from a mixing operation, contacts a waste exchange and is referred to another company which willingly purchases the sludge to use as a filler coat on cement blocks. Thus, the paint manufacturer avoids the high cost of disposal in a secure chemical landfill or controlled incinerator and also makes a modest profit on the sale of the waste. The buyer, too, is pleased with the arrangement because a needed raw material is obtained for a lower price than unused filler would have cost; and society is well served because a potentially hazardous substance has been prevented from entering the environment. The waste exchange concept originated in Europe where the first such program began in the Netherlands in 1972. The Midwest Industrial Waste Exchange, started in 1975 in St. Louis, was the first U.S. program, the forerunner of 45 government-subsidized materials exchange programs now operating in North America. By the late 1990s, several for-profit Web-based services also had emerged, charging companies a fee for listing their available wastes or waste material needs. The most common type of waste exchange is basically an information clearinghouse which publishes monthly, bi-monthly, or quarterly coded listings of waste items available or desired. Interested parties then contact the clearinghouse and negotiations between potential buyers and sellers are initiated. A smaller proportion of waste exchanges act as a direct brokerage service, sometimes actively seeking a buyer or seller for a particular waste material. Although waste exchanges were first developed exclusively for industrial hazardous waste trading, in recent years they have been increasingly involved in marketing nonhazardous solid waste materials as well (though solvents still remain the single most widely swapped item). As waste disposal costs continue to rise and as industries become more familiar with the opportunities for waste recycling, utilization of the services provided by waste exchanges is expected to increase significantly (Gruder, 1993).

Siting Problems: from "NIMBY" to "BANANA"

Everyone wants hazardous wastes to be managed in ways which present the least possible threat to health or the environment, but no one wants to live near the site chosen for such storage, treatment, or disposal. Get rid of such wastes in the next county, a neighboring state, out in the desert, anyplace else—but "Not In My Back Yard!" (referred to as the "NIMBY" problem in agency argot). This, in essence, is the siting dilemma which represents one of the most difficult obstacles faced by those trying to deal with municipal or hazardous wastes (not to mention *radioactive* refuse!) in a safe and responsible manner. Certainly waste disposal horror stories from Love Canal and countless other places across the nation have made citizens understandably nervous at the prospect of seeing hazardous waste management facilities locate in their communities. Nevertheless, if society desires to continue using products whose manufacture entails the production of hazardous wastes, improved waste handling facilities are urgently needed. Inevitably, the best location for some of those facilities will be in someone's "back yard." Responsible decision-making demands that citizens carefully evaluate the pros and cons of a site under consideration before automatically rejecting it. Laws governing the siting of hazardous waste facilities provide for public information and public participation programs during the siting process, though the scope for public input into the decision-making process varies widely from state to state. Before opposing or supporting a proposed facility, citizens should gather information on the following points:

- characteristics of the wastes involved
- nature of the proposed waste management process
- the design and manner of operation of the proposed facility
- the topographical, hydrogeological, and climatic characteristics of the site
- transportation routes to the site

BOX 16-4
Phytoremediation: Using Plants to Clean Up Pollution

During the hot, drought-plagued summer of 1999, residents of a low-income neighborhood in Hartford, Connecticut, watched with bemusement as six undergraduate students from nearby Trinity College labored over the mustard plants and sunflowers growing on an abandoned lot. No ordinary inner-city garden, the 1.2 acre plot was the former site of a now-defunct paint store that had contaminated the premises with dangerous levels of lead. Demolition of the building and burial of the rubble on-site simply added to the pollution problems. The city of Hartford assumed ownership of the land and licensed it for use as a community garden—a plan that was scuttled when the lead contamination problem was discovered. Unlike similar situations in so many other blighted urban areas, the story didn't end with the posting of "No Trespassing" signs around the lot. Two Trinity professors soon recognized the opportunity for a research project which would support their institution's commitment to forming academic-community partnerships emphasizing civic responsibility and educational innovation. Their plan was to use the small plot of wasteland to see if certain easily grown plant species could be successfully and cost-efficiently used to remediate lead-contaminated soil.

Not a wild pipe dream, the technique of phytoremediation has been rapidly gaining adherents in recent years as laboratory tests and field experiments alike demonstrate the potential of certain plants to extract toxic metals from soil or water. Not only that, they do so at a fraction of the cost of conventional methods, which typically involve excavation, acid-washing, and landfill disposal of contam-inated soils. By selectively removing only the troublesome pollutants, phytoremediation accomplishes the task economically and without massive environmental disruption.

At present, over 400 plant species have been identified as possessing the natural ability to take up quantities of metals such as lead, zinc, cadmium, and uranium from soils and accumulate them in quantities that would kill most other species. Referred to as **hyperaccumulators,** such plants can store as much as 2.5% of their dry weight in heavy metals in leaves without suffering any reduction in yields. Researchers have now identified the gene that produces phytochelatins, the substance that allows plants to detoxify heavy metals and hope to use this information to enhance further the natural ability of hyperaccumulator plants to take up toxic metals. Field studies are currently underway in a number of countries to identify which plants are best suited for phytoextraction purposes. The Trinity students in Hartford are concentrating their attention on Indian mustard (*Brassica juncea*), white mustard (*B. hirta*), Sudan grass (*Sorghum sudanense*), and sunflowers (*Helianthus sp.*). It is already known that Indian mustard excels at absorbing lead from soil, but the students want to determine the potential effectiveness of the other species as well.

Indian mustard is also being used to remove selenium from contaminated soils in California's San Joaquin Valley, where toxic selenium in agricultural drainage water has severely disrupted the ecosystem at Kesterson Reservoir. The state has set a high priority on remediating high-selenium soils and on minimizing movement of the chemical from soil to irrigation effluent. Since most of the conventional methods investigated were either very costly or only marginally effective, phytoremediation has attracted considerable interest as an economical, environmentally friendly alternative. Long-term field studies have shown that the top 24 inches of soil experienced nearly a 40% reduction in selenium content when planted with Indian mustard. Most of the selenium taken up was incorporated into plant tissue, while some was biologically volatilized into the air, primarily via the roots. Mustard plants with elevated concentrations of selenium have the potential to become a high-value crop for farmers, as well as a cheap method of soil improvement. Because selenium is an essential trace element for mammals, selenium containing mustard could be blended with alfalfa and feed to produce nutritious livestock forage—a win-win situation.

For cleanup of soils contaminated with zinc or cadmium, the humble Alpine pennycress (*Thlaspi caerulescens*) appears to be one of the most promising candidates. The plant has long been recognized in Europe as a good biological indicator of metal ore deposits. Recent studies have shown that pennycress takes up 35 times more zinc than other plant species growing in the same vicinity, concentrating the metal in its shoots. If properly fertilized and cared for, pennycress can uptake zinc from soils at the rate of 108 pounds per acre (125 kg/hectare).

Sunflowers have proven effective in remediating water tainted with low-level uranium, a situation where other methods either don't work or are prohibitively expensive. In a pilot project at a former uranium processing plant in Ashtabula, Ohio, researchers with Phytotech, Inc., a New Jersey-based firm specializing in phytoremediation, sunflowers were effective in reducing uranium in wastewater to

concentrations below EPA water quality standards. The uranium taken up by the plants remains localized in the roots, simplifying waste disposal since only the roots need to be managed as low-level wastes, generally by incineration and land disposal of the residual ash. Estimates for the cost of using sunflowers to remove radionuclides from water are in the $2–$6 per 1,000-gallons range, compared to $80 for conventional treatment methods.

Another plant successfully employed in wetlands systems to treat wastewaters contaminated by heavy metals is water hyacinth (*Eichhornia crassipes*). Water hyacinth multiplies rapidly, absorbing dissolved metals and accumulating them in plant tissues, especially the roots. Since *E. crassipes* floats on the water's surface, the plant can easily be harvested and, following incineration, its toxic metal component either recovered for reuse or land disposed. Water hyacinth is regarded as having good potential for *in-situ* remediation of hexavalent chromium, as well as a number of other toxic metals contaminating industrial wastewaters or sediments.

At the University of Georgia, researchers are striving to improve upon nature by inserting a gene that enables bacteria to tolerate high levels of mercury into the genetic code of tulip poplar (*Liriodendron tulipifera*). Thus modified, the trees experience a ten-fold increase in tolerance to mercury and an ability to take up methyl mercury from soils, reducing it to a less toxic form and releasing it from the trees' leaves into the air. Scientists hope the fast-growing tulip tree will prove a viable, inexpensive means of cleaning up polluted industrial sites or surface mining areas—and serve to beautify such locations at the same time.

At a time when the estimated cost of remediating the nation's hazardous waste legacy using conventional technologies exceeds $200 billion, phytoremediation has the potential to revolutionize our approach to cleanups. Although not every type of chemical contamination problem is amenable to a phytoremediation approach, a large number are. Among the top 20 Superfund site contaminants (see Table 16-3) arsenic, mercury, cadmium, and hexavalent chromium—are toxic metals that interact with phytochelatins. Phytoremediation's chief drawback is time; reducing concentrations of toxic metals to safe levels may require several years, depending on initial levels of contamination. Researchers hope that in the not-too-distant-future genetically engineered hyperaccumulators will be developed, capable of accomplishing the cleanup task more expeditiously. Nevertheless, for nonemergency situations where toxins are not immediately threatening human health, phytoremediation holds great promise as an affordable, effective, non-intrusive way to restore contaminated sites.

References

Banuelos, G.S., et al. 1997. "Phytoremediation of Selenium-Laden Soils: A New Technology." *Journal of Soil and Water Conservation* 52, no. 6 (Nov/Dec):426-31.

Bond, V. 1996. "Pint-Sized Plants Pack a Punch in Fight Against Heavy Metals." *Environmental Protection* (May):38-39.

- safeguards to be employed at the facility
- potential for human or ecological exposure to hazardous chemicals released into the air, water, or soil
- location of the site in reference to population centers, farmland, or valuable natural areas (e.g. wetlands, endangered species' habitat, etc.)
- possible uses of site after closure

Public opposition has brought acquisition of new hazardous waste management sites to a virtual standstill in recent years, with objectors mobilizing from far beyond the locality directly affected. Indeed, the sentiment prevailing among many activist groups at present has moved well beyond the familiar NIMBY protests to encompass the ultimate in negative responses: BANANA (Build Absolutely Nothing Anywhere Near Anything!). Unless society is willing to adopt a lifestyle in which no wastes whatsoever are generated (assuming this is even possible), a more reasonable, middle-ground approach to waste management decisions must be adopted. Protection of public health requires a new willingness on the part of citizens to sanction the siting of new facilities when a thorough review of site and operational considerations indicate that such facilities will not present serious environmental health problems.

Hazardous Waste Management Legislation: RCRA

An evaluation of the types of hazardous waste incidents that have occurred indicate that we are basically dealing with two different categories of hazardous waste problems: how to manage the new volumes of chemical wastes being generated daily by American industry and what to do about wastes improperly disposed of years ago which are only now beginning to make their presence known.

In order to tackle the first of these issues, the problem of newly created wastes, Congress in 1976 enacted the **Resource Conservation and Recovery Act (RCRA**—pronounced "rickra" in bureaucratese) which mandates that EPA:

- define which wastes are hazardous
- institute a **"manifest system"** to track the movement of hazardous wastes from the place they were generated to any off-site storage, treatment, or disposal facility
- set performance standards to be met by owners and operators of hazardous waste facilities
- issue permits for operation of such facilities only after technical standards have been met (operating licenses specify which types of wastes may be managed at that facility; thus most hazardous waste disposal sites are authorized to accept only certain classes of wastes)
- help states to develop hazardous waste management programs of their own which may be more stringent than the federal program, but which cannot be less so.

RCRA took effect in 1980 when EPA finally issued its generator and transporter regulations (i.e. manifest requirements) and marked an important step forward in responsible hazardous waste management. However, it soon became apparent that the 1976 law featured some glaring loopholes which needed to be plugged. There was also mounting sentiment in Congress and elsewhere that land disposal of hazardous wastes is the least desirable method of managing these substances and that legislation should encourage reliance on alternatives. Accordingly, when RCRA came before Congress for reauthorization in 1984, the original legislation was substantially strengthened with the enactment of the **Hazardous and Solid Waste Amendments (HSWA).** Among the key provisions of this law are mandates which 1) significantly reduce the types of hazardous wastes which can be buried in landfills; 2) strengthen requirements for landfill design and operation; 3) bring into the

---

Table 16-2   The ABC's of Waste Disposal
(Wall poster seen at the Environmental Protection Agency)

NIMBY	**Not In My Back Yard**
NIMFYE	**Not In My Front Yard Either**
PIITBY	**Put It In Their Back Yard**
NIMEY	**Not In My Election Year**
NIMTOO	**Not In My Term Of Office**
LULU	**Locally Unwanted Land Use**
NOPE	**Not On Planet Earth**

Source: A Dictionary of Environmental Quotations, Barbara K. Rodes and Rice Odell, eds., Simon & Schuster, 1992.

BOX 16-5

Pollution Prevention

Just as municipal waste management strategies emphasize the value of waste prevention as opposed to cleanup, so does national policy for hazardous waste management stress the importance of reducing the amount and toxicity of waste generated—an approach referred to among waste managers as **P2 ("pollution prevention")**. P2 is a concept that has gradually been winning adherents for more than a decade. In its 1984 Hazardous and Solid Waste Amendments to RCRA, Congress decreed that "the generation of hazardous waste is to be reduced or eliminated as expeditiously as possible." EPA was told to issue waste minimization regulations designed to increase awareness among industrial managers of waste reduction possibilities and to encourage voluntary initiatives aimed at lowering the amounts of waste generated. In 1990, pollution prevention became an official environmental policy of the United States when Congress enacted the **Pollution Prevention Act.** Although the initial response to such urgings was tentative within a corporate world still focused on traditional, end-of-pipe controls, during the past decade P2 has become a buzzword among savvy managerial types who recognize that implementing effective pollution prevention programs is a key to economic competitiveness. Not simply a public-relations ploy to appease the "green faction," corporate policies to reduce waste at the source—to prevent pollution before it's created—constitutes an economically sound business decision, since in today's highly regulated world it is far cheaper and more efficient to avoid the generation of waste rather than try to clean it up after the fact. Not only can effective P2 strategies save money on pollution abatement costs but by using raw materials more efficiently they also contribute to lower production costs. Fears of potential liability under the federal Superfund program have also been a strong motivating force for the adoption of pollution prevention programs— the fewer wastes shipped off-site for disposal, the less a company needs to fret about being cited as a "potentially responsible party" when a land disposal facility springs a leak!

The opportunities for significantly reducing the industrial waste stream are numerous—and often require little or no capital investment. Methods which can be employed with significant results include:

1. *Changing manufacturing processes* By switching from an acid spray to a mechanical scrubber using pumice and rotating brushes to clean copper sheeting at its electronics plant in Columbia, Missouri, the 3M Corporation reduced its generation of liquid hazardous wastes by 40,000 lbs. annually. Similarly, American Cyanamid modified a process it had long used for manufacturing yellow dye, thereby totally eliminating the need for a nitrobenzene solvent and its associated wastestream.

2. *Reformulating the product*—In a plastics factory in New Jersey, Monsanto changed the formula for an industrial adhesive it was producing; in doing so, it eliminated the need for filtering the product and thus no longer had any hazardous filtrate or filters requiring disposal.

3. *Substituting a nonhazardous chemical for a hazardous one in the manufacturing process*—In Memphis, Cleo Wrap, the world's largest producer of holiday gift-wrapping paper, switched from using solvent-based printing inks to water-

based materials. In so doing, the company virtually eliminated its generation of hazardous wastes.

4. *Changing equipment*—Simply by adding a condenser to an existing piece of equipment, a USS Chemicals plant in Ohio was able to capture escaping emissions of cumene, returning them to the phenol process unit. By so doing, the company solved an air quality problem and recaptured a major raw material. To recover product being lost during the drying stage for its salicylaldehyde process, Rhône-Poulenc installed in-line condensers which increased product yield by 10 pounds per batch.

5. *Altering the way hazardous wastes are handled in-plant*—Basically housekeeping changes, efforts at minimizing spills and using chemicals more conservatively can make a considerable difference in the amount of hazardous wastes generated. Segregating wastes to reduce contamination can also have a major impact. In Fremont, California, the Borden Chemical Company reduced the phenol content of its wastewater by 93% simply by separately collecting and reusing rinsewaters used to clean resin-contaminated filters. Formerly the company had allowed this rinsewater to flow into floor drains where it contaminated all the wastewater which flowed from the factory to a sewage treatment plant.

Not only do the approaches just described reduce the amounts of hazardous waste requiring disposal, they also save the companies which utilize them a great deal of money. The catch-phrase "Pollution Prevention Pays," coined by the 3M Corporation, rings true in case after case. In one year after changing its process for cleaning copper sheeting, 3M saved $15,000 in raw materials and in waste disposal and labor costs; the $100,000 which American Cyanamid invested in equipment modification to allow in-process recycling of another solvent substituted for nitrobenzene resulted in $200,000 in annual savings, thanks to reduced costs for energy and waste disposal; by switching to water-based inks, Cleo Wrap recouped $35,000 annually in waste disposal costs; by recovering 400,000 pounds of cumene after installation of a $5,000 condenser, USS Chemicals saved $100,000 in raw materials; Rhône-Poulenc's capital costs for its in-line condensers amounted to $10,000—repaid threefold by first-year savings of $30,000.

Until recently, many companies failed to take a comprehensive view of their waste streams—pinpointing precisely where wastes were generated and the exact management cost of each waste. By lumping all waste treatment, disposal, and oversight expenses together, corporate accountants denied themselves the opportunity of identifying specific process control points where considerable savings could be achieved. More recently, assisted and encouraged by state and federal programs as well as by enlightened self-interest, a growing number of firms are conducting intensive waste audits, instituting cost-accounting procedures, and involving employees at all levels to identify opportunities for pollution prevention. While wholehearted endorsement of P2 principles within conservative corporate boardrooms is by no means universal yet, the transition is now well underway.

References

Dorfman, Mark H., et al. 1992. "Environmental Dividends: Cutting More Chemical Wastes." *Inform*.

State of the Environment: A View Toward the Nineties. 1987. Conservation Foundation.

World Resources Institute. 1994. *World Resources 1994–95*. Oxford University Press.

regulatory framework hundreds of thousands of previously exempt "small quantity generators"—those who produce 100 kg (220 lbs.) per month or more of hazardous wastes (under the original law, only those generators producing 1,000 kg or more per month were subject to regulation); and 4) create a whole new program for detecting and controlling leakage of hazardous liquids (mainly petroleum products) from underground storage tanks. Implementation of these new requirements, while making hazardous waste management considerably more expensive than it had been previously, gave new impetus to safer, more environmentally responsible waste management strategies.

While confronting the issue of newly generated wastes with an array of regulatory approaches, RCRA does nothing to deal with the serious problem posed by leaking abandoned dumpsites. Even in the relatively few cases where the owners can be found, they often lack the financial resources to clean up the site, making litigation a futile exercise. Since EPA estimates there may be anywhere between 30,000–50,000 abandoned hazardous waste dumps in the United States—more than 2,000 of which are thought to present public health risks, the potential for future problems is obviously very great.

"Superfund"

Spurred by public demands that something be done to alleviate problems caused by old, leaking dumpsites, Congress in December of 1980 enacted the **Comprehensive Environmental Response, Compensation, and Liability Act (CERCLA**, dubbed the "Superfund"), authorizing the expenditure of $1.6 billion over a five-year period for emergency cleanup activities and for the more long-term containment of hazardous waste dump sites (the legislation, however, did not include funds to compensate victims for health damage incurred by exposure to such sites—an issue which was the focus of considerable debate). EPA, in cooperation with the states, was charged with compiling a **National Priority List (NPL)** of sites considered to be sufficiently threatening to public health or environmental quality to make them eligible for Superfund cleanup dollars. These funds can be used either to remove hazardous substances from the site (a process which may also include temporary relocation of people in the area and provision of alternative water supplies) or for remedial measures such as storage and confinement of wastes, incineration, dredging, or permanent relocation of residents.

The original Superfund bill expired in September 1985, and in spite of public demands for speedy reauthorization so that cleanup work could proceed

Table 16-3 "Top 20" Most Prominent Toxic Substances Found at NPL Sites

Lead	Cadmium	Trichloroethylene	DDE
Arsenic	PCBs	DDT	Arochlor 1242
Mercury (metallic)	Benzo(a)pyrene	Arochlor 1254	Dibenzo(a,h)anthracene
Benzene	Chloroform	Hexachlorobutadiene	Hexavalent chromium
Vinyl chloride	Benzo(b)fluoranthene	Arochlor 1260	Dieldrin

Ranking based on: 1) frequency at NPL sites, 2) toxicity, 3) exposure hazard to humans.
Source: Agency for Toxic Substances and Disease Registry.

Table 16-4   States with the Most NPL Sites (1998)

New Jersey	110	Florida	56	Indiana	34
Pennsylvania	104	Wisconsin	40	Ohio	31
New York	82	Washington	39	Texas	27
Michigan	77	Minnesota	37	South Carolina	25
California	71	Illinois	35	Massachusetts	23

without interruption, the law was not renewed until late the following year. Extreme congressional dissatisfaction with the excruciatingly slow rate of progress during Superfund's first years led to several significant changes in the 1986 **Superfund Amendments and Reauthorization Act** (SARA). Realizing that 1980 funding levels were inadequate, Congress in 1986 increased Superfund allocations to $8.5 billion to be spent over the next five years (in 1990 Congress once again reauthorized Superfund until September 1994, allocating an additional $5.1 billion for the program). EPA was given mandatory deadlines for initiating site-specific cleanup plans and remediation activities. Concerned that previous cleanup actions represented little more than moving contaminated wastes from one site to another site, which would itself then become eligible for Superfund status, Congress specified a preference for cleanup actions which "permanently and significantly" reduce the volume, toxicity, or mobility of hazardous substances. This mandate has given a major impetus to development of treatment or disposal technologies (e.g. mobile incinerators which can be moved from one Superfund site to another) which permit hazardous wastes to be destroyed or detoxified on site, thereby avoiding the risks of transporting such wastes to another facility where they might cause future problems.

While Americans (60 million of whom live within four miles of a Superfund site) generally support the concept of cleaning up our hazardous waste mistakes of the past, there has been considerable criticism regarding the pace of site cleanups. By mid-1999, the number of officially listed or proposed NPL sites had grown from an original 400 to 1,225. However, after more than a decade and a half of on-site work and the expenditure of many billions of dollars by government and industry, construction had been completed (i.e. all cleanup equipment was in place) at 432 sites and just 176 others had been completely remediated and taken off the NPL, indicating they no longer present a threat to human health or the environment.

Passionate disputes also rage over the extent of remediation necessary—"How clean is clean enough?" Critics complain that it makes no sense to spend millions of dollars to remove every last trace of contamination on a site destined to be paved over for a parking lot; it is quite likely that future amendments to the law will permit cleanup decisions to be based, at least in part, on the probable future use of the site. As EPA Administrator Carol Browner once remarked, ". . . there will be different levels of clean." Undoubtedly, the most controversial feature of the Superfund program has been its liability provisions, based on the philosophically sound "the polluter pays" principle, but which has resulted in fully one-quarter of all Superfund dollars spent thus far going to pay legal fees. While business interests are demanding fundamental

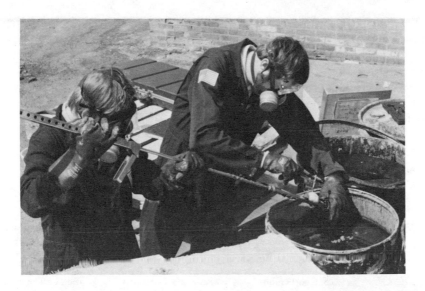

Cleanup of hazardous waste dump sites begins with careful sampling and identification of the abandoned material so that an appropriate disposal method can be chosen. Personnel carrying out the investigation wear protective "moon suits" and respirators to guard against personal injury. *[Illinois Environmental Protection Agency]*

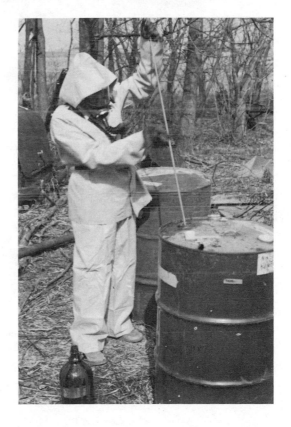

Table 16-5 Who Is Responsible for Hazardous Wastes?

At the national level there are a variety of agencies responsible for the control of hazardous wastes. Which agency is responsible and under what legislation is dependent upon whether the wastes are being transported, stored, disposed of, the type of wastes, and where they were found in the ecosystem. The following is a brief summary of federal responsibilities:

AREA	AGENCY	LEGISLATION	PROVISIONS
TRANSPORTATION	Department of Transportation	Hazardous Materials Transportation Act P.L. 93-633	Regulates interstate commerce of hazardous materials
	U.S. Environmental Protection Agency	Resource Conservation and Recovery Act of 1976 P.L. 94-580	Sets standards for manifests (shipping tickets and transporters)
	U.S. Coast Guard	Ports and Waterways Safety Act of 1972	The question of bulk shipment of oil and other hazardous materials on the lakes
WASTE DISPOSAL	U.S. Environmental Protection Agency	Resource Conservation and Recovery Act of 1976 P.L. 94-580	Sets standards and issues permits for producers, transporters, and disposal sites
AIR QUALITY	U.S. Environmental Protection Agency	Clean Air Act of 1970 P.L. 91-604 Amended 95-95	Sets emission standards for hazardous air pollutants
WATER QUALITY	U.S. Environmental Protection Agency	Clean Water Act of 1977 P.L. 95-217	Sets standards for toxic discharges through NPDES permits to achieve fishable and swimmable water
SPILLS	U.S. Environmental Protection Agency	Clean Water Act of 1977 P.L. 95-217	Prepares national contingency plan for spills, coordinates spill response, levies penalties and recovers costs
NUCLEAR WASTES	Nuclear Regulatory Agency	Atomnic Energy Act P.L. 87-703	Sets standards and licenses nuclear waste disposal sites
DRINKING WATER	U.S. Environmental Protection Agency	Safe Drinking Act of 1974 P.L. 93-523	Sets national standards for safe drinking water
			Regulates the underground injection of wastes which could contaminate drinking water

AREA	AGENCY	LEGISLATION	PROVISIONS
FOOD	Food and Drug Administration	Food, Drug, and Cosmetic Act P.L. 75-717	Sets, enforces tolerances for contaminants in food for interstate commerce, bans unsafe foods
OTHER CONSUMER PRODUCTS	Consumer Product Safety Commission	P.L. 92-573 Consumer Product Safety Act Hazardous Substances Act	Sets and enforces tolerances for household products, requires labelling, bans unsafe products
FISH AND WILDLIFE	Department of the Interior Fish and Wildlife Service	Fish and Wildlife Coordination Act of 1965	Research, technical assistance, spill response, monitoring for contaminants and effects on fish and wildlife
OCCUPATIONAL SAFETY	Occupational Safety and Health Administration	Occupational and Safety Health Act P.L. 91-596	Sets and enforces standards for worker exposure
CHEMICALS	U.S. Environmental Protection Agency	Toxic Substances Control Act	Obtains industry data on product use and health effects of chemicals
		P.L. 94-469	Regulation of manufacturer, use, distribution, and disposal of chemical substances
PESTICIDES	U.S. Environmental Protection Agency	Federal Insecticide Fungicide and Rodenticide Act as amended in 1975 P.L. 94-140	Registration and classification of all pesticides

changes in what they regard as inherently unfair provisions, environmental advocates strongly support the status quo, insisting that concerns about "Superfund liability" alone have caused generators to be much more conscientious about managing their wastes in a responsible manner and have given major impetus to serious efforts toward pollution prevention. As evidence, such advocates point to the fact that between 1987 and 1991, the chemical industry alone reduced its output of toxic wastes by 35%, largely in response to future liability considerations.

Finally, there is the question of cost. Close to one-quarter of EPA's entire budget has been allocated to Superfund. The Agency estimates it will cost at least $28 billion to clean up the sites currently on the NPL—and sees an additional 4,800 sites as likely candidates for listing in the years ahead. Although Superfund legislation mandates that 10% of site cleanup costs be paid by the state in which the site is located and requires that an attempt be made to find the **"potentially responsible party" (PRP)** who caused or contributed to the problem in order to recover cleanup expenses through litigation, the federal government will continue to bear much of the financial burden for site remediation efforts. The ultimate future of the Superfund program obviously will depend on the continued willingness of taxpayers to support the detoxification of America's hazardous waste dumpsites.

Household Hazardous Wastes

Comforting references to "Home Sweet Home" are slightly less reassuring today than in years past. The invisible hazards posed by radon and other indoor air pollutants make us wonder if we'd be safer inhaling deeply at a busy intersection than in our panelled family room. More recently, the righteous indignation directed at corporate polluters who disregard public well-being by careless disposal of their toxic by-products is being tempered somewhat by the realization that all of us—whatever our occupations—contribute to the nation's hazardous waste woes through our use, misuse, and thoughtless disposal of hundreds of potentially dangerous household chemicals.

It is estimated that the average American generates about 20 pounds of household hazardous waste each year. Typical examples of such discarded materials include pesticides, paints and varnishes, brush cleaners, ammonia, toilet bowl cleaners, bleaches and disinfectants, oven cleaners, furniture polish, swimming pool chemicals, batteries, motor oil, outdated medicines, and many others. Although these substances may be every bit as toxic, corrosive, flammable, or explosive as the industrial wastes regulated under RCRA, federal and state hazardous waste laws do not apply to the comparatively minor household sources. Nevertheless, the cumulative environmental impact of even small amounts of these materials being carelessly discarded by millions of individuals can be significant.

Household hazardous waste disposal presents a variety of concerns:

1. Stored inside the home, hazardous chemicals pose poisoning risks, particularly for children; some, such as paints and solvents, pose problems of indoor air pollution; others, ammonia and chlorine bleach, for example, can result in highly toxic emissions when inadvertently mixed; still others pose serious fire hazards.

2. The welfare of public employees can be threatened by hazardous household products. Home fires involving hazardous chemicals can result in explosions or the generation of toxic fumes which can kill or seriously injure firefighters. Refuse collectors frequently suffer injury when they throw garbage bags into compactor trucks, unaware that they contain corrosive or flammable materials.

3. The environment itself can be seriously degraded when householders pour hazardous liquids into drains and flush them down toilets or into septic systems. People who pour waste motor oil into storm sewers or dump paint cans in the woods can cause long-lasting damage to ground and surface water supplies.

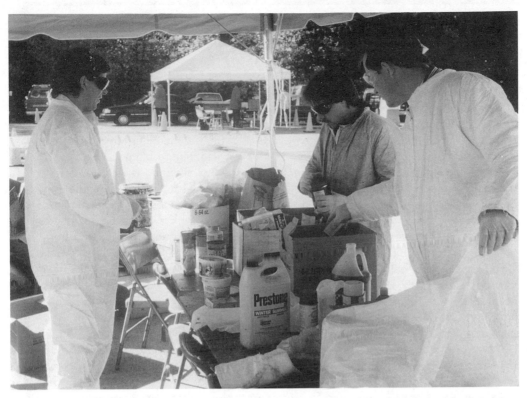

Hazardous household waste collection day: after residents have deposited their old paint cans, motor oil containers, discarded cleaning products, outdated medicine, and the like, workers from the Illinois EPA separate the wastes and prepare them for shipment to a licensed facility for disposal, treatment, or recycling. [Illinois Environmental Protection Agency]

A worker in protective gear examines potentially toxic containers at a hazardous household waste disposal center in Seattle. [© Steve Schneider/Greenpeace 1994]

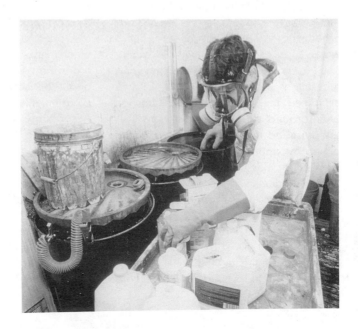

BOX 16-6

Underground Storage Tanks

In the early 1980s, as citizens became increasingly alarmed by the widespread scope of hazardous waste problems, people consoled themselves with the assumption that the threat was largely confined to industrial sites, leaky landfills, or out-of-the-way illegal dumps. It came as a shock, therefore, to discover that virtually every community in the land, no matter how small, harbored invisible sources of potential contamination in the form of **underground storage tanks (USTs)** containing petroleum or other hazardous liquids. By 1984 the extent of the problem was regarded as so serious that when Congress enacted the Hazardous and Solid Waste Amendments (HSWA) to the Resource Conservation and Recovery Act, it created a whole new federal program to deal with the situation. "Subtitle I," the Underground Storage Tank Program, required EPA to develop comprehensive regulations to protect public health and the environment from leaking underground storage tank systems. Groundwater pollution was the primary concern, since even small amounts of pollution can render groundwater supplies unusable without expensive treatment. At the time the new regulations were issued in 1988, EPA estimated the U.S. had over 2 million underground storage tank systems (i.e. underground tanks with their associated piping) at approximately 700,000 locations nationwide. Of those, between 25–30% were believed to be leaking their contents into the surrounding soil and aquifers; an additional 50% posed a significant threat of leakage and environmental harm. This sorry state of affairs stemmed from the fact that, until the mid-1980s, most tanks were made of bare steel without any form of corrosion protection and hence were subject to gradual deterioration. Subtitle I banned the installation of any new unprotected tanks as of 1985, but the older tanks remained an overwhelming problem.

Today that situation is well on its way to being resolved. Final UST regulations adopted in September of 1988 required that existing tank systems be replaced, upgraded, or closed (i.e. removed from the ground or filled with sand) by 1998. Owners failing to meet this deadline were advised they would face stiff fines for not complying with the law. The regulations further stipulated that all new tanks must conform with minimum standards that required corrosion protection as well as spill and overflow prevention equipment for the great majority of USTs that contain petroleum. In addition, secondary containment (i.e. essentially a double lining) and interstitial monitoring to detect potential leaks are mandated for the estimated 25,000 USTs that contain hazardous substances.

Most tank owners lacked the financial resources to comply with these requirements, since upgrading a tank can cost more than $12,000 while a new one is about $30,000. Simply closing a tank carries a tab of $5,000–11,000. Accordingly, in 1986 Congress created the Leaking Underground Storage Tank Trust Fund, providing funds for cleanups at sites where the owner of a tank is deceased or can't be located, is financially incapable of responding, or in cases requiring emergency action. Many state governments similarly have created special funds to expedite tank removals. By the time the federal deadline expired in December 1998, the majority of tank owners had complied with EPA regulations. During the preceding ten-year period, a million USTs had been closed or replaced, while an additional 600,000 were upgraded to prevent leakage. Enforcement actions then got underway, first targeting the remaining out-of-compliance facilities deemed most likely to present an environmental threat.

Tank removal and replacement are only partial solutions to USTs' past legacy of pollution, however. Expensive cleanup efforts at thousands of sites where corroding tanks silently leaked their contents into soil and groundwater undetected for years will undoubtedly continue for another several decades. A study conducted in 1992 concluded that the cost of remediating the damage caused by leaking underground storage tanks could well exceed $41 billion and take over 30 years. Nevertheless, notable progress has been made in the decade and a half since attention first focused on the "ticking time bombs" buried in every community across the land.

Reference Nardi, Karen J. 1995. "Underground Storage Tanks." In *Environmental Law Handbook, 13th edition,* Thomas FP Sullivan, ed. Government Institutes, Inc., pp. 76-100.

Throwing such hazardous materials in the trash may ultimately result in the threat of contaminated incinerator ash and air pollution or, alternatively, in the formation of toxic leachates at municipal landfills.

In an effort to raise public awareness about these problems and to provide concerned citizens with a safe and responsible way of getting rid of hazardous household wastes, an increasing number of communities and public interest groups have been sponsoring household hazardous waste collection programs in recent years. These events have attracted large numbers of householders who are happy to take advantage of the opportunity to clean out the basement or garage and safely get rid of those old bottles of pesticides, paints—even ammunition—that may have been sitting on a shelf gathering dust for 20 years or more. Once wastes are brought to a collection center, they must be separated by type, packaged, and manifested as RCRA hazardous wastes by trained personnel (usually licensed hazardous waste transporters). They are then taken to a licensed facility for treatment, disposal, or recycling. The cost of running such programs, as well as concerns about legal liability, have limited their more widespread adoption. Nevertheless, these widely publicized efforts have had an impact far beyond the city limits of their sponsoring communities, enhancing public awareness of the fact that each one of us is a part of America's solid waste problem and pointing the way toward safer, more responsible ways of managing the hazardous by-products of our national lifestyle.

BOX 16-7

Revitalizing Communities Through "Brownfields" Redevelopment

In cities across America, particularly in the industrial Northeast and Midwest, aging cities are pockmarked by boarded-up gas stations, abandoned factories, and rubble-strewn lots. Although located in close proximity to transportation services, utilities, and a willing workforce, these properties have been bypassed by developers and constitute a visual and economic blight on urban neighborhoods. Known as **brownfields**, these under-used, idled, or abandoned sites are shunned because of actual or suspected environmental contamination. Fearing legal liability for cleanup costs, prospective buyers have chosen to avoid any potential headaches, opting instead for construction on "greenfields" in the suburbs. In doing so, they have thwarted inner city residents' dreams of economic development, put still-clean lands at risk of future contamination, and exacerbated concerns about urban sprawl. Far from being irrational or discriminatory, developers' decisions have been based on the reality that, under CERCLA's "strict, joint and several" liability provisions, property owners could find themselves responsible for multimillion dollar cleanups, even though the contamination problems were caused by a previous owner many decades earlier. In addition, a developer's likelihood of being able to obtain financing for construction on a brownfield property was virtually negligible, as lending institutions have been extremely reluctant to finance development for fear that they, too, could incur unlimited liability under Superfund if the property owner were to default or disappear.

This seemingly intractable dilemma was confronted head-on in January 1995, when EPA launched its **Brownfields Action Agenda**. A visionary and aggressive program for restoring blighted properties to productive use while promoting job development and community participation in decision-making, the brownfields initiative has brought entrepreneurial activity and a new sense of hope to urban areas long mired in depression and decay.

The potential scope of brownfields reclamation efforts is immense. The U.S. Department of Housing and Urban Development (HUD) estimates there could be upwards of 450,000 contaminated sites nationwide. On most of these properties levels of contamination are low to moderate; Superfund-type sites that present a serious environmental health risk are not included in the brownfields program. A sizeable portion of brownfields are sites contaminated by gasoline leaking from underground storage tanks—half the brownfields in Illinois fall into this category. Others may be old dry-cleaning establishments where solvents were dumped on a back lot or abandoned factories with heavy metals contamination. Although most designated sites are urban, brownfields can also be found in suburban and rural areas as well.

The Brownfields Action Agenda includes four major initiatives:

1. **Grants for brownfields pilot projects.** To assist in evaluating site conditions, determining the extent of contamination so that cleanup costs can be estimated, the federal government funds brownfields pilot projects at amounts up to $200,000 each. By July 1999, over $69 million in grants had been awarded to states, cities, and tribal councils across the U.S.

2. Clarification of liability and cleanup issues. Since uncertainty regarding future liability for cleanup at polluted sites has been the main deterrent to restoration of brownfields, several important actions have been taken under this initiative. A major step was EPA's removal of approximately 25,000 locations from the list of potential Superfund sites. The sites deleted were ones already designated by the Agency as "no further response action planned," meaning they were not sufficiently contaminated ever to make the NPL. Nevertheless, the fact that they had been retained in the Superfund archives was a deterrent to potential developers, making their deletion from the list a symbolically reassuring action. Secondly, both EPA and many states have acted to limit the potential liability of brownfields purchasers to cleanup costs known at the time of purchase. This policy frees developers from the worry that unpleasant surprises discovered later could entail large, unanticipated expenses for remediation. Directives to those whose property lies above an aquifer contaminated by groundwater flow from an adjacent polluted site guarantees them freedom from liability for groundwater cleanup so long as they did not cause or contribute to the pollution. To reassure lenders and encourage the financing of brownfields projects, Congress in 1996 enacted legislation guaranteeing financial institutions from Superfund liability so long as they are not involved in routine management decision-making at a contaminated site.

One of the most critical issues addressed by the Brownfields Initiative was the "How clean is clean enough?" question. Insistence on the near-pristine standards required for remediated Superfund sites would doom the brownfields program by making such ventures cost-prohibitive. Accordingly, EPA and many state environmental agencies have introduced the concept of **risk-based corrective action** (RBCA referred to in Agency jargon as "Rebecca"). Originally applied to the remediation of petroleum-contaminated UST sites, RBCA is a decision-making process in which the required level of cleanup is based on real-life exposure risks, rather than on the assumption that the entire population of an area will be exposed to the maximum level of contamination present. Thus the degree of cleanup is based on the intended future use of a site. For example, a piece of land where trace amounts of lead remain in the soil could be covered with asphalt and used as a shopping mall parking lot without endangering anyone. If the same property were intended for use as a children's playground, higher cleanup standards would be in order.

3. Partnerships and outreach. Every brownfields project aims to establish a cooperative working relationship among federal agencies, states, cities, and community groups. Issues of environmental justice and the empowerment of brownfields area residents, encouraging their participation in decision-making, are key elements in this initiative.

4. Job development and training. A report issued in 1998 by the Northeast-Midwest Institute categorically stated that "Brownfields and employment problems go together." EPA emphasizes the importance of ensuring that brownfields redevelopment benefits area residents by providing both short- and long-term employment opportunities. To guarantee the availability of a locally based, well-trained labor pool, the Brownfields Action Agenda is establishing partnerships with local educational institutions, striving to develop long-term programs for worker training.

Since 1995 over 300 brownfields projects have been launched, with more than 2,000 new jobs created as a result. Geographically, these projects span the nation and include a computer-controlled greenhouse for tomato production in Buffalo, New York; a supermarket-apartment-office complex in Trenton, New Jersey; an upscale shopping and restaurant district in Charlotte, North Carolina; and two Dick Nugent-designed golf courses near downtown Chicago. All were built on abandoned, contaminated sites long viewed as worthless.

Brownfields initiatives throughout the country are revitalizing American communities by restoring degraded sites to new uses, increasing property values, stimulating tax revenues, and improving the quality of life in hundreds of low-income neighborhoods. As EPA Administrator Carol Browner remarked in a press release on June 21, 1999:

"There is no greater example of the environment and the economy working hand-in-hand to benefit the American people than the Administration's efforts to clean up and revitalize brownfields. Across the nation, our cities are coming back to life, due in part to the new jobs and new opportunities created by brownfields revitalization."

References

Berenyi, Eileen Brettler. 1999. "Whither MRF-based Recycling?" *Resource Recycling* 18, no. 4 (April):12–17.

Boerner, Christopher, and Kenneth Chilton. 1994. "False Economy: The Folly of Demand-Side Recycling." *Environment* 36, no. 1 (Jan/Feb).

Environmental Protection Agency (EPA). 1998. *Characterization of Municipal Solid Wastes in the United States: 1997 Update*. Office of Solid Waste, Report No. EPA530-R-98-007 (May).

Glenn, Jim. 1999. "The State of Garbage in America." *BioCycle* 40, no. 4 (April):60-71.

Greczyn, Mary. 1994. "Researchers and Community Reps Call for More Bioaerosol Research." *Environmental Health Letter* 33, no. 7 (March).

Greenhouse, Linda. 1994. "Justices Decide Incinerator Ash Is Toxic Waste." *New York Times,* May 3.

Gruder, Sherrie. 1993. "Matchmakers: Materials Exchange Programs." *Resource Recycling* 12, no. 12 (Dec.).

League of Women Voters Education Fund. 1993. *The Garbage Primer*. Lyons & Burford, Publishers.

Levine, Adeline G. 1982. *Love Canal: Science, Politics, and People*. Lexington Books, D. C. Heath & Company.

Melosi, Martin V. 1981. *Garbage in the Cities: Refuse, Reform, and the Environment, 1880-1980*. Texas A&M University Press.

Miller, Chaz. 1998. "Profiles in Garbage: Old Newspaper." *Waste Age* 29, no. 8 (August):79-80.

Newton, Lisa H., and Catherine K. Dillingham. 1994. "Toxin's Halloween." In *Watersheds: Classic Cases in Environmental Ethics*. Wadsworth Publishing Company.

Stolting, W. H. 1941. *Food Waste Material, A Survey of Urban Garbage Production, Collection, and Utilization*. U.S. Department of Agriculture.

Appendix A

Environmental Agencies of the Federal Government

National policy-making regarding environmental health issues has been delegated among several different federal agencies and cabinet-level departments. Among the more important groups dealing with issues discussed in this book are:

Environmental Protection Agency (EPA)
401 M Street, N.W., Washington, D.C. 20460

Created by President Nixon in December 1970, the EPA is an independent agency formed to coordinate the administration of a wide range of environmental programs which, prior to that time, had been scattered among a number of governmental agencies and departments, several of which frequently worked at cross-purposes. EPA has been charged with setting and enforcing standards pertaining to air and water pollution, solid and hazardous waste management, noise, public water supplies, pesticides, and radiation (excluding that associated with nuclear power plants). The agency also administers the municipal sewage treatment plant construction grant program authorized by Congress in the 1972 Clean Water Act. All EPA actions are published in the *Federal Register* as "proposed regulations," with time being allowed for public comment prior to their adoption as legally enforceable "final regulations."

The Administrator of the EPA is appointed by the President of the United States, as are five assistant administrators who head the five major divisions within the agency: the Office of Planning and Management, the Office of Enforcement, the Office of Air and Waste Management, the Office of Water and Hazardous Substances, and the Office of Research and Development. All six presidential appointments must be confirmed by the U.S. Senate. Although EPA headquarters are in the nation's capital, the agency has ten regional offices, each with its own regional administrator, responsible for the states within its region.

The Council on Environmental Quality (CEQ)
722 Jackson Place, Washington, D.C. 20006

Established by the National Environmental Policy Act signed by President Nixon on January 1, 1970, the CEQ operates within the Executive Office

683

of the president. Consisting of three members appointed by the president, one of whom functions as chairperson, the CEQ employs a professional staff of scientists and attorneys. Prior to the Reagan Administration, this professional staff consisted of about 30 people; all were dismissed by Reagan (the first time any staff member had been discharged by an incoming administration) and replaced by approximately six new staff people. The CEQ coordinates the environmental impact statements required by the National Environmental Policy Act and assists the president in preparing environmental legislation. It also had conducted extensive studies on the environmental effects of governmental policies and is charged with preparing annual reports for the president on the current state of the nation's environmental quality. Unfortunately, the drastic budget cuts imposed on the CEQ and the dismissal of all experienced staff members under the Reagan Administration seriously limited the council's previously valuable activities.

Nuclear Regulatory Commission (NRC)
1717 H Street, N.W., Washington, D.C. 20555

A five-member civilian board, this agency was created in 1974 by the National Energy Reorganization Act which broke up the old Atomic Energy Commission (AEC) into the research-oriented Energy Research and Development Administration (ERDA-subsequently absorbed by the Department of Energy) and the NRC. The Nuclear Regulatory Commission has jurisdiction over the licensing and regulation of nuclear reactors and also over the processing, transportation, and security of nuclear materials.

Office of Science and Technology Policy
Executive Office Building, Washington, D.C. 20500

Established within the Executive Office of the president, this agency advises the president on scientific and technological considerations involved in a wide range of national concerns, including health and the environment.

Consumer Product Safety Commission
1111 Eighteenth Street, N.W., Washington, D.C. 20207

This independent regulatory agency seeks to reduce unreasonable risks of injury associated with consumer products by encouraging the development of voluntary standards related to consumer product safety, requiring the reporting of hazardous consumer products and, if justified, recall for corrective action of hazardous products already on the market. The commission conducts research on consumer product hazards, can establish mandatory standards, and, if necessary, has the authority to ban hazardous consumer products.

Public Health Service
200 Independence Ave., S.W., Washington, D.C. 20201

An office within the Department of Health and Human Services, the U.S. Public Health Service assists states and communities in developing local health resources, conducts and supports medical research, and overseas other public health functions. Among the various subdivisions within the Public Health Service which are of particular environmental health interest are:

Centers for Disease Control and Prevention (CDC)
1600 Clifton Road, N.E., Atlanta, GA 30333

This agency is charged with protecting public health by providing leadership and direction in the prevention and control of disease. It administers programs related to communicable and vectorborne diseases, urban rat control, control of childhood lead-based paint poisoning, and a range of other environmental health problems. CDC also participates in a national program of research, information, and education regarding smoking and health. The nine major offices of the CDC are those dealing with epidemiology, international health, laboratory improvement, prevention services, environmental health, occupational safety and health, health promotion and education, professional development and training, and infectious diseases.

Food and Drug Administration (FDA)
5600 Fishers Lane, Rockville, MD 20857

The FDA's activities are aimed at protecting public health against impure and unsafe foods, drugs, cosmetics, and other possible hazards such as radiation. In carrying out its responsibilities, the FDA conducts research and develops standards for food, drugs, medical devices, veterinary medicines, and biologic products. Through its National Center for Toxicological Research, the FDA studies the biologic effects of potentially toxic chemicals in the environment.

Occupational Safety and Health Administration (OSHA)

Operating within the Department of Labor, OSHA develops and promulgates safety and health standards and regulations for the American workforce. It conducts investigations and inspections of workplaces to ensure compliance with those regulations and can issue citations and propose penalties for employers who violate such standards.

Fish and Wildlife Service

A bureau within the Department of the Interior, the Fish and Wildlife Service has jurisdiction over matters regarding endangered species, certain marine mammals, wild birds, inland sports fisheries, and wildlife research. The bureau carries out biological monitoring for effects of pesticides, heavy metals, and thermal pollution; it maintains wildlife refuges, enforces game laws, and carries out programs to control livestock predators and pest species. The bureau maintains a number of fish hatcheries, conducts environmental education and public information programs, and provides both national and international leadership regarding endangered fish and wildlife species.

Office of Surface Mining Reclamation and Enforcement

Another agency within the Interior Department, this office is charged with assisting states in developing a nationwide program to protect society and the environment from the harmful effects of coal mining, while simultaneously ensuring an adequate coal supply to meet the nation's energy needs.

Bureau of Land Management (BLM)

The BLM is responsible for managing the nation's 341 million acres of public lands, most of which are located in the Far West. In doing so, the bureau manages the timber, minerals, rangeland vegetation, wild and scenic rivers, wilderness areas, endangered species, and energy resources of these lands. BLM also is involved in watershed protection, development of recreational opportunities, and programs to protect and manage wild horses and burros. The bureau provides for the protection, orderly development, and use of public lands and resources under principles of multiple use and sustained yield. Criticism in recent years has focused on the bureau's overemphasis on permitting exploitation of public resources for private gain and insufficient protection and conservation of these resources.

Natural Resources Conservation Service (NRCS)

An agency of the Department of Agriculture, the NRCS develops and carries out soil and water conservation programs in cooperation with landowners and operators, land developers, and community planning agencies. NRCS also is active in programs aimed at controlling agricultural pollution and in effecting environmental improvement.

Appendix B

Environmental Organizations

American Lung Association
1740 Broadway, New York, NY 10019
www.lungusa.org

Basel Action Network
c/o Asia Pacific Environmental Exchange
1827 39th Ave. E, Seattle, WA 98112
www.ban.org

Center for Health, Environment and Justice
150 S. Washington, Suite 300
P.O. Box 6806, Falls Church, VA 22040
www.essential.org/cchw/

Center for Science in the Public Interest
1875 Connecticut Ave., NW, Suite 300, Washington, DC 20009
www.cspinet.org

Defenders of Wildlife
1244 19th St., NW, Washington, DC 20036
www.defenders.org

Ducks Unlimited, Inc.
One Waterfowl Way, Memphis, TN 38120-2351
www.ducks.org

Environmental Defense
257 Park Ave. South, New York, NY 10010
www.environmentaldefense.org

Friends of the Earth
1025 Vermont Ave., NW, Washington, DC 20005
www.foe.org

Greenpeace USA, Inc.
1436 U St., NW, Washington, DC 20009
www.greenpeaceusa.org

League of Conservation Voters
1707 L St., NW, #750, Washington, DC 20036
www.lcv.org

League of Women Voters of the United States
1730 M St., NW, Suite 100, Washington, DC 20036
www.lwv.org

National Audubon Society
700 Broadway, New York, NY 10003-9562
www.audubon.org

National Environmental Health Association
720 S. Colorado Blvd., Suite 970-S, Denver, CO 80246
www.neha.org

National Wildlife Federation
8925 Leesburg Pike, Vienna, VA 22184
www.nwf.org

The Nature Conservancy
4245 N. Fairfax Dr., Suite 100, Arlington, VA 22203
www.tnc.org

Natural Resources Defense Council
40 West 20th St., New York, NY 10011
www.nrdc.org

Pesticide Action Network North America
49 Powell St., Suite 500, San Francisco, CA 94102
www.panna.org

Population Action International
1120 19th., NW, Suite 550, Washington, DC 20036
www.populationaction.org

The Population Institute
107 Second St., NE, Washington, DC 20002
www.populationinstitute.org

Population Reference Bureau, Inc.
1875 Connecticut Ave., NW, Suite 520, Washington, DC 20009-5728
www.prb.org

Sierra Club
85 Second St., Second Floor, San Francisco, CA 94105-3441
www.sierraclub.org

The Wilderness Society
900 17th St., NW, Washington, DC 20006-2596
www.wilderness.org

Worldwatch Institute
1776 Massachusetts Ave., NW, Washington, DC 20036-1904
www.worldwatch.org

World Wildlife Fund
1250 24th St., NW, Washington, DC 20077-7180
www.worldwildlife.org

Zero Population Growth, Inc.
1400 Sixteenth St., NW, Suite 320, Washington, DC 20036
www.zpg.org

Index